HANDBOOK OF
SMALL ANIMAL ORTHOPEDICS & FRACTURE TREATMENT

SECOND EDITION

WADE O. BRINKER, D.V.M., M.S.
Diplomate, American College of Veterinary Surgeons
Professor Emeritus
Department of Small Animal Surgery and Medicine
Michigan State University
College of Veterinary Medicine
East Lansing, Michigan

DONALD L. PIERMATTEI, D.V.M., Ph.D.
Diplomate, American College of Veterinary Surgeons
Professor
Department of Clinical Sciences
College of Veterinary Medicine and Biomedical Sciences
Colorado State University
Fort Collins, Colorado

GRETCHEN L. FLO, D.V.M., M.S.
Professor
Department of Small Animal Surgery and Medicine
Michigan State University
College of Veterinary Medicine
East Lansing, Michigan

Illustrations by Richard M. Fritzler, A.M.I., and F. Dennis Giddings, A.M.I.

1990
W.B. SAUNDERS COMPANY
Harcourt Brace Jovanovich, Inc.

Philadelphia   London   Toronto   Montreal   Sydney   Tokyo

W. B. SAUNDERS COMPANY
Harcourt Brace Jovanovich, Inc.

The Curtis Center
Independence Square West
Philadelphia, PA 19106

Library of Congress Cataloging-in-Publication Data

Listed here are the latest translated editions of this book together
with the language of the translation and the publisher.

German (1st Edition)—F. K. Schattauer, Stuttgart, Germany

Portuguese (1st Edition)—Editora Manole LTDA, RUA 13 de Maio, Bela Vista, São Paulo, Brazil

Japanese (1st Edition)—Buneido Co. LTD., No. 27–18, Hongo 2-Chome, Bunkyo-ku, Tokyo, Japan

French (1st Edition)—Editions Le Point Veterinaire, 25 Rue Bourgelat, 94700 Maisons-Alfort,
France

Editor: Linda E. Mills
Developmental Editor: Roseanne Hallowell
Designer: W. B. Saunders Staff
Production Manager: Carolyn Naylor
Manuscript Editor: W. B. Saunders Staff
Illustration Coordinator: Lisa Lambert
Indexer: Maria Coughlin

Handbook of Small Animal Orthopedics and Fracture Treatment   ISBN   0–7216–2808–7

Printed in the United States of America.

Last digit is the print number: 9   8   7   6   5   4   3   2   1

PREFACE

Since the first edition of this book was published in 1983, many new orthopedic conditions have been recognized, and a variety of new procedures and treatments, based on well-grounded scientific data, have been developed in various areas of orthopedics and fracture treatment. These have been gleaned, sorted, prioritized, and presented here in keeping with the authors' experience.

In compiling this second edition, the central theme of rapid return of ambulation and complete functional recovery following treatment of locomotor impairment has been maintained. With this objective in mind, and with the results of several thousand documented cases, the most rewarding methods of treatment have been assembled and presented.

A special attempt has been made to present this material in a straightforward and readily understandable manner, usable by both the student and the practicing surgeon. The text is profusely illustrated for clarity and easy reference. Richard Fritzler has produced many new drawings as well as a number of revisions and additions to previous drawings. No attempt has been made to provide an exhaustive coverage. Truly rare and unusual conditions have been omitted, and only absolutely necessary references have been cited.

The index has been expanded to make it easier and faster to locate specific conditions, and the page layout has been redesigned to make headings more distinctive and recognizable. We thank the entire editorial and production staff at W. B. Saunders Co. for their help and patience during this revision process.

Wade O. Brinker
Donald L. Piermattei
Gretchen L. Flo

CONTENTS

PART I

Fractures

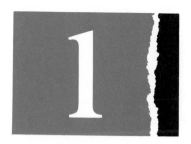

Fractures: Classification, Diagnosis, and Treatment

A fracture is a complete or incomplete break in the continuity of bone or cartilage. A fracture is accompanied by various degrees of injury to the surrounding soft tissues, including blood supply, and by a compromise of locomotor system function. The examiner handling the fracture must take into consideration the patient's local and overall conditions.

CLASSIFICATION OF FRACTURES

Fractures may be classified on many bases, and all are useful in describing the fracture.[1-3] These bases include causes, presence of a communicating external wound, extent of damage, direction and location of the fracture line, and stability of the fracture following replacement in the normal anatomical position.

Causes

Direct Violence Applied to the Bone ■ Statistics indicate that at least 75 to 80 percent of all fractures are caused by car accidents or motorized vehicles.[4]

Indirect Violence ■ The force is transmitted through bone or muscle to a distant point where the fracture occurs (e.g., fracture of the femoral neck, avulsion of the tibial tubercle, fracture of the condyles of the humerus or femur).

Diseases of Bone ■ Some bone diseases cause bone destruction or weakening to such a degree that trivial trauma may produce a fracture (e.g., bone neoplasms, or nutritional disturbances affecting the bone).

Repeated Stress ■ Fatigue fractures in small animals are most frequently encountered in bones of the front or rear foot (e.g., metacarpal or metatarsal bones in the racing greyhound).

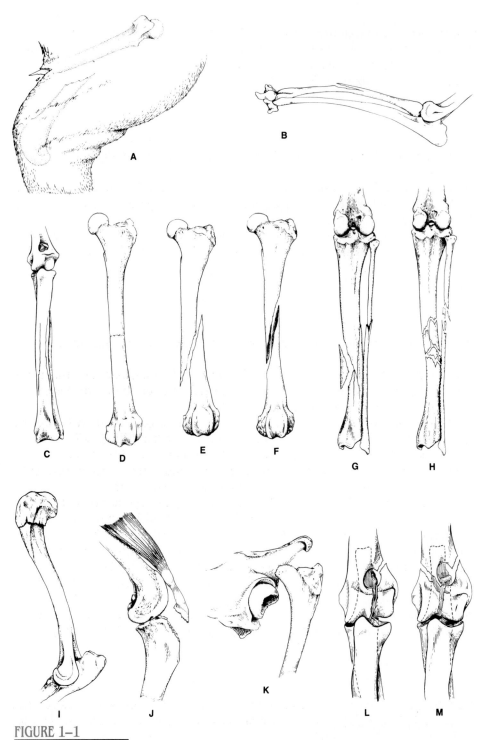

FIGURE 1–1

Types of fractures. *(A)* Open. *(B)* Green-stick. *(C)* Fissure. *(D)* Transverse. *(E)* Oblique. *(F)* Spiral. *(G)* Comminuted. *(H)* Multiple or segmental. *(I)* Impacted. *(J)* Avulsion. *(K)* Physeal. *(L)* Unicondylar. *(M)* Bicondylar.

Presence of a Communicating External Wound

Closed Fracture ■ The fracture does not communicate to the outside.

Open Fracture ■ The fracture site communicates to the outside. These fractures are very apt to be contaminated or infected, and healing at best may be complicated and delayed (Fig. 1–1A).

Extent of Damage

Complete Fracture ■ There is a total disruption of the bone, usually accompanied by marked displacement.

Green-stick Fracture ■ One side of the bone is broken, and the other is bent (Fig. 1–1B). This type of fracture is usually seen in the young growing animal. Displacement is minimal, and healing is rapid.

Fissure Fracture ■ One or more fine cracks penetrate the cortex, often in a spiral or longitudinal direction. The periosteal covering is usually still intact (Fig. 1–1C).

Direction and Location of Fracture Line

Transverse Fracture ■ The fracture occurs at right angles to the axis of the bone (Fig. 1–1D).

Oblique Fracture ■ The line of fracture is diagonal to the long axis. The fragments tend to slip by each other as a result of spastic contraction of muscles unless stability is maintained by fixation (Fig. 1–1E).

Spiral Fracture ■ The line of fracture is a curve. The fragments tend to slip by each other and rotate unless fixation measures are taken (Fig. 1–1F).

Comminuted Fracture ■ Splintering or fragmentation is present (Fig. 1–1G).

Multiple or Segmental Fracture ■ The bone is broken into three or more segments; the fracture lines do not meet at a common point (Fig. 1–1H).

Impacted Fracture ■ The bone fragments are driven firmly together (Fig. 1–1I).

Avulsion Fracture ■ A fragment of bone, which is the site of insertion of a muscle, tendon, or ligament, is detached as a result of a forceful pull (Fig. 1–1J).

Physeal Fracture ■ The fracture-separation occurs at the epiphyseal line or growth plate. This type occurs only in the young growing animal (Fig. 1–1K).

Unicondylar or Condylar Fracture ■ The fracture line passes through a condyle (e.g., humerus, femur) (Fig. 1–1L).

Bicondylar Fracture ■ The fracture is situated between two condyles and the diaphysis and at least three fracture fragments are present (Fig. 1–1M).

Stability Following Replacement in Normal Anatomical Position

Stable Fracture ■ Fragments interlock and resist shortening forces (e.g., transverse, green-stick, impacted). The primary objective of fixation is to prevent angular and/or rotational deformity.

Unstable Fracture ■ The fragments do not interlock and thus slide by each other and out of position (e.g., oblique, spiral, multiple). Fixation is indicated to maintain length and alignment and to prevent rotation.

BLOOD SUPPLY AND HEALING OF BONE

Until about 1940, almost all fractures were reduced, closed, and stabilized by external means such as coaptation splints, plaster of Paris casts, and Thomas splints. The various methods of internal fixation were introduced and developed in the same time period as were aseptic technique in veterinary surgery, open approaches to the various bones and joints, and open reduction of fractures. In order to properly handle tissues and implement reduction and fixation to best advantage, an understanding of blood supply and bone healing is essential.

Normal Vascularization of Bone

An adequate blood supply is necessary for bone to carry out its normal physiological function. Clinically, most vascular problems arise in the long bones. Blood supply to these bones is derived from three basic sources: the afferent vascular system, the intermediate vascular system of compact bone, and the efferent vascular system.[5, 6] The afferent system carries arterial blood and consists of the principal nutrient artery, the metaphyseal arteries, and the periosteal arterioles at muscle attachments (Fig. 1–2). The periosteal arterioles are minor components of the afferent system and supply the outer layers of the cortex in the vicinity of firm fascial or muscle attachments.

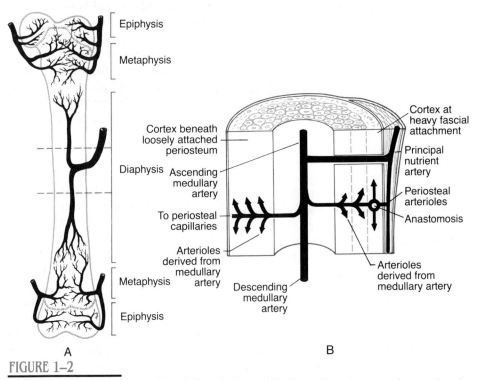

FIGURE 1–2

Normal blood supply to bone. (A) Schema of afferent blood supply to immature bone. After the growth plate closes (adult bone), the metaphyseal and epiphyseal vessels anastomose. (B) Section of diaphysis showing schema of normal afferent blood supply to compact bone. (From Rhinelander F, et al, 1968.)[6]

The vessels in compact bones are intermediate between the afferent and efferent systems and function as the vascular lattice where critical exchange between the blood and surrounding living tissue occurs. This system consists of the cortical canals of Havers and Volkmann and the minute canaliculi, which convey nutrients to the osteocytes.

Venous drainage (the efferent system) of cortical bone takes place at the periosteal surface. Blood flow through the cortex is essentially centrifugal, from medulla to the periosteum. Other venous drainage from the marrow cavity is present; however, this is connected with the hematopoietic activity of the marrow cavity.

Response of Vascularization Following Fracture

Disruption of the normal blood supply to bone varies with the complexity of the fracture. The afferent vascular components are stimulated and respond by hypertrophy, increasing in both diameter and number. In addition, a new blood supply is developed, termed the extraosseous blood supply of healing bone,[5, 6] from the immediate surrounding soft tissues. This is separate from the normal periosteal arterioles. It furnishes blood to detached bone fragments, devitalized cortex, and the developing periosteal callus. When stability at the fracture site and continuity of the medullary circulation are established, the extraosseous blood supply regresses. Fortunately, the regenerative powers of the medullary arterial supply are rapid and enormous under favorable circumstances, since this must be re-established for healing of cortical bone.

Some of the factors that may deter vascular response and, thus, bone healing are (1) trauma in connection with the original accident, (2) careless or improper surgical handling of the soft tissues, (3) inadequate reduction, and (4) inadequate stabilization of bone fragments. Intramedullary nails may temporarily damage the medullary afferent system, whereas plates may block the venous outflow. Either blood supply to the bone may be partially compromised, but both must be present to an adequate degree for bone healing.

Bone Healing

The sequence of events following fracture may be very briefly stated as (1) hemorrhage in the area, (2) clot formation, (3) inflammation and edema, followed by (4) proliferation of cells, (5) cartilage and bone formation, and (6) remodeling of the callus back to normal bone.

Callus formation may be subdivided on the basis of location as (1) medullary bridging callus, (2) periosteal bridging callus, and (3) intercortical bridging callus (Fig. 1–3). The pattern of callus formation will vary markedly in response to circumstances and stimuli present.[7] In general, stabilization of fractures by external splintage, the external fixator, and intramedullary pins is characterized by the formation of callus in all three areas. Stabilization of fractures by use of plates and screws is characterized by intercortical callus and some medullary bridging callus. Other than in the young growing animal, the amount of callus is in inverse relation to the degree of stability at the fracture site. Healing depends on and is influenced by blood supply, reduction, and stabilization of the fracture fragments.

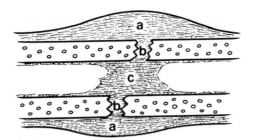

FIGURE 1–3

Callus formation in bone healing. *(A)* Periosteal bridging callus. *(B)* Intercortical bridging callus. *(C)* Medullary bridging callus.

DIAGNOSIS OF FRACTURES AND PRINCIPLES OF TREATMENT

The history and clinical signs usually indicate the presence of a fracture; however, radiographs are essential for precise determination of its nature.

The first consideration is preserving the patient's life; repair of tissues and restoration of function are secondary. Treatment for shock, hemorrhage, and wounds of the soft tissues, if present, should be instituted immediately, and the patient should be made as comfortable as possible.

Examination of an animal with a fracture or suspected fracture should include:

1. Assessment of the animal's general health.

2. Determination of whether tissues or organs adjacent to the fracture or other parts of the body have been damaged and to what extent.

3. Examination to ascertain whether fractures or dislocations are present in other parts of the body.

4. Precise evaluation of the fracture or fractures. (See Chapter 15 for a more complete discussion on physical examination of the locomotor system.)

Clinical Signs

Even though they are not always readily detectable, visible signs at the fracture area include one or more of the following:

1. Pain or localized tenderness.

2. Deformity or change in angulation.

3. Abnormal mobility.

4. Local swelling. This may appear almost immediately or not until several hours after or a day following the accident. It usually persists for 7 to 10 days owing to disturbed flow of blood and lymph.

5. Loss of function.

6. Crepitus.

Radiographic Examination

Radiographs of at least two views at right angles to each other are essential for accurate diagnosis and selection of the best procedures for reduction and immobilization. In the immature or deformed animal, interpretation of the radiograph may present special problems because of the presence and stages of development of various osseous growth centers. Radiographs of the opposite limb are usually helpful.

Treatment

The goal of fracture treatment is early ambulation and complete return of function. Reduction and fixation of the fracture should be undertaken as soon as the patient's condition permits.[8, 9] Delay makes reduction more difficult because of spastic contraction of the muscles and inflammatory thickening of the soft tissue. In some cases, fixation can be accomplished when the patient is presented; in others, it may be advisable to delay for a day or longer until the patient becomes an acceptable anesthetic risk. It is inadvisable to wait until the swelling has subsided before going ahead with reduction and fixation. By this time, organization of the hematoma and callus formation are well under way. The latter also obscures fracture lines, nerves, and blood vessels. Surgical hemorrhage is also markedly increased as a result of increased circulatory response in the area. This circulatory response is usually evident around the fourth day post-trauma. Surgery prior to this time is accompanied by less hemorrhage.

RATE OF BONE UNION AND CLINICAL UNION

The moment a fracture occurs, changes in the tissue in the immediate area set the stage for its repair, and the rapidity of the process of repair may be influenced by many factors. The surgeon can do little to alter such factors as age, character of the fracture, state of the soft tissues in the surrounding area, and certain systemic or local bone diseases. Unfavorable factors such as poor reduction, inadequate immobilization, excessive trauma, or lack of aseptic procedures in surgery, however, are within the control of the surgeon. These factors may slow or even interrupt the healing process. When all other factors are equal and the fracture is optimally treated, age of the patient is the most influential single factor affecting the rate of healing.

Clinical union refers to that period of time in the recovery process of a fracture when healing has progressed to the point in strength so that the fixation can be removed. Average periods of anticipated healing time for the typical uncomplicated fracture treated in optimal fashion are listed in Table 1–1. These healing times vary somewhat, depending on the type of fixation

TABLE 1–1

Rate of Union in Terms of Clinical Union[3]

AGE OF ANIMAL	EXTERNAL, SKELETAL, AND INTRAMEDULLARY PIN FIXATIONS	FIXATION WITH BONE PLATES
Under 3 months	2–3 weeks	4 weeks
3–6 months	4–6 weeks	2–3 months
6–12 months	5–8 weeks	3–5 months
Over 1 year	7–12 weeks	5 months–1 year

used. Fractures immobilized with external fixation, skeletal fixation, and intramedullary pins heal with the development of an external and internal bridging callus. The bridging callus does give added early strength to the fracture site. Fractures immobilized with rigid fixation (bone plate) heal primarily by direct union and some internal callus, and fractures treated by this method should have the fixation in place for a longer period of time.

Table 1–1 is not to be interpreted as an indication that one method of fixation is superior to another. Each method has its place, indications, and contraindications. Bone plates and screws have been a most welcome addition to the armamentarium of the orthopedic surgeon, particularly in the treatment of the more complicated unstable fractures.

Factors to be considered when evaluating union of a fracture are:

1. Age of the patient.
2. Location and type of fracture.
3. History of fracture—infection, single or multiple surgeries, interrupted or inadequate fixation, impaired circulation, inadequate reduction.
4. Lapse of time since reduction and fixation.
5. Functional use of limb.
6. Type of fixation—less than optimum, optimum, or too rigid.
7. Radiographic examination—two views.

REDUCTION OF FRACTURES

Reduction of a fracture refers to the process of replacing the fractured segments in their original anatomical position. Bones with their muscles attached may be likened to a system of levers with springs attached. Muscles are constantly contracting (normal tonus). Flexors oppose extensors, counterbalancing the part at the joint. When a bone is fractured, all opposing muscles contract maximally, and overriding and shortening of the bone occur. Spastic contraction of the muscle is intensified by injury to soft tissues of the region. The pull caused by the muscle spasm is constant and continuous, even under general anesthesia. Initially, the contraction and overriding are primarily muscular and are responsive to general anesthesia, countertraction, and some of the muscle-relaxing drugs. After several days, inflammatory reaction in the area with its accompanying proliferating changes brings about contraction of a more permanent nature; thus, more difficulty is encountered when attempting reduction.[2, 3]

Gas anesthesia (halothane, methoxyflurane, or isoflurane) is superior to use of the barbiturates in bringing about relaxation of muscle spasm. The addition of muscle relaxants is helpful in overcoming spastic contraction when used in addition to general anesthesia and within the first 3 days after a fracture occurs. Succinylcholine (.44 mg/kg) or pancuronium (.05 to .1 mg/kg) has been used in small animals. The former drug is preferred. At these doses, they also produce respiratory paralysis, and assisted respiration is a necessity. The duration of action is about 20 to 30 minutes.

To a large extent, healing is influenced by the handling of the soft tissues, blood supply to the fracture segments, accuracy of reduction, and efficiency of immobilization. All may be influenced or altered by the surgeon.

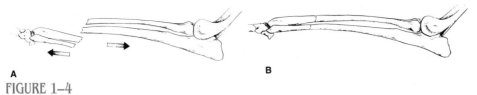

FIGURE 1–4

(A, B) Application of traction, countertraction, and manipulation.

The ideal is anatomical replacement of the fracture segments because this gives the possibility of maximum stability when fixation is applied. Anatomical apposition is always preferred but not always necessary, particularly in fractures of the diaphysis. Faulty alignment and rotation should be avoided. When a joint surface is involved in a fracture, the articular fragments must always be reduced anatomically to restore joint congruency and thus to eliminate or at least minimize abnormal wear and secondary osteoarthrosis. Reduction may be achieved closed (without opening the skin) or open (with surgical exposure). The secret of reduction is the application of continual steady pressure over a period of time. This fatigues the muscles, bringing about relaxation and lengthening.

Closed Reduction

Closed reduction is usually accomplished by manipulation along with the application of traction and countertraction. This is ideal, provided that it can be accomplished and maintained with minimal tissue trauma. The procedure is usually limited to recent fractures, certain stable fractures, and animals that are easily palpated (e.g., cats, small dogs).

METHODS OF CLOSED REDUCTION

Some suggested methods follow.[2, 3]

1. Application of traction, countertraction, and manipulation (Fig. 1–4).
2. Application of traction, countertraction, and bending (Fig. 1–5).
3. Use of the animal's weight to apply traction and countertraction to fatigue the spastically contracted muscles (Fig. 1–6). Ten to 30 minutes may

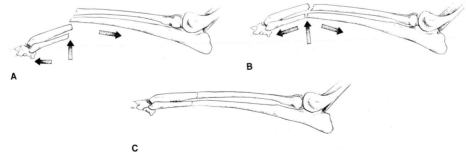

FIGURE 1–5

(A–C) Application of traction, countertraction, and bending.

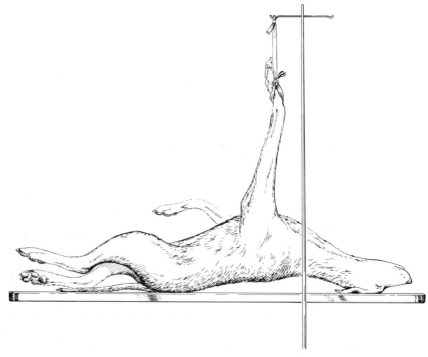

FIGURE 1–6

Use of the animal's weight to apply traction and countertraction in fatiguing spastically contracted muscles.

be necessary to fatigue the muscles so that the fracture may be manipulated and reduced.

4. Use of the Gordon extender (Fig. 1–7). Fatiguing the muscles and relaxation are best accomplished by a slow progressive increase in pressure application over a period of time (e.g., 10 to 30 minutes).

Open Reduction

Open reduction is a method of choice in many cases. The fragments are reduced under direct vision, and usually some type of internal fixation is applied to ensure that the position is maintained. (Internal fixation is discussed under the section on immobilization and treatment of specific fractures.)

Open reduction technique is usually used in a high percentage of fracture cases, particularly in those that are unstable and more complicated, those of more than several days' duration, those involving an articular surface, and those for which internal fixation is indicated. Many of the more common open approaches are described in connection with the treatment of fractures involving the various bones. The reference book *Atlas of Surgical Approaches to the Bones and Joints in the Dog and Cat* is a must for the orthopedic surgeon.[14] The surgeon should strive continually to improve soft tissue handling techniques. The following are some of the principal points to follow:

1. Attain strict hemostasis. Active bleeding must be controlled if the operative field is to be clearly visualized. Control of hemorrhage may also be

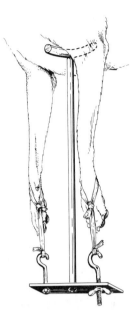

FIGURE 1–7

Use of the Gordon extender. Gradual turning down of the wing nut increases traction on the affected limb. The wing nut is tightened at about 5-minute intervals to increase traction.

critical in preserving the life of the animal, and it reduces some of the possible complications in postoperative healing.

2. Follow normal separations between muscles and fascial planes.

3. If a muscle needs to be severed for exposure, do this near its origin or insertion to minimize trauma and hemorrhage, facilitate closure, and minimize loss of muscular function.

4. Know the location of major blood vessels and nerves. Locate these structures and work around them.

5. Avoid putting excess traction on nerves because this may bring about temporary or permanent injury.

6. Preserve soft tissue attachments (and, therefore, blood supply) to bone fragments in the process of exposure, reduction, and application of fixation.

7. Avoid periosteal stripping.

8. Use suction, rather than blotting, to minimize soft tissue trauma.

9. When necessary, blot with moist gauze sponges (Ringer solution) to help clear the area. Avoid wiping.

Each fracture is unique and may require a different maneuver or combination of maneuvers to bring about reduction. Again, the preferred technique in most cases is the application of gradual progressive pressure over a period of time to fatigue the muscles and bring about sufficient relaxation to allow the reduction of bone fragments.

Disposition of Bone Fragments at the Fracture Site

The presence of various bone fragments in the fracture area is frequently encountered. As a general rule, all fragments are kept whether or not they have soft tissue attachment. All fragments with soft tissue attachments are carefully handled to maintain this attachment. The pieces that are too small for internal fixation with bone screws, wires, or Kirschner wires are maneuvered back into position as best possible. In most cases, the surrounding soft tissue maintains or even improves the position of these pieces as the process of healing begins. Large fragments, with or without soft tissue attachment, are usually fixed in place with bone screws, wires, or Kirschner wires.

As a general rule, these fragments aid in restoring the original bone substance and function as an autogenous bone graft. They only form sequestra when contamination or infection is present, and even under these circumstances, they may enter into callus formation.

Removal of fragments in many cases results in delayed union, nonunion, or a decrease in diameter of the bone in that area. Generally, if removed, they should be replaced by a bone graft. This is particularly true if rigid fixation (plate) is applied, or if any conditions are present (aged animal, devitalized surrounding tissue, architectural deficits after reduction, and so forth) that result in slow healing.

METHODS OF OPEN REDUCTION

The following are presented as suggestions:

1. Application of levering by use of some instrument such as an osteotome, bone skid, spay hook handle, or scalpel handle (Fig. 1–8).

2. Application of direct force (using bone-holding forceps) on one or more of the bone fragments (Fig. 1–9).

3. Direct application of force on both of the bone fragments (Fig. 1–10). After they are reduced by the application of traction, countertraction, and corrective rotation, self-holding bone forceps may be used to temporarily maintain reduction while fixation is applied.

4. Direct application of force on both of the bone fragments combined with the use of levering (Fig. 1–11).

Note: Bone fragments must be handled with care because too much force may result in additional fragmentation.

IMMOBILIZATION (FIXATION)

Immobilization involves fixing the bone fragments so that they are motionless with respect to each other during the healing process. The objectives are to stabilize the fragments in their normal anatomical position and to prevent

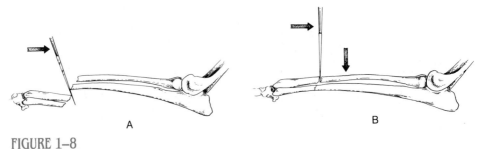

FIGURE 1–8

(A, B) Application of levering by use of an osteotome.

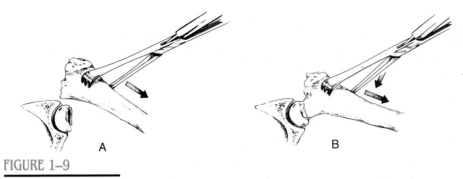

FIGURE 1–9

(A, B) Application of direct force (using bone-holding forceps) on one or more bone fragments.

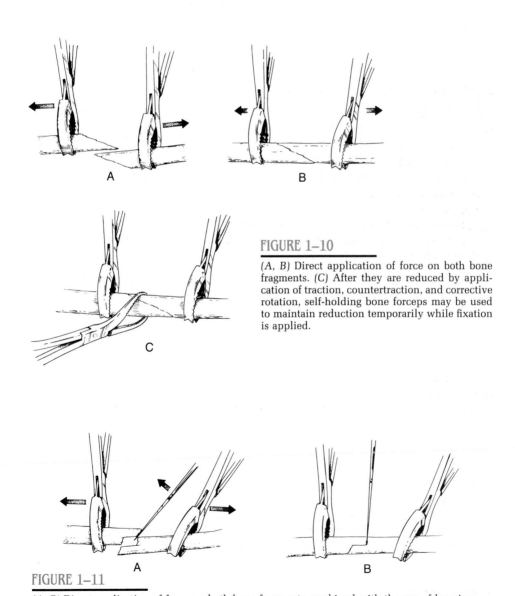

FIGURE 1–10

(A, B) Direct application of force on both bone fragments. *(C)* After they are reduced by application of traction, countertraction, and corrective rotation, self-holding bone forceps may be used to maintain reduction temporarily while fixation is applied.

FIGURE 1–11

(A, B) Direct application of force on both bone fragments combined with the use of levering.

displacement, angulation, and rotation. Ideally, the method used should (1) accomplish rigid uninterrupted stabilization at the time of the original surgery, (2) permit early ambulation, and (3) permit the use of as many joints as possible during the healing period.

The peculiarities of each fracture will dictate or suggest the method of immobilization to be employed. Some fractures lend themselves to a variety of methods, whereas in others, the methods may be very limited for a successful outcome.

Methods of Fixation

The methods of fixation may be classified as follows:

1. Limb splintage principle (coaptation splints, casts, modified Thomas splint).

2. Bone splintage principle (external fixator/Kirschner splint, intramedullary pins, bone plates, bone screws, tension band wires, cerclage and hemicerclage wires, or combinations). This principle is preferred for most fractures because it usually allows early ambulation and the use of all joints.

TEMPORARY SPLINTAGE

If for some reason there is a delay in reduction and fixation, temporary splintage (e.g., Robert Jones dressing, coaptation splint, Thomas splint) of the limb may be indicated to reduce additional trauma. This is true particularly for fractures distal to the elbow and stifle. In most other fractures, the animal is more comfortable with cage rest. The objective in most fracture cases is early reduction and fixation.

COAPTATION SPLINTS AND CASTS

These devices[2, 3, 10] consist of a mold of material that surrounds the affected part and thus has the potential of holding fracture segments or dislocated bones in the reduced position until healing occurs. The basic objective is immobilization of the joint above the fracture and all joints below the fracture. As the sole method of fixation, the coaptation splint functions primarily as a "limb splint." Included in this group are:

1. Plaster of Paris casts.
2. Various fiber glass and plastic casts.
3. Mason metasplints.[2]
4. Various semicasts made from plastics, wood, or other rigid material.

Coaptation splints may be used:

1. For fractures distal to the elbow, tibia, tail, and ribs. In Figure 1–12, a, b, and c indicate the region of location of the fracture; a', b', and c' indicate the height of the splint or cast if it is to function optimally.
2. For stable fractures.
3. In combination with other methods as auxiliary fixation.
4. As a temporary splint.

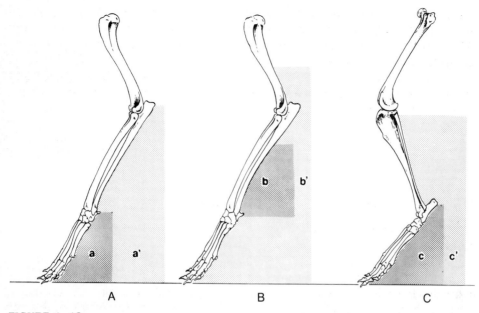

FIGURE 1-12

(A–C) Optimal splint or cast length indicated by a′, b′, and c′ for fractures.

When a coaptation splint is used, the following points should be considered:

Padding ■ If closed reduction is used, the hair is usually not clipped. A light padding (cast padding, stockinette, cotton, sheet wadding, felt) should be applied to protect the soft tissues, with particular emphasis given to bony prominence (e.g., accessory carpal pad, tuber calcis, olecranon process, dewclaw). This is best accomplished by increased padding in the depressed areas and less over the prominences. Avoid overpadding because it may allow movement of bone fragments inside the coaptation splint or cast.

Fixation ■ Anchor in place to avoid shifting on the limb. This is particularly applicable if the leg is swollen when the cast is applied. This may be accomplished with use of adhesive tape and by molding the cast to the contour of the limb.

Radiographs ■ Check reduction radiographically before and after application and again in several days.

Extent ■ Distally, the toes may be covered or preferably the center two digital pads exposed.

Patient's Tolerance ■ Usually, coaptation splints are reasonably well tolerated by the animal, if they are accomplishing their mission, the cast is kept dry, and activity is limited. Indications of complication include pain, elevation of temperature, swelling, edema, numbness, foul odor, cyanosis of digits, loss of appetite, systemic depression, irritated areas, and chewing on the cast. For more details on coaptation splint application see Chapter 19.

MODIFIED THOMAS SPLINT

In the past, this splint was widely used for small animals.[11–13] Today, however, its use is quite limited because better methods have been developed. Its most common uses concern:

1. Immobilization of stable fractures distal to the elbow or stifle joint. It is not used as the sole method of fixation for fractures of the humerus and femur.

2. Occasionally, acting as an additional immobilizing device in connection with internal fixation.

3. Immobilization secondary to joint surgery.

4. Immobilization in the treatment of tendon and nerve injuries.

5. Temporary splinting.

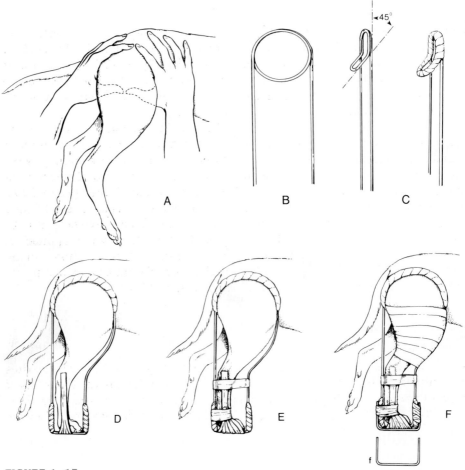

FIGURE 1–13

Fabrication of the modified Thomas splint. After the diameter of the thigh is approximated (A), the aluminum alloy rod is bent, forming one and one-half circles (B). (C) The lower half of the ring is bent at a 45° angle to accommodate the thickness of the thigh and to avoid femoral vessel pressure; Styrofoam, cotton, or cast padding is added, followed by gauze and tape. (D) With the splint pushed firmly up in the inguinal region, the caudal bar is first bent to approximate the length of the leg with the limb in normal standing angulation and the toes flexed to simulate standing. Next the cranial rod is bent to approximate normal angulation of the limb with the toes flexed to simulate standing. The distal ends of the bars are then taped securely together. (E) Splint is again pushed firmly up in the inguinal region; foot is anchored with adhesive tape. (F) If a dog weighs more than 25 pounds, a walking bar (f) is applied. A layer of cotton is placed around the upper leg, then both are anchored as one to the cranial bar with a layer of gauze and tape. Anchoring the tape to the bar in the inguinal area holds the padding for the thigh in place; otherwise it slips distally and serves no useful purpose.

The splint is usually designed and applied so that the leg is in the angulation of the standing position, including the toes. It is used primarily to restrict movement; however, it may be applied to combine limited traction with fixation.

The splint should be kept dry and the animal's activity restricted. Modified Thomas splints should be checked regularly and repaired as indicated. In general, they are too cumbersome for use with medium-size and large dogs. Commercially made splints are available, but those made for the individual animal serve best.

Fabrication

Aluminum alloy rods are available in 6' lengths and assorted diameters (⅛", ³⁄₁₆", and ⅜"). After the diameter of the thigh is approximated (Fig. 1–13A), the rod is bent, forming one and one-half circles (Fig. 1–13B, C). The lower half of the ring is bent at a 45° angle to accommodate the thickness of the thigh and to avoid femoral vessel pressure. It is then padded with Styrofoam, cotton, or cast padding, followed by gauze and tape.

With the splint pushed firmly up in the inguinal region (Fig. 1–13D), the caudal bar is first bent to the approximate length of the leg with the limb in normal standing angulation and the toes flexed to simulate standing. Next, the cranial rod is bent to approximate the normal angulation of the limb with the toes flexed to simulate standing. If the leg is extended, the splint will be too long, leading to disuse and discomfort. The splint is again pushed firmly up in the inguinal region and the foot is anchored with adhesive tape (Fig. 1–13E). If the dog weighs more than 25 pounds, a walking bar is applied. A layer of cotton is placed around the upper leg, then the leg is anchored to the cranial bar with a layer of gauze and tape. The tape should be attached firmly to the ring in the inguinal or axillary region (Fig. 1–13F).

EXTERNAL FIXATOR

Use of the external fixator for immobilization of long bone fractures requires transcutaneous insertion of two to four pins in each of the proximal and distal bone fragments, which are then connected by one or more external bars (Figs. 1–14, 1–20, 1–21, 1–22, and 1–23).[2, 3, 15–22] Fixators can be used on all of the long bones and the mandible.

Indications or Uses [2, 3, 15–39]

The external fixator is adaptable to:

1. Stable and unstable fractures
2. Open fractures
3. Gunshot fractures
4. Osteotomies
5. Delayed unions and nonunions

The advantages of the external fixator include (1) ease of application; (2) its usefulness in treating open or closed reduced fractures; (3) if applied in

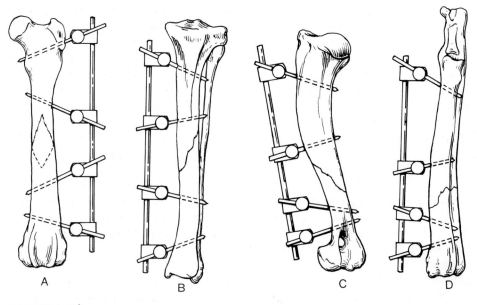

FIGURE 1-14

Preferred location of the unilateral external fixator in relation to the bone surface and associated soft tissue. *(A)* Lateral surface of femur. *(B)* Medial surface of tibia. *(C)* Craniolateral surface of humerus. *(D)* Craniomedial or medial surface of radius.

connection with an open approach, minimization of the approach; (4) fixation pins that can usually be inserted proximal and distal to the wound; (5) a wound that is readily accessible for dressing; (6) its compatibility for use in conjunction with other internal fixation devices; (7) toleration by both dogs and cats; (8) in most cases, removal without placing the animal under general anesthesia; and (9) reasonable cost.

Fundamentals in Application

These guidelines should be followed:[2, 3, 19]

1. *Use aseptic technique.* This includes preparation of the patient, the operating room, the equipment, the surgeon, and aftercare.

2. *Use proper bone surface location.* Complications can be minimized if the splint is located on the bone surface that allows insertion of the fixation pins through the skin and directly into the bone. This minimizes the length of pin between the fixation clamp and bone thus keeping maximum pin stiffness. It also minimizes soft tissue irritation; pins penetrating through muscle and skin are more irritating than those penetrating skin alone. The proper surface for the unilateral splint on the tibia is medial, for the radius is craniomedial or medial, for the humerus is craniolateral, and for the femur is lateral (Fig. 1–14). In order to insert the pins in the humerus and femur, it is necessary to penetrate both skin and underlying muscle; however, the aforementioned surfaces keep muscle thickness to a minimum.

3. *The fracture should be reduced and maintained in reduction during application of splint.* With the fracture reduced, the soft tissues are restored to their normal anatomical position, and the pins can be inserted without

binding the soft tissues. This helps to minimize tissue irritation and discomfort to the animal. If at any time reduction is lost during pin insertion, it should be regained before proceeding.

4. *Auxiliary fixation should be used when indicated.* The goals of fracture treatment are early ambulation and full return of function. In order to accomplish these goals, rigid uninterrupted stabilization of the main fracture fragments must be accomplished. Auxiliary fixation (which may include use of lag screws, intramedullary pins, and cerclage, hemicerclage, or one of the various wire configurations) may be helpful in maintaining reduction during insertion of the fixation pins and in aiding rigid stabilization (Fig. 1–15).

5. *Use an acceptable mode of pin insertion.*[2, 3, 19, 29–31] Use of the hand chuck or slow-speed power drill (150 rpm or less) is acceptable (Fig. 1–16). After insertion, each pin should be checked to make sure it is solidly anchored in the bone. A high-speed power drill creates an undue amount of heat, which can cause bone necrosis and pin loosening. Trocar pointed pins are favored, and those with a relatively long point are preferred because they penetrate the bone faster and are easier to insert (Fig. 1–17).

6. *Insert the pins at an angle of 70° to the long axis of the bone* (Fig. 1–18).[27, 41] Pins inserted at this angle give maximum stiffness to the fixator along with maximum pull-out resistance from the bone.[19, 22, 34]

7. *Insert all fixation pins in the same plane.* This has two advantages: (1) all pins can be attached to a common connecting bar, and (2) if postoperative swelling occurs, the fixation clamps can be loosened and readily adjusted without affecting reduction at the fracture site. The procedure for application using one connecting bar is shown in Fig. 1–19.

8. *Insert pins in the proper location of the bone fragment.*[35, 36] Experimental and clinical studies indicate that maximum stability is accomplished

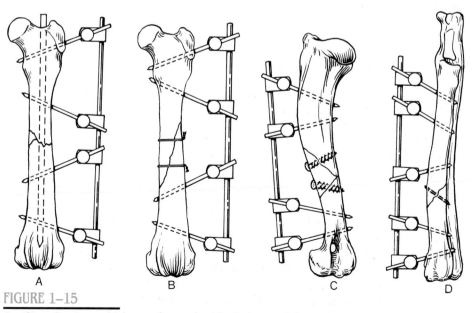

A   B   C   D

FIGURE 1–15

Auxiliary fixation, which may be used with the external fixator. (A) Intramedullary pin. (B) Cerclage wire. (C) Lag screws. (D) Diagonally inserted Kirschner pin.

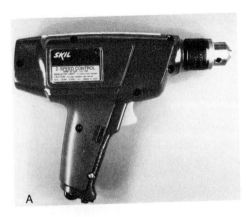
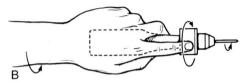

FIGURE 1–16

Trocar pointed Steinmann pins are inserted with a low-speed power drill (150 rpm or less) *(A)* or by use of a hand chuck *(B)*. The correct method of holding the hand chuck or pin drill to minimize wobbling is with the wrist straight and the elbow flexed. The forearm, pin chuck, and pin are rotated as one unit.

by inserting the pins near the proximal and distal ends of the bone fragment rather than by inserting both pins near the ends or near the fracture site (Fig. 1–20). Because the cortex is normally thinner near the proximal and distal ends, it is advantageous to avoid placing pins in these areas if possible. Cancellous bone has very little holding power on the pins.

9. *Insert two to four pins in each major bone fragment.*[19, 29, 35–39] Until the early 1970s, two pins per bone fragment were used in most cases. Studies since that time definitely indicate that three or four pins per fragment increase the stiffness of the fixator (Figs. 1–21, 1–22). How much stiffness is needed to heal various types of fractures is unknown. Clinically, it appears that one of the major advantages of using more than two pins per fragment is better distribution of the forces to which the pins are subjected during healing. This appears to hold true in clinical use because bent pins and loosening are much less frequently encountered when three to four pins per fragment are used. All fractures require a minimum of two pins on each segment. If healing is anticipated to be slow as a result of comminution, contamination, old age, and so forth, more pins per segment are useful.

10. *Choose optimal size of the fixation pins and connecting bar.* The appropriate size of both varies with the size of the bone involved. In the United States, the Kirschner splint is the make of apparatus used almost exclusively in small animals. The medium-size fixation clamps accommodate

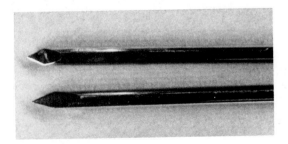

FIGURE 1–17

Trocar pointed Steinmann pins. The relatively long point is preferred over the short point; it penetrates faster and easier.

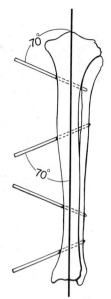

FIGURE 1–18

For maximum stiffness, the fixation pins should be inserted at a 70° angle to the long axis of the bone.

a ³⁄₁₆″ connecting bar. The use of two connecting bars (Fig. 1–21) approximately doubles the stiffness of the splint and may be indicated for use in some of the very large or giant breed dogs. The medium-size fixation clamps accommodate ⅛″ and ³⁄₃₂″ fixation pins. The ⅛″ pins are used most frequently; however, the ³⁄₃₂″ pins may be used on animals in the 18-to-25 pound range. The miniature

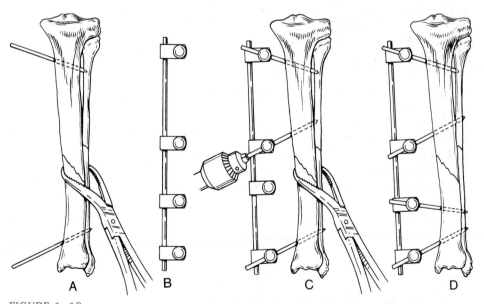

FIGURE 1–19

Unilateral external fixator, one connecting bar, 2/2 pins. (A) The fracture is first reduced, and reduction is maintained during the application procedure. The proximal and distal pins are inserted. (B) The fixation clamps are assembled on the connecting bar. (C) The fixation clamps are attached to the proximal and distal pins. The remaining two pins are inserted through the center clamps and bone. (D) All clamps are tightened, and the incision is closed.

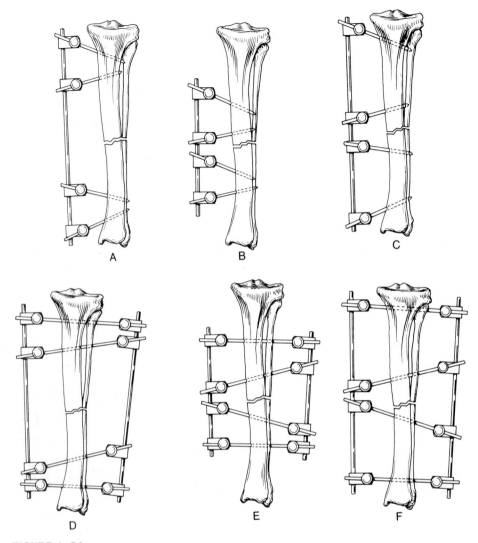

FIGURE 1–20

Unilateral configuration (A–C) and bilateral configurations (D–F). Maximum stability is accomplished by inserting the pins near the proximal and distal ends of the bone fragment (C, F) in preference to both pins near the proximal end (A, D) or the fracture site (B, E).

clamps accommodate a ⅛″ connecting bar and fixation pins can range up to ¹⁄₁₆″ in diameter. In clinical settings, the largest practical pin size is used because this gives stiffness to the apparatus, bends less at the pin-bone interface on cyclic loading, and is less apt to loosen during the healing period. However, in general, the fixation pin should not exceed one third of the diameter of the bone because weakening and fracture can occur.

11. *Insert pins through both cortices of the bone.* Invariably, any pin that is not inserted through both cortices loosens and thus does not accomplish its mission (Fig. 1–14). With few exceptions, the pin point can be palpated on penetration of the far cortex. The pin should penetrate about the length of the trocar point. If pins should penetrate too far on insertion, they can be backed out to the proper depth.

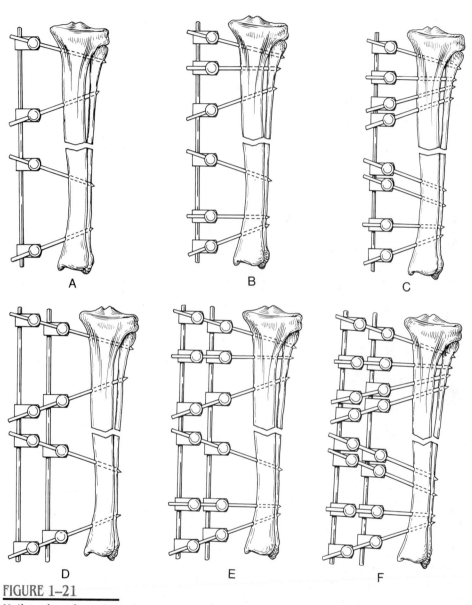

FIGURE 1–21

Unilateral configurations. One connecting bar: (A) 2/2 pins/fragment, (B) 3/3 pins/fragment, (C) 4/4 pins/fragment. Two connecting bars: (D) 2/2 pins/fragment, (E) 3/3 pins/fragment, (F) 4/4 pins/fragment. Using two connecting bars approximately doubles the stiffness of the splint; however, this is usually only indicated in the very large dog. *Note*: The "fracture gap" is for artistic clarity.

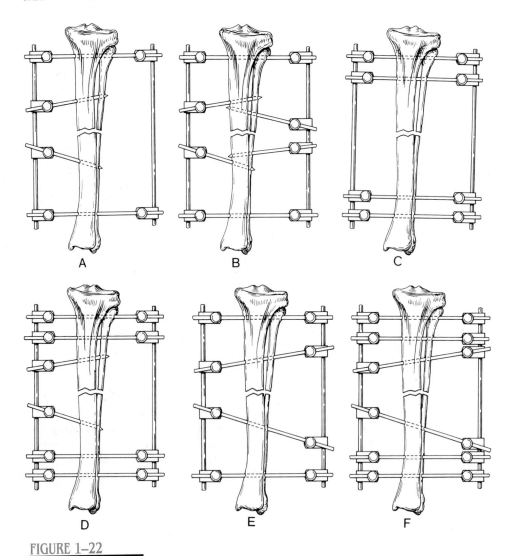

A   B   C

D   E   F

FIGURE 1–22

Various bilateral configurations. On the basis of stiffness response, starting from the least and progressing upward, the ranking is A through F. Stiffness is improved by through-and-through pins instead of half pins, using angled pins, or increasing the number of pins. *Note:* The "fracture gap" is for artistic clarity.

12. *Use the more suitable configuration of the splint.*[16–19, 27–30, 35–38] The four most common configurations used in veterinary orthopedics are unilateral (Fig. 1–21), bilateral (Fig. 1–22), biplanar (Fig. 1–23), and the original Kirschner design (Fig. 1–24). The original Kirschner design and the unilateral configuration can be used on all of the long bones and the mandible. The biplanar and bilateral configurations are limited in use to fractures of the tibia, radius and ulna, and mandible to avoid interfering with the body wall. Static strength and stiffness evaluations of the four configurations, starting from the lowest, places them approximately in the order of (1) the original Kirschner design, (2) unilateral, (3) biplanar, and (4) bilateral. This cannot be made as a definite statement because stiffness and clinical performance are dependent on the diameter of the connecting bars, diameter and number of pins, angle and location of pins in the cortical bone, length of the pins from the fixation

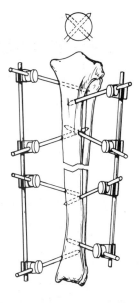

FIGURE 1-23

Biplanar configuration. One unilateral external fixator is placed on the medial surface of the tibia or radius, and another is placed on the cranial surface. Their connecting bars may be bridged by two or more connecting bars; however, this is usually not necessary. Modifications of this configuration work well to bridge joints when fixation of the joint is indicated. *Note:* The "fracture gap" is for artistic clarity.

clamps to the bone, and the inherent stability at the fracture site. The addition of auxiliary fixation at the fracture site can significantly increase stability of the fractured bone.

Past clinical experience supports the statement that the stiffness produced by the original Kirschner design with two connecting bars and that produced by the unilateral configuration, one connecting bar with two to four pins per bone fragment, are adequate in most cases. Because fractures vary widely in type, stability, condition of soft tissue, animal activity, and size of the patient, no single configuration is best suited for all fractures; however, the simple configurations serve very well on most fractures.

FIGURE 1-24

Original Kirschner configurations using one *(A)* or two *(B)* connecting bars. With clinical patients, two connecting bars are used in most cases because this markedly increases splint stiffness and stability. *Note:* The "fracture gap" is for artistic clarity.

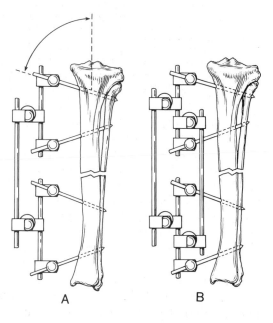

A   B

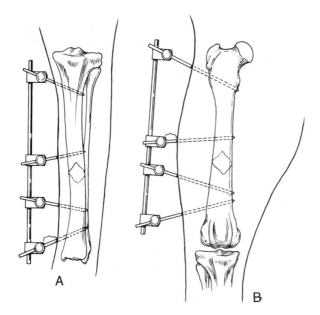

FIGURE 1–25

The distance between the fixation clamps and the skin is usually ⅜″ to ½″. (A, B) This distance varies with the size of the animal and anticipated postsurgical swelling. If swelling causes the skin to press against the fixation clamps, readjustment and movement of the clamps outward on the pins are indicated because contact pressure will result in necrosis of the soft tissue.

13. *Bone graft architectural deficits.* Because rigidity of fixation using the external fixator is usually less than that when using plates, the body is stimulated to produce more bridging callus. If there are definite architectural deficits present, however, they should be filled with a bone graft. This is particularly true in mature and older animals, certain osteotomies, and nonunions.

14. *Place the pins an optimal distance between the fixation clamps and the skin.* This distance at the time of application varies with both the size of the animal and the anticipated postsurgical swelling. The distance is usually ⅜ to ½″ (Fig. 1–25). Postsurgical swelling, which usually occurs within the first 10 days, may necessitate readjustment and moving the fixation clamps outward on the pins because contact pressure will result in necrosis of the soft tissue. Regions of tissue movement (e.g., near joints) swell more than do regions of little motion.

15. *Use proper aftercare.* Following application, the external fixator is usually covered by a dressing of cotton (particularly between the skin and fixation clamps), gauze, and tape. Redressing is usually indicated in 1 week or less and at 2-week intervals thereafter. If seepage develops around any of the pins, the dressing is removed and left off. Rarely is any treatment beyond removal of the bandage indicated for seepage around the pins. Some limitation of activity is indicated depending on the overall evaluation of the patient and the fracture area.

Most of the complications that have been attributed to use of the external fixator can be minimized or eliminated if these basic guidelines in its application are meticulously followed and if it has not been used on fractures beyond its capability.

INTRAMEDULLARY PINS

There are many different types of pins available; however, the round pins (Steinmann, Kirschner drill wire) are most commonly used.[2, 3, 40–43] Pins with other than a round cross-sectional diameter (diamond, cloverleaf, V-shaped) have been developed to engage the inner surface of the cortex and thus improve stability. As a result of variations in the diameter of the marrow cavity and of the length and curvature of the long bones in dogs, their insertion is difficult and may be accompanied by complications.

Intramedullary pins may be used for stable fractures; in unstable fractures, they are used in combination with other methods of fixation.

As the sole method of fixation, round intramedullary pins are used primarily on stable fractures in small dogs and cats. Angular stability and maintenance of length are achieved by rigid fixation of the pin in both ends of the bone, with impingement of the pin by the inner surface of the cortex at the fracture site. The pin should approximate the diameter of the marrow cavity at the fracture site; however, curvature of the bone, variations in cross-sectional diameter of the shaft, and the nature of the fracture may necessitate a compromise in pin diameter, particularly in the canine. In the feline, the long bones are relatively straight, and the pin can more nearly approximate the diameter of the marrow cavity. Rotational stability is aided by muscle forces and the interlocking of the serrated edges at the fracture site.

Intramedullary fixation with Steinmann (round) pins may be accomplished by an open or closed method. The closed technique is restricted to simple fractures, those of recent origin, and those that can be reduced with ease and accuracy. This technique may be applied to the femur, tibia, humerus, ulna, and some of the other small bones. Refer to the specific bone for points of insertion. The open technique is used for the more complex fractures, those requiring an open reduction, those requiring additional internal fixation, nonunions, and so forth.

AUXILIARY FIXATION WITH INTRAMEDULLARY PINS

When the intramedullary pin alone does not give sufficient rigid stability, which is usually the case, the use of auxiliary fixation is indicated to help protect against rotation and shortening. The following are among the methods of the auxiliary fixation.[2, 3]

1. Cerclage or hemicerclage wire (Fig. 1–26A, B).

2. Unilateral fixator, 1/1 pin per fragment is used on relatively stable fractures (Fig. 1–26C); 2/2 pins per fragment are used on unstable fractures. In addition, cerclage wires may be used to further improve stability in certain unstable fractures (Fig. 1–26D).

3. Bone screws inserted with a lag effect (Fig. 1–26E). With the fracture reduced and held in position, the intramedullary pin is inserted first and then the lag screw is inserted in an off-center position.

4. Use of two or more pins, or what is usually referred to as stacking pins (Fig. 1–26F).

5. Use of interfragmentary orthopedic wire inserted to secure the cortical segments to each other and the intramedullary pin at the fracture site (Fig. 1–26G, H).

6. Any combination of the above may be used when indicated to obtain stability.

Note: Proximal pin migration postoperatively is a definite indication of movement and insufficient stability at the fracture site. Distal pin migration

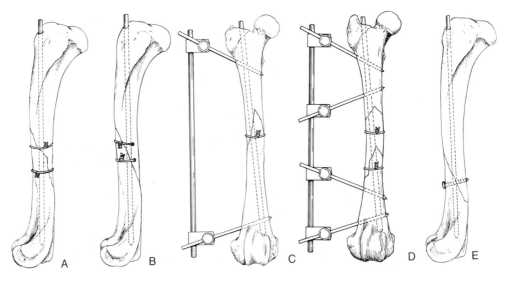

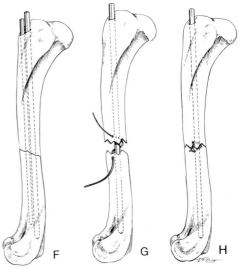

FIGURE 1–26

Auxiliary fixation used with an intramedullary pin. *(A)* Two cerclage wires. *(B)* Two hemicerclage wires. *(C)* External fixator 1/1 pin (half Kirschner splint) and a cerclage wire. *(D)* External fixator, 2/2 pins, and cerclage wires used in a multiple fracture. *(E)* Lag screws. Their use is usually limited to larger dogs. *(F)* Two intramedullary pins used in a serrated short oblique fracture. *(G, H)* Interfragmentary wire crossed around intramedullary pin as auxiliary fixation in a serrated transverse fracture.

into the joint, with very few exceptions, means that the pin penetrated the distal articular cartilage at the time of insertion. Usually, this can be corrected at the time of surgery by retracting the pin so that the point is in the marrow cavity, then by reangling the distal segment slightly before advancing the pin into the distal segment.

TENSION BAND WIRE

According to the tension band wire principle, active distracting forces are counteracted and converted into compressive forces.[44, 45, 47] The tensile forces exerted by contraction of muscles on fractures such as those involving the olecranon process, trochanter major, tuber calcis, or detached tibial tubercle can be overcome and converted to compressive forces by inserting two Kirschner wires and a tension band wire (Fig. 1–27).

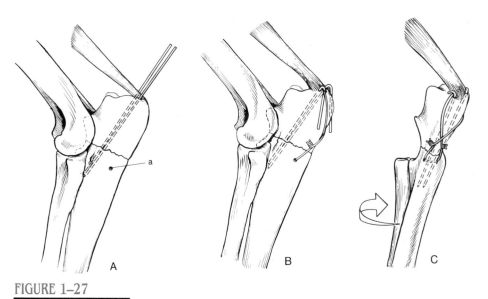

FIGURE 1-27

Tension band wire and Kirschner wire fixation. (A) Olecranon fracture. Kirschner wires placed at caudomedial and lateral corners of triceps tendon insertion. Ideally, the pins contact the cranial ulnar cortex distal to the coronoid process. A transverse hole (a) is drilled through the caudal cortex. (B) The tension band wire is positioned and twisted tight on both sides of the figure "8." The wire should pass through the triceps tendon close to the olecranon proximally. The Kirschner wires are bent caudally, cut, and (C) rotated 180° so that the ends are buried in soft tissue. If the fragments of the above fracture do not interlock or if comminution is present, plate fixation is indicated.

Technique

The usual procedure in repairing a fracture or osteotomy of the olecranon process requires first reducing the fracture, then inserting two pins that are started on the caudomedial and lateral corners. Such placement interferes less with the triceps tendon, and bending of the pins can be accomplished more effectively. If the pins can be inserted diagonally to engage the cranial cortex distally, they do a better job of securing the fragments and countering rotational and shearing forces than if they just go down the medullary canal. The pins should be as parallel to each other as possible. A transverse hole is then drilled through the diaphysis distal to the fracture site (Fig. 1–27A). The wire is inserted in a figure-8 fashion and tightened by twisting. Avoid overtightening, because this will create a gap at the articular notch if the fracture is in this area (Fig. 1–27B). The individual Kirschner drill wires are then bent down the caudal surface of the ulna cut (Fig. 1–27B), and rotated so that the ends are buried in soft tissue (Fig. 1–27C). If properly inserted, most of these do not interfere with movement of soft tissue and usually do not need to be removed after healing.

Other situations in which the tension band wire principle can be used to advantage include the following:

1. Avulsion fracture or osteotomy of the trochanter major of the femur (Fig. 1–28A).
2. Avulsion fracture of the tibial tubercle (Fig. 1–28B).
3. Fracture or osteotomy of the medial malleolus of the tibia (Fig. 1–28C).
4. Fracture of the tuber calcanei (Fig. 1–28D).

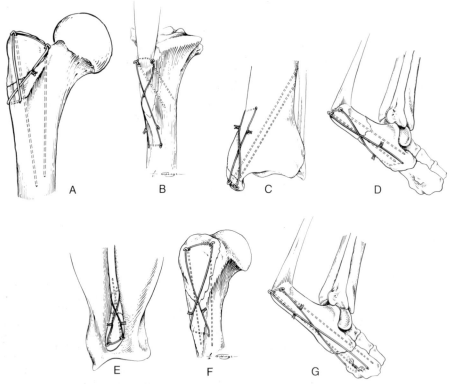

FIGURE 1–28

Conditions in which the tension band wire principle can be used to advantage. *(A)* Avulsion fracture or osteotomy of the trochanter major of the femur. *(B)* Avulsion fracture of the tibial tubercle. *(C)* Fracture or osteotomy of the medial malleolus of the tibia. *(D)* Fracture of the tuber calcanei. *(E)* Fracture or osteotomy of the acromion process of the scapula. *(F)* Fracture or osteotomy of the greater tuberosity of the humerus. *(G)* Arthrodesis of the intertarsal joint for fracture separation.

    5. Fracture or osteotomy of the acromial process of the scapula, usually in large dogs (Fig. 1–28E).

    6. Fracture or osteotomy of the greater tuberosity of the humerus (Fig. 1–28F).

    7. Arthrodesis of the intertarsal joint for fracture separation (Fig. 1–28G).

CERCLAGE OR HEMICERCLAGE WIRE

This procedure refers to a circle of wire that completely (Fig. 1–29A) or partially (Fig. 1–29B) goes around the circumference of a bone.[3, 46–48] Cerclage or hemicerclage wire is not used as the sole method of fixation on any type of long bone fracture.

Indications

These wires are used primarily on long oblique, spiral, and certain comminuted or multiple fractures. They are used in auxiliary fixation (Figs. 1–29A,

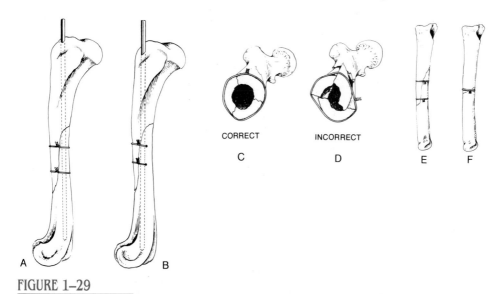

FIGURE 1–29

Uses of cerclage and hemicerclage wires. *(A)* Double cerclage wires. *(B)* Double hemicerclage wires. *(C)* Cerclage wires used to reconstruct a comminuted fracture. The fragments are anatomically reduced. *(D)* Failure to reduce fracture anatomically allows fragments to collapse despite cerclage wire. *(E)* When cerclage wires are used on oblique fractures, the fracture line must be at least twice as long as the bone diameter, i.e., the fracture line is 45° or less. This allows interfragmentary compression. In keeping with the length of the obliquity, the cerclage wires are usually placed about 1 to 1.5 cm apart. Cerclage wire should not be placed closer than 5 mm from the proximal or distal tip of the obliquity. *(F)* If the fracture line is greater than 45°, tightening the cerclage wires produces shear force rather than compression force.

B and 1–32*B*) and aid in holding the fracture segments in the reduced position while primary fixation is applied (Fig. 1–32A–C).

Technique

Several fundamentals must be observed if these wires are to be used with optimal success.

1. Use stainless steel wire of sufficient strength for immobilization. Wire of about 22 gauge (.025″, 0.635 mm) is suitable for toy breeds and cats, 20 gauge (.032″, 0.812 mm) for average dogs, and 18 gauge (.040″, 1.02 mm) diameter for large breeds. A number of wire tighteners are available; most are satisfactory if used properly (Fig. 1–30).

2. Apply the wire tightly to bring about rigid fixation of the fracture segments. (Anything short of this allows movement, devascularization, and demineralization of bone.)

3. In applying the wire, avoid destruction of blood supply (resulting from detachment of soft tissue). The wire passer (Fig. 1–31) serves very well for placing the wire around the bone with a minimum of trauma.

4. Restrict use of wires primarily to areas where the cylinder of bone can be reconstructed anatomically; they should not be used to surround multiple unreduced fragments (Fig. 1–29C, D).

5. When used with oblique fractures, wire fixation should be restricted to those with a fracture line approximately twice the diameter of the bone or

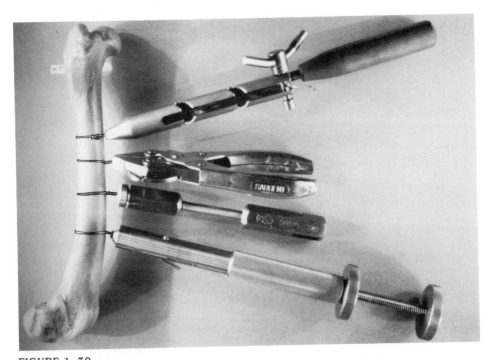

FIGURE 1-30

Various types of wire tighteners that may be used for twisting and tightening cerclage wires.

longer (Fig. 1–29E, F). (The same principle applies for the use of a lag screw in oblique fractures.)

6. Above all, stabilize the main bone fragments with rigid, uninterrupted primary fixation (Figs. 1–29A, B and 1–32C). Depending on the type of fracture, this may be accomplished with an intramedullary pin, an external fixator, or a plate.

7. If a relatively long fracture area is to be covered, the cerclage wires should be spaced approximately 1 to 1.5 cm apart. Placement closer than this may result in unnecessary devitalization of the bone (caused by detachment of soft tissue in placing the wires) and delay of union and does not increase the fixation stability. The number of cerclage wires used is in direct relation to the length of the fractures. When placing a full cerclage on a bone that is conical in shape (e.g., proximal femur), precautions may need to be taken to avoid distal slipping. This can be accomplished by notching the bone or driving a small Kirschner wire perpendicular to the bone. One end of the Kirschner wire is bent 90° to discourage late migration of the implant.

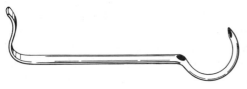

FIGURE 1-31

Wire passer. This instrument makes it possible to insert the cerclage wire around the bone with a very minimum of soft tissue detachment.

FIGURE 1–32

Cerclage wire and bone plate. *(A)* Comminuted fracture of the femur. *(B)* Comminuted area reconstructed and compressed using cerclage wires and a lag screw. *(C)* Neutralization plate applied.

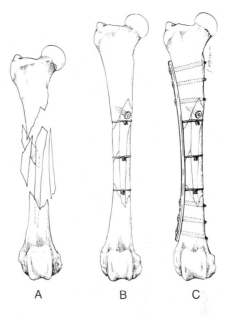

A   B   C

BONE SCREWS

There are two basic types of bone screws: cancellous (Fig. 1–33A) and cortical (Fig. 1–33D).[44, 45] Cancellous screws are used to compress fragments of epiphyseal and metaphyseal bone. The screw may be partially or completely threaded with relatively few threads per unit length; threads are quite deep, and the pitch of the threads is relatively high. Cortical screws are used primarily in the diaphyseal bone. The screw is fully threaded with more threads per unit length than cancellous screws; threads are shallower and more flatly pitched than cancellous screws.

Indications for Use

PRIMARY FIXATION IN CERTAIN FRACTURES ■ These fractures are usually in the metaphyseal or articular areas of the bone rather than in the diaphysis. To accomplish interfragmental compression, cancellous screws are inserted so that the thread of the screw does not cross the fracture line (Fig. 1–33B, C). The fracture segments are first reduced; after the hole is drilled, the thread is cut using the appropriate tap. Some cancellous screws are self-tapping and thus do not require pretapping. Tightening the screw produces compression of the fracture segments as the near fragment glides on the smooth shank of the screw.

INTERFRAGMENTAL COMPRESSION ■ A cortical screw will bring about interfragmentary compression (Fig. 1–33E) when it is inserted to accomplish a lag effect. This requires that an oversized hole equal to the diameter of the screw threads ("gliding hole") be drilled in the near cortex and that a hole equal in size to the diameter of the screw core ("thread hole") be drilled in the far cortex and tapped so that the screw thread becomes engaged on insertion. Tightening the screw allows compression to be exerted between the two cortices. For best

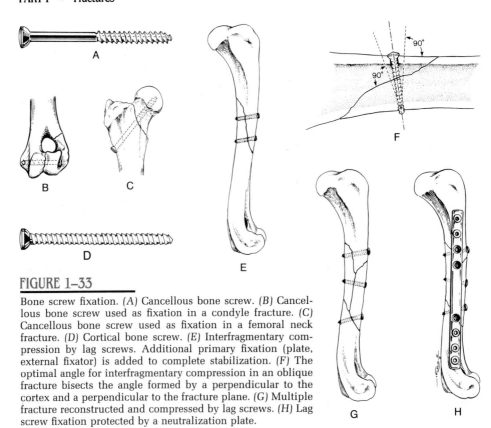

FIGURE 1–33

Bone screw fixation. *(A)* Cancellous bone screw. *(B)* Cancellous bone screw used as fixation in a condyle fracture. *(C)* Cancellous bone screw used as fixation in a femoral neck fracture. *(D)* Cortical bone screw. *(E)* Interfragmentary compression by lag screws. Additional primary fixation (plate, external fixator) is added to complete stabilization. *(F)* The optimal angle for interfragmentary compression in an oblique fracture bisects the angle formed by a perpendicular to the cortex and a perpendicular to the fracture plane. *(G)* Multiple fracture reconstructed and compressed by lag screws. *(H)* Lag screw fixation protected by a neutralization plate.

mechanical advantage, the hole is drilled so that it bisects the angle formed by a perpendicular fixation to the cortex and a perpendicular fixation to the fracture plane (Fig. 1–33F). Screws are never used as the primary fixation in shaft fractures. They are always supplemented with a plate, pin, or external fixator splint.

AID IN REDUCTION AND AUXILIARY FIXATION ■ With long oblique, spiral, or multiple fractures of the diaphysis, cortical bone screws inserted with a lag effect to accomplish interfragmentary compression may be used as an aid in accomplishing reduction and serve as auxiliary fixation (Fig. 1–33, G). Two adjoining fragments are reduced and usually held in the reduced-compressed position during drilling, tapping, and insertion of the bone screw. The bone screw should be inserted at a distance from the fracture line at least equal to the screw diameter. When the fracture is multiple in nature and the bone segments are of sufficient size, the entire bone or portions of it may be reconstructed anatomically by reducing and fixing two fragments at a time until reconstruction is complete (Fig. 1–33G). A "neutralization" plate is then applied for final fixation (Fig. 1–33H).

Whenever possible, lag screws should be used in preference to cerclage wire to accomplish interfragmental compression and to aid in reduction and auxiliary fixation. Clinical documentation of fracture treatment clearly substantiates this statement.[4]

One of the primary objectives in the treatment of fractures is early return to full function of the injured limb. Bone plates are ideal for accomplishing this goal because they have the potential to restore rigid stability to the reconstructed fractured bone when properly applied.[44, 45, 49-56] Although different designs and sizes of plates are available, the ASIF* system (see Figure 1–42) is used to illustrate the principles.[44, 45]

For optimum results in the use of bone plates, a scientific understanding of the following areas is a prerequisite:

1. Anatomy (e.g., structure of bone; location of blood and nerve supply; muscle separations; and attachments of muscles, tendons, and ligaments).

2. Principles of active forces (knowledge of compression, tension, and torsional and bending forces as they affect the bone).

3. Understanding of the mechanics of fixation in detail and viewing and planning its application in three dimensions.

4. Proper selection of a surgical approach and method of internal fixation best suited for the individual fracture.

5. Bone healing (biological response with rigid fixation and interpretation of radiographic findings, primary bone union versus development of a cloudy irritation callus; the latter is a warning sign and indicates some movement occurring at the fracture site).

When two vascular, anatomically reduced bone fragments are rigidly fixed under compression so that no shearing or torsional forces can act on them, no resorption of bone at the fracture line takes place, and a direct bony union occurs without any radiologically visible periosteal callus (so-called primary bone union).

Terminology

Plates may be inserted to function as a compression plate, a neutralization plate, or a buttress plate.

COMPRESSION PLATE ■ When the plate is applied so that it is under tension and the fracture fragments are under compression, it is referred to as a compression plate. It is vital that the plate be applied on the side of the bone that is most frequently under a distracting or tension force (e.g., lateral surface of the femur, medial or cranial surface of the tibia, cranial or lateral surface of the humerus, craniomedial or cranial surface of the radius). This function may be accomplished by use of a regular plate and tension device (Fig. 1–34), the self-compressing plate (DCP) (see Figures 1–40 and 1–41), or a semitubular plate (see Figure 1–39). Axial compression is accomplished at the fracture site. Compression plates are used on stable fractures, osteotomies, and arthrodeses.

NEUTRALIZATION PLATE ■ The plate is applied on the tension side of the bone to neutralize or overcome those forces (torsional, bending, compressive, distraction) to which the fractured bone may be subjected during the healing process. If possible, the plate is applied to exert some axial compression. However, the

---

*Association for the Study of Internal Fixation, Synthes Ltd. (USA), Wayne, PA.

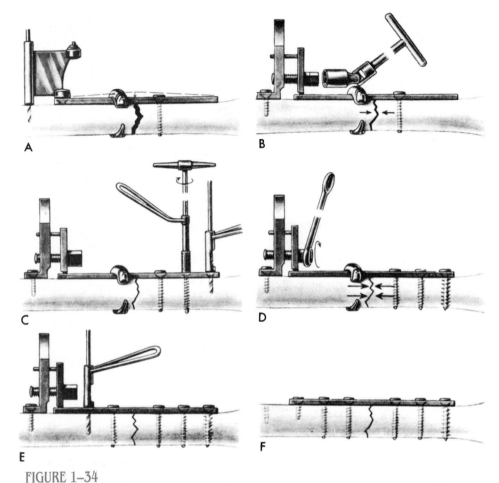

FIGURE 1-34

Application of a regular plate to accomplish axial compression by using a tension device. *(A)* The plate is first attached to one of the bone segments. *(B)* The tension device is attached and lightly tightened. *(C)* The remaining screws are inserted in the first segment. *(D)* The tension device is tightened. *(E, F)* The remaining screws are placed in the adjoining segment, and the tension device is removed. (From Müller, et al: Manual of Internal Fixation, 2nd ed. Translated by J. Schatzker. New York, Springer-Verlag, 1979, p 55.)

major interfragmentary compression is supplied by lag screws and cerclage or hemicerclage wire (Fig. 1–33H). Neutralization plates are used on unstable fractures or osteotomies that can be anatomically reconstructed using lag screws or cerclage wire.

BUTTRESS PLATE ■ The plate is used to shore up a fragment of bone, thereby maintaining length and the proper functional angle in fractures such as those involving the proximal tibial plateau (Fig. 1–35B). It also may be considered to splint or bridge the fracture area to maintain length of the bone (Fig. 1–35C).

Note: The various names given to plates refer to function only. The same plate can be used in any of the described manners.

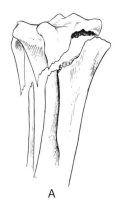

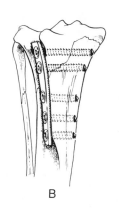

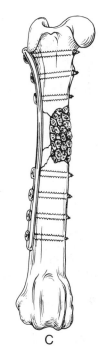

FIGURE 1–35

Buttress plate. *(A)* Fracture of the proximal tibial plateau. *(B)* Buttress plate fixation shores up the fragment, maintaining length and proper functional angle. *(C)* Buttress plate bridges a defect filled with bone graft.

Indications

Bone plates are adaptable for these situations:

1. Most bone fractures.
2. Multiple and complex fractures.
3. Fractures in the larger dogs and semidomesticated animals (because postoperative complications are less frequent when the fixation apparatus is covered with soft tissue and skin).

Tension Band Plate Principle (Compression Plate)

Long bones (e.g., the femur) are subject to eccentric loading and may be compared to a bent column. The lateral side is subject to distracting or tension forces; the medial side, to impacting or compressive forces (Fig. 1–36*A, B*). When a plate is applied to the lateral surface, it counteracts all tension forces and creates compressive forces along the fracture line, thus providing rigid internal fixation (Fig. 1–36*C*). If it were applied on the medial surface, it would not give long-lasting fixation because the plate would be under excessive bending stress and subject to fatigue fracture (Fig. 1–36*D*).

Number of Screws

Clinical data indicate that an absolute minimum of two screws (four cortices) should be used in the bone segments on each side of the fracture in small animals. However, a minimum of three to four screws (six to eight cortices) is ideal and mandatory in many of the larger small animals (Fig. 1–37).

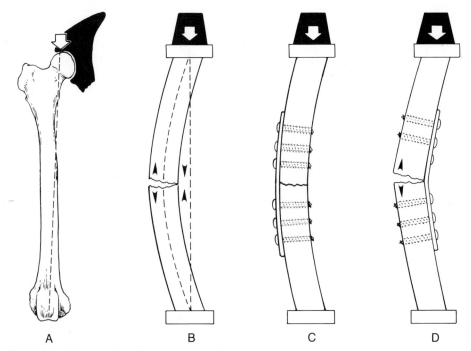

FIGURE 1–36

Principle of a compression plate. Insert the plate only on the tension side of the bone so that the bone will receive compressive forces. Because long bones are subject to eccentric loading, the side of the bone to be under tension must be known to determine where to apply the plate. The femur *(A)*, for example, can be compared to a bent column *(B)*. The plate that is applied to the outer or convex side can then counteract all tension forces *(C)* and provide rigid internal fixation. If it were applied on the inner or concave surface, it would not provide fixation *(D)*; such a plate would come under excessive bending stresses and would soon show a fatigue fracture.

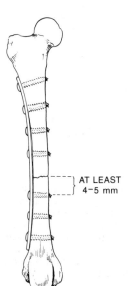

AT LEAST
4–5 mm

FIGURE 1–37

Plate fixation: number of screws and screw placement. Although two screws (four cortices) are an absolute minimum on each side of the fracture line, three to four screws (six to eight cortices) are more ideal and are mandatory for larger breeds. Minimal distance between fracture lines and screws is 4 to 5 mm.

Placement of Screws

Clinical and experimental data indicate that the minimal distance between screw hole and fracture line should be 4 to 5 mm, or at least the diameter of the screw used (Fig. 1–37).[4, 44, 45]

Length and Size of Bone Plate

A long plate is much more effective than a short plate in neutralizing forces to which the fractured bone may be subjected. The ideal in most cases is to use a plate that is just short of the entire length of the bone (Fig. 1–37). (See Figure 1–43 for plate size guidelines.) Because the number of screw holes is directly proportional to the length of the plate, with the longer plate, more screws are used.

Contouring the Plate

If anatomical reduction of the bone fragments is to be maintained during application of the bone plate, it is mandatory that the plate be contoured to closely fit the bone surface to which it is to be applied. In some cases, this is accomplished by bending; in others, by a combination of bending and twisting. The plate should be bent between the screw holes (Fig. 1–38A). Prestressing (underbending) the plate is advisable in most cases because it aids in mini-

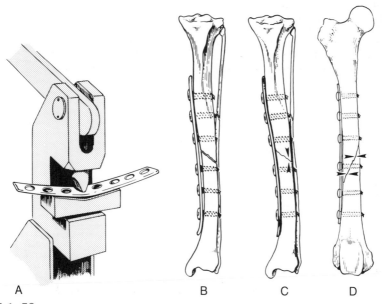

A　　　　　　　　B　　　C　　　D

FIGURE 1–38

Plate fixation: contouring the plate. *(A)* The plate must be contoured so that it approximately fits the bone surface to which it is applied. Using the bone plate bending press, gently bend the plate between the screw holes. *(B)* Prestressing (underbending) the plate supplies added compression to the far cortex. In a curved bone, the plate is contoured to leave a 1-mm gap between plate and bone at the fracture site. In a straight bone, the plate is bowed slightly to produce the 1-mm gap. *(C)* Tightening the prestressed plate causes added compression on the cortex opposite the plate. *(D)* Lag screw through the plate. When the fracture line allows, interfragmentary compression can be applied by a lag screw through the bone plate. The plate then functions as a neutralization plate.

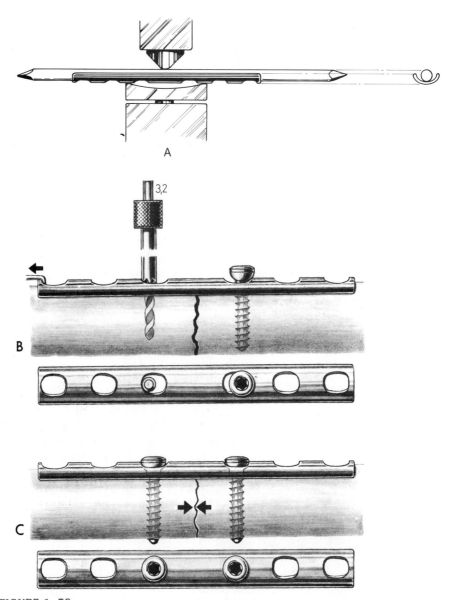

FIGURE 1–39

Semitubular plate. (A) A large Steinmann pin is placed in the concave side of a semitubular plate to accomplish slight bending without flattening. (B) Eccentrically located holes are drilled on either side of the fracture line, and screws are inserted. (C) Tightening the screws compresses the bone fragments at the fracture site. The remaining screws are usually inserted in the neutral position. (From Müller, et al: Manual of Internal Fixation, 2nd ed. Translated by J. Schatzker. New York, Springer-Verlag, 1979, p 67.)

mizing the gap on the far cortex and aids in compression when the screws are finally tightened. This usually amounts to a 1-mm gap between the bone and plate at the fracture site (Fig. 1–38B, C).

Insertion of a Lag Screw Through the Plate

In some cases, the fracture line lends itself to interfragmentary compression by inserting the lag screw through the bone plate (Fig. 1–38D).

Semitubular Plate

These plates are relatively thin and gain their strength by being semitubular in construction. They should be used as straight plates or with a minimum of bending. If minimal bending is indicated, this can best be accomplished by incorporating a ³⁄₁₆″ Steinmann pin in the process (Fig. 1–39A). This minimizes flattening of the plate in the bending process.

⁚ The holes in the plate are oval. Thus, when the first hole on each side of the fracture is drilled off center (i.e., away from the fracture line), compression takes place at the fracture site when the screws are tightened (Fig. 1–39B, C). The remaining screws are usually inserted by drilling in the center of the oval and placing them in the neutral position. Semitubular plates are used most frequently for fractures of the radius and ulna in dogs under about 50 pounds and for fractures on the radius, femur, and tibia of cats because their bones are relatively straight. The dynamic compression plate (DCP) is superior in construction and most frequently used.

Dynamic Compression Plate (DCP)

The design of the screw holes in this plate is based on the spherical gliding principle developed by the ASIF and patented by Synthes. As the screw is tightened, the spherical screw head glides toward the center of the plate until the deepest portion of the hole is reached (Fig. 1–40A, B). The result is that the bone fragment into which the screw is being driven is displaced at the same time and in the same direction—toward the center of the plate and the fracture line. By alternate tightening of the screws on each side of the fracture line, the fragments are compressed (Fig. 1–40C). The tension device may be used for additional compression (Fig. 1–40D).

Two drill guides (neutral, load) are used in drilling the holes in the proper position. The load guide has the potential of moving the fragment 1.0 mm and the neutral guide 0.1 mm in the 4.5-mm plate (Fig. 1–41A, B).

In general, all of the principles that apply to the insertion of regular plates apply to the DCP; however, the DCP[44, 45] has these additional advantages:

1. Cancellous bone screws may be inserted in each plate hole.
2. Plate screws may be applied at varying angles when used as lag screws (Fig. 1–41C).
3. With a fracture of three or more segments, the plate has the potential of compression at each of the fracture lines (Fig. 1–41D–F).

Selection of Proper Bone Plate and Screw Sizes

One of the problems confronting the surgeon is the choice of the size of implant to use on the various fractures in patients of different sizes. Various

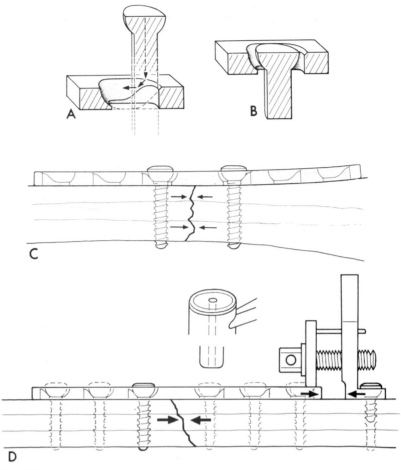

FIGURE 1–40

Self-compressing plate (DCP). (A, B) Sagittal sections of a screw and screw hole in a DCP show the mechanical principle. (C) The first screws on either side of the fracture line are inserted eccentrically (load position) and alternately tightened to produce compression. (D) If there is a wide fracture gap, additional compression can be accomplished by the use of a tension device. (From Müller, et al: Manual of Internal Fixation, 2nd ed. Translated by J. Schatzker. New York, Springer-Verlag, 1979.)

factors may be considered in choosing the size of implant, such as type and location of the fracture, age, activity, size of bone, weight of animal, and condition of soft tissue.[45, 55, 59] However, when the basic fundamentals of implantation are observed, the most consistent factor in choosing the size of the implant is the weight of the patient.

To provide guidelines in selecting proper bone plate and screw size, data were compiled on approximately 1000 bone plate cases and 300 screw fixation cases (Fig. 1–42) in which they were used as the primary method of fixation. The summation of data collected is presented in Figure 1–43. Corrections have been made and included for implants that were too weak (resulting in breaking or bending) or too strong (resulting primarily in stress protection). As expected, there is some overlapping of appliance sizes for given weights. In addition to the size of the implant, some of the more common causes of failure include bone plates that are too short in length, an insufficient number of bone screws, vascular impairment, infection, and failure to bone graft.

Removal of Bone Plates in Small Animals

INDICATIONS FOR REMOVAL

Bone plates should be removed under certain conditions[45, 56]:

1. When the plates become nonfunctional (e.g., loose, broken, or bent), they are no longer serving a useful purpose and some cause discomfort.

2. The plate may be acting as a thermal conductor. A small number of owners have observed that their animals show some favoring of the leg after being out in the cold for a period of time. However, normal functions return after the animal comes back into the house. This is thought to be caused by a difference in expansion and contraction of the plate and bone when subjected to change in temperature. Removal of the bone plate, after clinical union, has corrected the temporary lameness. Lameness has been most frequently noted with plate fixation of the radius and tibia.

3. The bone plate may cause stress protection. Bone plates are much more rigid than bone. When applied to bone for fixation of fractures, the plate prevents the bone from responding to normal physiological stimuli and thus may bring about alterations in architecture as visualized on the radiograph and in histological sections. These changes may be in part a result of a local

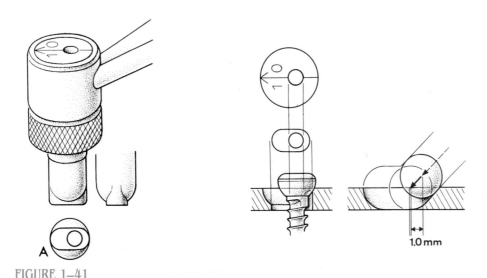

FIGURE 1–41

Drill guides for insertion of the self-compressing plate (DCP). (A) Load guide. The guide is inserted in the screw hole of the plate with the arrow pointing to the fracture line. The screw is located eccentrically so that in tightening, it moves 1 mm (it also moves the bone fragment 1 mm). (B) Neutral guide. The screw is located slightly eccentrically so that in tightening it moves 0.1 mm. (C) For oblique fractures, a lag screw may be inserted at an angle through the plate. (D–F) When multiple fracture lines are present, the first fracture line is compressed as the second screw in the load position is tightened. The second fracture line is compressed as the third screw in the load position is tightened. (From Allgöwer M, et al: The Dynamic Compression Plate. New York, Springer-Verlag, 1973, pp 15, 24, 34.)

Illustration continued on following page

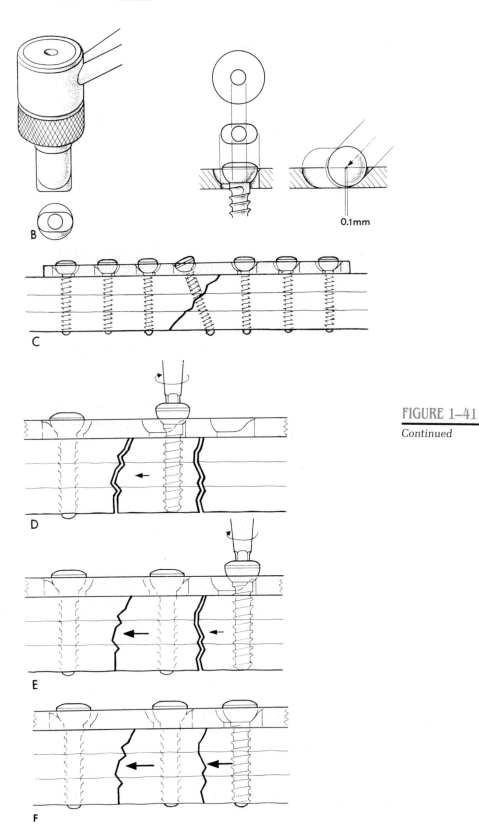

B

C

D

FIGURE 1–41

Continued

E

F

0.1mm

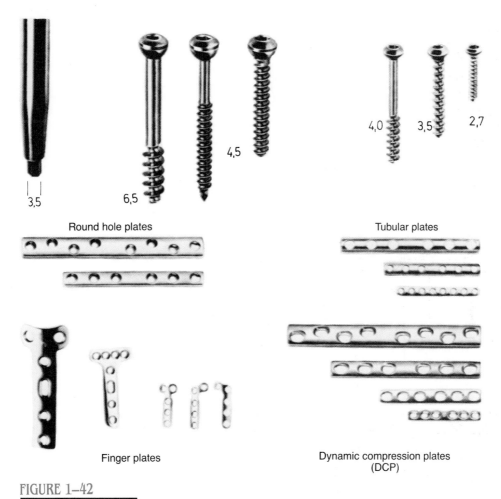

Round hole plates

Tubular plates

Finger plates

Dynamic compression plates
(DCP)

FIGURE 1–42

Bone plate and screw implants. (From Müller, et al: Manual of Internal Fixation, 2nd ed. New York, Springer-Verlag, 1979, pp 35, 49.)

periosteal circulatory disturbance brought about by plate/bone contact. The number in this category that give rise to a clinical problem is small and can usually be traced to using an implant that was too large and rigid or to leaving the plate in place for a prolonged period of time.

4. Interference with bone growth may occur in the young animal. Although many shaft fractures in the young can be treated by closed reduction and fixation since they heal rapidly, and because most axial deformities correct themselves during bone remodeling growth, open reduction and internal fixation are indicated when congruent articular surfaces or leg length cannot be obtained and maintained by conservative means. In our experience, altered bone growth in the young has not been a problem when bone plates have been removed at the time of clinical union.

5. The plate may cause irritation. Occasionally, an implant just beneath the skin gives rise to a lesion characteristic of a lick granuloma. Plate removal after clinical union has occurred has cleared up the condition.

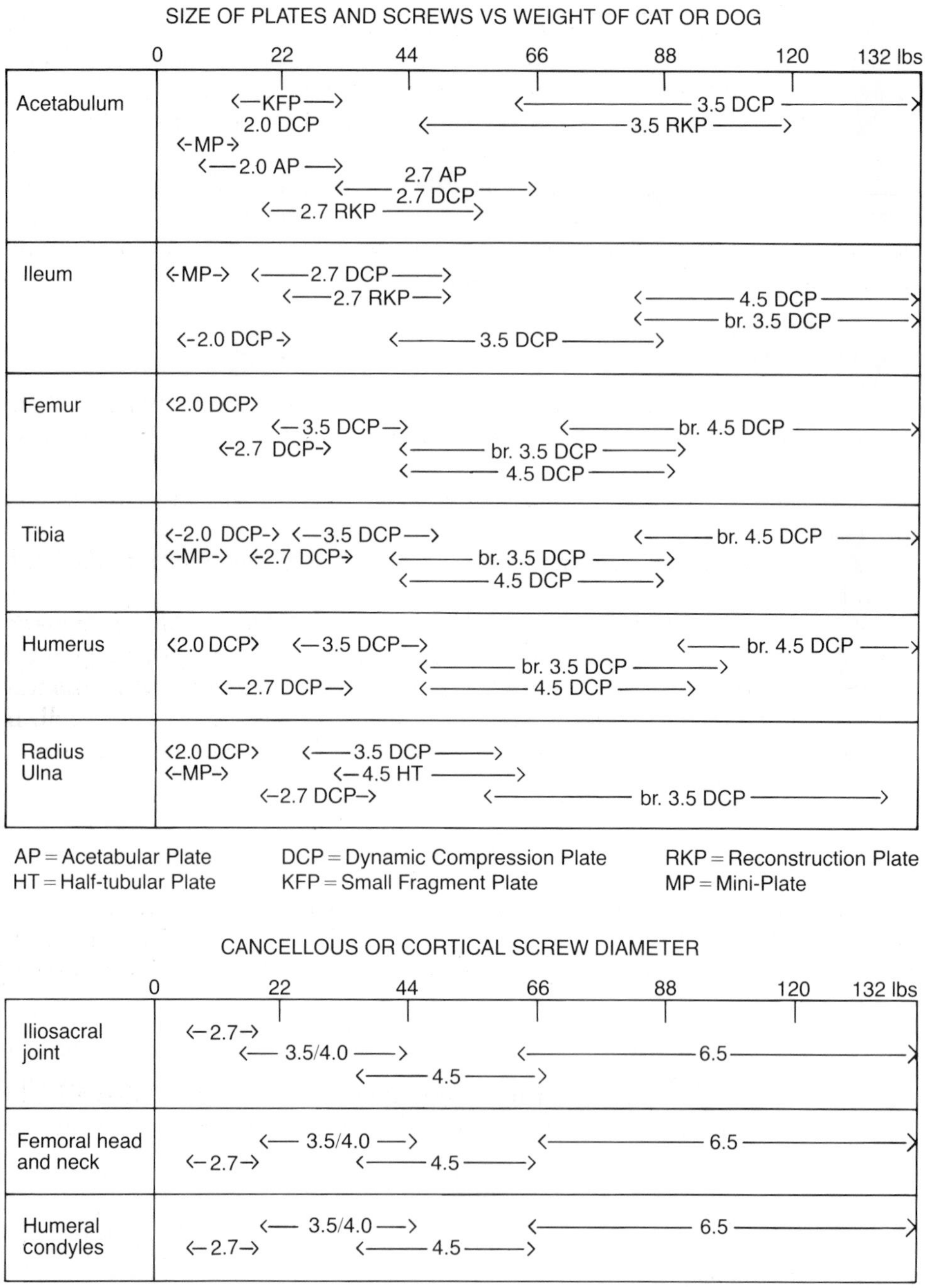

SIZE OF PLATES AND SCREWS VS WEIGHT OF CAT OR DOG

	0	22	44	66	88	120	132 lbs
Acetabulum		<—KFP—> 2.0 DCP <-MP-> <—2.0 AP —> <— 2.7 RKP ——>	2.7 AP 2.7 DCP	<———————— 3.5 DCP ————> <———————— 3.5 RKP ———>			
Ileum	<-MP-> <-2.0 DCP->	<——2.7 DCP——> <——2.7 RKP——>	<———— 3.5 DCP ————>	<——————— 4.5 DCP————> <——————— br. 3.5 DCP ————>			
Femur	<2.0 DCP>	<— 3.5 DCP—> <-2.7 DCP->	<——— br. 3.5 DCP ———> <————— 4.5 DCP ———>	<————— br. 4.5 DCP —————>			
Tibia	<-2.0 DCP-> <-MP->	<—3.5 DCP——> <-2.7 DCP->	<——— br. 3.5 DCP ———> <——— 4.5 DCP ———>	<——— br. 4.5 DCP ——>			
Humerus	<2.0 DCP> <—2.7 DCP—>	<—3.5 DCP—>	<——— br. 3.5 DCP ———> <——— 4.5 DCP ———>	<—— br. 4.5 DCP ——>			
Radius Ulna	<2.0 DCP> <-MP-> <-2.7 DCP->	<——3.5 DCP——> <—4.5 HT ——>	<——————— br. 3.5 DCP ———————>				

AP = Acetabular Plate   DCP = Dynamic Compression Plate   RKP = Reconstruction Plate
HT = Half-tubular Plate   KFP = Small Fragment Plate   MP = Mini-Plate

CANCELLOUS OR CORTICAL SCREW DIAMETER

	0	22	44	66	88	120	132 lbs
Iliosacral joint	<—2.7—>	<— 3.5/4.0 —> <——— 4.5 ——>		<——————— 6.5———————>			
Femoral head and neck	<-2.7->	<— 3.5/4.0 —> <——4.5——>		<——————— 6.5 ———————>			
Humeral condyles	<-2.7->	<— 3.5/4.0 —> <——4.5——>		<——————— 6.5 ———————>			

FIGURE 1–43

The plate and screw names and sizes are given in terms of ASIF equipment. (Association for the Study of Internal Fixation, Synthes Ltd., Wayne, PA (USA).

6. Infection may occur. If infection is present, it is difficult to clear it up totally until the plate is removed. As a rule, if the plate is not loose, it is left in place as long as immobilization is indicated. When clinical union is achieved, it is removed and the infection usually clears up. This is particularly indicated because most fracture-associated sarcomas in animals have a history of a metallic implant, infection, and a disturbed fracture healing pattern.[57]

7. After the fractured bone reaches the stage of clinical union, the plate serves no further purpose and, in fact, removes normal tensile, compressive, and torsional forces resulting in changes of the inner architecture of the bone. After clinical union and removal of an implant, return to approximately normal strength is relatively rapid. The plate may also impede full functional performance in field and racing animals.

SUGGESTED POLICY IN REGARD TO PLATE REMOVAL

1. Leave all pelvic plates in place unless specific complications indicate removal. Relatively small plates are used, and to date no evidence of stress protection has been noted.

2. Leave plates in place in older animals (older than 8 to 10 years) unless otherwise indicated.

3. In immature animals, remove all plates on the long bones at the time of clinical union.

4. Ideally, it is best to remove all plates on long bones. Call an owner's attention to the reasons for removal at the time of discharge and give an approximate time for recheck and plate removal. Needless to say, it is difficult to get an animal back for plate removal when all appears to be going well. If complications occur after clinical union, it is best to have talked to the owner about recheck and plate removal.

SUGGESTED TIME FOR PLATE REMOVAL

Data were collected covering patient age and plate removal time in more than 300 cases. Table 1–2 suggests time for removal of bone plates. The time until removal may need to be increased in more complex cases or problem cases.

SURGICAL REMOVAL OF IMPLANT

Radiographs should be taken prior to and after plate removal. This will add to one's knowledge of bone healing and radiographic interpretation, and it

TABLE 1–2
Removal of Bone Plates

AGE	POSTOPERATIVE TIME FOR PLATE REMOVAL
Under 3 months	4 weeks
3–6 months	2–3 months
6–12 months	3–5 months
Over 1 year	5–14 months

will help to avoid repeating surgical errors. The procedure is performed as follows:

    1. The cicatrix is opened over the length of the bone plate.

    2. In some animals, a portion of the plate will be covered with a layer of bone. An osteotome is usually required for its removal over the surface of the plate.

    3. Following bone plate removal, active hemorrhage (which is usually minimal) is controlled, the wound is closed in layers, and a pressure dressing is applied. To date, cerclage wires and lag screws have been routinely left in place.

REFRACTURE

Refracture is a fracture of normal bone occurring in the region of a previous fracture that appears to have undergone sound union both clinically and radiographically.[45, 56–59] An incidence of less than 1 percent has been encountered in our fracture documentation series.[4] Most refractures result from premature implant removal, poor anatomical reduction, or osteoporotic bone. They can be kept very minimal if the basic fundamentals of applying and removing implants are followed, with particular emphasis on anatomical reduction, proper implant size, and bone grafting of architectural deficits.

POSTOPERATIVE CARE FOLLOWING REMOVAL

The appearance of the radiographs and the activity of the patient are usually the determining factors in postoperative care. Treatment usually involves the following:

    1. Application of a compression bandage over the operative area for 2 to 3 days to help prevent possible hematoma or seroma formation.

    2. Supportive measures (such as a coaptation splint, external fixator, or plate replacement) if bone healing on the radiograph following plate removal appears to be less than adequate or if the bone appears to be markedly osteoporotic under the plate. If the size or composition of the bone in the fracture area is markedly altered, bone grafting may be indicated.

    3. Restriction of activity for 1 to 4 weeks. This may range from confinement to the kennel or house, walking on a leash, or restricting play.

OPEN FRACTURES

Open fractures usually occur in about 5 to 10 percent of the total fracture cases seen. The term "compound fracture" is obsolete, and its use should be discouraged. An open wound overlying a fracture practically always means contamination, reduction in local host defense mechanism by the presence of foreign material and debris, devitalized necrotic tissue, and dead space. All these factors increase the potential for infection in the open wound.

Classification

Open fractures are classified as:

First Degree ■ One occurring from within, with the fractured bone penetrating the skin at the time of injury. The bone may still be protruding or may have retracted under the skin.

Second Degree ■ A wound inflicted from the outside with contusion of the skin and underlying soft tissue.

Third Degree ■ Extensive skin, muscle, and possible nerve damage with a comminuted fracture. The wound occurs from the outside and may show considerable loss of skin, muscle, and bone. The damage is extensive and potentially difficult to treat.

Treatment

BASIC PRINCIPLES

The following principles apply to the treatment of open fractures.[3, 45, 60]

    1. Prevention or minimization of contamination from time of occurrence of injury until initiation of surgical treatment.
    2. Thorough cleaning and aseptic surgical debridement.
    3. Preservation of vascularity (soft tissue and bone).
    4. Uninterrupted immobilization of fracture segments.

EMERGENCY TREATMENT

First aid by the owner is usually directed toward stopping hemorrhage and preventing contamination. Covering the area with a clean bandage applied with minimal pressure usually accomplishes this objective. Further evaluation and first aid are carried out on arrival at the hospital. An open fracture is always considered an emergency and is treated as such.

    Particular attention is given to the cardiovascular system—perfusion and circulating red blood cell volume. It is a good rule to take chest radiographs of all fracture patients as soon as their general condition permits. A thorough physical and radiographic orthopedic examination is essential for diagnosis, prognosis, and determination of the type of treatment.

SURGICAL TREATMENT

Preparation of the Surgical Area

Utmost care in aseptic technique is indicated because surveys of human wound infections indicate that most strains of bacteria found in wounds are indigenous to the hospital in which treatment was performed rather than to the scene of the accident. Preparation of the surgical area is carried out in the operative preparation room with the patient under anesthesia. The surgeon is capped, masked, and gloved. The open area is covered with sterile gauze, and the surrounding surgical area is clipped and surgically scrubbed.

    Mechanical cleaning, debridement, and flushing with lactated Ringer solution or isotonic saline solution are performed. Enlargement of the wound, if indicated, should be kept at a minimum.

    First- and second-degree wounds seen within 6 to 8 hours ("golden period") may be considered noninfected and can be treated by primary closure following cleaning and debridement. Third-degree and more seriously involved second-degree wounds are handled as open wounds followed by delayed primary or secondary closure. Infected wounds are treated as open wounds and are never closed primarily.

Fracture Fixation

The following types of fixation may be used; each has its indications and limitations.

1. Splints and casts are usually reserved for those cases with minor puncture wounds, those treated within the first 6 to 8 hours, and stable fractures of the distal half of the radius and ulna, carpus, tarsus, and foot.
2. Internal fixation involves these methods:
   a. Intramedullary pins are usually restricted to stable, contaminated fractures treated within 6 to 8 hours. Secondary fixation (such as an external fixator) may be added for more stability.
   b. Bone screws and/or plates have the advantage of rigid uninterrupted fixation; however, an extensive open approach is required for application. They are particularly applicable when the fracture involves an articular surface.
   c. Skeletal fixation with the external fixator has the advantage of minimal application time, and the fixation pins can usually be applied proximally and distally to the involved area. Thus the traumatized area is freely accessible for repeated dressing. This type of fixation is particularly adaptable to infected fractures, gunshot fractures, and the more severely traumatized cases.

Whatever type of fixation is used should remain in place until clinical union is achieved, as long as it is secure and accomplishing stabilization of the fracture segments. Loose implants should be replaced.

Bone Grafting

Bone grafting is usually indicated in open fracture cases in which bone is missing and in some of the more severely comminuted fractures. For more complete details, refer to Chapter 3.

Autogenous cancellous grafts can be used at the time of surgery, after debridement, reduction, and fixation. If infection and questionable vascularity are present, however, it is usually advisable to delay grafting for about 2 weeks until these have improved. If the graft cannot be covered with soft tissue, it is usually covered with petroleum-impregnated gauze.

Cortical grafts should not be used in an infected area because they are slow in becoming vascularized and usually lead to sequestration. If a cortical graft is indicated, the procedure should be delayed until the infection has cleared.

Case Studies

CASE 1 ■ Figure 1–44A shows a grade 2 open comminuted fracture in a 1-year-old, 55-pound dog that was struck by a car bumper. The open area was covered with a clean bandage immediately and presented for treatment within

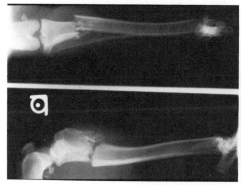
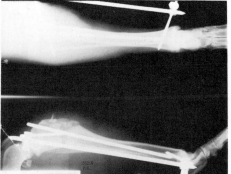
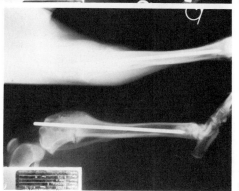

FIGURE 1–44

(A) Grade 2 open comminuted fracture that resulted when a 55-pound, 1-year-old dog was struck by a car bumper. Open area was covered with a clean bandage immediately and presented for treatment within 8 hours. (B) Fixation using an intramedullary pin and unilateral external fixator, 1/1 pin. (C) Intramedullary pin shown at time of clinical union (7 weeks). The external fixator was removed at 4 weeks and the intramedullary pin at 7 weeks.

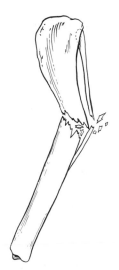
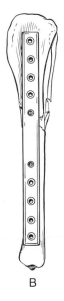
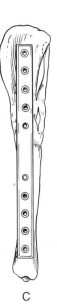
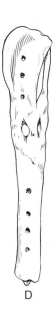

A   B   C   D

FIGURE 1–45

(A) Grade 2 open gunshot fracture in a 60-pound dog. (B) Fixation using a bone plate. (C) Fracture had healed (11 months after injury); however, intermittent minor draining tracts were still present. (D) After removal of the plate and sequestra, the draining tracts disappeared. The defect in the diaphysis was the site of sequestra. In retrospect, a better choice of stabilization would have been a unilateral external fixator.

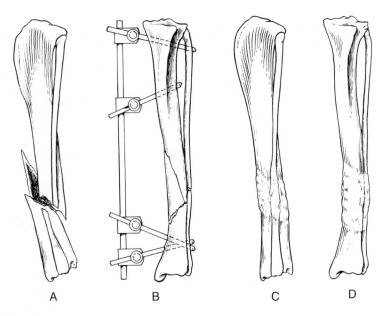

A   B   C   D

FIGURE 1–46

(A) Grade 3 open infected fracture, 6 days after trauma, in a 15-pound dog 8 months of age. End of distal segment still protruding from skin, temperature 105° F. *(B)* Unilateral external fixator was applied. *(C, D)* Local and systemic infection cleared; healing was delayed, although without sequestra formation. Splint removed at 4 months.

8 hours. Fixation was performed using an intramedullary pin and a unilateral fixator, 1/1 pin (Fig. 1–44*B*). The wound was treated as an open lesion with nitrofurazone dressings. The skin lesion closed within 2 weeks (Fig. 1–44*C*). The external fixator was removed in 1 month, and the intramedullary pin was removed at the time of clinical union (2 months).

CASE 2 ■ Figure 1–45*A* shows a grade 2 open gunshot fracture in a 2-year-old, 60-pound dog. Fixation was done using a bone plate (Fig. 1–45*B*). The fracture healed; however, minor fistulous tracts opened up intermittently during the healing period (Fig. 1–45*C*). These cleared up promptly after removal of the bone plate and a sequestrum 11 months after injury. The defect in the shaft was the sequestrum site (Fig. 1–45*D*).

CASE 3 ■ Figure 1–46*A* depicts a grade 3 open infected fracture in an 8-month-old, 15-pound dog 6 days after trauma. The end of the distal segment was still protruding from the skin; the dog's temperature was 105° F. An external fixator was applied, and the local area was treated with numerous nitrofurazone dressings. The animal was placed on a systemic antibiotic (Fig. 1–46*B*). The local and systemic infection cleared, and healing was delayed, although without sequestra formation (Fig. 1–46*C*, *D*). The splint was removed at 4 months.

PRINCIPLES OF JOINT FRACTURE TREATMENT

Intra-articular fractures are potentially devastating injuries that require prompt and aggressive surgical treatment. Open reduction and rigid internal fixation offer the best hope for uninterrupted function.

Failure to adequately stabilize joint fractures leads to malarticulation. Irregularities in the articular surface cause grinding of cartilage from the opposing surfaces. Liberation of intracellular proteoglycans is followed by inflammatory and degenerative changes within the joint, and varying degrees of degenerative joint disease (arthritis) follow. A certain amount of instability is also present as a result of malarticulation, which further adds to the degenerative joint disease (DJD).

PRINCIPLES OF SURGICAL TREATMENT

Step 1: Intra-articular surgery

Step 2: Extra-articular surgery

Step 3: Cancellous bone grafting, if needed

Step 4: Repair of soft tissue injuries—ligamentous instability, musculotendinous disruption

Intra-Articular Surgery

1. Wide surgical exposure is needed. Consider osteotomy of ligamentous/tendinous attachments to allow generous exposure.

2. In the presence of open wounds, it may be necessary to enter the joint through the wound, with appropriate debridement. If possible, however, enter through normal tissues.

3. Make a general inspection of the joint to assess the damage and to correlate it with the radiographs. Identify all fracture lines and bony fragments.

4. Remove cartilage chips and foreign bodies, and debride nonviable tissue.

5. Save cartilage fragments that have subchondral bone attached.

6. In reconstructing/reducing the fracture, handle cartilage gently. Use pointed reduction forceps, Schroeder vulsellum forceps, or Kirschner wires to hold pieces in reduction. Small gaps are better tolerated than stairstep defects.

7. Size of fragments may dictate the fixation method. Some fragments are too small for anything but a small Kirschner wire. Where these are placed on gliding surfaces, they should be countersunk beneath the cartilage surface. Lag screw fixation is generally the most versatile and reliable method of fixation. The interfragmentary compression produced generally is the most effective method of preventing shearing forces from disrupting the reduction. Use of plastic spiked washers (Synthes)* can be useful in distributing the compression load of the screw head more evenly over small, thin fragments. When tension loads are the primary consideration, the pin/tension band wire technique may be useful, especially with small fragments. Lag screws are useful in large fragments if the screw can be positioned so that it is loaded only in the axial direction and is not subjected to bending loads. Positioning lag screws may be influenced by the type of fixation required when extra-articular fractures are present (see below).

---

*Synthes Ltd. (USA), Wayne, PA.

8. Know anatomy well. It is easy to misdirect a screw and not secure adequate fixation. The use of an aiming device (Synthes) can be very helpful. In some cases, it may be better to excise small fragments that cannot be adequately reduced and stabilized. For example, fractures of the distal one third of the patella are best treated by excision of the fragments and reattachment of the patellar ligament to the remaining patella.

Extra-Articular Surgery

Many intra-articular fractures have an extra-articular component, such as the T-Y fractures of the distal humerus and femur. Fixation of the extra-articular fracture should be completed at this time. Plates and external skeletal fixators are most widely applicable in these situations, although occasionally certain forms of pinning, especially with Rush pins, are applicable.

Cancellous Bone Grafting

Both intracapsular and extracapsular bone deficits may be present after reduction and fixation. Such defects can lead to loss of stability as a result of delayed bony bridging by callus formation. Autogenous cancellous bone grafts will greatly speed callus formation. Do not place the graft where it is exposed to synovial fluid or where graft fragments could become free floating within the joint.

Repair of Soft Tissue Injuries

Ligamentous instability due to the fracture-producing trauma is the most common soft tissue problem. Appropriate reconstructive surgery should be done at this time because the instability is deleterious to the joint, and any additional insult to the fractured joint is definitely not needed at this point. Examine carefully for musculotendinous injuries, especially in gunshot fractures and those produced by sharp trauma.

AFTERCARE

Aftercare varies with the joint involved, the security of fixation achieved, and the size and activity level of the animal. The major question to be resolved is the necessity for cast or sling immobilization. Often, the fixation is less than adequate to allow weight bearing before some degree of fracture union is achieved.

As a general rule, immobilization of the elbow and stifle joints is best avoided. Both of these joints are susceptible to periarticular fibrosis and intra-articular cartilaginous degeneration, leading to loss of motion. If the fixation is so tenuous as to require external immobilization, try to delay applying the cast or splint for several days postoperatively until the animal starts to use the limb. Even the slight passive motion involved in nonweight-bearing activity gives the joint a chance to clear some of the hemarthrosis and inflammatory debris. Flexion bandages of the carpus and tarsus are often effective in allowing some motion while preventing weight bearing.

The shoulder and hip joints and the joints of the carpus and tarsus tolerate immobilization better and can be safely supported in the appropriate cast, splint, or sling. Generally 3 to 4 weeks of external support is sufficient to allow restricted activity throughout the rest of the healing period. Most animals can be returned to moderate levels of activity by 12 weeks postoperatively.

The determination of implant removal must be approached on a case-by-case basis. If bone plates have been used, they are often relatively short and end in the mid-diaphysis. This is a good situation for a pathological fracture to develop at the end of the plate after the animal returns to normal activity and is a good argument for plate removal at about 6 months. Screws can usually be left in place with no ill effects. Pin and tension band wire fixation, unless very carefully applied, often cause irritation of overlying soft tissues and will need to be removed as soon as practical. Twelve to 20 weeks is usually adequate to allow good healing in this situation.

REFERENCES

1. Adams JC: Outline of Fractures, 7th ed. Edinburgh, F&S Livingstone Ltd, 1978, pp 4–8.
2. Brinker WO: Fractures in Canine Surgery. Santa Barbara, American Veterinary Publications Inc. Ed 2, 1952, pp 548–643; Ed 3, 1957, pp 548–640; First Archibald Ed, 1965, pp 777–849; Second Archibald Ed, 1975, pp 957–1048.
3. Brinker WO: Small Animal Fractures. East Lansing, Mich., Department of Continuing Education Services, Michigan State University Press, 1978.
4. Brinker WO: Fracture Documentation Studies. East Lansing, Mich, Michigan State University. Unpublished data, 1971–1978.
5. Rhinelander F: The normal microcirculation of diaphyseal cortex and its response to fracture. J Bone Joint Surg 50-A:784, 1968.
6. Rhinelander F, Phillips RS, Steel WM, et al: Microangiography in bone healing. J Bone Joint Surg 50-A:643, 1968.
7. Parren SM, Boitzy A: Cell differentiation and bone biomechanics during the consolidation of a fracture. Anat Clin 1:13–28, 1978.
8. Seibel R, LaDuca J, Border JR, et al: Blunt multiple trauma, femur traction, and the pulmonary state. Ann Surg 202:283–395, 1985.
9. Allgower M: The scientific basis of aggressive traumatology in lesions of the locomotor system. Dialogue 1:2–3, 1985.
10. Swaim SF: Management and bandaging of soft tissue injuries of the dog and cat. J Am Anim Hosp Assoc 21:329–340, 1985.
11. Schroeder EF: Fractures of the femoral shaft of dogs. North Am Vet 14:38–46, 1933.
12. Schroeder EF: The traction principle in treating fractures and dislocations in the dog and cat. North Am Vet 14:32–36, 1933.
13. Schroeder EF: The treatment of fracture in dogs. North Am Vet 14:27–31, 1933.
14. Piermattei DL: Atlas of Surgical Approaches to the Bones of the Dog and Cat, 3rd ed. Philadelphia, WB Saunders Co, in preparation.
15. Stader O: A preliminary announcement of a new method of treating fractures. North Am Vet 18:37–38, 1937.
16. Stader O: Treating fractures of long bones with a reduction splint. North Am Vet 20:55–59;62, 1939.
17. Ehmer FA: Bone pinning in fractures of small animals. J Am Vet Med Assoc 110:14–19, 1947.
18. Brinker WO, Flo GL: Principles and application of external skeletal fixation. Vet Clin North Am 5:197–208, 1975.
19. Brinker WO: Update of fundamentals on application of the external fixator. Tidschrift Voor Diergeneeskunde 111:1189–1196, 1986.
20. Wa JJ, Shyr HS, Chao EY, et al: Comparison of osteotomy healing with different stiffness characteristics. J Bone Joint Surg 66-A:1258–1264, 1984.
21. Lewallen DG, Chao EY, Kelly PJ, et al: Comparison of the effects of compression plates and external fixators on early bone healing. J Bone Joint Surg 66-A:1084–1091, 1984.
22. Seligson D, Pope M: Concepts in External Fixation. New York, Grune & Stratton, Inc, 1982, pp 13–109.
23. Clancey GJ, Hansen JT: Open fractures of the tibia: a review of 102 cases. J Bone Joint Surg 60-A:118–122, 1978.

24. Edge AS, Denham RA: External fixation for complicated tibial fractures. J Bone Joint Surg 63-B:92–97, 1981.

25. Chapman MW, Mahoney M: The role of early internal fixation in the management of open fractures. Clin Orthop 138:120–131, 1979.

26. Rittman WW, Schibli M, Matter P, et al: Open fractures: long-term results in 200 consecutive cases. Clin Orthop 138:132–140, 1979.

27. Etter C, Burri C, Kuner K, et al: Treatment by external fixation of open fractures associated with severe soft tissue damage of leg. Clin Orthop 178:81–88, 1983.

28. Behrens F, Searls K: External fixation of tibia: basic concepts and prospective evaluation. J Bone Joint Surg 68-B:246–254, 1986.

29. Egger EL, Histland MB, Blass CE, et al: Effect of pin insertion on bone pin interface. Vet Surg 15:246–252, 1986.

30. Pettit GD: Kirschner fixation splint. In Pettit GD (ed): Kirschner Catalog, Aberdeen MD, Kirschner Co, 1980, pp 96–99.

31. Gumbs JM, Brinker WO, DeCamp CE, et al: Comparison of àcute and chronic pull out resistance of pins used with the external fixator (Kirschner splint). J Am Anim Hosp Assoc 24:231–234, 1988.

32. DeCamp CE, Brinker WO, Sautas-Little RW: Porous titanium-surfaced pins for external skeletal fixation. J Am Anim Hosp Assoc 24:295–300, 1988.

33. Matthews LS, Green CA, Goldstein SA: The thermal effect of skeletal fixation—pin insertion in bone. J Bone Joint Surg 66-A:1077–1083, 1984.

34. Evans M, Kenwright J, Lanner K: Analysis of Single-Sided External Fracture Fixation. Engineering in Medicine, Vol 8, No 3, pp 133–137, 1979.

35. Boltze NH, Chiquer C, Niederer PG: Der fixateur externe stabililatsprofung. Berne, AO Bulletin, 1978.

36. Brinker WO, Verstraete ME: Unpublished data, 1985.

37. Brinker WO, Verstraete ME, Soutas-Little RW: Stiffness studies on various configurations and types of external fixators. J Am Anim Hosp Assoc 21:280–288, 1985.

38. Egger EL: Static strength evaluation of six external skeletal fixation configurations. Vet Surg 12:130–136, 1983.

39. Egkher E, Martiner KH, Wielke B: How to increase the stability of external fixation units, mechanical tests and theoretical studies. Arch Orthop Trauma Surg 96:35–43, 1980.

40. Brinker WO: The use of intramedullary pins in small animal fractures: a preliminary report. North Am Vet 29:292–297, 1948.

41. Carney JP: Rush intramedullary fixation of long bones as applied to veterinary surgery. Vet Med 47:43, 1952.

42. Jenny J: Kuntscher's medullary nailing in femur fractures of the dog. J Am Vet Med Assoc 17:381–387, 1950.

43. Rudy RL: Principles of intramedullary pinning. Vet Clin North Am 5:209–228, 1975.

44. Muller ME, Allgower M, Schneider R, et al: Manual of Internal Fixation, 2nd ed. Schatzker J (transl). New York, Springer-Verlag, 1979, pp 29–82.

45. Brinker WO, Hohn RB, Prieur WD: Manual of Internal Fixation in Small Animals. Heidelberg, W Germany, Springer-Verlag, 1984, pp 29–79; 104–107.

46. Gambaradella PC: Full cerclage wires for fixation of long bone fractures. J Comp Cont Ed 2:665–671, 1980.

47. Birehard SJ, Bright RM: The tension band wire for fracture repair. J Comp Cont Ed 3:37–41, 1981.

48. Withrow SJ, Holmberg DL: Use of full cerclage wires in the fixation of 18 consecutive long bone fractures in small animals. J Am Anim Hosp Assoc 13:735–743, 1977.

49. Perren SM, Russenberger M, Steinemann S, et al: A dynamic compression plate. Acta Orthop Scand (Suppl) 125:31, 1969.

50. Perren SM, Allgower M, Ehrsam R, et al: Clinical experience with a new compression plate—DCP. Acta Orthop Scand (Suppl) 125:45, 1969.

51. Perren SM, Hutzschenreuter P, Steinemann S: Some effects of rigidity of internal fixation on the healing pattern of osteotomies. Z Surg 1:77, 1969.

52. Matter P, Brennwald J, Rüter A, et al: The effect of static compression and tension on internal remodeling of cortical bone. Helvetica Churugica Acta (Suppl 12) 5–43, 1975.

53. Uhthoff J, Duduc H: Bone structure changes in the dog under rigid internal fixation. Clin Orthop 81:165, 1971.

54. Woo SL, Akeson WH, Coutts RD, et al: A comparison of cortical bone atrophy secondary to fixation with plate with large differences in bending stiffness. J Bone Joint Surg 58-A:190–195, 1976.

55. Brinker WO, Flo GL, Lammerding JJ, et al: Guidelines for selecting proper implant size for treatment of fractures in dog and cat. J Am Anim Hosp Assoc 13:476–477, 1977.

56. Brinker WO, Flo GL, Braden TD, et al: Removal of bone plates in small animals. J Am Anim Hosp Assoc 11:577–586, 1975.

57. Stephenson S, Hohn RB, Pohler OEM, et al: Fracture-associated sarcomas in the dog. J Am Vet Med Assoc 180:1189–1196, 1982.

58. Noser GA, Brinker WO, Little RW, et al: Effect of time on strength of healing bone with bone plate fixation. J Am Anim Hosp Assoc 13:559–561, 1977.

59. Jiunn-Jerr W, Shyr HS, Chao EYS, et al: Comparison of osteotomy healing under external fixation devices with different stiffness characteristics. J Bone Joint Surg 66-A:1258–1264, 1984.

60. Nunamaker DM: Treatment of open fractures in small animals. Princeton Junction, NJ, Veterinary Learning Systems Co, Inc, J Comp Cont Ed 1:66–75, 1979.

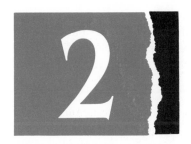

Treatment of Acute and Chronic Bone Infections

Osteitis or *osteomyelitis* is defined as a bone inflammation involving the haversian spaces, Volkmann canals, and generally, the medullary cavity and periosteum. Bone infection is usually associated with open fractures, bone surgery, or systemic illness.

Acute infection is diagnosed by a supportive history, localized pain, heat, swelling, and elevation of body temperature. In many early cases, radiological signs may not be evident.

Chronic infection is diagnosed by a supportive history, draining tracts, lameness, and positive radiographic changes. These changes may include bone lysis; disuse osteoporosis; rough, thick periosteum; new bone formation; formation of sequestra and involucra; soft tissue swelling; and sclerosis.[1, 2] A *sequestrum* is a piece of dead bone that has become separated from sound bone during the process of necrosis and is surrounded by a pool of infected exudate. An *involucrum* is a covering or sheath of new bone formation and fibrous tissue covering a sequestrum.

Most commonly, osteomyelitis implies *bacterial* infection; however, fungi or viruses can also infect bone and marrow. The organism most commonly found in all studies was *Staphylococcus aureus*.[3–8] Other common organisms include *Streptococcus*, *E. coli*, *Proteus*, *Pasteurella*, and *Pseudomonas*. About 50 percent of infections are caused by a single organism; others are caused by multiple organisms.

ROUTES OF INFECTION

The routes of infection, in order of occurrence, are as follows:

1. Direct contamination from open fractures, surgical intervention in treatment of a fracture, and puncture wounds. The highest percentage of infected fractures follow either open fracture repair or open repair of closed fractures.[3–8]

2. Direct extension from infected adjacent tissue.

3. The blood stream, from such conditions as vertebral osteomyelitis,

discospondylitis (*Brucella, Staphylococcus,* and so forth), and bacterial endocarditis. This source of osteomyelitis by comparison is rare.[3–6, 9–11]

TISSUE CHANGES

Infection in the proximity of bone produces vascular congestion, edema, and an inflammatory exudate that spreads through the bone, killing osteocytes and marrow cells. Sometimes the involvement is confined to a localized area; in other cases, large areas are involved. Spread of infection is easiest along the medullary canal; however, it also occurs beneath the periosteum and in the cortex. With subsidence of the acute phase, pyogenic granulation tissue attacks and absorbs dead spongiosa and separates as sequestra those parts of the cortex that are necrotic. The periosteum lays down new bone, the so-called *involucrum.* Even though the repair process is active, it is seldom completely successful. With repeated cycles of infected exudate formation and stripping of the periosteum, a thick, multilayered involucrum, penetrated here and there by cloacae, builds up. Many involucra develop sinus tracts to the outside.[1–5, 14]

Surgical or medical intervention frequently seems to arrest infection, leading to its elimination, followed by gradual reworking of the involucrum into a shaft that may surprisingly look like the original one. This process of healing is best discussed by considering (1) changes in necrotic bone, (2) formation of new bone, and (3) changes in old, living bone.

Necrotic Bone

Dead bone is absorbed by the action of granulation tissue that develops about its surface. If the dead bone is cancellous, it may be removed entirely, leaving a cavity behind. Dead cortex in any appreciable amount is gradually detached. After sequestration, the bone is less readily attacked and more slowly absorbed due to the physical barrier imposed by the scar tissue walls of the cavity surrounding the sequestrum. Cortical sequestra may take years or even the lifetime of the animal to be completely absorbed. Some sequestra are never absorbed and will continue to cause drainage until they are surgically removed.

New Bone

New bone forms from primitive mesenchymal cells in the surviving portions of periosteum, endosteum, and cortex. Recurrence of infection may result in the formation of superimposed layers of involucrum.

Old, Living Bone

In osteomyelitis, surviving bone usually becomes osteoporotic during the active period of infection because of disuse atrophy and decalcification resulting from inflammatory hyperemia. After subsidence of infection and resumption of function of the part, bone density increases again.

CLINICAL APPROACH

History, signs, and radiographic findings are essential in making a diagnosis and in determining the extent of the lesion.[1-8] If possible, the next logical step is to culture and determine the antibiotic sensitivity of the causative organisms.[3-8, 11] It is imperative that the culture be taken from the infected area and not from the draining sinus tracts. The latter are commonly contaminated with skin organisms. In acute cases, it is best to perform needle aspiration from the infected area. In chronic cases, culture at the time of sequestrectomy is indicated.

Factors that increase the incidence of postoperative infection include breaks in sterile technique during surgery, increased duration of surgical procedure, soft tissue trauma (ischemia), and presence of a remote infection. Fractures will heal in the presence of infection; however, every precaution should be taken to avoid it.

Acute Infection

Treatment varies, but usually involves one or more of the following:

1. Placing the animal on the indicated systemic antibiotic.[3-8, 11]

2. Establishing rigid uninterrupted stability of the fracture if necessary.[3-8, 12]

3. Complete and careful debridement of wound if indicated.

4. Establishing surgical drainage to the area if exudate is present. This may necessitate nonclosure after debridement or use of drains with or without suction or irrigation.[12-14] Because of the difficulty of maintaining drains in animals, many advocate leaving the wound entirely open. In this method, the open wound can be covered with a bandage that is changed daily until the defect is filled with granulation tissue. At this time, it may be indicated to fill the bone defect with an autogenous cancellous bone graft.[16] Another technique involves primary closure of the wound over drains to allow irrigation and suction. The drains are placed into the wound bed and exit the skin at a distant site.[15] The tubes are used to flush the wound bed with fluids containing the appropriate antibiotic based on culture and sensitivity results.

Chronic Infection

Treatment usually involves:

1. Placing the animal on the indicated antibiotic.

2. Removing sequestra if present. In most instances, it is advantageous to follow the same surgical approach used in open reduction of the fracture rather than following the sinus tract if there is one present. As a rule, it is not necessary to curette the area or sinus tract or to use chemical or proteolytic enzymes following removal of sequestra that are walled off with granulation tissue.

3. Evaluating fracture stability. If the fracture is healed and implants are present, they are removed. If implants are secure and stabilizing the fracture,

they should be left in place until the fracture is healed. If instability is present and implants are loose, they should be removed and replaced by suitable fixation. Use of the external fixator or plates and screws is preferred over intramedullary pins. Once the fracture is healed, removal of implants is generally required to completely clear the infection.

If a draining tract persists, it is most probable that all sequestra have not been removed and a second or even a third attempt may be in order.

There is an exception to the rule that dead bone should be removed as soon as it is separated. This occurs when the sequestrum comprises the whole thickness of the shaft of a long bone. If these large fragments are removed at the time of the original surgery—shortly after injury or within a few weeks—the surrounding tube of periosteum may collapse and the subperiosteal

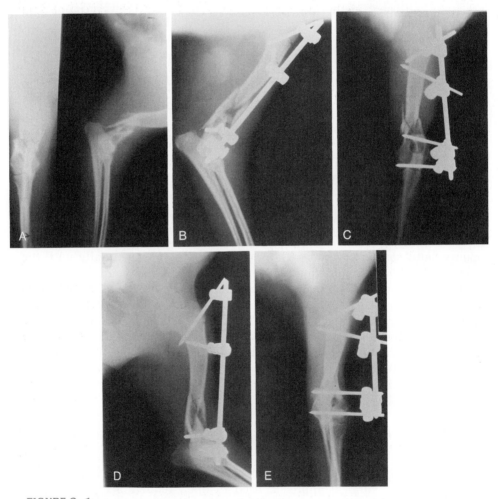

FIGURE 2–1

(A) Radiographic views of a distal humeral fracture, 5 days' duration, with an open suppurating wound. The dog's temperature was 104.5° F. (B, C) Lateral and craniocaudal views of the unilateral external fixator consisting of 2/2 pins applied for fixation. The draining area was treated as an open wound. It closed in about 2 weeks. (D, E) Lateral and craniocaudal views at 9 weeks; clinical union was present, and the splint was removed.

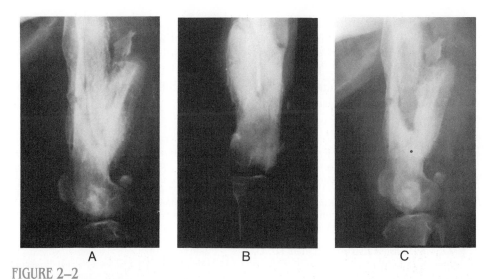

FIGURE 2–2

Fractured femur that had been treated 5 months previously; draining sinus tracts were present near the popliteal lymph nodes. (A, B) Lateral and craniocaudal views indicating a walled-off sequestra. (C) One large and two small sequestra were removed surgically using a lateral approach to the femur. The sinus tracts disappeared in 1 week.

hematoma may be obliterated. There is no longer a continuous hematoma between the fragments, and the fracture cannot unite. In such a case, it is better to defer sequestrectomy for several months until the surrounding involucrum of subperiosteal bone has been laid down, thereby ensuring continuity of the shaft. Bone grafting with autogenous cancellous bone is usually indicated after removal of sequestrum of this magnitude.

Case Studies

Case 1 ■ Figure 2–1 depicts acute bone infection. In (A), a cocker spaniel struck by a car 5 days previously presented with an open draining area with bone protruding on the medial surface and a temperature of 104.5° F. The immediate objectives in treatment were to minimally flush the area with Ringer solution, apply rigid fixation, and place the animal on systemic antibiotics. The area was prepared for surgery, including a minimal flushing of the area. In (B, C), fixation was accomplished by application of a unilateral external fixator, 2/2 pins. Because the distal bone segment was too short for placement of two pins proximal to the supracondylar foramen, the distal pin was placed in a transcondylar position. The proximal pin was inserted next, followed by application of the connecting bar and clamps, then the two center pins. This arrangement allowed full use of the leg during the healing period. The draining area was treated as an open wound, and it closed in about 2 weeks. Healing was uneventful. In (D, E), clinical union was present at 9 weeks, and the external fixator was removed.

Case 2 ■ Figure 2–2 depicts the history of a fractured femur, which had been treated 5 months previously. Infection had been a constant problem from the time of surgery. Several draining tracts were present in the region of the popliteal lymph nodes, and a walled-off sequestrum was present.

Culture study indicated *Staphylococcus pyogenes*, which was sensitive to chloramphenicol, oxytetracycline, and chlortetracycline. In Figure 2–2C, one large and two small sequestra have been removed surgically by a lateral approach to the femur. The bone was well healed, and the infection was walled off in the local area. The animal was placed on systemic antibiotics, and the draining tract disappeared in 1 week.

REFERENCES

1. Hodges PC: Normal bone, diseased bone, dead bone. Am J Roentgenol 71:925–940, 1954.
2. Walker MA, Lewis RE, Kneller SK, et al: Radiographic signs of bone infection in small animals. J Am Vet Med Assoc 166:908, 1975.
3. Caywood DD, Wallace LJ, Braden TD: Osteomyelitis in the dog: a review of 67 cases. J Am Vet Med Assoc 172:943, 1978.
4. Smith CW, Schiller AG, Smith AR, et al: Osteomyelitis in the dog: a retrospective study. J Am Anim Hosp Assoc 14:589, 1978.
5. Aron DN: Pathogenesis, diagnosis, and management of osteomyelitis in small animals. J Comp Cont Ed 1:824–830, 1979.
6. Nunamaker DM: Management of infected fractures—osteomyelitis. Vet Clin North Am 5:259, 1975.
7. Hirsh DC, Smith TM: Osteomyelitis in the dog: microorganisms isolated and susceptibility to antimicrobial agents. J Small Anim Pract 19:679, 1978.
8. Wingfield WE: Surgical treatment of chronic osteomyelitis in dogs. J Am Anim Hosp Assoc 11:568, 1975.
9. Hurov L, Troy G, Turnwald G: Discospondylitis in the dog: 27 cases. J Am Vet Med Assoc 173:275, 1978.
10. Smeak DP, Olmstead ML, Hohn RB: *Brucella canis* osteomyelitis in two dogs with total hip replacements. J Am Vet Med Assoc 191:986–989, 1987.
11. Mackowiak PA, Jones SR, Smith JW: Diagnostic value of sinus tract cultures in chronic osteomyelitis. J Am Med Assoc 239:2772, 1978.
12. Etter C, Burri C, Claes L, et al: Treatment by external fixation of open fractures associated with severe soft tissue damage of the leg. Clin Orthop 178:80–88, 1983.
13. Keely JP, Martin WJ, Coventry MB: Chronic osteomyelitis II: treatment with closed irrigation and suction. J Am Med Assoc 213:1843, 1970.
14. Petty W, Spanier S, Shuster JJ, et al: The influence of skeletal implants on incidence of infection. J Bone Joint Surg 67A:1236–1244, 1985.
15. Clawson DK, Davis FJ, Hansen ST: Treatment of chronic osteomyelitis with emphasis on closed suction-irrigation technique. Clin Orthop 96:88, 1973.
16. Bardet JF, Hohn RB, Basinger BS: Open drainage and delayed autogenous cancellous bone grafting for treatment of chronic osteomyelitis in dogs and cats. J Am Vet Med Assoc 183:312–317, 1983.

3

Bone Grafting

Bone grafting was introduced into general surgical practice in 1915,[1] and the principles of grafting have been well established. Use of banked bone (frozen, freeze-dried, and irradiated) came into general usage in the late 1940s.[2, 3]

Infection associated with bone grafting in animals has been minimal, particularly when aseptic procedures have been used and the bone has not been introduced into a contaminated or infected area.[2, 9] We have not encountered outright rejection by the body or bone sequestrum formation when autogenous or frozen allografts are used. Introduced bone does undergo osteoconduction (creeping substitution) and is replaced by the host. When problems are encountered, they are usually caused by failure to follow the fundamentals of grafting or by misuse of the procedure.

INDICATIONS FOR GRAFTING

Bone grafting is recommended in several circumstances:

1. To promote healing in delayed unions, nonunions, and osteotomies.
2. In arthrodesis of joints.
3. To bridge major defects in multiple or comminuted fractures by establishing continuity of bone segments and filling architectural deficits.
4. To fill cavities or defects resulting from cysts, tumors, and corrective procedures.

FUNCTIONS OF BONE GRAFTS

Bone grafts serve as a source of osteogenesis and may also serve as a mechanical support.[2, 4–9] New bone that is formed on or about a graft is either of graft origin, i.e., from cells that survive the transfer and are capable of forming bone, or from cells of host origin. At best, survival of osteoblasts from the graft is estimated at 10 percent when a fresh autogenous cancellous graft is used and handled under optimum conditions. The second way in which the bone graft may function as a source of osteogenesis is by recruitment of mesenchymal or pleuropotential cells in the area, which then differentiate into cartilage and bone-forming cells. This is called osteoinduction.

When placed in large deficits resulting from trauma or resection of neoplastic bone, bone grafts and implants serve as weight-bearing fillers and act as a scaffold for the ingrowth of new host bone. The term *osteoconduction* is given to the three-dimensional process of ingrowth of sprouting capillaries, perivascular tissue, and osteoprogenitor cells from the recipient bed into the structure of an implant or graft.

CHARACTERISTICS OF BONE GRAFTS

Sources

Grafts originate from three sources:

1. *Autograft* or *autogenous graft*—from the same animal. Autografts give maximum stimulation and earliest response, but they can increase operative time and may subject the animal to increased operative risk.[2, 8–11]

2. *Allograft* or *homogenous graft*—from the same species. Formerly known as *homografts*, these grafts are collected and held in the bone bank (freezer) for future use. Experimentally and clinically, an allograft has about the same stimulative effect as autogenous bone; however, there is no direct growth and there is an initial delay in response of about 2 weeks in comparison with the response of an autograft.[9, 12] Availability is the main advantage.[2, 7–12]

3. *Xenograft* or *heterogenous graft*—from a different species. This graft is the least stimulative and is most likely to cause a foreign body reaction. The term *heterograft* is obsolete.

Structure

Grafts may be either *cancellous or cortical*. Cancellous grafts have many advantages such as rapid stimulation, early vascularization, and early osteoin-duction.[2, 5, 12] Cortical grafts are usually a combination of cortical and cancellous bone. Vascular invasion and osteoconduction occur much more slowly, but a cortical graft has the advantage of affording some rigidity to the area.

CLINICAL APPLICATION OF BONE GRAFTS

Collection of Bone for Grafting

Strict aseptic technique is mandatory in all grafting procedures.

AUTOGENOUS CANCELLOUS BONE

Figure 3–1A–D shows the most common areas for collection in small animals, namely the humerus, the femur, the tibia, and the crest of the ilium. The area is approached through a 2- to 3-cm skin incision. The cortical bone is opened with a trephine or a trocar-pointed Steinmann pin, and cancellous bone is scooped out with a curette (Fig. 3–1E). The material is usually held in a small

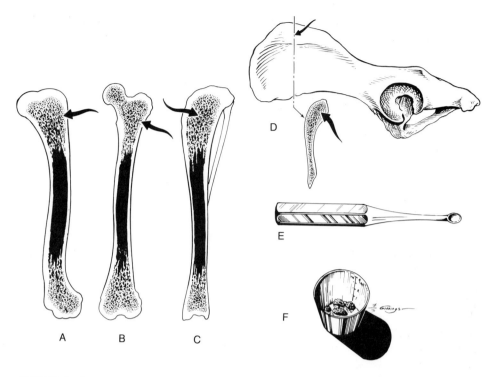

FIGURE 3–1

Collection of autogenous cancellous bone for grafting. *(A–D)* Sagittal sections of a humerus, femur, tibia, and ilium indicating location for collection of bone graft. *(E)* Curette used to scoop out cancellous bone. *(F)* Receptacle used for temporarily holding collected graft.

container (covered with a gauze sponge moistened with lactated Ringer solution) until time for transfer to the new area (Fig. 3–1F).[2, 9, 11] Do not immerse the graft in the fluid and do not apply antibiotics.

BONE BANK

Bone is collected from a healthy donor animal of the same species under strict aseptic procedure (Fig. 3–2A).[2, 9, 11, 13] Usually, all soft tissue is removed from the bone at time of collection. In canines, it is preferable to use a donor from one of the large breeds approximately 4 to 6 months of age. Ribs are the most common source of bone because they have a relatively high proportion of cancellous bone.

The harvested bone is placed in a sterile test tube or similar container. A small amount of Ringer solution may be added to keep the bones moist and to prevent freezer burn (dehydration) in storage. Each bone is usually placed in an individual container for convenient usage (Fig. 3–2B). The sealed and labeled containers are placed in a deep freezer and held at 0° F (−18° C) or lower. Bone preserved in this fashion may be held for approximately 1 year.

Types of Grafts

The types most commonly used are bone-chip, onlay, tubular, and sliding inlay grafts (Fig. 3–3).

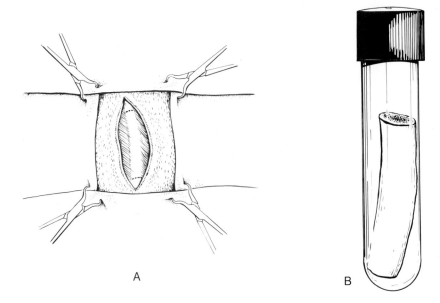

FIGURE 3–2

Collection of rib grafts for bone bank. *(A)* Ribs are aseptically collected from a donor animal and cleaned of all soft tissue. *(B)* Each rib is placed in a sterile test tube or similar container.

BONE CHIPS

Bone chips of 2 to 5 mm in diameter (Fig. 3–3A) are added to fill deficient areas in fresh fractures. The bone chips are created by using a rongeur. In delayed unions or nonunions, the sclerotic tissue and periosteum are peeled off the host bone segments at the fracture site. This is usually accomplished by using a periosteal elevator or osteotome and mallet (see Figure 4–2B). The bone segments are compressed, if possible, and rigidly immobilized. The finely cut donor bone is placed around the fracture site between the elevated periosteum and cortex.

ONLAY BONE GRAFT

Figure 3–3B shows the onlay graft. The sclerotic tissue and periosteum are elevated and reflected off the host area. The bone segments are compressed, if possible, and rigidly immobilized. One or more onlay grafts are placed on the bone, spanning the fracture site. The graft may be secured in place by bone screws or stainless steel wires or by suturing the patient's tissue over the area. Rigid fixation of bone segments in the host is much more important than fixation of the transplant. It is usually a good procedure to place bone chips around the remaining uncovered portion of the fracture site.

TUBULAR OR FULL-CYLINDER DIAPHYSEAL GRAFT

Tubular grafts[6, 13–15] (Fig. 3–3C, D) are indicated chiefly for:

1. Severe multiple or comminuted shaft fractures that do not lend themselves to anatomical reconstruction.
2. Fractures with missing bone segments.

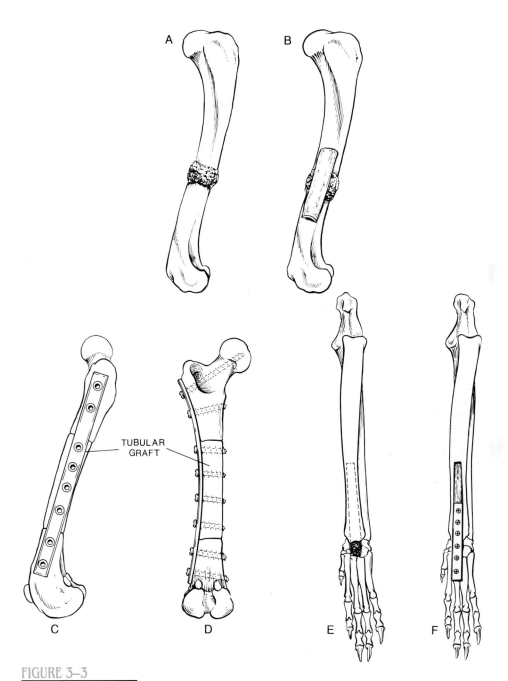

TUBULAR
GRAFT

A   B

C   D   E   F

FIGURE 3–3

Types of bone grafts. *(A)* Bone chips created by use of a rongeur are packed around the fracture site. *(B)* Onlay graft (usually a split rib) spans the fracture, and chips are packed around the fracture site. *(C, D)* Tubular allograft used to replace a section of the diaphysis. *(E, F)* Sliding inlay graft from the cranial surface of the distal radius is freed and moved distally for panarthrodesis of the carpus. The graft is attached with bone screws.

3. Replacement of surgically removed segments of neoplastic bone.

4. Reconstruction of certain atrophic nonunion fractures.

The procedure usually consists of squaring off the ends of the viable bone segments, inserting the proper size and length of cylindrical diaphyseal allograft, and immobilizing it under compression by using a dynamic compression plate. Functionally, most animals respond in the same fashion as the patient with an average multiple fracture stabilized with a bone plate. Replacement of the allograft is slow, and it may take 2 years, more or less, for the graft to be replaced by new living bone. In most cases, bone plates can be removed in 18 months.

SLIDING INLAY GRAFT

The sliding inlay graft (Fig. 3–3E, F) is most often used in arthrodesis. After the area is surgically exposed, two parallel cuts are made so that the graft is about two thirds the width of the bone. The articular surfaces are curetted free of cartilage. Next, the graft is loosened from its bed, moved distally to span the adjoining segments, and anchored in the previously prepared bed. Autogenous cancellous bone graft is placed around the bone surfaces to be healed. Fixation of the adjoining bone segments should be rigid and uninterrupted until there is good union, as confirmed by radiographs.

REFERENCES

1. Crenshaw AH: Campbell's Operative Orthopaedics, Ed 7. St. Louis, CV Mosby Co., 1987, pp 12–21.
2. Brinker WO: Fractures in Canine Surgery. Santa Barbara, American Veterinary Publications, Ed 2, 1952, pp 548–643; Ed 3, 1957, pp 546–640; First Archibald Ed 1965, pp 777–849; Second Archibald Ed 1975, pp 957–1048.
3. DeVries PN, Kempel K, Brinker WO: Sterilization of bone transplants by cobalt 60 radiation. Univ of Mich Bull 21:29–33, 1955.
4. Stevenson S: Bone grafting. In Slatter DH (ed): Textbook of Small Animal Surgery, Vol II. Philadelphia, WB Saunders Co, 1985, pp 2035–2048.
5. Hulse DA: Pathophysiology of autologous cancellous bone grafts. J Comp Cont Ed 2:378, 1973.
6. Mankin HJ, Fogelson FS, Trasher AZ, et al: Massive resection and allograft transplantation in the treatment of malignant bone tumors. N Engl J Med 294:1247, 1976.
7. Ray RD: Vascularization of bone grafts and implants. Clin Orthop 87:43, 1972.
8. Gambardella PC: Bone grafts in small animal orthopedics: a review. J Comp Cont Ed 1:596–603, 1979.
9. Brinker WO: Small animal fractures. Dept of Continuing Education Services, East Lansing, MI, Michigan State University, 1978.
10. Olds RB, Sinibaldi KR, DeAngulus M: Autogenous cancellous bone grafting in problem orthopedic cases. J Am Anim Hosp Assoc 9:430–435, 1973.
11. Schena CJ: The procurement of cancellous bone for grafting in small animal orthopedic surgery: a review of instrumentation, technique and pathophysiology. J Am Anim Hosp Assoc 19:695–704, 1983.
12. Rhinelander FW: Circulation of bone. In Bourne G (ed): Biochemistry and Physiology of Bone, Vol 2, 2nd ed. New York, Academic Press, 1972, pp 2–76.
13. Schena CJ, Mitten RW, Haefle WD: Segmental freeze-dried and fresh cortical allografts in canine femur: A sequential radiographic comparison over a one-year time interval. J Am Anim Hosp Assoc 20:911–925, 1984: A sequential histological comparison over a one-year time interval. J Am Anim Hosp Assoc 21:193–206, 1985.
14. Wadsworth PL, Henry WB: Entire segmental cortical bone transplant. J Am Anim Hosp Assoc 12:741–745, 1976.
15. Henry WB, Wadsworth PL: Retrospective analysis of failures in the repair of severely comminuted long bone fractures using large diaphyseal allografts. J Am Anim Hosp Assoc 17:535–546, 1981.

Delayed Union and Nonunion

Delayed union refers to a fracture that has not healed in the usual time. *Nonunion* refers to a fracture in which all evidence of osteogenic activity at the fracture site has ceased, movement is present at the fracture site, and union is no longer possible without surgical intervention. The most common causes of these two conditions are:

1. Inadequate immobilization, or failure to maintain immobilization for a sufficient length of time.
2. Inadequate reduction.
3. Impairment of the blood supply resulting from the original trauma or traumatic surgery.
4. Infection. A fracture may heal in the presence of infection; however, at best, healing is delayed.
5. Loss of bone or bone fragments from open trauma or surgery.

DELAYED UNION FRACTURES

The most common cause of delayed union is inadequate or interrupted fixation of the fracture segments.[1] On radiographic examination, the fracture line is evident, callus formation may be minimal, and the fracture site has a "feathery" or woolly appearance. Evidence of osteogenic activity is visible.

Clinical evaluation and treatment of delayed union fractures may be approached by various means:[2, 3]

1. If reduction is satisfactory, rigid uninterrupted fixation should be ensured and maintained for an extended period of time (Fig. 4–1A, B).
2. If there is good end-to-end bone contact with malalignment or bending at the fracture site, the bone should be straightened and rigid uninterrupted fixation should be applied. Usually, straightening can be accomplished by careful but forceful pressure with the hands or by applying pressure over a fulcrum point. This is preferable to doing an open surgical breakdown and saves many weeks of healing time (Fig. 4–1C, D).
3. If reduction is unsatisfactory, surgical intervention is indicated to correct the deficiencies of reduction and fixation (Fig. 4–2A–D).

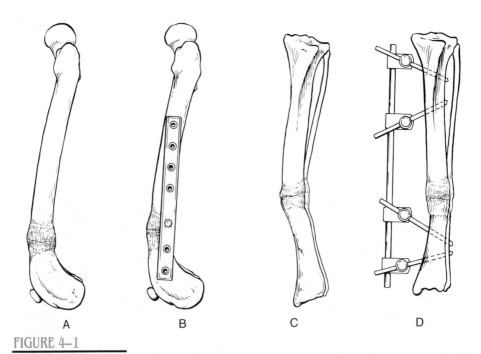

FIGURE 4–1

Delayed union fractures. *(A)* Satisfactory reduction of delayed union femoral fracture previously treated with an intramedullary pin. *(B)* Rigid internal fixation provided by a compression plate. *(C)* Delayed union fracture of a tibia with good contact of bone fragments but with valgus deformity. *(D)* Bone straightened manually, without surgical exposure. A unilateral external fixator consisting of 2/2 pins was applied for fixation.

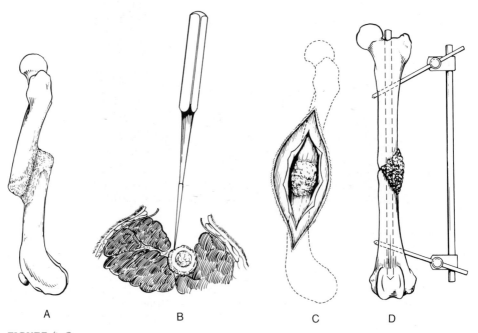

FIGURE 4–2

(A) Delayed union fracture with evidence of osteogenic activity, movement at fracture site, overriding of fracture segments, shortening, and favoring the leg. *(B–D)* Open approach, modified periosteal callus layers were reflected away from the cortex as one layer. Reduction and stabilization were achieved by inserting an intramedullary pin and unilateral external fixator (1/1 pins). A cancellous bone graft was added around the fracture site. In cases like this, the medullary space is filled with internal callus; thus, the intramedullary pin fits very snugly and affords excellent stability. The external fixator was added to stabilize against rotation. The other alternative is to use a plate for fixation.

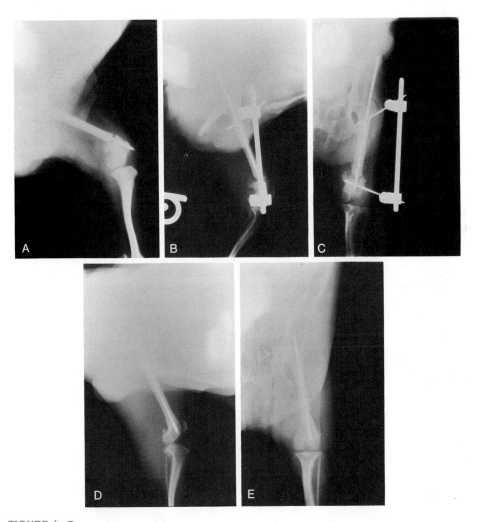

FIGURE 4–3

Nonunion of a supracondylar fracture in a small Yorkshire terrier immobilized by use of an improperly placed intramedullary pin. There was rotation at the fracture site. (A) Radiographic appearance at 3 months. Clinically, the area was very painful, and the animal totally refused to use the leg. (B, C) A lateral open approach was used, and an intramedullary pin and unilateral external fixator (1/1 pin) were applied for stabilization. The external fixator was removed in 6 weeks because there was sufficient callus to stabilize against rotation. (D, E) Clinical union was present at 3 months, and the intramedullary pin was removed. The animal regained a full range of movement and function.

NONUNION FRACTURES; PSEUDOARTHROSIS

There are two basic types of nonunion fractures.[4-7]

1. *Vascular* or *"elephant type" pseudoarthrosis*. This type is characterized by a proliferative bone reaction with interposed cartilage and fibrous tissue, which is evidenced radiographically and histologically. If reduction is satisfactory, most patients will respond to rigid fixation with compression at the fracture site, e.g., with a compression plate.

An alternate method of treatment (Fig. 4–3) is to perform an open approach, reflect the covering thickened periosteum with a periosteal elevator or osteotome, remove the fibrous soft tissue between the bone ends, fill the space between the reflected periosteum and bone with cancellous bone chips, and apply rigid fixation, e.g., with a bone plate, external fixator, or an intramedullary pin and external fixator (Kirschner splint).

2. *Atrophic* or *biologically inactive pseudoarthrosis*. In this type, there is no radiographic or histological evidence of bone reaction, and union is primarily by fibrous tissue. The ends of the bone segments are rounded, and the marrow cavity is sealed with dense trabecular bone (Fig. 4–4A).

Treatment consists of performing an open approach, reflecting the thickened periosteum overlying the cortical bone, removing sclerotic tissue between the bone ends (Fig. 4–4B), re-establishing the medullary canal by reaming, filling the space between the reflected periosteum and cortex with cancellous bone chips, and applying rigid fixation. In some cases, the combination of an onlay bone graft and bone chips is advantageous. Rigid, uninterrupted fixation

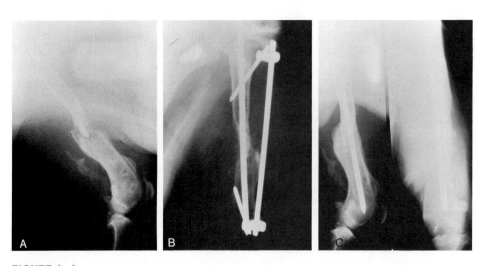

FIGURE 4–4

Nonunion of a fracture of the femur. The markedly comminuted fracture was originally fixed by use of a plate; however, the fracture site deficits were not filled with bone graft. At 15 months, when the animal returned for plate removal, he was favoring the leg. *(A)* Radiograph of femur following plate removal, lateral view. *(B)* Following reflection of the modified periosteum in the fracture site area, an intramedullary pin and a unilateral external fixator (1/1 pin) were applied for fixation, lateral view. A bone graft was applied in the fracture area. *(C)* Clinical union at 4½ months, lateral view. Demineralized bone such as this one responds faster if subjected to stresses; therefore, the intramedullary pin and external fixator were chosen for stabilization.

may be accomplished with a bone plate, an intramedullary pin and external fixator, or an external fixator alone. Healing is slow and the fixation will need to remain in place for a prolonged period of time (4 to 6 months). Some of the more indolent conditions may necessitate grafting procedures a second or third time.

REFERENCES

1. Watson-Jones R: Fractures and Joint Injuries, Vol 1. Baltimore, Williams & Wilkins, 1976, pp 13–48.
2. Brinker WO: Fractures in Canine Surgery, 2nd Archibald ed. Santa Barbara, American Veterinary Publications Inc, 1974, pp 949–1048.
3. Brinker WO: Small Animal Fractures. East Lansing, MI, Depart Cont Ed Serv, Michigan State University, 1978.
4. Rosen H: Compression treatment of long bone pseudoarthrosis. Clin Orthop 138:154, 1979.
5. Weber BG, Cech D: Pseudoarthrosis, Pathology, Biomechanics, Therapy, Results. Bern, Switzerland. Hans Huber Medical Publisher, 1976.
6. Brinker WO, Hohn RB, Prieur WD: Manual of Internal Fixation in Small Animals. Heidelberg, Springer-Verlag, 1984, pp 241–254.
7. Cechner PF, Knecht CD, Chaffee VW: Fracture repair failure in the dog. J Am Anim Hosp Assoc 13:613–615, 1977.

5

Fractures of the Pelvis

Fractures of the pelvis are relatively common, and in many veterinary practices they constitute 20 to 30 percent of all fractures. Most fractures are multiple in that three or more bones are involved. Rarely are they open or compound.

ANATOMY

Structurally, the pelvis roughly forms a rectangular box and is made up of the ossa coxae (ilium, ischium, and pubis), sacrum, and first coccygeal vertebra (Figs. 5–1 and 5–2). The structure is well covered with muscles and soft tissues. In fractures with minimal displacement, the muscles serve very effectively in supporting the bones. If there is gross displacement of the fracture segments, spastic contraction of the muscles increases the difficulty of surgical reduction and fixation.

HISTORY AND EXAMINATION

The patient's history usually includes traumatic injury and a sudden onset of symptoms. Because of the degree of trauma necessary to fracture the pelvis or cause a fracture dislocation, adjacent tissue and surrounding organ systems must be carefully evaluated. Fractures of the pelvis are always multiple in nature and, if displacement is present, at least three or more bones are assumed to be fractured.

Examination should include:

1. Physical examination and evaluation of the entire body.

2. Special emphasis on some of the more common complicating injuries—traumatic lung syndrome, pneumothorax (chest radiographs are taken routinely), rupture of the bladder or urethra, fractures of the spine, fractures of the femoral head and neck, and neurological deficits. Neurological examination of the rear limbs should include observation of voluntary leg movement while supporting the trunk, deep pain reflexes on all four toes of each foot, femoral nerve reflex (knee jerk), sciatic nerve reflex (withdrawal), as well as observations of the rectum and perineal reflex.

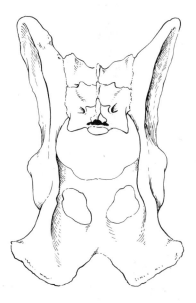

FIGURE 5–1

Pelvis, caudodorsal aspect.

3. Palpation of the pelvic area including a digital rectal examination.

4. Radiographs including ventrodorsal and lateral views. A lateral radiograph is taken with the affected side down, the lower hip flexed, and the upper hip extended. Tilting the pelvis to produce a slightly oblique view helps to separate the two sides.

TREATMENT

In regard to treatment, pelvic fractures may be divided into two groups—nonsurgical and surgical.[1, 2]

Nonsurgical Group

Included in the nonsurgical group are patients with little or no displacement of the fracture segments, an intact acetabulum, and continuity of the pelvic ring remaining essentially intact. The pelvic musculature serves very effectively in immobilizing the fracture segments. Perfect anatomical alignment of fractures involving the bones of the pelvis (other than articular surfaces) is

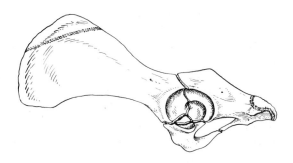

FIGURE 5–2

Left os coxae of young dog, lateral aspect, showing the acetabulum made up of the ilium, ischium, pubis and acetabular bones, and physis of ilium and ischium.

not necessary for healing or function. Management of the patient usually consists of cage rest, limitation of activity, and measures to ensure regular urination and defecation. To help prevent the development of decubital ulcers, a well-padded kennel is needed, particularly for those patients who are temporarily nonambulatory; many patients are able to stand up and move around within a day or two or, in the case of multiple fractures, in a week or two. Healing time for bones of the pelvis is approximately the same as for other bones in the body.

Surgical Group

Surgical intervention should be considered in animals with pelvic fractures characterized by one or more of the following:[2]

1. Marked decrease in the size of the pelvic canal.
2. Fracture of the acetabulum (displacement of articular surfaces).
3. Instability of the hip (e.g., fracture of ilium, ischium, and pubis on the same side).
4. Unilateral or bilateral instability, particularly if accompanied by coxofemoral dislocation or other limb fractures.

Careful study of the radiographs can show the type and location of the fractures involved and can suggest the appropriate surgical approach. In some multiple fractures, it may be necessary to use a combination of approaches to expose the involved areas and accomplish reduction and fixation.

Most pelvic fractures are accompanied by extensive muscle trauma, hemorrhage, and soft tissue injury. Such conditions usually result in increased surgical risk. The condition of the patient may prohibit carrying out all of the surgery that may be indicated. Traumatic lung syndrome may complicate anesthesia and delay surgery for 3 to 6 days.

Reduction and fixation are accomplished much more easily and accurately if undertaken within the first four days of injury. Each day's delay adds to the injuries to major nerves and blood vessels and to the time involved in obtaining reduction of the bones. In some instances, a prolonged delay may limit or prevent surgical repair. The chief advantages of early reduction and fixation are minimal hospitalization time, early ambulation, and minimization of fracture disease.

The various means of fixation for pelvic fractures may include intramedullary pins, Kirschner wires, external fixators, bone plates, bone screws, Lee clamps, stainless steel wires, or a combination of two or more of these techniques. Clinical data indicate that the highest percentage of successful cases have been treated with bone plates and screws.[3]

For surgical treatment of pelvic fractures, major emphasis is placed on the sacroiliac joint, ilium, and acetabulum. If these three areas are properly reduced and fixed, the other areas (ischium, pubis) as a rule fall into place and, with very few exceptions, need no specific surgical treatment. In most cases, it is to the surgeon's advantage to proceed in the order of sacroiliac joint, ilium, and acetabulum if all three are involved. If the ilium and acetabulum are involved, reduction and fixation of the ilium first give stability to a portion of the acetabulum; thus, there is a stable segment to build on for reduction and fixation of the remaining portion.

TYPES OF FRACTURES

Fracture-Dislocation of the Sacroiliac Joint

In this condition, the ilium is usually displaced craniodorsally. Displacement is always accompanied by fractures of the pubis and ischium or by separation along the pelvic symphysis, making half of the os coxae unstable. Adduction of the rear limb may present a problem in some cases. In many animals, this condition is accompanied by considerable discomfort and a prolonged period of favoring the involved rear limb, particularly when the lumbosacral nerve trunk is traumatized. Reduction and stabilization speed healing of the nerve trunk. Minor luxations of the sacroiliac joint with little or no displacement may be treated conservatively with restricted activity.

OPEN APPROACH PROCEDURE

The sacroiliac area may be exposed by either the dorsolateral approach[1, 2, 4, 5] (Fig. 5–3) or the ventrolateral approach[6] (Fig. 5–4). Either approach may be used; the dorsolateral lends itself to fracture separations alone or in conjunction with acetabular fractures and to fractures of the opposite os coxae; the ventrolateral approach lends itself to fracture separations alone or in conjunction with fractures of the ilium on the same side.

REDUCTION AND FIXATION

From the dorsolateral approach, the articular surface on the medial side of the ilium lies just ventral to the dorsal iliac spine in the caudal half of the wing (Figs. 5–5, 5–6C). After location or visualization of the fracture separation surface on both the ilium and sacrum, reduction is accomplished by grasping the edge of the iliac wing with a bone-holding forceps and moving it into position. A countering force on the sacrum by use of a hemostat is helpful in accomplishing reduction (Fig. 5–5). Because the reduction is always unstable, a Kirschner wire is inserted through the wing and into the sacrum for temporary fixation (Fig. 5–6A, E). It is highly recommended that the surgeon visualize these areas on a cadaver specimen and also compare the anatomical positions of the ilium and sacrum with a bone specimen. Anatomical reduction is essential.

After reduction, the ideal is to insert a lag screw into the body of the sacrum. Looking at the lateral surface of the ilium, the area for insertion of the screw through the wing and into the sacral body is indicated by the + mark on Fig. 5–6C. This is located by first dividing the length of the straight portion of the dorsal iliac crest into two equal parts. The craniocaudal location of + lies in the center of the caudal half. The dorsoventral location of + lies in the center of the ilial width in this area. The first screw goes into the sacral body (Fig. 5–6B). If a second screw is inserted, it is usually located just cranial and slightly dorsal to the first, and the length is just short of the neural canal (Fig. 5–6A). Screw length is measured on the dorsoventral view of the radiograph. A second screw gives two-point fixation and may be desirable, particularly where a portion of the sacrum is fractured or the first screw is not ideally placed in the body of the sacrum.

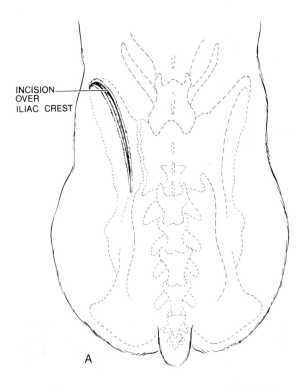

INCISION
OVER
ILIAC CREST

A

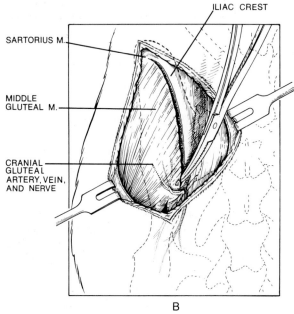

ILIAC CREST

SARTORIUS M.

MIDDLE
GLUTEAL M.

CRANIAL
GLUTEAL
ARTERY, VEIN,
AND NERVE

B

FIGURE 5–3

Dorsolateral approach for sacro-iliac fracture-separations. *(A)* A skin incision is made over the crest of the ilium and extended caudally along the dorsal iliac spine. *(B)* The cutaneous trunci muscles and subcutaneous fat are incised to expose the dorsal and upper half of the cranial border of the wing of the ilium and the origin of the middle gluteal muscle. The middle gluteal muscle is incised at its origin just inside the cranial and dorsal borders of the wing. Subperiosteal reflection of the middle gluteal muscle is then begun. As one approaches the caudal end of the straight portion of the dorsal iliac spine, a curved hemostat is used to run along the dorsal iliac spine to locate the caudal border of the sacrum. The cranial gluteal vessels and nerve pass from medial to lateral over the caudal iliac spine and enter the middle and deep gluteal muscles. The inserted hemostat helps to locate this area and also helps to avoid severing the cranial gluteal vessels and nerve.

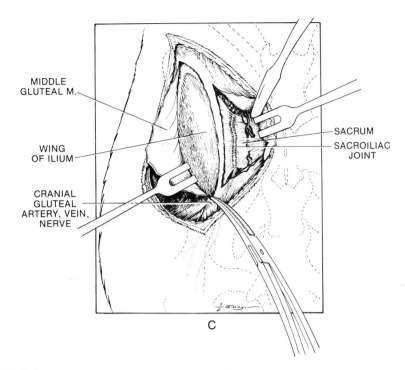

MIDDLE
GLUTEAL M.

WING
OF ILIUM

CRANIAL
GLUTEAL
ARTERY, VEIN,
NERVE

SACRUM
SACROILIAC
JOINT

C

FIGURE 5–3

Continued (C) The hemostat is retained in place and the subperiosteal reflection stops just short of this area, thus avoiding injury to the gluteal vessels and nerve. In most cases, the tissue between the iliac crest and adjoining sacrum is separated and little additional cutting or blunt dissection is necessary to expose the opposing surfaces of the sacrum and wing of the ilium. Additional soft tissue is reflected off the dorsal surface of the sacrum to expose the sacroiliac joint. The hemostat remains in place during the entire procedure, including dissection, reduction, and fixation because it helps to protect the cranial gluteal vessels and nerve and serves as an aid in keeping anatomical landmarks in mind.

FIGURE 5–4

Ventrolateral approach for a sacroiliac fracture-separation is the same as the lateral approach for the ilium (see Fig. 5–15). In addition, the iliacus muscle is incised and subperiostally elevated along the ventromedial border of the iliac body as needed to allow insertion of one finger in the pelvic inlet. The inserted finger is used to palpate the area of synchondrosis of the ilium and sacrum for reduction and screw placement. The Kern bone-holding forceps is used to move the ilium into reduction on the sacrum. The arrow and dot indicate the approximate location for inserting the lag screw through the ilium and into the body of the first sacral vertebrae.[6] This is the same location for placement of the lag screw as in a dorsolateral approach.

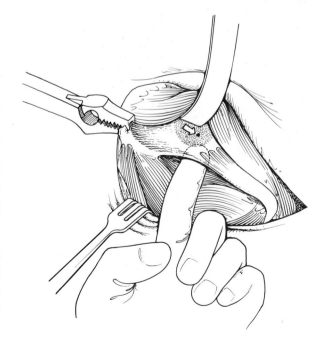

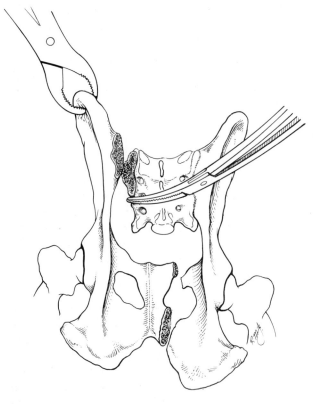

FIGURE 5–5

In a fracture-separation of the sacroiliac joint, the wing of the ilium lies in a craniodorsal position in relation to the sacrum. From a dorsolateral approach, reduction is usually accomplished by grasping the wing of the ilium with a bone-holding forceps and exerting a caudal and downward force. This is countered by a directly opposite force exerted on the sacrum by a curved hemostat or scissors.

Another approach to reduction and fixation from the craniodorsal exposure is to visualize the notch on the lateral surface of the sacrum (Fig. 5–6D). Pulling the wing ventrally and laterally aids in locating this area.[7, 8] The screw hole into the sacral body should always be drilled just caudal to this notch and cranial to the crescent-shaped auricular cartilage. The clear area on Fig. 5–6D shows the area in which the screw can be inserted for maximum holding and that is free of important structures.[7] The area for drilling the glide hole through the wing is the same as in Fig. 5–6A, E. The screw is advanced through the ilial hole and, when the tip appears on the medial side, the fracture is reduced and the screw is directed and inserted into the predrilled sacral hole. Many surgeons prefer this procedure over the aforementioned technique.

From the ventrolateral approach, the inserted finger is used to palpate the area of synchondrosis on the ilium and the ventral portion of the sacrum.[6] A bone-holding forceps placed on the iliac wing (Fig. 5–4) is used to accomplish reduction. A Kirschner wire is inserted through the ilial wing and into the sacrum for temporary stabilization until one or two lag screws are inserted through the wing into the sacrum. It is recommended that the surgeon visualize and palpate these areas as well as review the anatomical position of the ilium and sacrum on a bone specimen.

In some cases (e.g., in markedly overweight dogs, in impacted fractures involving a portion of the sacrum, and in some bilateral fractures), an additional stabilizing bolt will improve stability. It passes transversely through the iliac wings and dorsally to the seventh lumbar vertebra. This is a partially threaded Steinmann pin, bent at the smooth end and with a nut placed on the threaded end (Fig. 5–6F).

Note: Accurate reduction and placement of screws are at times challenging, especially if a week or more has elapsed since the traumatic episode. A common error involves screw placement in lumbar articular processes, the lumbosacral disc space, or the 7th lumbar vertebra, or missing the sacrum entirely.

CASE STUDIES

CASE 1 ■ Figure 5–7A shows a mature St. Bernard with a unilateral fracture-separation of the sacroiliac joint and fractures of the ischium and pubis.[2] On the fourth day after the trauma occurred, the animal still exhibited considerable pain on attempting to move and was unable to rise. Two cancellous bone screws were used for fixation (Fig. 5–7B). Reduction and fixation of the sacroiliac joint also aided in stabilization of the other fractures. The animal was able to stand and walk on the first postoperative day.

CASE 2 ■ Figure 5–8A depicts a large mixed-breed dog with bilateral sacroiliac separations, a coxofemoral dislocation, and fractures of the pubis and ischium. The animal was unable to rise and lay in the spread-eagle position. Reduction and fixation were done using two cancellous bone screws on each side (Fig. 5–8B). It is necessary to stabilize the acetabulum before reduction of the hip joint can be maintained. An open approach was performed to reduce the hip joint and suture the joint capsule. The legs were tied together for 6 days (see Figure 5–25A) to protect against abnormal abduction.

Fractures of the Acetabulum

When fractures of the acetabulum show no displacement on ventrodorsal and lateral radiographs, they are usually treated conservatively, with marked restriction of activity indicated for a period of time. In some cases, it may be advantageous to place the leg in a single (Ehmer) sling for a period of 7 to 10 days.

Reduction and fixation are indicated for those cases in which dislocation or instability of the fractured segments is present.[1–3, 5, 9–11] Crepitation is usually felt on movement of the hip joint. If these cases are untreated, pain and permanent lameness follow as a result of abnormal wear and ensuing osteoarthritis. Another reason for surgical treatment is that the animal frequently lies on the affected side, which further displaces the fracture fragments.

OPEN APPROACH AND REDUCTION

Figure 5–9 shows the dorsal open approach to the hip joint.[2, 4] The method of reduction varies with the type and location of the fracture. In many patients, reduction consists of a combination of traction, countertraction, levering, and rotation. Insertion of a Steinmann pin through the skin and tuber ischii is one way of grasping and moving the caudal segment (Fig. 5–10A). Rarely is the

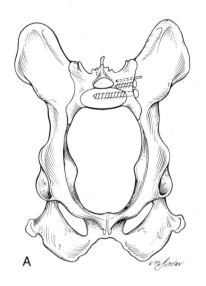

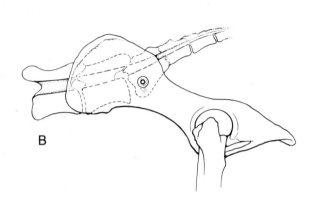

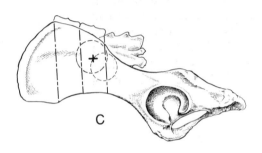

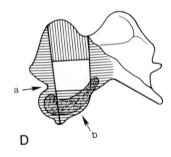

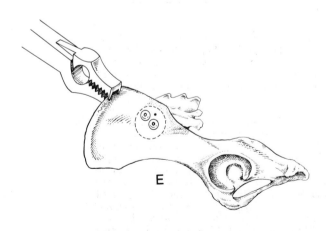

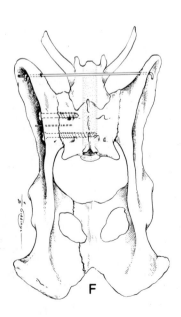

FIGURE 5–6

See legend on opposite page

fracture stable after reduction. The fracture must be held in the reduced position while fixation is being applied. Use of reduction forceps that straddles the trochanter major and anchor on the cranial and caudal rims of the acetabulum is helpful in maintaining reduction and compression in a stable fracture (Fig. 5–10B) (see Figures 5–11 through 5–13). If the fracture is oblique, the compression forceps is placed at right angles to the fracture line (Fig. 5–10B).

In many cases, a bone hook moved down along the medial surface of the caudal segment is helpful in the reduction procedure (Fig. 5–10C). The use of a small bone-holding forceps to grasp the ischium and move the caudal segment into reduction can be helpful (Fig. 5–10B). Utmost care must be taken to avoid injury to the sciatic nerve. Anatomical reduction is a must in acetabular fractures. Final reduction is checked by observing the fracture line, the acetabular rim, and the articular cartilage inside the acetabulum.

FIXATION

The method of fixation varies with the type of fracture. Bone plates and screws have yielded the best percentage of success.[1–3, 5, 9–14] The various types of bone plates that may be contoured and used on acetabular fractures include regular, acetabular,* reconstruction,* and small fragment plates. The reconstruction and acetabular plates lend themselves to easy contouring. Some fractures can be managed with pin fixation; however, the pins have a tendency to work loose prior to healing in many cases. Tension band wire fixation can be used only on interlocking stable fractures. (See Chapter 1, Fig. 1–43 for suggestions of plate size to use in relation to the weight of the animal.) The dorsal side of the acetabulum is used for tension band fixation.

---

*Synthes, Wayne, PA, manufacturer.

FIGURE 5–6

Reduction and fixation. (A) Craniocaudal view of the pelvis showing proper position of the lag screw into the sacral body. Penetration is usually about 60% of the width of the sacral body. A second screw may be inserted for two-point fixation. (B) Schema of lateral view of pelvis with screw inserted into the body of the sacrum. (C) Lateral view of the ilium; + marks the spot for drilling and inserting the lag screw. Craniocaudally, the + is located in the center of the caudal half, and proximal-distally, it is located in the center of the ilial width. (D) The area of the lateral surface of the body of the sacrum available for proper screw placement is only slightly larger than 1 cm in the average-size dog, as denoted by the clear area in D. The cross-hatched area represents a thinner portion of the sacral wing, which can only accommodate short screws. This means that for many cases, there is only room for placement of one screw within the area of the sacral body. The notches (a) along the cranial border of the sacrum and the crescent-shaped auricular cartilage (b) are used as landmarks in locating the area for screw insertion into the sacral body. (E) After reduction, a Kirschner wire is inserted for temporary stabilization. The first lag screw is inserted through the ilium and into the sacral body. When a second screw is inserted, it is usually located slightly cranial and proximal. The depth for drilling this hole and length of the lag screw to be inserted are determined from the ventrodorsal radiograph. The drill hole and screw should stop just short of the neural canal. The authors prefer two-point fixation in most cases. (F) If additional fixation is indicated for stabilization, a transilial bolt passing through the wings and over the dorsal surface of L7 may be inserted.

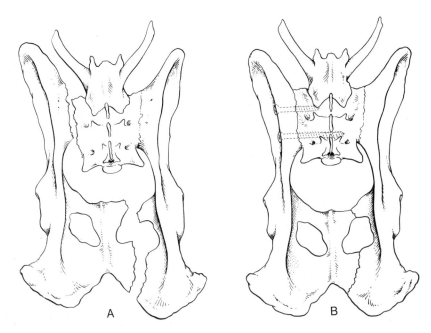

FIGURE 5–7

(A) Mature St. Bernard with a unilateral fracture-separation of the sacroiliac joint and fractures of the ischium and pubis. *(B)* Postoperative view showing two cancellous bone screws used for fixation.

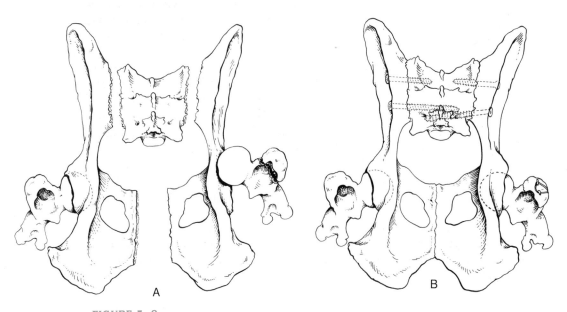

FIGURE 5–8

(A) Large dog with bilateral sacroiliac separations, a coxofemoral dislocation, and fractures of the pubis and ischium. *(B)* Postoperative view showing two cancellous bone screws on each side used for fixation. The acetabulum must be stabilized before reduction of the hip joint can be maintained. A dorsolateral approach was used to expose the hip joint; after reduction, the ruptured joint capsule was sutured in place.

Closure is important in restoring good stability to the hip joint. This consists of suturing the joint capsule, the severed internal obturator and gemellus muscles, and the deep gluteal muscle. The osteomized tip of the trochanter major is fixed with the tension band wire technique. The remaining muscles— the superficial gluteal, the biceps femoris, and tensor fasciae latae—are sutured in place, followed by the gluteal fascia, subcutaneous tissue, and skin.

CASE 1 ■ Figure 5–11A, B show a serrated transverse fracture of the acetabulum along with fractures of the ischium and pubis. With bone plate fixation, at least two screws should be inserted on each side of the fracture line (Fig. 5–11C, D). Care must be taken in contouring the plate so that it fits the surface to which it is applied. In most cases, reduction and fixation of the acetabular fracture realign the accompanying fractures of the ischium and pubis and afford satisfactory stability to them.

CASE 2 ■ Figure 5–12 shows an oblique fracture through the cranial part of the body of ilium and acetabulum (Fig. 5–12A). One or more Kirschner wires are inserted to help maintain reduction prior to lag screw insertion. Two screws are preferable if there is room for insertion (Fig. 5–12B). This fracture is also very amenable to plate fixation.

CASE 3 ■ In Fig. 5–13A, an oblique fracture has occurred through the caudal part of the body of the ischium and caudal acetabulum. Two screws have been inserted for fixation (Fig. 5–13B). Reduction can be aided and maintained by use of self-locking compression forceps while the screws are being inserted.

CASE 4 ■ Figure 5–14 shows multiple fractures of the acetabulum. As the pieces were reduced, they were skewered into place with Kirschner wires, one at a time (Fig. 5–14A). The reconstruction bone plate was then contoured and applied (Fig. 5–14B). The two center fragments were too small for screw fixation. Following closure, the leg was placed in a single (Ehmer) sling for 10 days to prevent weight bearing (see Figure 5–24B).

Fractures of the Ilium

Most fractures of the ilium[1–3, 5, 10, 14] are oblique in nature, and the caudal segment is depressed medially, resulting in a decreased size of the pelvic canal. Some fractures are multiple, and most are accompanied by fractures of the ischium and pubis.

Figure 5–15 shows an approach to the lateral surface of the ilium.[1, 2, 4, 15] Reduction usually consists of a combination of levering, traction, and rotation. The caudal segment generally needs to be levered out from underneath the

Text continued on page 93

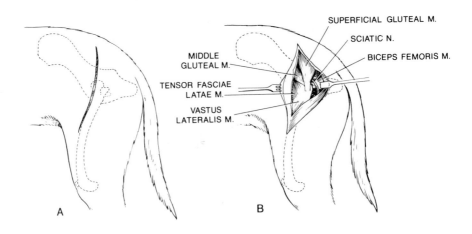

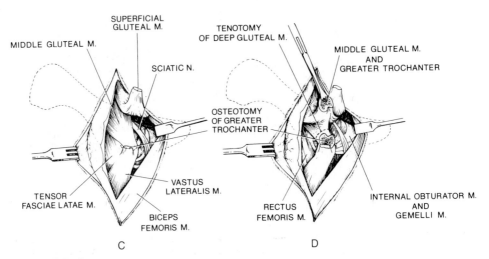

FIGURE 5–9

Dorsal open approach to the hip joint with osteotomy of the tip of the trochanter major. (A) A slightly curved skin incision is made over the lateral surface of the trochanter major and is extended toward the midline of the back proximally and toward the patella distally. (B) The fascia uniting the biceps femoris and tensor fasciae latae muscles is incised; the biceps muscle is retracted caudally. (C) The superficial gluteal muscle is severed ¼″ from its insertion on the lateral surface of the trochanter major and reflected proximally. The proximal end of the trochanter major is cut with an osteotome to include the entire insertion of the middle gluteal muscle only. (D) Insertion of the deep gluteal muscle is severed ¼″ from its attachment on the facet on the craniolateral surface of the trochanter major.

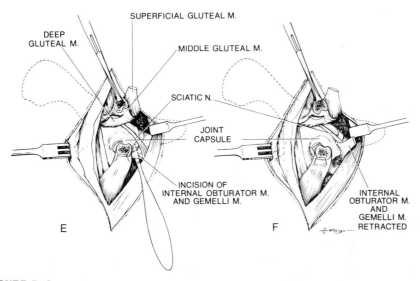

FIGURE 5–9

Continued (E, F) With the use of an osteotome or periosteal elevator, subperiosteal reflection of these muscles continues dorsally and cranially to expose the rim of acetabulum, the bone dorsal and medial to it, and the shaft of the ilium. Cutting of the insertion and reflection of the severed internal obturator and gemellus muscles expose the caudal portion of the acetabulum and shaft of the ischium.

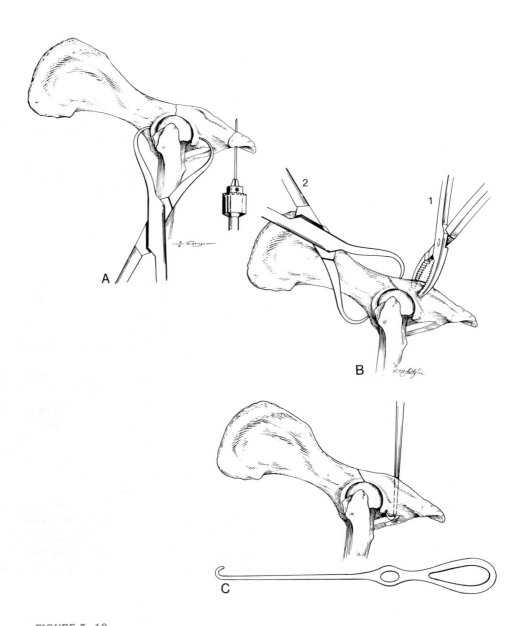

FIGURE 5–10

(A) Reduction of an acetabular fracture facilitated by driving a Steinmann pin vertically through the tuber ischii. The pin can then be used to apply traction and rotation. *(B–1)* In some cases, grasping the ischium with a bone-holding forceps can be helpful in maneuvering the fragment into reduction. *(B–2)* In oblique cases, a sharp-pointed reduction forceps placed at right angles to the fracture line is helpful in maintaining reduction. *(C)* In many cases, a bone hook slid down along the medial surface of the ischium is helpful in maneuvering the caudal fragment into reduction.

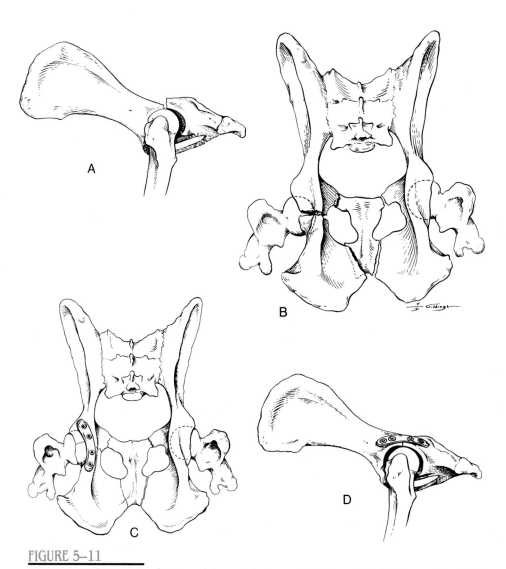

FIGURE 5–11

(A, B) Serrated transverse fracture of the acetabulum and fracture of the ischium and pubis. (C, D) With bone plate fixation, at least two screws should be inserted on each side of the fracture line. The plate should be contoured so that it fits the surface to which it is applied. In cases such as this, any one of the various types of plates could have been used: reconstruction, acetabular, regular, or small fragment.

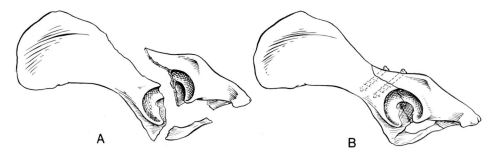

FIGURE 5–12

(A) Oblique fracture through the cranial part of the body of the ilium and acetabulum. *(B)* Two lag screws are preferable if there is room for insertion.

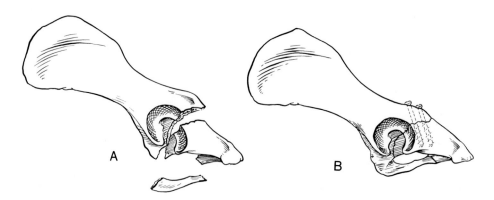

FIGURE 5–13

(A) Oblique fracture through the caudal part of the body of the ischium and acetabulum. *(B)* Two lag screws are inserted for fixation.

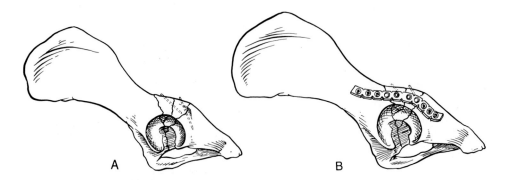

FIGURE 5–14

(A) Multiple fractures of the acetabulum; as pieces were reduced, they were skewered into place with Kirschner wires, one at a time. *(B)* Bone plate contoured and applied; the center two fragments are too small for screw fixation. A reconstruction plate contours very easily and is very adaptable to fractures of this type.

cranial segment. Use of a Steinmann pin inserted through the ischiatic tuberosity may be helpful in maneuvering and realigning the caudal segment. Self-retaining bone forceps (e.g., compression, speed-lock, or Verbrugge forceps) is helpful in accomplishing and maintaining reduction while fixation is applied (Fig. 5–16D). The fracture is semireduced (Fig. 5–16B). The ilial plate must be bent concave. This is essential to help restore the normal size of the pelvic canal. An effort should be made to place the cranial part of the plate with a screw hole over the center of the sacral body for increased purchase of screws (see Figure 5–16B, C, D). The cranial part of the wing of the ilium is thin, and screws may strip easily. The plate is attached to the caudal segment first. Lateral traction is exerted on the trochanter major along with medial pressure on the cranial end of the plate prior to and during insertion of the bone screws into the cranial segment. This aids in lining up and stabilizing fractures of the ischium and pubic bones (Fig. 5–16C).

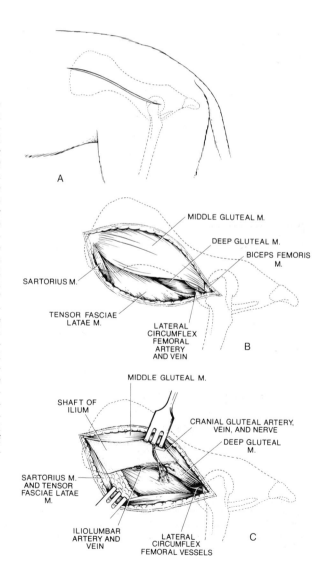

FIGURE 5–15

Approach to the lateral surface of the ilium. *(A)* A skin incision starts at the iliac crest and extends caudally over the lateral surface of the trochanter major toward the ischial tuberosity. *(B)* Subcutaneous fat and the fascia are incised to expose muscle separation between the gluteus medius (dorsally) and the tensor fasciae latae (ventrally) and the sartorius (cranially). *(C)* Subperiosteal reflection upward of the middle and deep gluteal muscles exposes the ventral border and lateral surface of the body and wing of the ilium. The primary structures of importance encountered in this approach are the lateral circumflex femoral vessels (just cranial to the acetabulum), the cranial gluteal nerve (midway), and the iliolumbar vessels (located at the caudal iliac spine). The iliolumbar vessels are cut and ligated in carrying out the approach. The cranial gluteal vessels and nerve may be cut if necessary to obtain adequate exposure.

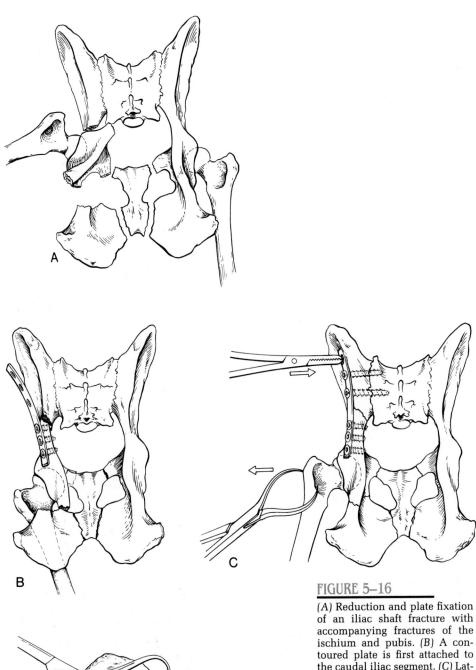

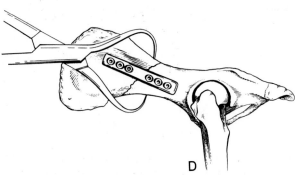

FIGURE 5–16

(A) Reduction and plate fixation of an iliac shaft fracture with accompanying fractures of the ischium and pubis. (B) A contoured plate is first attached to the caudal iliac segment. (C) Lateral traction by way of the trochanter major and medial pressure on the cranial end of the bone plate bring about reduction of all of the fractures. Cranial screws are then placed. (D) Bone-holding forceps maintains reduction while cranial screws are placed.

Many methods of fixation for fractures of the ilium have been presented and used. The highest percentage of successful cases can be attributed to the use of bone plates and screws.[3] Pins have a tendency to become loose or back out prior to clinical union. At times, they are very difficult to insert in an effective position. The Lee clamp and, in most cases, the Kirschner splint all too frequently become loosened, and reduction is lost prior to clinical union.

In certain cases (e.g., oblique fractures and fractures in large dogs and relatively lean animals), the insertion of two cancellous lag screws is very effective; however, they may be difficult to insert properly (see Figure 5–20D). In multiple fractures of the ilium, they may be combined with the use of a bone plate for fixation.

CASE STUDIES

Cases 1 through 3 describe treatment with bone plates and screws.

CASE 1 ■ Figure 5–17A shows an oblique fracture of the ilium along with fractures of the ischium and pubis and sacroiliac separation on the opposite side. If attention is directed toward reduction and fixation of the sacroiliac separation and the fractured ilium, the rest of the fractures will usually align in a satisfactory manner.

The separated sacroiliac joint was treated first and stabilized with the use

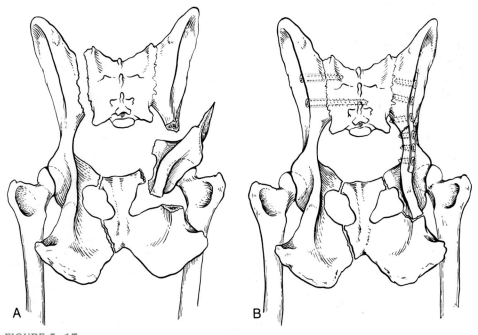

A   B

FIGURE 5–17

(A) Oblique fracture of the ilium, along with fractures of the ischium and pubis; sacroiliac separation on opposite side. *(B)* The sacroiliac is stabilized by two cancellous screws; a lateral approach exposes the ilium, which was fixed by use of a bone plate.

of two cancellous screws. This made reduction easier on the opposite side. The lateral approach was used to expose the ilium, which was fixed by the use of a bone plate.

Note: The plate is contoured in a concave fashion. This restores the pelvic canal to normal size and realigns the fractured ischium.

CASE 2 ■ Figure 5–18*A*, *B* depict oblique fractures of the ilium, ischium, and acetabulum. In this case, the lateral view is most helpful in determining the direction of the fracture line through the acetabulum and in planning the surgical approach.

The ilium was reduced and fixed first (Fig. 5–18*B*, *C*). This rigidly stabilizes one segment of the acetabulum, thereby making reduction of the acetabular fracture easier. A pin through the tuber of the ischium and compression forceps were used to assist and maintain reduction while the lag screws were inserted.

CASE 3 ■ Combination fractures as shown in Fig. 5–18 and Fig. 5–19*C*, *D* are best approached by using a combined lateral exposure to the ilium and dorsal approach to the hip joint (Fig. 5–19*A*, *B*).[1–4] This exposes both fracture areas at the same time and aids in reduction.

An oblique fracture of the ilium and a serrated short oblique fracture through the acetabulum on the same side are shown in Fig. 5–19*C*. Usually, the iliac fracture is first reduced and fixed with a bone plate. The acetabulum is then reduced and stabilized. A DCP plate is particularly advantageous in gaining compression in serrated interlocking fractures.

Figure 5–20 gives some examples of ilial and acetabular fractures sur-

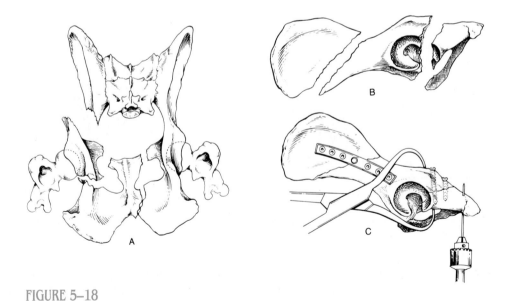

FIGURE 5–18

(A, B) Oblique fractures of the ilium, ischium, and acetabulum. *(B, C)* Reduction and fixation of the ilium rigidly stabilized one segment of the acetabulum, thereby facilitating reduction of the acetabular fracture. A pin through the tuber ischii and compression forceps assisted and maintained reduction while lag screws were inserted.

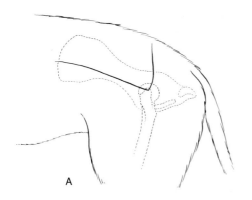

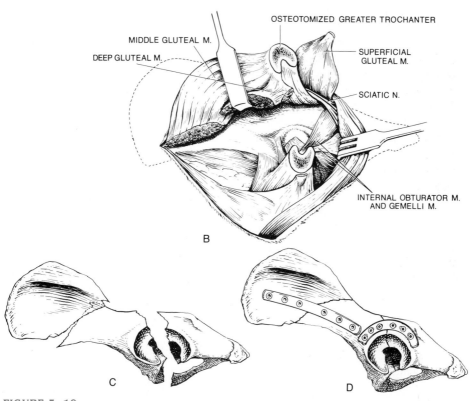

FIGURE 5–19

Example of a surgically treated case. *(A, B)* Combination fractures may be exposed by a combined lateral exposure to the ilium and dorsal approach to hip joint. *(C)* Lateral view of an oblique fracture of the ilium and a serrated short oblique fracture through the acetabulum on the same side. *(D)* The ilial fracture is reduced and fixed with a bone plate; the acetabulum is then reduced and stabilized with an acetabular plate.

gically stabilized using methods other than bone plate fixation. All of the various methods depicted have been used. However, plates and screws are much easier to apply and, with few exceptions, are far superior in stabilizing the fractures shown. Pins have a definite tendency to loosen and migrate to other parts of the body. Frequently, this occurs before healing has taken place, and reduction is lost. These are only offered as alternatives when plates and screws are not available.

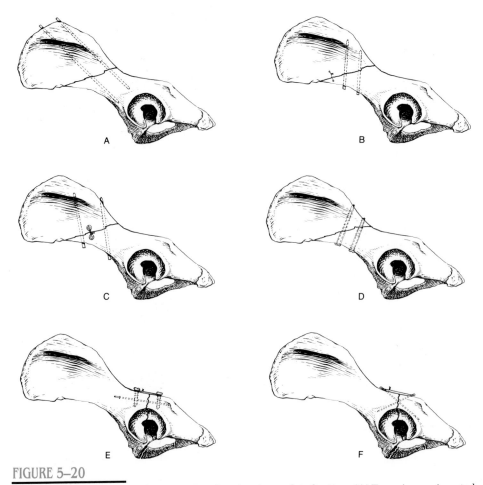

FIGURE 5–20

Example of surgically treated cases using other than bone plate fixation. *(A)* Two pins are inserted to give sufficient stability, to prevent rotation of fracture segments, and to maintain tightness. *(B)* Fixation is achieved with two pins inserted from the ventral border or with double-pointed pins inserted in a retrograde fashion. Interfragmentary wire is added for stability. *(C)* Oblique fracture stabilized with two pins and two screws with a connecting wire. *(D)* Two screws inserted with a lag screw effect are superior to the methods used in *A, B,* and *C. (E)* Serrated transverse fracture of the acetabulum. Tension band fixation using two screws and wire. Following reduction, a Kirschner wire can be inserted first to help maintain reduction and stabilize the fracture. *(F)* Fixation with Kirschner wires inserted diagonally; the wire is twisted tightly between pins to provide compression and rigidity. This method is usually only applicable in a serrated transverse fracture. Plates and screws are much easier to apply and, with few exceptions, are far superior in stabilizing the fracture.

Fractures of the Ischium

Most fractures of the ischium[1–3, 5] accompany other fractures (e.g., in the ilium or acetabulum or sacroiliac separation). If these fractures are properly reduced and immobilized, the ischium may need no further treatment. When an ischial fracture is of primary concern (e.g., fracture of the ischial shaft and pubis with marked dislocation), reduction and fixation may be indicated, but ordinarily these are not repaired. By modifying and abbreviating the dorsal approach to the hip, the shaft of the ischium can be exposed (Fig. 5–21).[4, 5]

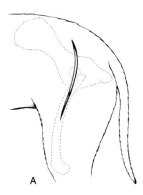

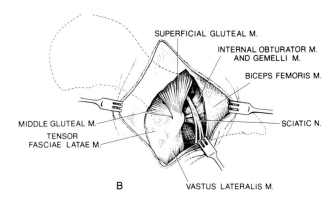

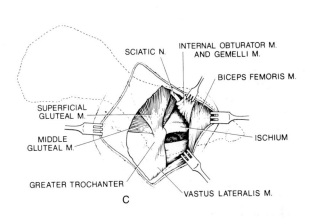

FIGURE 5–21

Approach to the shaft of the ischium. *(A)* A slightly curved skin incision over the lateral surface of the trochanter major extends toward the midline of the back dorsally and the patella ventrally. The fascia uniting the biceps femoris and tensor fasciae latae muscles is incised. *(B)* The biceps femoris is retracted caudally. *(C)* The conjoined tendon of the internal obturator and gemelli muscles is undermined and severed close to its insertion in the trochanteric fossa. This approach may also be used to expose, reduce, and apply fixation to certain caudal acetabular fractures. Levering the gluteal muscles cranially with a Hohmann retractor markedly increases the exposure.

FIXATION

Fixation is usually accomplished by the use of an intramedullary pin, Kirschner wire, stainless steel wire, or small bone plate.

Following open reduction, the pin is usually inserted in the region of the tuber ischium, and insertion is continued cranially beyond the fracture site until good anchorage is obtained (Fig. 5–22A). The addition of an interfragmentary or tension band wire aids in stability; thus, the pin is less apt to loosen and work itself out prior to clinical union. The wire is usually inserted first, the pin next, and the wire then tightened.

In some cases, a stainless steel wire suture affords sufficient fixation (Fig. 5–22B). Space in this area is usually very limited because of the location of the sciatic nerve. In some larger dogs, however, a small, short bone plate adds to the rigidity of the fixation (Fig. 5–22C).

Fractures of the Ischiatic Tuberosity

Most fractures of the ischiatic tuberosity[1–3, 5] respond satisfactorily to conservative treatment. In some patients, a sizable bone segment is fractured and

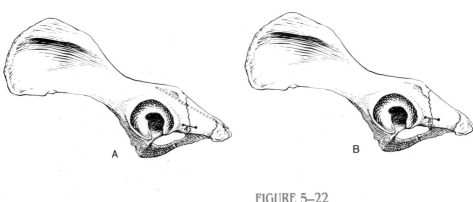

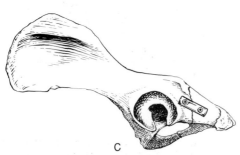

FIGURE 5–22

(A) Following open reduction, the pin is usually inserted in the region of the tuber ischii and moved cranially beyond the fracture site until good anchorage is obtained. The addition of a wire suture aids stability. *(B)* Stainless steel wire suture used alone for fixation. *(C)* Small bone plate used for fixation. In most cases, there is only space for the insertion of one screw in each fragment. Ordinarily, these fractures need no repair unless the fragment is markedly dislocated, is very painful, or has a definite cosmetic effect on a show animal.

pulled distally, causing considerable discomfort. In these instances, surgical treatment may be indicated.

OPEN APPROACH PROCEDURE

A longitudinal skin incision is made over the ischial tuberosity. This is continued down through the subcutaneous fat and fascia. Muscle attachments are subperiosteally elevated to expose the fracture area.

REDUCTION AND FIXATION

The ventral surface of the ischiatic tuberosity gives rise to the powerful hamstring muscles—the biceps femoris, the semitendinosus, and the semi-membranosus. Contraction of these muscles pulls the fracture segment distally (Fig. 5–23A). The tuberosity fragment is fixed in place with pins, and a dorsal tension band wire is looped over a screw, or the fragment is fixed with screws alone (Fig. 5–23B). Small Kirschner wires are used to hold the fragment in the reduced position while the fixation is inserted.

Fractures in the Region of the Pelvic Symphysis

As a result of traumatic injury, the os coxae may become separated at the pelvic symphysis.[1, 2] This may be accompanied by separation at the sacroiliac articulation. When this occurs, the animal loses the ability to adduct the legs;

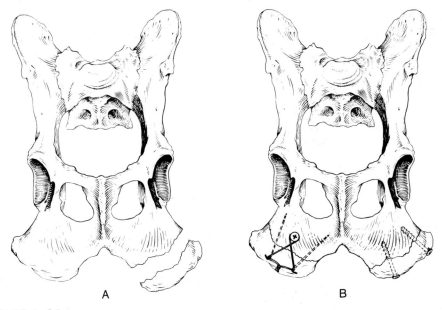

FIGURE 5–23

(A) Ventral surface of the ischial tuberosity gives rise to powerful hamstring muscles—the biceps femoris, the semitendinosus, and the semimembranosus. *(B)* Tuberosity fragment fixed in place with pins and a dorsal tension band wire looped over a screw or with a screw alone. Small Kirschner wires hold fragment in reduced position while screws are inserted.

the rear legs abduct, and the patient is unable to stand. The condition is seen most frequently in an immature animal before the symphysis has ossified. If other fractures are present (e.g., in the ilium or acetabulum, or if there is fracture-separation of the sacroiliac articulation), proper treatment of these fractures usually gives sufficient stability so that surgery in the pelvic symphysis area is not necessary. Another method of reduction and stabilization

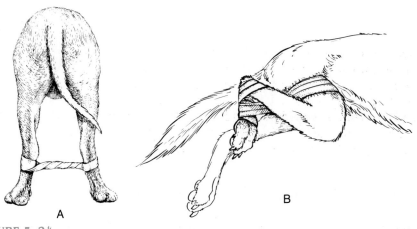

FIGURE 5–24

(A) Rear legs tied together to restrict abduction until healing is under way and power of adduction is recovered. *(B)* A single (Ehmer) sling keeps the animal from weight bearing and helps to protect fractures and prevent dislocation in the region of the hip joint.

is to use a ventral midline approach and insert hemicerclage wires (Fig. 5–25).

CASE STUDIES

CASE 1 ■ In Figure 5–24A, the rear legs are tied together to prevent uncontrolled abduction until healing is under way and the power of adduction is recovered. A single (Ehmer) sling (Fig. 5–24B) is applied primarily to keep the animal from weight bearing and to help protect fractures and prevent dislocation in the region of the hip joint.

CASE 2 ■ Figure 5–25 depicts fracture-separation of the pelvic symphysis and sacroiliac articulation and gross dislocation of the os coxae. Reduction and fixation were accomplished by two stainless steel wires (Fig. 5–25B). Reduction and fixation of the symphysis improved stability at the sacroiliac separation. Another method of fixation is to insert two lag screws at the sacroiliac articulation.

Healed, Unreduced Fractures Collapsing the Pelvic Canal

Healed fractures of the pelvis resulting in a marked decrease in size of the pelvic cavity are shown in Figure 5–26. This condition may be accompanied by constant or intermittent constipation or obstipation. A midline ventral approach is used to expose the pelvic symphysis area (Fig. 5–26B). The symphysis is split longitudinally with an osteotome, the two halves are carefully spread, and an allograft (body of ilium) is inserted and fixed in place

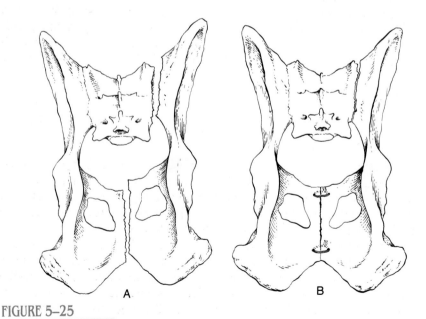

A   B

FIGURE 5–25

(A) Fracture-separation of pelvic symphysis and sacroiliac articulation; gross dislocation of the os coxae. *(B)* Reduction and fixation by use of two stainless steel wires. Two lag screws inserted to stabilize the sacroiliac articulation would achieve the same effect.

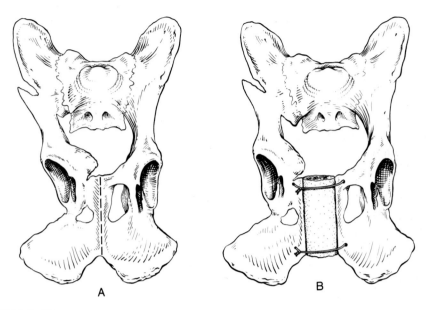

FIGURE 5–26

Healed, unreduced fractures collapsing the pelvic canal. (A) Healed fractures of the pelvis resulting in marked decrease in size of pelvic cavity, accompanied by constant or intermittent constipation or obstipation. (B) A midline ventral approach exposes pelvic symphysis area. The symphysis is split longitudinally with an osteotome. The two halves are spread, and an allograft (body of ilium) is inserted and fixed in place using two wires. This increases the diameter of the pelvic canal and facilitates defecation.

using two stainless steel wires. This markedly increases the diameter of the pelvic canal and returns defecation to normal,[1, 2, 5] provided neurological control of defecation is normal. Occasionally, it may be necessary to osteotomize the ilial shaft unilaterally to allow adequate spreading of the pelvis. Caution must be taken because the lumbosacral trunk may be incorporated in the bony callus on the medial side of the ilium. Plate fixation is used on the ilium.

POSTOPERATIVE MANAGEMENT OF PELVIC FRACTURES

Hemostasis prior to closure creates a smoother recovery period and minimizes complications in the operative area. The wound is closed in layers. A good anatomical closure, particularly in the hip area, aids in rapid restoration of function and stability of the hip joint. A good skin closure is mandatory. Stainless steel and nylon are preferred suture materials.

Rarely is avascular necrosis of skin a problem. If it occurs, however, it may be caused by the original trauma in the area, by unnecessary subcutaneous dissection in the operative process, or by a combination of both. Conservative treatment is usually sufficient for a small area of necrosis, but debridement followed by secondary closure may be indicated if a large area is involved.

Good nursing is an essential part of the aftercare. Particular attention must be paid to the patient's appetite, urination, defecation, and cleanliness. If the patient is temporarily nonambulatory, decubital ulcers may become a secondary complication. A dry, well-padded bed and frequent turning from side to side are good preventive measures.

Movement and restriction of activity will vary greatly with the individual case, the degree of trauma, and the stability of fixation. If good, rigid stability can be achieved, limited restricted movement should be encouraged. Local restriction of activity in the form of a single or Ehmer sling for 5 to 10 days is usually indicated in fractures involving the acetabulum and femoral head and neck or in a reduced coxofemoral dislocation (Fig. 5–24B).

If adduction is a problem resulting from multiple fractures in the pelvic symphysis area or from muscle trauma, a restriction bandage or hobble is indicated for 5 to 7 days to limit abduction (Fig. 5–24A). Marked restriction of activity is always indicated when many fractures are present.

Fractures of the pelvis require the usual span of time for healing, which is normally 6 to 10 weeks. Some alteration in gait can be expected during this period.

In general, bone plates and bone screws are not removed unless specifically indicated. Long-term follow-ups often show no radiological indications of loosening, alteration in bone density, or stress protection. If other means of fixation are used (e.g., intramedullary pins or external fixator), removal is indicated after the fracture has reached clinical union.

REFERENCES

1. Brinker WO: Fractures in Canine Surgery, 2nd Archibald ed. Santa Barbara, American Veterinary Publications, Inc, 1974, pp 949–1048.
2. Brinker WO: Small Animal Fractures. East Lansing, MI, Depart Cont Ed Serv, Michigan State University, 1978.
3. Brinker WO: Fracture Documentation Studies. East Lansing, MI, Michigan State University, Unpublished material, 1971–1978.
4. Piermattei DL: An Atlas of Surgical Approaches to the Bones of the Dog and Cat, 3rd ed. Philadelphia, WB Saunders Company, in preparation.
5. Brinker WO, Hohn RB, Prieur WD, et al: Manual of Internal Fixation in Small Animals. New York, Springer-Verlag, 1984, pp 152–165.
6. Montavon PM, Boudrieu RG, Hohn RB: Ventrolateral approach for repair of sacroiliac fracture-dislocation in the dog and cat. J Am Vet Med Assoc 186:1198–2001, 1985.
7. DeCamp C, Braden TD: The surgical anatomy of the canine sacrum for lag screw fixation of the sacroiliac joint. Vet Surg 14:131–134, 1985.
8. DeCamp C, Braden TD: Sacroiliac fracture-separation in the dog: a study of 92 cases. Vet Surg 14:127–130, 1985.
9. Wheaton L, Hohn RB, Harrison J: Surgical treatment of acetabular fractures in the dog. J Am Vet Med Assoc 162:385–392, 1973.
10. Denny HR: Pelvic fractures in the dog: a review of 123 cases. J Small Anim Pract 19:151, 1978.
11. Hulse DA, Root CR: Management of acetabular fractures: a long-term evaluation. J Comp Cont Ed 2:189, 1980.
12. Wadsworth PL, Henry WB: Dorsal surgical approach to acetabular fractures in the dog. J Am Vet Med Assoc 165:908, 1975.
13. Hinko PJ: The use of a precontoured pelvic bone plate in the treatment of comminuted pelvic fractures: a preliminary report. J Am Vet Med Assoc 14:229–232, 1978.
14. Bild C: Practice tips. Presentation at 3rd Annual Meeting of the American College of Veterinary Surgery. Park City, Utah, February 1969.
15. Hohn BH, James JM: Lateral approach to canine ilium. J Am Anim Hosp Assoc 2:111–113, 1966.

Fractures of the Femur and Patella

The incidence for fractures of the femur is about 20 to 25 percent in most veterinary practices; this rate is higher than for any of the long bones in the body. The femur also has the highest incidence of nonunion and osteomyelitis in most practices. Proper surgical intervention is indicated in practically all femoral fractures.[1-3] This chapter suggests ways of treating various types of fractures at the proximal end, shaft, and distal end.

FEMORAL FRACTURES

Classification

FRACTURES AT THE PROXIMAL END

a. Avulsion fracture and dislocation of the femoral head (Fig. 6–1A).
b. Fracture-separation of the proximal femoral epiphysis (Fig. 6–1B).
c. Fractures of the femoral head (Fig. 6–1C).
d. Fractures of the femoral neck (Fig. 6–1D).
e. Fractures or fracture-separation of the trochanter major with or without dislocation of the femoral head (Fig. 6–1E).
f. Combination of any of these with or without fractures of the femoral shaft (Fig. 6–1F).

SHAFT FRACTURES

(See Figs. 6–13 through 6–20.)

FRACTURES AT THE DISTAL END

a. Supracondylar fracture (see Fig. 4–3), fracture-separation of distal femoral physis (see Figs. 6–21 through 6–23).
b. Bicondylar fracture (see Fig. 6–24).
c. Unicondylar fracture (see Fig. 6–25).

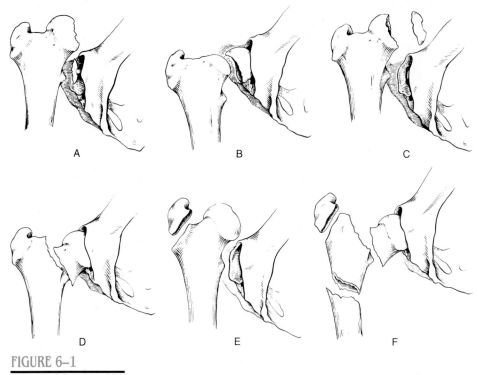

FIGURE 6–1

Fractures of the proximal femur. (A) Avulsion fracture and dislocation of the femoral head. (B) Fracture-separation of the proximal femoral physis. (C) Fracture and dislocation of the femoral head. (D) Fracture of the femoral neck. (E) Fracture-separation of the trochanter major physis with coxofemoral luxation. (F) Subtrochanteric shaft fracture of the femur with fractures of the trochanter major and femoral neck.

Proximal Femoral Fractures

AVULSION FRACTURE OF THE FEMORAL HEAD

With this fracture, a small portion of the femoral head remains attached to the round ligament, and the femoral head is dislocated in the craniodorsal position (Fig. 6–2A). The fracture segment remaining attached to the round ligament varies in size and is usually visible on a radiograph.

Treatment

Treatment varies with the individual case. Presented here are five suggestions of courses that may be followed.

REPLACEMENT OF THE DISLOCATED FEMORAL HEAD BY CLOSED REDUCTION ■ A single sling is applied for approximately 2 weeks, and activity is restricted for an additional 2 to 4 weeks. Success of this procedure depends on perfect reduction at the fracture site and maintenance of the reduction until the fracture segments have healed. Both of these conditions must be met if this procedure is to be successful, but this is difficult to accomplish.

SURGICAL REMOVAL OF THE AVULSED PIECE OF BONE AND REPLACEMENT OF THE DISLOCATED FEMORAL HEAD ■ The avulsed segment is removed through an open approach to expose the hip joint. The femoral head is replaced; following closure, the leg is immobilized for approximately 7 to 14 days (e.g., by means of a single sling). If the removed avulsed segment is too large, the remaining portion of the femoral head may not remain stable in the acetabulum, and dislocation will occur.

OPEN REDUCTION AND FIXATION OF THE FRACTURE SEGMENTS[1, 2, 4] ■ A dorsal open approach by cutting the tip of the trochanter major is used to expose the hip joint (see Fig. 5–9).[2, 5] A small threaded pin, starting in the center of the fracture surface of the femoral head, is passed retrograde through the head and neck, emerging at the base of the trochanter major (Fig. 6–2B). The pin is inserted until it is flush with the fracture surface, and the chuck is attached on the opposite end at a distance from the bone corresponding to the thickness of the avulsed

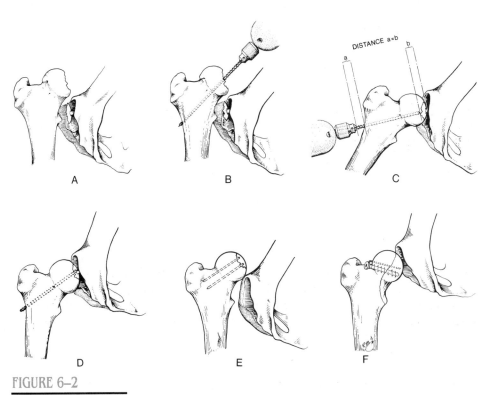

FIGURE 6–2

Fixation of an avulsion fracture of the femoral head. *(A)* Avulsion fracture with dislocation of the femoral head. *(B)* A small double-pointed thread pin is inserted in the center of the fracture surface and passed retrograde through the head and neck, emerging at the base of the trochanter major. *(C)* A pin chuck is attached at a distance from the bone (a) corresponding to thickness of avulsed segment (b); fracture segments are reduced and compression is applied during insertion of the pin. *(D)* About ⅛" of the pin is left protruding so that removal is possible. *(E)* Alternate method is to cut the round ligament, reduce the fracture, and stabilize by inserting two or more countersunk Kirschner wires. *(F)* Occasionally, a portion of the femoral head and neck is fractured off in an oblique fashion. If the fragment is large enough, it may be fixed using a small screw and Kirschner wire.

fragment (Fig. 6–2C). The fracture is held in reduction and compressed during insertion of the threaded pin. The pin is then cut off about ⅛″ beyond the bone (Fig. 6–2D). If the fracture segment is large enough, two pins are inserted. Following closure, the leg is immobilized in a nonweightbearing position (e.g., by means of a single sling for about 10 to 14 days). Exercise is restricted until healing is complete.

Another method of fixation worth consideration is to cut the round ligament, reduce the fracture fragments, and stabilize by use of two or more small countersunk Kirschner wires (Fig. 6–2E). In some cases, the ventral portion of the head and neck is fractured obliquely and may be reduced and fixed in place using a small screw and Kirschner wire (Fig. 6–2F).[4]

TOTAL HIP REPLACEMENT ■ When the femoral head cannot be reconstructed and saved, total hip replacement should be considered as an option.

EXCISION OF THE FEMORAL HEAD AND NECK ■ This procedure is usually considered a last resort because the intact joint should be maintained if possible. (See Chapter 20.)

FRACTURE OF THE PROXIMAL FEMORAL EPIPHYSIS

The condition is limited to young animals in which the physis is still present. It usually occurs between the ages of 4 and 11 months. In most cases, it is primarily a separation at the epiphyseal line (Salter-Harris I or II); however, minor fractures may also be present (see Figure 6–3A). The joint capsule can be attached to the epiphysis, partially detached, or completely stripped off, which undoubtedly affects healing. Fortunately in most cases there is some attachment.

If reduction and fixation are to be done, they should be performed as soon as possible—preferably within the first 24 hours—to avoid the danger of thrombosis occurring in the kinked capsular vessels at the junction of the femoral head and neck. The femoral neck also undergoes demineralization quite rapidly, and this change is usually evident on the radiograph within 7 to 10 days. The percentage of success decreases with each day's delay. A good healing response is possible for patients treated within 4 days. Success has been achieved in patients treated within 10 days; however, after this period of time, rigid fixation is difficult to obtain because of demineralization of the femoral neck.

Treatment

The primary goal of treatment is to save the hip joint. The craniolateral (see Fig. 20–11) or dorsal open approach may be used. The authors prefer the former because it affords better visualization of the involved area.[1, 2, 5, 6]

KIRSCHNER WIRE OR PIN FIXATION ■ Figure 6–3 shows the surgical procedure for fixation of a proximal femoral epiphyseal fracture.[1, 2, 14] The exposure of the area should be conservative to minimize destruction of blood supply.

Reduction of the fracture is best accomplished by grasping the trochanter major with vulsellum forceps and moving the femur distally and medially

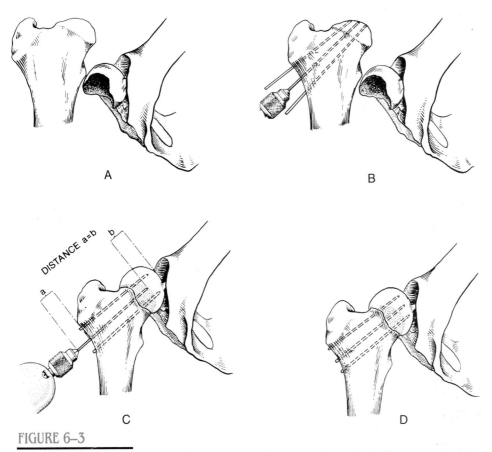

FIGURE 6–3

Normograde fixation of a proximal femoral physeal fracture with multiple Kirschner wires. *(A)* Physeal fracture. *(B)* Two to four Kirschner wires are driven from the base of the trochanter major up through the femoral neck to the fracture surface. *(C)* After reduction, a pin chuck is set at a distance from the bone corresponding to the thickness of the epiphysis; pins are driven into the epiphysis. *(D)* All pins are deeply seated into the epiphysis but do not penetrate the articular cartilage.

into position (see Fig. 1–9*A*, *B*). Occasionally, the epiphyseal end may be rotated in relation to the neck and may cause some difficulty in reduction. Medial pressure on the trochanter while flexing and extending the hip joint will usually cause the epiphysis to derotate and lock into the femoral neck in the reduced position. Applying medial pressure will maintain reduction while fixation is applied.

Note: A review of the contour of the epiphysis and epiphyseal line is most helpful prior to undertaking anatomical reduction.

Two to four small smooth pins are inserted for immobilization. Pin size corresponds with the size of bone and may range from a 0.035″ Kirschner wire to a 1/16″ Steinmann pin. The pins may be inserted in antegrade (Fig. 6–3) or retrograde (Fig. 6–4) fashion. The former is preferred by the author in most cases. The pins may be inserted parallel or in a converging-diverging fashion. The main objective is to have them well distributed at the fracture surface.

The pin chuck is set on the pin so that the distance from the chuck to the

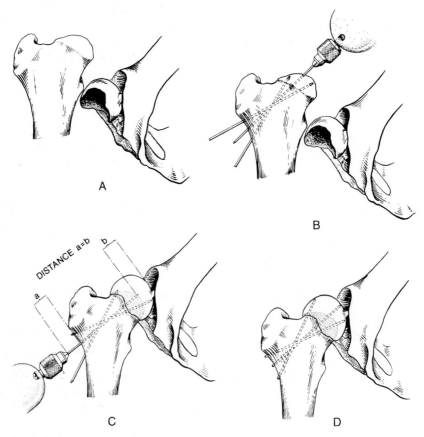

FIGURE 6–4

Retrograde fixation of a proximal femoral physeal fracture with multiple Kirschner wires. *(A)* Physeal fracture of the proximal femur. *(B)* Two to four double-pointed Kirschner wires are driven retrograde from the fracture to exit distal to the trochanter major on the lateral femoral surface. *(C)* After reduction, a pin chuck is set at a distance from the bone corresponding to the thickness of the epiphysis; pins are driven into the epiphysis. *(D)* All pins are deeply seated in the epiphysis but do not penetrate the articular cartilage.

lateral femoral cortex corresponds with the thickness of the epiphysis (Figs. 6–3C; 6–4C). With the fracture compressed in the reduced position, the pins are inserted into the epiphysis one at a time (Figs. 6–3C, D; 6–4C, D). The pins should not penetrate the articular cartilage. Pin penetration can be checked by careful movement of the femoral head in the acetabulum after each pin is inserted and by palpation of the femoral head using a small curved hemostat. The various tissues, starting with the joint capsule, are closed in layers.

Note: At the completion of surgery, radiographs should be taken from two ventrodorsal views; one view should show the legs flexed at the hip (frog-leg), and the second should show the rear legs extended. Follow-up radiographs should be taken at about 6 weeks. At this time, they should reveal healing or any complications.

Aftercare ■ A single sling is applied to the leg for about 7 to 10 days. Exercise should be limited for the next 5 weeks. The pins are usually left in place unless indicated otherwise.

Prognosis of this procedure depends on early accomplishment of surgery, preservation of blood supply in the operative procedure, accurate reduction at the fracture site, rigid uninterrupted fixation, and restriction of early weight bearing. If the above can be complied with, the prognoses for healing and return of function are favorable.

LAG SCREW FIXATION ■ In those animals approximately 7 months of age or older, the epiphysis may be reattached by use of lag screw fixation (Fig. 6–5).

The pin techniques described in Figures 6–3 and 6–4 are preferable to use of a lag screw in most cases and particularly in younger animals because they are less apt to bring about premature closure of the physeal plate and resultant femoral neck shortening.

ALTERNATE PROCEDURES ■ In lieu of these operative procedures or in the presence of unfavorable complications, excision of the femoral head and neck with false joint formation or total hip replacement may be recommended.

FRACTURE OF THE FEMORAL NECK

In this kind of fracture, the fracture line varies and is usually simple; however, it may be multiple in nature. Various degrees of embarrassment to the blood supply of the head and neck may occur in connection with the original injury.[7–14, 23]

Studies indicate that the incidence of unfavorable complications can be markedly reduced by (1) early surgery, (2) accurate reduction with compression at the fracture site, (3) rigid uninterrupted fixation, and (4) careful supervision of the postoperative care. In general, if these points can be complied with, the prognosis is favorable.

An impacted fracture with no displacement may heal with external immobilization and restricted exercise. The safer and preferred procedure is to apply fixation using a bone screw or threaded pin without further disturbing the position. Fractures showing various degrees of displacement respond best to an open approach with reduction and fixation. Excision of the femoral head and neck or replacement by a prosthesis is usually considered a second choice in most fresh fractures of the femoral neck.

Note: Repair of a fractured femoral neck or of a fracture of the proximal femoral epiphysis in a young growing animal, which results in shortening of the femoral neck and instability of the hip joint, may give rise to alterations of the hip joint characteristic of hip dysplasia.

FIGURE 6–5

Lag screw fixation. Care must be taken in tightening the screw because the threads in the epiphyseal end are in cancellous bone.

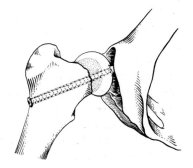

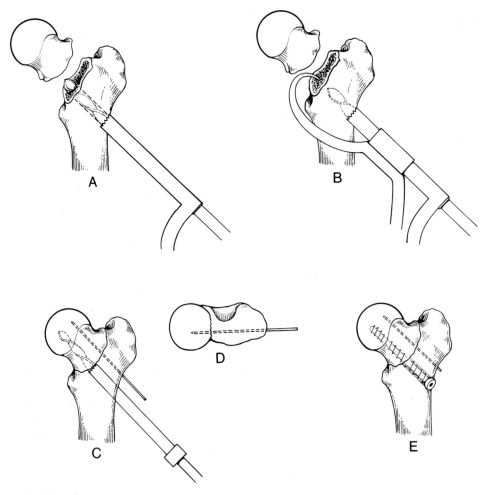

FIGURE 6–6

When a cortex screw is used, the gliding hole is drilled up through the femoral neck before reduction so that the hole is properly placed. *(A)* Drilling the hole using regular drill guide. *(B)* Drilling the hole using a pointed drill guide. This is advantageous in placing the hole properly. *(C, D)* The fracture is next reduced, and small Kirschner wire is inserted to aid in stabilizing the fragments. The appropriate drill sleeve is inserted into the femoral gliding hole. This functions as a guide for drilling the appropriate size hole in the femoral head. *(E)* After the hole is measured and tapped (unless a self-tapping screw is used), the appropriate size and length of screw is inserted. This serves as a lag screw in compressing the fragments.[2, 14] A cancellous screw could be used to accomplish the same objective if all of the threads are on the far side of the fracture line.

Operative Treatment Using a Bone Screw

A craniolateral approach (see Fig. 20–11) is normally used because it gives the best visualization of the fracture area.[2, 5, 6] A dorsal approach may be used, but this is usually a second choice because in most cases there is more destruction of the blood supply to the head and neck and poorer visualization of the fracture line.

After making the approach, temporary reduction is usually carried out to see if reduction and fixation are feasible. This usually can be accomplished by grasping the trochanter major with vulsellum forceps and manually maneuvering the fracture segments back into position (see Fig. 1–9A, B).

When a cortical lag screw is used for fixation, the gliding hole is first drilled through the femoral neck (Fig. 6–6A, B). With the fracture segments compressed and reduced, one or more Kirschner wires are inserted through the trochanter, femoral neck, and head. For maximum holding power, the Kirschner wire should traverse the bridge of bone between the trochanter major and femoral head and not the trochanteric fossa (Fig. 6–6C, D). The pin is positioned proximally so that it does not interfere with insertion of the bone screw. It will assist in maintaining reduction and will help keep the femoral head from turning during the drilling, tapping, and insertion of the bone screw. Maintenance of reduction is assisted by applying pressure at the fracture site using vulsellum forceps attached to the trochanter major.

An appropriate size drill sleeve is next inserted through the glide hole; this serves as a guide for drilling the appropriate size hole in the femoral head. Ideally, the depth of the hole should be to the subchondral bone; this depth can be estimated by visualizing and measuring the head and neck segment. The depth of the hole is measured, tapped, and the appropriate size cortical (lag) screw is inserted (Fig. 6–6E). The Kirschner wire is usually left in place. Following closure of the tissue layers, the leg is usually placed in a single sling (Ehmer) for 7 to 10 days.

Note: A common mistake is to insert the bone screw in a more or less transverse fashion instead of in the oblique upward position through the femoral neck. The former is more apt to work loose or fracture prior to clinical union.

At the completion of surgery, radiographs should be taken from two ventrodorsal views; one view should show the legs flexed at the hips, and another should show the rear legs extended. Follow-up radiographs should be taken at about 6 weeks.

Operative Treatment Using Kirschner Wires

An alternate method is to insert three or more Kirschner wires for fixation (Fig. 6–7). This method has the disadvantage of no compression at the fracture site.[2, 14] It is usually reserved for cats and small dogs.

Aftercare ■ The single sling is maintained in position for approximately 7 to 10 days. Exercise is restricted for the next month or until the stage of clinical union is reached as evaluated radiographically. The bone screw and pin are not usually removed.

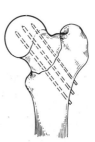

FIGURE 6–7

Fixation of a femoral neck fracture using Kirschner wires. This method is used primarily for small dogs and cats.

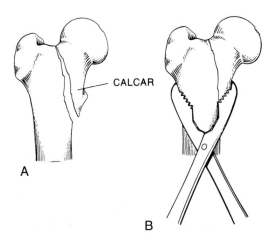

FIGURE 6–8

(A) Oblique fractures of the femoral neck require care (B) to reduce and compress the calcar region prior to bone screw fixation.

Long Oblique Fractures of the Femoral Neck

Special attention must be paid to reduction on long oblique fractures because there may not be good contact at the distal part. Elevation of a portion of the vastus lateralis off the fractured neck allows visualization of the reduction. Application of reduction forceps during fixation in the distal calcar area is essential in most cases of this type (Fig. 6–8).

FRACTURE OF THE TROCHANTER MAJOR WITH OR WITHOUT DISLOCATION OF THE FEMORAL HEAD

In most cases, this is a physeal separation accompanied by dislocation of the femoral head (Fig. 6–9A).[1, 2] With the animal under anesthesia, a closed reduction of the femoral head is usually attempted first. If this can be accomplished and the reduction feels stable, fixation of the fracture is next in order. If the dislocation cannot be reduced or is unstable on reduction, the open approach should include the coxofemoral joint.

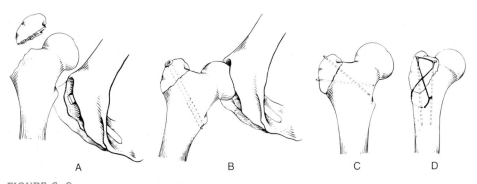

FIGURE 6–9

(A) Fracture of the trochanter major with dislocation of the femoral head. (B) Fixation of the trochanter major with a cancellous bone screw. (C) Fixation by two small pins. (D) Fixation by tension band wire; this is usually the method of choice.

The following steps are observed:

1. Make a longitudinal skin incision over the lateral surface of the proximal femur, and extend it toward the midline on the back (see Fig. 5–9A).

2. Incise the fascia separating the biceps femoris muscle and fascia lata.

3. If there is no indication to open up the coxofemoral joint, proceed with fixation of the trochanter major (Fig. 6–9B–D).

4. When survey and repair of the coxofemoral joint capsule are indicated, proceed with the approach to the hip joint.

5. Some of the origin of the vastus lateralis muscle is usually still attached to the lateral surface of the fractured trochanter major. Sever this origin with a tag end remaining attached to the trochanter major. (This will be sutured on closure.)

6. After replacing the femoral head, obtain stability by closing the joint capsule. Abduction of the leg allows for easier and tighter closure of the joint capsule.

7. Apply fixation of the trochanter major (Fig. 6–9B–D).

8. Following closure, place the leg in a single sling for 5 to 7 days, and limit exercise during the healing period.

Figure 6–9 shows a fracture-separation of the trochanter major with dislocation of the femoral head.

Fixation with a cancellous bone screw is usually used only for animals approximately 4½ months of age or older (Fig. 6–9B). The trochanter major may be fixed by using two small pins (Fig. 6–9C). Fixation by use of a tension band wire is usually the procedure of choice, particularly in larger dogs (Fig. 6–9D). In our experience, this procedure has not significantly altered anatomical growth of the femur (length or shape) in dogs over 4½ months of age.

FRACTURES OF THE FEMORAL NECK, TROCHANTER MAJOR, AND FEMORAL SHAFT

For these fractures,[1, 2, 14] reduction is accomplished by performing an open approach. The exposure of choice is usually a combination of the craniolateral approach to the hip joint and the lateral approach to the femur.[14] Fixation can best be accomplished using a bone plate and bone screws. Fractures of this type in some of the larger dogs are amenable to the use of a hook plate.[39]

In Figure 6–10, a craniolateral approach to the hip joint and a lateral approach to the femur are performed to expose the fracture site. The approach procedure is modified to fit the individual fracture. Reduction is usually accomplished by starting at the proximal end and working toward the distal end. Bone-holding forceps, Kirschner wires, lag screws, and cerclage wire help hold the fragments in the reduced position.

The bone plate is contoured. An easy and helpful procedure is to pre-bend the plate to the curvature of the lateral surface of the opposite femur, as

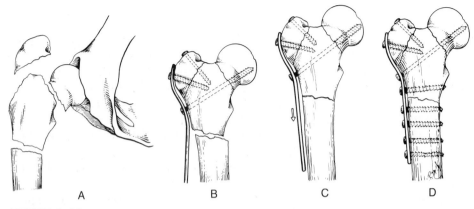

A   B   C   D

FIGURE 6–10

Fixation of fractures of the femoral neck, trochanter major, and femoral shaft. *(A)* Fracture as seen in a craniocaudal radiograph. *(B)* The plate is contoured, and a long lag screw is placed in the femoral neck. The trochanter major is reduced and fixed. *(C)* The subtrochanteric fracture is reduced. A tension device or dynamic compression plate (DCP) is used to obtain compression. *(D)* Fixation plate in place.

shown from a craniocaudal view on the radiograph. The use of a compression plate (DCP) has the added advantage of allowing oblique insertion of the bone screw proximally into the femoral neck and head along with affording compression of the various fracture segments.

Usually, the first bone screw is inserted through the base of the trochanter major and neck, and into the femoral head. The trochanter major is then reduced and fixed in position (Fig. 6–10A, B). The remaining bone screws are inserted as indicated. In some cases, additional bone screws that produce a lag effect may be used advantageously to assist in compressing at the fracture site (Fig. 6–10C, D).

Aftercare ■ Following closure, a single sling to keep the leg off weight bearing may be indicated for 3 to 7 days. Exercise is restricted for 4 to 6 weeks.

COMPLICATIONS IN FRACTURES OF THE FEMORAL HEAD AND NECK

Most complications in femoral head and neck fractures are caused by:

1. Embarrassment of the blood supply to the femoral head and neck that occurs at the time of the initial injury or during the surgical procedure.
2. Poor bone reduction.
3. Inadequate fixation.
4. Premature weight bearing.

The most frequently occurring complications are:

1. Delayed union or nonunion.
2. Avascular necrosis.
3. Secondary osteoarthritis.
4. Cessation of neck growth in young animals as a result of premature closure of the physis, leading to subluxation of the hip.

Radiographic evidence of a complication may show up as a loss of density in the femoral neck or along the fracture line in contrast to the surrounding bony tissue. Such a sign points toward disturbance in blood supply, demineralization, and possible movement at the fracture site. In long-standing cases, a mottled appearance of the femoral head indicates replacement of some areas of necrotic bone by new bone. In some instances, the femoral neck may disappear partially or completely in 3 to 6 weeks.

In most cases, clinical and radiographic evidence of complications is evident within 6 weeks. However, about 6 months should elapse before the clinician attempts to determine the ultimate fate of the femoral head and neck, even in those patients that appear to be healing initially.

Most cases of coxofemoral dislocation, physeal separation, or femoral neck fracture that made a good recovery show some temporary demineralization and slight narrowing of the femoral neck.

If reduction and fixation are satisfactory, restricted activity and more healing time are indicated. In some cases, a more rigid internal fixation with restriction of activity is indicated. Those beyond salvaging with a good hip joint are subjects for excision arthroplasty of the femoral head and neck or for total hip replacement.

This topic is addressed in Chapter 20.

Fractures of the Femoral Shaft

These fractures are usually the result of direct trauma and are accompanied by various degrees of soft tissue damage and hematoma.[1, 2, 14-31] The fracture pattern may be quite variable: transverse, oblique, spiral, multiple, comminuted, or, occasionally, green-stick in the young animal. If reduction is to be maintained until clinical union, external fixation is rarely adequate. The internal methods of fixation include use of:

1. Intramedullary pin alone.
2. Intramedullary pin plus auxiliary fixation.
3. Unilateral external fixator with an intramedullary pin and other auxiliary fixation as indicated.
4. Plate with or without lag screws or cerclage wires.

Femoral fractures can be treated successfully with various methods of fixation. The multiple and very unstable fractures, in general, respond best to bone plate and screw fixation. In large dogs, almost all femoral shaft fractures make a better functional response and are accompanied by fewer complications with bone plate and screw fixation.

The various methods of fixation as they apply to femoral fractures are presented as suggested methods of treatment. Some of the stable and uncom-

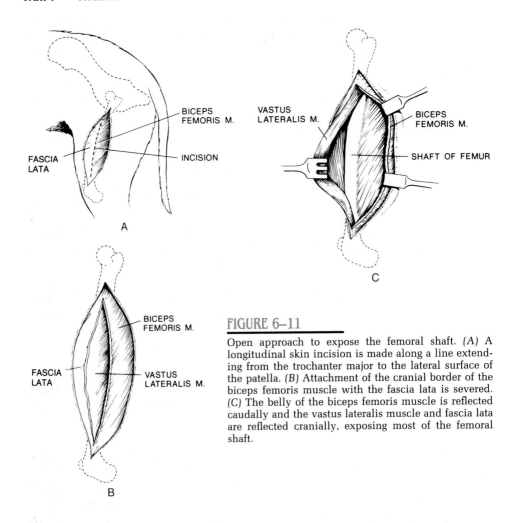

FIGURE 6–11

Open approach to expose the femoral shaft. *(A)* A longitudinal skin incision is made along a line extending from the trochanter major to the lateral surface of the patella. *(B)* Attachment of the cranial border of the biceps femoris muscle with the fascia lata is severed. *(C)* The belly of the biceps femoris muscle is reflected caudally and the vastus lateralis muscle and fascia lata are reflected cranially, exposing most of the femoral shaft.

plicated fractures can be treated by closed methods; however, in most femoral fractures, an open approach is advantageous.

In mid to proximal femoral fractures, the proximal fragment rotates caudally, allowing excessive anteversion of the femoral head. This must be remembered when applying fixation, especially in comminuted fractures (see Fig. 6–18A).

OPEN APPROACH

With few exceptions, a lateral approach (see Fig. 20–11) is used to expose the femoral shaft for reduction and internal fixation (Fig. 6–11).[1, 5]

FIXATION

Modified Thomas Splint

For a period of about 20 years, starting in the early 1930s, the modified Thomas splint[2, 15, 16] was the most commonly used method of immobilizing femoral fractures. With the advent of internal fixation (intramedullary pins, external fixator, and bone plate), this splint has rapidly faded from common usage as the sole method of immobilizing femoral fractures. There are better methods available and, in keeping with good practice procedures, these should be used.

When used as the sole method of fixation, the modified Thomas splint is usually confined to green-stick fractures, fissure fractures, and fractures with minimal displacement in the very young patient. One must keep in mind that the ring, when properly applied, lies at the proximal third of the femur and may act as a fulcrum at the fracture site resulting in more harm than good.

The leg may be attached to the modified Thomas splint with the joints in various angles to exert the best mechanical advantage on the fracture. In most cases, however, the leg is splinted in the angulation of the normal standing position (see Fig. 14–6). Placing the leg in full extension over a period of time may lead to a decrease in range of joint movement in the stifle and to some loss of function or total dysfunction if fibrous ankylosis occurs in the hyper-extended position.

The splint must be frequently checked for pressure points, readjusted, and repaired during the healing period. It must be protected against moisture, both inside and out. Exercise must be restricted to help protect the splint from becoming loose or damaged.

Intramedullary Pinning

There are numerous types of intramedullary pins available with various types of points.[1, 2, 20] The round pins (Steinmann, Kirschner drill wire) are by far the most commonly used.

STEINMANN PIN ■ When the Steinmann pin is used as the sole method of fixation, it should be reserved primarily for stable fractures. It may be used for unstable fractures only with supplemental fixation such as an external fixator, cerclage wire, stacking pins, lag screws, and so forth. Pin diameter should approximate the size of the marrow cavity. This is possible in the cat and toy dog breeds because the femur is straight (Fig. 6–12F); however, it is not quite applicable in most dogs because of the cranial bowing of the femur (Fig. 6–12C, D). In the dog, the pin should occupy about 50 to 70 percent of the marrow cavity diameter.

The pin may be inserted from the proximal end (normograde) by entering at the trochanteric fossa (Fig. 6–12A) or by passing it retrograde proximally through the medullary canal (Fig. 6–12B). Normograde pin insertion is preferred because it has the advantage of sliding close to the medial surface of the trochanter major (thus further away from the femoral head and sciatic nerve), trapping less soft tissue. It also facilitates cutting the pin shorter, which minimizes seroma formation and decreases patient discomfort (Fig. 6–12Ab). Before and during the insertion process, the proximal femur is held in the angulation and rotation of the normal standing position. If the retrograde technique is used, care should be taken to have the proximal fracture fragment adducted and in the angulation and rotation of the normal standing position. On passing the pin up through the proximal segment, it is directed along the lateral surface of the marrow cavity (Fig. 6–12Ba). All of these precautions help keep emergence of the pin away from the femoral head and sciatic nerve.

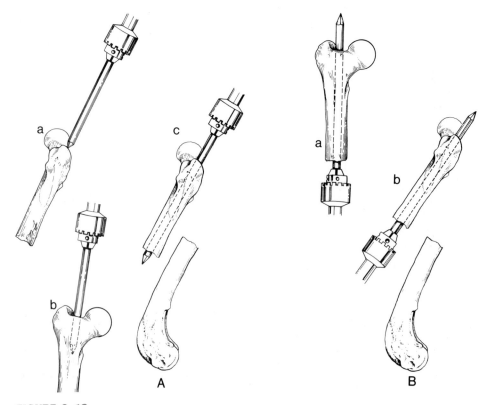

FIGURE 6–12

Intramedullary pinning technique using Steinmann pin. Normograde technique with the proximal femur in the angulation posture and rotation of the normal standing posture *(A a, b, c)*. The pin is inserted through the skin and underlying soft tissue at the tip of the trochanter major. The pin slides along the medial surface of the trochanter major into the trochanteric fossa, through the cortical bone, and down the medullary cavity. The pin is held in axial alignment, and the bone fragment is held with bone-holding forceps to prevent rotation during pin insertion. Retrograde technique *(B a, b)*. The distal end of the proximal bone fragment is grasped with bone-holding forceps, and the pin is inserted up the medullary canal, making an effort to direct it along the lateral surface of the marrow cavity. The proximal bone fragment is adducted and held in the rotation and angulation of the normal standing position.

As the pin enters the distal segment, it is best to angle the segments slightly caudally. This allows for deeper insertion of the pin in the cancellous bone of the distal metaphysis and for more rigid fixation (Fig. 6–12E).

After the pin is inserted to the full depth with the point of the pin near, but not penetrating, the subchondral bone, it is cut as short as possible or it may be retracted ¼", cut off, then driven back into position by means of a countersink and mallet. A long pin in the gluteal area can lead to discomfort and seroma formation as well as to increasing the possibility of sciatic nerve entrapment by the tissue reaction incited by the pin.

Depth of insertion is best checked by taking a radiograph prior to cutting the pin. In practice, the incision may be closed, the radiograph taken, and adjustments made prior to cutting the pin.

Horizontal shearing and rotary instability are the most common complications when a round pin is used. Additional supplemental fixation should

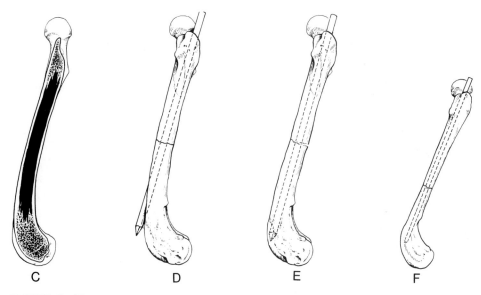

C   D   E   F

FIGURE 6–12

Continued (C) Sagittal section through a canine femur showing the cortical bone, cancellous bone, and marrow cavity. *(D)* The canine femur has some cranial curvature, and the intramedullary pin cannot be inserted to a sufficient depth with the fracture reduced in perfect apposition. *(E)* With the fracture segments bent caudally at the fracture site, the intramedullary pin can be passed along the caudal cortex into cancellous bone at the distal end. This anchorage in cancellous bone markedly improves stability. *(F)* Anatomical reduction of a cat femur and insertion of a straight Steinmann pin for fixation. The diaphysis of a cat femur is straight.

be added to guard against instability and movement at the fracture site. Supplemental fixation is described later in this chapter.

Note: Rarely does the sciatic nerve become irritated or trapped over the top of the cut-off intramedullary pin during the convalescent period if the precautions stated are observed. If this occurs, however, there is an acute onset of extreme pain, and the proprioceptive reflex of the foot is diminished or lost. This is an emergency, and immediate surgical intervention is in order. After careful dissection down to the area, the pin is either cut shorter or removed. Injury to the sciatic nerve may be temporary or permanent.

If the pin has been driven too far distally and penetrates the stifle joint, simple pin retraction is not appropriate because it often migrates through the pin tract and re-enters the joint. The pin should be retracted to the fracture site, the fracture reangulated, and the pin driven distally into new or unpenetrated trabecular bone.

Postoperative Management ■ Activity must be restricted until the stage of clinical union is reached. Union should be checked radiographically before removal of the pin. After clinical union is achieved, the pin is removed by incising over its top and retracting it by pulling with quarter turns back and forth. This is usually done under a short-acting anesthetic, but in some cases, it may be removed under local anesthesia. Aseptic procedures are used for removal of the pin.

KÜNTSCHER NAIL ■ This nail has the advantage of affording rigid stability to both bending and torsion or rotation; however, insertion requires attention to the details in its use. Frequent complications include (1) the nail may jam in the medullary canal or split the bone, (2) longitudinal fracture lines already present may be opened up, or (3) if too small in diameter, it may not give sufficient stability. The Küntscher nail is rarely used in the United States for small animals because of aforementioned complications and the availability of other fixation methods.

Intramedullary Pin and External Fixator

The external fixator is added to help increase stability by reducing movement and rotation at the fracture site and helping to maintain length.[1, 2, 24, 25] The unilateral external fixator, 1/1 pins (Fig. 6–13C), is used primarily for transverse and short oblique fractures. The unilateral external fixator, 2/2 pins (Fig. 6–13D), is used on comminuted fractures.

TECHNIQUE ■ The procedure for inserting the intramedullary pin (Fig. 6–13A, B) is the same as described earlier. In addition, a fixation pin of appropriate diameter for the external fixator clamps is inserted in the proximal and distal fragments. Following are the steps to use:

1. Start the pin insertion with the soft tissue in its normal position. The pin should pierce intact skin and preferably not enter on the incision line.

2. Insert the pins near the proximal and distal ends to obtain the best mechanical advantage (Fig. 6–13B, C).

3. Insert slightly off center to miss the intramedullary pin.

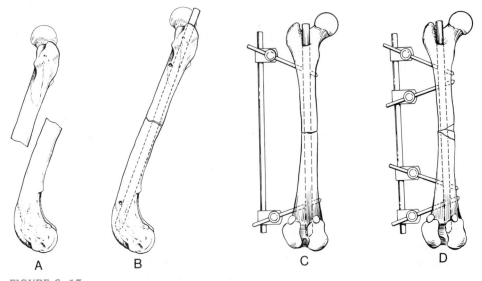

A   B   C   D

FIGURE 6–13

Insertion of an intramedullary pin and external fixator, 1/1 pins for fixation. (A) Transverse fracture of the femur. Fractures of this type have a tendency to rotate. (B) Self-locking bone-holding forceps holds fracture reduced during insertion of the Steinmann pin into the distal segment. Holding both fracture segments so that they do not rotate during the insertion process makes for a tighter fitting pin. The two circles show approximate location of pins. (C) Caudocranial view of reduced and fixed fracture. (D) Comminuted fracture (caudocranial view) immobilized by use of an intramedullary pin and external fixator, 2/2 pins. Four pins are inserted for added stability.

4. Place the fixation pins at approximately a 70° angle to the long axis of the bone, and penetrate both cortices and connect the pins with single clamps and a connecting bar (Fig. 6–13C).

5. When 2/2 pins are used (Fig. 6–13D), four single clamps are assembled on the connecting bar, and the remaining third and fourth pins are inserted through the clamps into the bone.

The wound may be closed before or after application of the external fixator. Closure after application has the advantage of enabling visualization of the fracture site until all fixation is in place. In fractures in large dogs and in comminuted fractures, the added stability gained by use of an external fixator, 2/2 pins (Fig. 6–13D), is essential.

Postoperative Management ■ Activity should be restricted during the healing period. The external fixator usually can be removed after a good primary callus has formed; this takes about 4 to 6 weeks. The intramedullary pin is removed when the fracture has reached the stage of clinical union.

Intramedullary Pin and Cerclage Wire or Lag Screw Supplemental Fixation[1, 2, 14, 26]

Rigid uninterrupted fixation is fundamental in treating all fractures. The trend in treatment is to splint the bone internally to facilitate early restoration of function.

CASE 1 ■ A long oblique fracture of the femur is shown in Figure 6–14A. Following a lateral open approach, the intramedullary pin is inserted in the proximal segment, the fracture is reduced and maintained by using self-retaining bone forceps, and the pin is then inserted into the distal segment (Fig. 6–14B). In long oblique fractures, cerclage wires are inserted at about 1-cm intervals (Fig. 6–14C). After clinical union, the intramedullary pin is removed, and the cerclage wires are left in place.

CASE 2 ■ Figure 6–15A presents another instance of a long oblique femoral fracture. After reduction and insertion of the intramedullary pin, one or more lag screws may be inserted to bring about interfragmentary compression (Fig. 6–15B, C). In this case, an intramedullary pin slightly smaller in diameter was used. The lag screws were inserted off center to avoid the intramedullary pin. The procedure is more applicable to medium- and large-size dogs. After clinical union, the intramedullary pin is removed, and the lag screws are left in place.

CASE 3 ■ In the multiple fracture of the femur shown in Figure 6–16, rigid fixation was accomplished by use of an intramedullary pin, three cerclage wires, and an external fixator, 2/2 pins. The splint was removed after approximately 1 month, the intramedullary pin was removed at time of clinical union, and the cerclage wires were left in place. In fractures of this type, bone plate fixation may be more appropriate, particularly in medium- and large-size dogs.

External Fixator

One is restricted to use of the unilateral configuration on the femur. In general, the splint is well tolerated by the patient.[1, 2, 24, 25, 27] Because the splint is

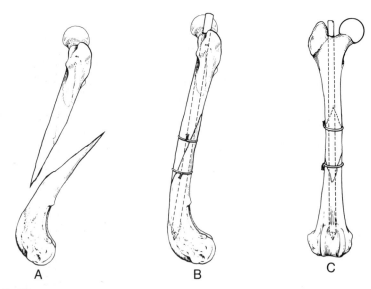

A   B   C

FIGURE 6–14

(A) Long oblique fracture of the femur. *(B)* Following a lateral open approach, an intramedullary pin is inserted into the proximal segment. The fracture is reduced and maintained by self-retaining bone forceps; the pin is inserted into the distal segment. *(C)* In long oblique fractures, cerclage wires are inserted at 1- to 2-cm intervals; after clinical union, the intramedullary pin is removed and cerclage wires are left in place. If there is any doubt in regard to stability after applying the above, an external fixator may be added at the time of surgery.

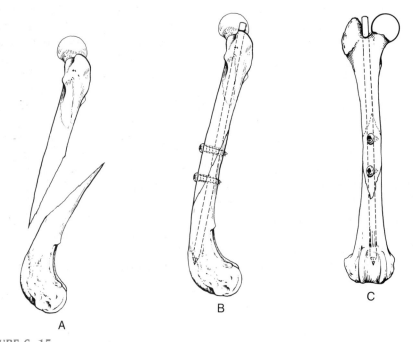

B   C   A

FIGURE 6–15

(A) Long oblique fracture of the femur. *(B)* After reduction and insertion of an intramedullary pin, lag screws may be inserted to bring about interfragmentary compression. *(C)* Lag screws may be inserted off center to avoid the intramedullary pin. After clinical union, intramedullary pin is removed and lag screws are left in place.

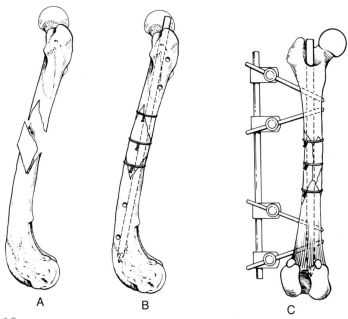

A   B   C

FIGURE 6–16

(A) Multiple fracture of the femur. (B, C) Rigid fixation by use of an intramedullary pin, three cerclage wires, and an external fixator.

inserted on the lateral surface of the femur and penetrates large muscles, however, it is vulnerable to trauma and premature loosening. This may occur in up to 50 percent of the cases.[40] The loosening can be partially overcome by inserting 3/3 or 4/4 pins. This, too, has a drawback because the pins are inserted through both the biceps femoris muscle (a flexor) and the vastus lateralis muscle (an extensor). This temporarily limits the range of stifle joint movement, which with the formation of adhesions may become a permanent limitation.

When the external fixator is applied on femoral fractures as the sole method of fixation, it is used primarily on small breeds of young dogs and cats. These in general heal quite rapidly. When used on other femoral fractures, it is combined with use of the intramedullary pin (Figs. 6–13D; 6–16).

The splint may be applied with the fracture site closed or open. The latter is preferable because the reduction can be visualized during the insertion procedure. If used in combination with an intramedullary pin, the external fixator can be removed when sufficient callus has been laid down to stabilize the area, which is usually after about 1 month, and the intramedullary pin is removed at the time of clinical union.

Bone Plate

A bone plate is adaptable to practically all types of shaft fractures and has the distinct advantage of providing uninterrupted rigid internal fixation. In most cases, it is the fixation of choice in large dogs.[14]

The plate is usually applied on the lateral surface and contoured to fit that surface. Usually, the curvature pattern for bending can be taken from a craniocaudal radiograph of the opposite femur, or the plate may be contoured at the time of reduction and application. A liberal exposure is necessary for application of the bone plate. Ordinarily, it is placed without stripping the periosteum.

At least two or preferably three or more bone screws (penetrating both cortices) should be placed in each of the proximal and distal bone segments. Whenever possible, the plate and screws should be inserted to develop compression at the fracture site. This has the distinct advantage of providing a more rigid fixation and making conditions more nearly optimal for healing.

CASE 1 ■ Figure 6–17 shows a femoral shaft fracture with a butterfly fragment. The butterfly segment was first reduced and then fixed in place using a lag screw for interfragmentary compression (Fig. 6–17B). The contoured bone plate was applied on the lateral surface of the femur (Fig. 6–17C, D). Use of a DCP plate has the advantage of adding axial compression.

CASE 2 ■ Figure 6–18 presents a multiple fracture of the femoral shaft with numerous fissure fractures. Reduction was accomplished by reducing the fracture segments one by one (Fig. 6–18B). Cerclage wires were used to immobilize the fragments and reconstruct the femur. The neutralization plate was then applied on top of the cerclage wires. Usually, the first screw to be inserted is the one going into the femoral neck and head. Next is the most distal screw; this aligns the plate with the femoral shaft. Screw holes in the plate directly overlying fracture lines are left empty.

CASE 3 ■ Figure 6–19 shows a four-segment, multiple femoral fracture. The fracture is first reduced to three segments by use of a lag screw, then to a two-

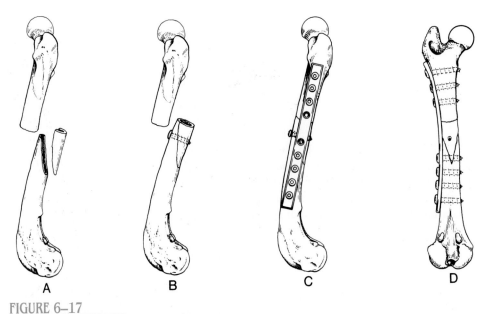

A   B   C   D

FIGURE 6–17

(A) Femoral shaft fracture with butterfly fragment. *(B)* Reduction of fracture and fixation in place using a lag screw for interfragmentary compression. *(C, D)* Contoured bone plate applied on lateral surface of the femur.

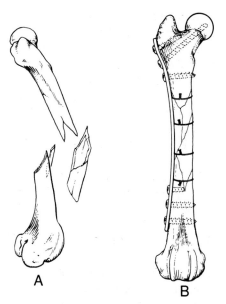

FIGURE 6–18

(A) Multiple fracture of the femoral shaft with numerous fissure fractures present. (B) Reduction of fracture segments, one by one. Cerclage wires immobilize fragments and reconstruct femur. Neutralization plate applied; screw holes in plate directly overlying fracture lines are left vacant.

segment and a one-segment fracture by the same procedure. In cases such as this, it is best to insert some of the lag screws through the neutralization plate. Whenever a screw crosses a fracture line, it should be inserted with a lag effect.

Interfragmentary compression is gained by use of lag screws, both through the bone alone and through the plate (Fig. 6–19B). The neutralization plate is applied to overcome rotary, bending, and compressive forces. In this case, placing the plate on the cranial surface appeared to be advantageous, although this is not standard procedure.

FIGURE 6–19

(A) Multiple (four-segment) fracture of the femur. (B) Fracture reduced; interfragmentary compression achieved by use of lag screws through the bone alone and through the plate. A neutralization plate is applied to overcome rotary, bending, and compressive forces. In this case, it was more advantageous to apply the plate on the cranial surface.

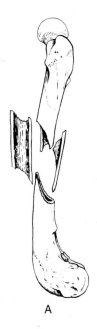
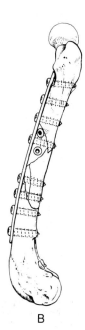

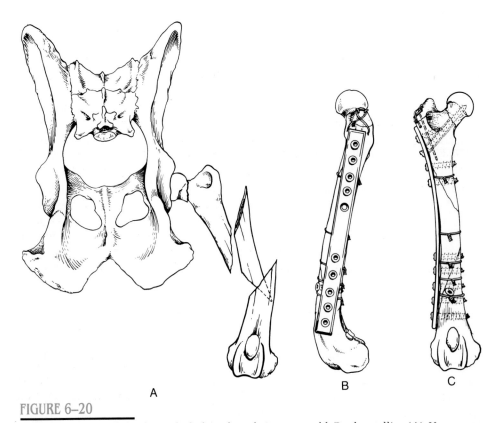

A   B   C

FIGURE 6–20

Multiple fracture of the femoral shaft and neck in 1-year-old Border collie. *(A)* Upon open approach, numerous fissures were noted in the various fracture segments. *(B, C)* The femoral shaft was first reconstructed and fixed together with one lag screw and four cerclage wires. A neutralization plate was applied with a 4.5-mm lag screw to immobilize the femoral neck fracture. The plate was removed at 7 months; shaft lag screw and cerclage wires were left in place.

CASE 4 ■ Figure 6–20 shows multiple fractures of femoral shaft and femoral neck in a 1-year-old Border collie. Upon open approach, numerous fissures were noted in the various fracture segments (Fig. 6–20A). The femoral shaft was first reconstructed and fixed together by using one lag screw and four cerclage wires (Fig. 6–20B). A neutralization plate was then applied with a 4.5-mm lag screw to immobilize the femoral neck fracture. The neutralization plate was removed at 7 months. The lag screw and cerclage wires were left in place.

Bone Screws

In immobilizing shaft fractures of the long bones, bone screws are rarely used as the sole method of fixation. They can be used advantageously for interfragmentary compression in oblique, spiral, and butterfly segments and in certain types of multiple fractures. If bone segments are large enough for bone screws to be used, then they are preferred to cerclage wire. When properly inserted, bone screws are superior for compression and rigid fixation.

Distal Femoral Fractures

SUPRACONDYLAR FRACTURE AND FRACTURE OF THE DISTAL FEMORAL EPIPHYSIS

Fractures involving the distal femoral epiphysis are relatively common, particularly in young animals, and are seen primarily between the ages of 4 and 11 months.[1, 2, 28–38] The distal segment is usually displaced caudally and accompanied by a sizable hematoma (Fig. 6–21A). The objectives of treatment should include (1) anatomical reduction or reduction with the distal segment placed slightly craniad, and (2) rigid uninterrupted fixation so that the animal is free to move the stifle joint during the healing period. Suggested methods of treatment include use of two small intramedullary pins, Rush pins, or pins inserted in a crossing pattern. In Salter II-type fractures in which a portion of the metaphysis is attached to the distal epiphysis, it may be advantageous to insert a screw to attach the metaphyseal portion. Supracondylar fractures are seen most frequently in the mature animal and require internal stabilization (e.g., intramedullary pin and external fixator [see Fig. 4–3] or bone plate).

Open Approach

The patient is placed in the dorsal recumbent position. A skin incision is made parallel to the lateral border of the patellar tendon and is extended proximally over the femoral shaft, as indicated, for exposure. The incision through the joint capsule is made along the lateral border of the patellar ligament and patella and is extended proximally through the fascia lata exposing the fracture site. At this stage, before proceeding it is advisable to check that reduction can be accomplished.

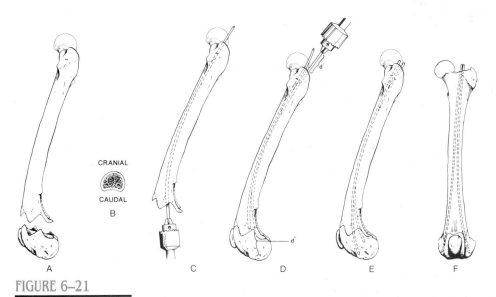

FIGURE 6–21

Intramedullary fixation of a distal femoral physeal fracture with two pins. *(A)* Salter-Harris Type I fracture of the distal femoral physis. *(B)* Cross-section of the metaphysis showing location of intramedullary pins. *(C)* Retrograde insertion of Kirschner wire or Steinmann pins. *(D)* Following reduction, the pin chuck is attached at a distance from the skin (d′) corresponding to the thickness of the physis (d″). *(E, F)* Pins are driven into the physis and cut proximally.

Reduction

Reduction is usually accomplished by levering the segments back into position. If a week or more has elapsed since fracture, it may be necessary to remove a small amount of bone from the distal end of the proximal segment. Perfect red·.ction is ideal; however, if this is not possible, the distal segment should be overreduced cranially to avoid patellar impingement during extension of the stifle.

Fixation Using Two Intramedullary Pins Inserted Retrograde

These pins enter the distal end of the proximal segment, one near the caudomedial border and the other near the caudolateral border (Fig. 6–21B, C). Pins of smaller diameter are used so that they can bend with the curvature of the bone when inserted retrograde. When the pins are inserted retrograde, the proximal segment of the femur must be adducted and in the angulation and rotation of the normal standing position. For a dog weighing about 50 pounds, size ³⁄₃₂″ pins are used. For the average-size cat, 0.062″ Kirschner wire is used.

The fracture is reduced and the leg extended at the stifle (Fig. 6–21D) to stabilize the distal segment and compress the fracture site. With the pin chuck attached to the proximal end of one of the pins (attached at a distance from the skin to correspond with the thickness of the distal segment at the point of insertion) (Fig. 6–21d′, d″), the pin is inserted well into the distal segment. The second pin is inserted in a similar manner (Fig. 6–21D–F). The pins should be inserted to the depth of subchondral bone.

Two pins stabilize against rotation, and the combination of weight bearing and muscle pull compresses the fracture segments. In the majority of cases, two-pin fixation is preferable to single-pin methods.

Aftercare ■ Activity should be restricted, and no additional fixation is usually indicated. If there is considerable trauma in the area, it may be advisable to have the owner apply 20 to 30 gentle passive flexion-extension movements of the stifle joint two to three times daily. The pins should be removed at clinical union (3 to 5 weeks).

Fixation Using Two Crossing Pins or a Reconstruction Plate

For exposure, the same approach is used as described above. When using cross pins, they are usually started in the metaphyseal area and extend distally into the condyles. This avoids penetration of the articular cartilage, thus no pin ends are in the joint (Fig. 6–22B, C).

In larger dogs that are close to maturity, a small contoured reconstruction plate may be used (Fig. 6–22D). Because it is inside the joint, joint irritation is a definite consideration. Use of one of the other methods of fixation should be seriously considered.

Fixation Using Two Rush Pins

Two Rush pins are inserted by first drilling a diagonal hole (20° to the sagittal plane of the femur) into the medial and lateral surfaces of the condyles (Fig.

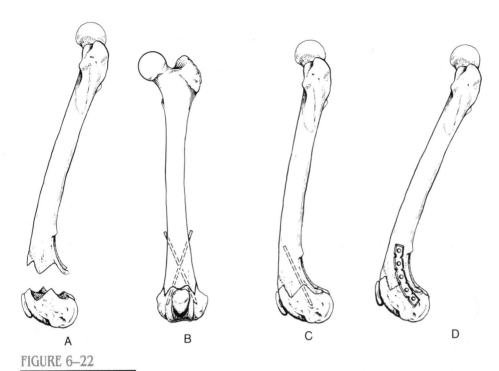

FIGURE 6–22

(A) Distal femoral physeal fracture separation. *(B, C)* After reduction, fixation may be accomplished by the use of two cross pins. These are inserted from proximal to distal and do not penetrate the subchondral bone and articular cartilage. *(D)* In the larger dogs that are close to maturity, a small contoured reconstruction plate may be used for fixation. This is a more costly method and takes longer to apply.

6–23B, C). The two pins are then inserted and driven into the femoral shaft simultaneously (Fig. 6–23D, E). Care must be taken so that the holes in the distal segment are not split out in the drilling and insertion process. In most cases, no additional fixation is necessary. Healing is rapid, and the pins are removed in 3 to 5 weeks, particularly if they are used in a young, growing animal. If the animal is near to skeletal maturity, the pins can be left in situ because they have very little tendency to loosen and migrate. This method is most applicable to large breeds of dogs. In cats and toy breeds of dogs, 0.045″ to 0.062″ Kirschner wires can be used in a manner similar to that for Rush pins.

Conservative Treatment

In early cases with minimal displacement, the fracture may be reduced by flexing the stifle joint with the tarsus extended and applying downward traction on the caudal surface of the proximal part of the tibia. Flexion of the stifle usually maintains the reduction if it is a stable fracture. Immobilization is applied, holding the stifle in flexion by means of a modified Thomas splint or single-sling (Ehmer) bandage.

Reduction should be confirmed radiographically. This treatment is likely to result in some stiffness of the stifle because the joint is not free to move during the healing period. Intra- and extra-articular adhesions are likely to

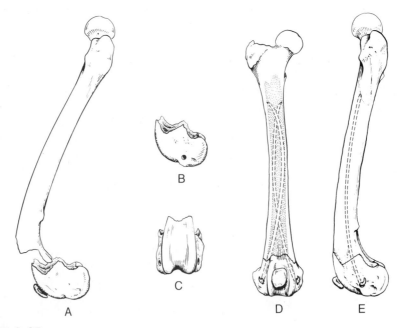

FIGURE 6–23

Rush pin fixation of distal femoral physeal fractures. *(A)* Salter-Harris type 1 fracture of the distal femoral physis. *(B, C)* Position on femoral condyles of entry holes for Rush pins. These holes should be the same diameter as Rush pins and placed in the caudal half of the physis (condylar area). *(D, E)* After reduction of the fracture, double Rush pins are driven into the femoral medullary canal. Pins should be two thirds to three fourths of the length of the femur. The pins bend in two planes as they are driven, thus storing energy that is transferred to the bone as compression.

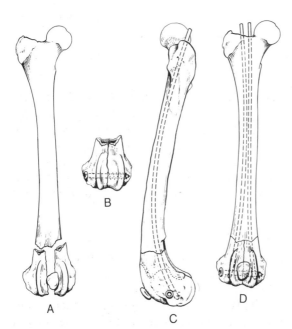

FIGURE 6–24

Fixation of a bicondylar fracture (T or Y) of the distal femur. *(A)* Fracture. *(B)* A transcondylar lag screw is applied first. *(C, D)* The supracondylar fracture is fixed with two small Steinmann pins inserted in retrograde fashion (see Fig. 6–21).

form during the period of immobilization of the joint. Removing the fixation at 2 weeks will minimize this problem.

BICONDYLAR FRACTURE OF THE FEMUR—T OR Y FRACTURE

This is a supracondylar and bicondylar fracture in combination.[2] In addition to the condyles being fractured at their junction with the shaft, there is a longitudinal split between the condyles (Fig. 6–24A). This fracture is relatively rare and is usually accompanied by displacement, extensive soft tissue damage, and hemarthrosis. The joint should be checked for ligament and meniscal damage. Anatomical reduction, rigid fixation of the fractured segments, and movement of the stifle joint are essential to ensure good return of function.

Operative Treatment

An open approach is performed as described earlier. The fractured condyles are reduced and held together by vulsellum or similar forceps. Because the fracture involves an articular surface, anatomical reduction is essential. A hole is drilled transversely through the condyles, and a bone screw is inserted. A cancellous or cortical screw inserted with a lag effect will compress the fracture site (Fig. 6–24B).

Essentially, the fracture has now been converted into a supracondylar fracture. The condyles are attached to the femoral shaft using two intramedullary pins (Fig. 6–24C, D), two cross pins (Fig. 6–22B, C), or two Rush pins (Fig. 6–23).

Postoperative Treatment

In some cases, some temporary additional support is indicated for the first 2 weeks. A modified Thomas splint or Robert Jones bandage works well as additional stabilization. Exercise is restricted until clinical union is reached. If intramedullary pins are used for fixation, they are removed.

CONDYLAR OR UNICONDYLAR FRACTURE OF THE FEMUR

Condylar fractures (Fig. 6–25A) are quite rare; when they occur, the medial condyle is the one must frequently involved. In most instances, the caudal cruciate ligament and the medial collateral ligament are attached to the fractured segment. In some cases, the fractured condyle is a single segment; in others, it is multiple in nature. The latter may be difficult to treat and restore to good function. A good functional recovery depends on anatomical reduction, rigid fixation, and movement of the joint during the healing period.

Operative Treatment

An open approach is performed as already described. If the fracture is primarily in one piece, and particularly if it includes attachments of the cruciate and collateral ligaments, reduction and fixation should be attempted. Reduction is usually accomplished by use of a hook to pull the segment cranially, and levering is used for final reduction. If reduction is impossible, especially if

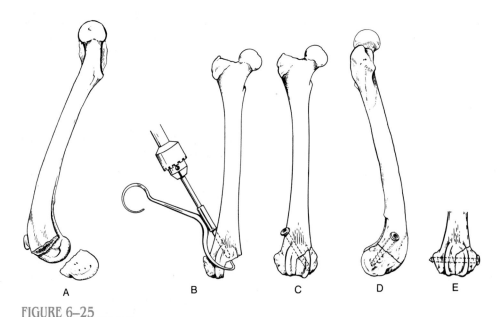

FIGURE 6–25

(A) Condylar fracture of the femur. (B) Fixation by drilling and inserting a cancellous bone screw diagonally from proximally into the fractured segment. (C, D) Anteroposterior and lateral views of the fracture reduced and cancellous bone screw in place. (E) If the fractured condylar segment is large enough, it may be immobilized by a transcondylar bone screw (cancellous or cortical screw with lag effect).

the injury is several days old, a partial horizontal capsulotomy in addition to the standard vertical parapatellar incision allows room for maneuvering the caudally displaced condyle. Exposure can also be improved by osteotomy of the origin of the collateral ligament.[5]

Fixation may be accomplished by drilling and inserting a cancellous bone screw diagonally from proximally in the metaphysis into the fractured condyle (Fig. 6–25B–D). In larger dogs, it is advantageous to insert two bone screws. If the segment is large enough, the screw may be inserted in a transcondylar fashion (Fig. 6–25E). Before closure, the joint should be inspected for any small fragment of loose bone that should be removed.

Postoperative Treatment

Temporary support, if indicated, is usually provided by a modified Thomas splint or Robert Jones bandage. Activity should be limited during the healing period.

PATELLAR FRACTURES

Fractures of the patella or rupture of the patellar ligament is rarely encountered in small animals. Tension band wiring is the preferred method of fixation because it allows early motion of the stifle joint and converts tensile forces into compression forces.[2, 14] When possible, the addition of Kirschner wires results in a more stable fixation. Severely comminuted fractures may be beyond satisfactory repair; in these, partial or total patellectomy is indicated.

Surgical Procedure for Fixation

TRANSVERSE FRACTURE

Figure 6–26 illustrates a transverse fracture fixed with one Kirschner wire and a tension band wire. A medial or lateral parapatellar incision is made for examination of the fracture line and articular surface (Fig. 6–26A). With a 1.5-

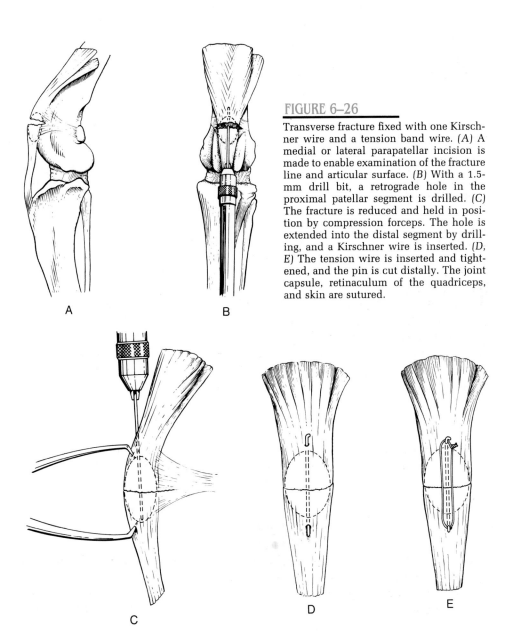

FIGURE 6–26

Transverse fracture fixed with one Kirschner wire and a tension band wire. *(A)* A medial or lateral parapatellar incision is made to enable examination of the fracture line and articular surface. *(B)* With a 1.5-mm drill bit, a retrograde hole in the proximal patellar segment is drilled. *(C)* The fracture is reduced and held in position by compression forceps. The hole is extended into the distal segment by drilling, and a Kirschner wire is inserted. *(D, E)* The tension wire is inserted and tightened, and the pin is cut distally. The joint capsule, retinaculum of the quadriceps, and skin are sutured.

A

B

C

D

E

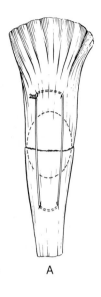
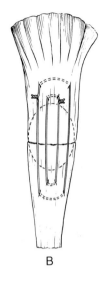

A

B

FIGURE 6–27

Fissure fracture of the patella immobilized by two tension wires. *(A)* One wire is inserted through the quadriceps tendon and patellar ligament close to the patella. Passage of the wire through the tissue can be facilitated by first passing a bent hypodermic needle and then inserting a wire through it. *(B)* The second wire is inserted in a similar or figure-8 fashion, but in a more cranial position. The wires are then tightened.

mm drill bit, a retrograde hole is drilled in the proximal patellar segment (Fig. 6–26*B*).

The fracture is reduced and held in position by use of one or two reduction forceps. The hole is extended into the distal segment by drilling, and a Kirschner wire is inserted (Fig. 6–26*C*). The tension band wire is inserted and tightened, and the pin is cut distally. The joint capsule, retinaculum of the quadriceps, and skin are sutured (Fig. 6–26*D, E*).

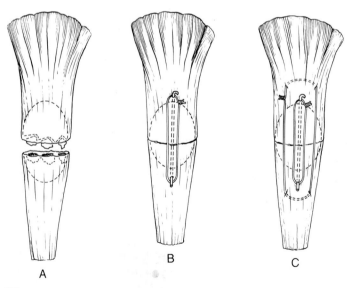

A

B

C

FIGURE 6–28

Comminuted fracture of the patella fixed with one Kirschner wire and two tension wires. *(A, B)* If indicated, the small chips are removed. A Kirschner wire is inserted after drilling a 1.5-mm hole. A tension wire is applied and tightened. *(C)* In many cases, an additional tension wire is inserted through the tendon of the quadriceps and patellar ligament for more stability.

FISSURE FRACTURE

Figure 6–27 shows a fissure fracture of the patella immobilized by use of two tension band wires.

The first wire is inserted through the quadriceps tendon and patellar ligament close to the patella. Passage of the wire through the tissue can be facilitated by first passing a bent hypodermic needle and then inserting a wire through it. The second wire is inserted in a similar or figure-8 fashion but in a more cranial position. The wires are then tightened (Fig. 6–27B).

COMMINUTED FRACTURE

Figure 6–28 shows a comminuted fracture of the patella fixed with one Kirschner wire and two tension band wires. If indicated, the small chips are removed. A Kirschner wire is inserted after drilling a 1.5 mm hole. A tension band wire is applied and tightened (Fig. 6–28A, B). In many cases, an additional tension band wire is inserted through the tendon of the quadriceps and patellar ligament for increased stability.

RUPTURE OF THE PATELLAR LIGAMENT

In this kind of injury, the ligament is sutured and a supporting figure-8 wire is inserted (Fig. 6–29B, C).

Postoperative Care

Additional auxiliary fixation, such as a modified Thomas splint, may be indicated in some cases to relieve the operative area of excessive tension

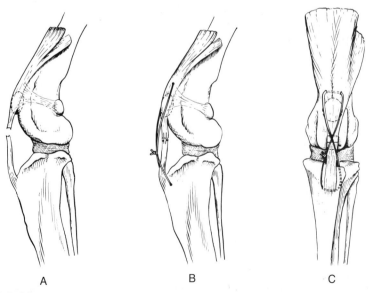

A   B   C

FIGURE 6–29

Rupture of the patellar ligament. (A) Lateral view of rupture. (B) Lateral view of ligament sutured, with a supporting figure-8 wire in place. (C) Cranial view with sutures in place.

during the early healing period (1 to 2 weeks). Activity should be restricted until clinical union. The Kirschner wires and tension wires may need to be removed at this time.

REFERENCES

1. Brinker WO: Fractures in Canine Surgery, 2nd Archibald ed. Santa Barbara, American Veterinary Publications, Inc, 1974, pp 949–1048.
2. Brinker WO: Small Animal Fractures. East Lansing, MI, Depart Cont Ed Press, Michigan State University, 1978.
3. Phillips IR: A survey of bone fractures in the dog and cat. J Small Anim Pract 20:123–126, 1983.
4. Vernon FF, Olmstead ML: Femoral head fractures resulting in epiphyseal fragmentation. Vet Surg 12:123–126, 1983.
5. Piermattei DL: An Atlas of Surgical Approaches to the Bones of the Dog and Cat, 3rd ed. Philadelphia, WB Saunders Co, in preparation.
6. Brown SG, Rosen H: Craniolateral approach to the canine hip: a modified Watson-Jones approach. J Am Vet Med Assoc 159:1117–1122, 1971.
7. Brindley HH: Avascular necrosis of the head of the femur: an experimental study. J Bone Joint Surg 45-A:1541, 1963.
8. Brinker WO: Factors influencing the results in fractures of the femoral neck. J Am Anim Hosp Assoc 2:160, 1966.
9. Cawley AJ, Archibald J, Ditchfield WJB, et al: A technique for repair of fractures for the femoral neck. J Am Vet Med Assoc 129:354, 1956.
10. Nilsson F: Operative treatment of fractures of the neck of the femur and epiphyseal separation of the head of the femur in the dog (abstr). North Am Vet 22:557, 1941.
11. Anderson WD, Schlotthauer CF, Janes JM, et al: Method for treatment of fractures of the femoral neck in the dog: an experimental study. J Am Vet Med Assoc 122:155, 1953.
12. Nunamaker DM: Repair of femoral head and neck fractures by interfragmentary compression. J Am Vet Med Assoc 162:569, 1973.
13. Kaderly RE, Anderson WD, Anderson BG: Extraosseous vascular supply to the mature dog's coxofemoral joint. Am J Vet Res 43:1208, 1982.
14. Brinker WO, Hohn RB, Prieur WD: Manual of Internal Fixation in Small Animals. Springer-Verlag, New York, 1984, pp 165–179.
15. Schroeder EF: Fractures of the femoral shaft of dogs. North Am Vet 14:38, 1933.
16. Leonard EP: Feline therapeutics and hospitalization. North Am Vet 19:58, 1938.
17. Kogan KG: Multiple intramedullary pin fixation of the femur of dogs and cats. J Am Vet Med Assoc 182:1251, 1983.
18. Brinker WO: The use of intramedullary pins in small animal fractures: a preliminary report. North Am Vet 29:292, 1948.
19. Lawson DD: The technique of Rush pinning in fracture repair. Mod Vet Pract 40:32, 1959.
20. Rudy RL: Principles of intramedullary pinning. Vet Clin North Am 5:209–228, 1975.
21. Cechner PE, Knecht CD, Chaffee VW, et al: Fracture repair failure in the dog: a review of 20 dogs. J Am Anim Hosp Assoc 13:613, 1977.
22. Fanton JW, Blass CE, Withrow SJ: Sciatic nerve injury as a complication of intramedullary pin fixation of femoral fractures. J Am Anim Hosp Assoc 19:687–694, 1983.
23. Daily WR: Femoral head and neck fractures in the dog and cat: a review of 115 cases. Vet Surg 7:29, 1978.
24. Brinker WO, Flo GL: Principles and application of external skeletal fixation. Vet Clin North Am 5:197–208, 1975.
25. Renegar WR, Leeds EB, Olds RB: The use of the Kirschner-Ehmer splint in clinical orthopedics. J Comp Cont Ed 4:381, 1982.
26. Gambordella PC: Full cerclage wires for fixation of long bone fractures. J Comp Cont Ed 11:665, 1980.
27. Egger ER, Runyon CL: Use of type I double connecting bar configuration of external skeletal fixation on long bone fractures in dogs: a review of 10 cases. J Am Anim Hosp Assoc 22:57–64, 1986.
28. Campbell JR: The technique of fixation of fractures of the distal femur using Rush pins. J Sm Anim Pract 17:323–329, 1976.
29. Milton JL, Horne RD, Goldstine GM: Cross pinning: a simple technique for treatment of certain metaphyseal and physeal fractures of the long bones. J Am Anim Hosp Assoc 16:891, 1980.
30. Shires SK, Hulse DA: Internal fixation of physeal fractures using the distal femur as an example. J Comp Cont Ed 2:854–861, 1980.
31. Grauer GF, Banks WJ, Ellison GW, et al: Incidence and mechanism of distal femoral physeal fractures in the dog and cat. J Am Anim Hosp Assoc 17:579–586, 1981.
32. Tarvin G, Fraehlich PS: Surgical management of supracondylar femur fractures. Calif Vet 35:17–22, 1981.
33. Parker RB, Bloomberg MS: Modified intramedullary pin technique for repair of distal femoral physeal fractures in the dog and cat. J Am Vet Med Assoc 184:1259–1265, 1984.
34. Hardies EM, Chambers JN: Factors influencing the outcome of distal femoral phy-

seal fracture fixation: a retrospective study. J Am Anim Hosp Assoc 20:927–931, 1984.

35. Lavack B, Flannagan JP, Hobbs S: Result of surgical treatment of patellar fractures. J Bone Joint Surg 67-B:416–419, 1985.

36. Whitney WO, Sehrader SC: Dynamic intramedullary cross pinning technique for repair of distal femoral fractures in dogs and cats: 71 cases (1981–1985). J Am Vet Med Assoc 191:1133–1138, 1987.

37. Sumner-Smith G, Dingwal JS: A technique for repair of the distal femoral epiphysis in the dog and cat. J Am Anim Hosp Assoc 9:171–174, 1973.

38. Berg RJ, Egger E, Blass CE, et al: Evaluation of prognostic factors for growth following distal femoral physeal injuries in 17 dogs. Vet Surg 13:1172–1180, 1984.

39. Lewis DD, Bellah JR: Use of the double-hook plate to repair a subtrochanteric femoral fracture in an immature dog. J Am Vet Med Assoc 191:440–442, 1987.

40. Brinker WD: Fracture documentation studies at Michigan State University. Unpublished material, 1971–1978.

41. Corb A: A partial patallectomy procedure for transverse patellar fractures in the dog and cat. J Am Anim Hosp Assoc 11:649–657, 1975.

7

Fractures of the Tibia and Fibula

CLASSIFICATION

Fractures of the tibia and fibula are classified as follows:[1-3]

1. Avulsion of the tibial tubercle (Fig. 7–1A).
2. Proximal fractures.
   a. Fracture-separation of the proximal epiphysis (see Fig. 7–2A, B).
   b. Fractures of the proximal end (see Figs. 7–3A and 7–4A).
3. Shaft fractures (see Figs. 7–6 through 7–11).
4. Distal fractures.
   a. Fracture-separation of the distal epiphysis (see Fig. 7–12).
   b. Fracture of the medial or lateral malleolus (see Fig. 7–13).

AVULSION OF THE TIBIAL TUBERCLE

This type of separation occurs infrequently and is limited to younger animals, usually under the age of 10 months. The tibial tubercle has a separate growth center and becomes fused to the tibia as the animal reaches maturity. In large dogs, the endochondral ossification process of the physis may be irregular as seen radiographically. Frequently, this is mistaken for a pathological process. The tibial tubercle serves as the insertion point of the quadriceps muscles.

Clinically, the detached tubercle can usually be palpated and is dislocated proximally. The patella also rides higher in the trochlear groove of the femur. Failure to return the tibial tubercle to its original position results in loss of power to the quadriceps muscles and in extension of the stifle joint. Reduction and rigid fixation should be accomplished early.

Operative Treatment

A longitudinal incision is made just medial or lateral to the patella, the patellar ligament, and the tibial tubercle. The blood and fibrin clot is removed from the original location of the tibial tubercle (Fig. 7–1A).

With the stifle extended and a hook or similar instrument attached to the ligament just above the tibial tubercle, the tubercle is slowly and gently pulled back into its original position. A pull is necessary to fatigue and overcome the spastic contraction of the quadriceps muscles. At this stage, the tibial tubercle is rather friable, and care must be taken to avoid fragmentation.

The tibial tubercle is then anchored in place using one of the methods shown in Figure 7–1:[1–6]

1. Ligament-bone suture technique using nonabsorbable suture material (Fig. 7–1B, C).
2. Two Kirschner wires (Fig. 7–1D).
3. Two stainless steel wire sutures (Fig. 7–1E).
4. Cancellous bone screw and pin (Fig. 7–1F).
5. Tension band wire[2, 5] (Fig. 7–1G).

The preferred technique is tension band wiring. If the animal has a considerable amount of growth potential remaining, the fixation should be removed as early as possible to help avoid premature closure of the growth center and disfiguration of the proximal tibia.

Postoperative Treatment

Additional support (e.g., a modified Thomas splint) is usually indicated for the first 2 weeks. Exercise should be restricted for an additional 2 to 3 weeks.

PROXIMAL FRACTURES

Fracture of the Proximal Tibial Epiphysis

The entire epiphysis is usually involved, and the tendency is for dislocation in a caudolateral direction in relation to the tibial shaft. This injury may be accompanied by damage to the ligamentous structures (collateral ligaments in particular), which may vary from a sprain to a complete rupture. If the fracture is not reduced and maintained in position, both function and appearance are affected.[1–3, 6]

CONSERVATIVE TREATMENT

In some cases, further reduction is not essential, or it can be accomplished by closed means. Immobilization is accomplished by the use of a modified Thomas splint for three weeks. The splint is usually applied with the leg in the angulation of the standing position. In addition, it is attached so that some outward force is exerted on the medial surface of the proximal tibia, which aids in maintaining reduction. If this technique is used, the modified Thomas

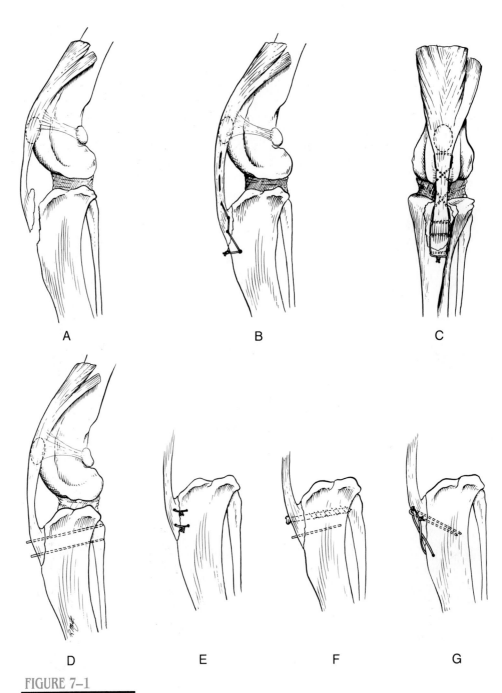

FIGURE 7–1

Operative treatment for the detached tibial tubercle. (A) Avulsion. (B, C) Ligament-bone suture technique using nonabsorbable suture material. (D) Two Kirschner wires. (E) Two stainless steel wire sutures. (F) Cancellous bone screw and pin. (G) Tension band wire.

splint must remain firmly attached and kept in good repair. Loosening invariably results in a crooked leg.

APPROACH AND REDUCTION ■ In most cases, an open approach is necessary for returning the epiphysis to its proper position (Fig. 7–2A, B). A longitudinal skin incision is made on the craniomedial surface of the proximal tibia and stifle. In some instances, it is advantageous to make the skin incision on the craniolateral surface of the proximal tibia and stifle. Reflection of the proximal belly of the tibialis cranialis muscle may aid in exposing the fracture to best advantage for reduction and fixation, particularly if a portion of the metaphysis remains attached to the epiphyseal end (Salter-Harris II, Fig. 7–2B).

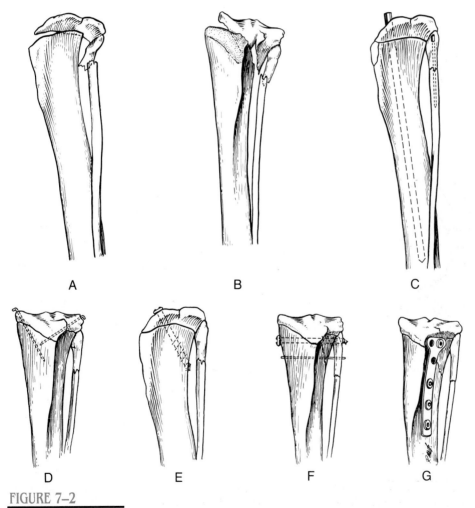

FIGURE 7–2

Fixation methods. *(A)* Epiphyseal separation of the proximal tibia and fracture of the fibula. *(B)* Fracture-separation of proximal tibia and fibular fracture. *(C, D)* Insertion of pins through the epiphysis distally into the tibia. If it is unstable, the fibula may also be pinned. *(E)* Insertion of a cancellous bone screw. *(F)* Insertion of bone screws in a transverse direction, indicated in some impacted fractures. *(G)* Use of a small **T** plate as a buttress plate.

The fascia and soft tissues are separated by blunt dissection to expose the fracture site. By gentle elevation of the epiphysis with an osteotome or similar instrument, the dislocated part can usually be levered back into position. It may be necessary to dislocate the proximal end further, remove the blood and fibrin clot, and reduce by levering. If the fibula is fractured and overriding, reduction and fixation of the fibula may be helpful in supporting and restoring length to the lateral surface.

FIXATION ■ The method of fixation varies. Usually, one of the techniques shown in Figure 7–2 will accomplish the objective.[1–5]

1. Insertion of one or more pins through the epiphysis and distally into the tibia in a Salter-Harris I fracture (Fig. 7–2C, D). If the fibula is unstable, it may also be pinned.
2. Insertion of a cancellous bone screw (Fig. 7–2E). This method is restricted to those patients that are close to maturity so that it does not interfere with growth.
3. Insertion of one or more cancellous bone screws in a transverse direction, indicated in some Salter-Harris II fractures (Fig. 7–2F).
4. Use of a buttress plate in Salter-Harris II fractures (Fig. 7–2G). Additional filling with bone chips may be indicated in some impacted fractures in which deficit remains after reduction.

Aftercare ■ Following closure, additional external immobilization and restricted activity may be indicated for most of the healing period.

Fracture of the Proximal End

Fractures occurring near the proximal end of the tibia and fibula are usually transverse, impacted, or short oblique in nature.[1–3] If the proximal end is dislocated, it will usually be tilted caudally. In many instances, reduction can be accomplished by closed manipulation. Fixation may be accomplished by use of a modified Thomas splint or an intramedullary pin that is inserted from the proximal end into the tibial shaft.

Most often, an open approach is indicated for reduction. In these cases, fixation is usually accomplished by the insertion of an intramedullary pin, a Rush pin, a bone plate, or a cancellous bone screw. Additional support, such as a modified Thomas splint, will depend on the stability of the individual fixation.

If the proximal end of the fibula is fractured and detached, it should be reattached by use of a bone screw because the lateral collateral ligament inserts on its lateral surface. Usually, no auxiliary immobilization is needed with intramedullary pinning, bone screw fixation, or bone plating with fractures of this type.

Figure 7–3 shows a fracture of the proximal metaphyseal area of the tibia and fibula. Reduction is performed, and an intramedullary pin is inserted.

In Figure 7–4, a short oblique fracture of the proximal end of the tibia and fibula is shown. Fixation can be accomplished by using one or more cancellous bone screws. A plate may be used if the proximal fragment is of sufficient length for inserting at least two bone screws in each fracture segment.

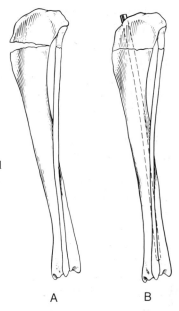

FIGURE 7–3

(A) Fracture of the proximal metaphyseal area of the tibia and fibula. (B) Fracture reduced and intramedullary pin inserted.

A   B

SHAFT FRACTURES

Because the fibular shaft is small and plays an insignificant part in support, for practical purposes it may be disregarded. If fractures of the tibia are treated properly, those of the fibula will heal with no special treatment. Occasionally, restoring the length of the fibula is helpful in determining if a severely comminuted fracture of the tibia has been restored to its proper length.

The incidence of open tibial fractures is higher than that of other long bones. Tibial fractures, if properly treated, appear to heal in approximately the same period of time as other long bones and are not more prone to delayed union and nonunion in small animals.

The various methods of stabilization that may be considered (in decision-making) include use of:[1–3, 7–10]

1. External splint (e.g., modified Thomas splint, coaptation splint).

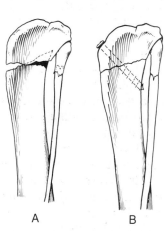

FIGURE 7–4

(A) Short oblique fracture of the proximal end of the tibia and fibula. (B) Fixation with a cancellous bone screw.

A   B

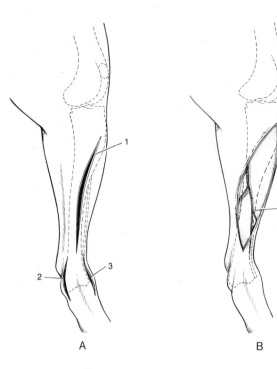

FIGURE 7–5

Surgical approach to the shaft of the tibia and malleoli. *(A)*, (1) For shaft fractures, a longitudinal craniomedial incision is made parallel to the crest of the tibia. (2) Incision to expose medial malleolus. (3) Incision to expose distal end of fibula (lateral malleolus). *(B)*, (1) Craniomedial approach to the tibial shaft showing approximate location of medial saphenous vessels and nerve. (2) With care, the saphenous vessels and nerve, which cross the field obliquely in the middle third of the tibia, can be avoided. This approach can expose the entire length of the tibia.

2. Intramedullary pin alone or with supplemental fixation (e.g., external fixator, cerclage wire, lag screw).

3. External fixator (Kirschner splint) alone or with supplemental fixation (e.g., intramedullary pin, cerclage wire, lag screw).

4. Plate alone or with supplemental fixation (e.g., cerclage wire, lag screw).

Conservative Treatment

Green-stick fractures, some stable fractures, and fractures in very young animals may be treated by the use of a modified Thomas splint, a coaptation splint, or a combination of both.

Figure 7–5 shows various surgical approaches to the tibial shaft and the malleoli.[1, 2, 9]

Internal Fixation

Rigid internal fixation offers many advantages, including allowing freedom of movement of the joints above and below during the healing period. Some of the more commonly used fixation methods that employ internal fixation are described.

INTRAMEDULLARY PINS

The main shortcoming of an intramedullary pin as the sole method of fixation is that it permits rotation at the fracture site. This method of fixation is particularly adaptable to transverse, short oblique, and minimally comminuted fractures of the tibia in smaller dogs and cats.

The pin should be inserted from the proximal end of the tibia. Retrograde pinning must be avoided because the pin will emerge in the immediate proximity of or in the stifle joint. Closed pinning may be used for those fractures that can be reduced closed with a minimum of manipulation and trauma to the soft tissue in the area. Otherwise, an open reduction is indicated. More difficult fractures may be handled by the combined use of an intramedullary pin and supplementary fixation (see discussion later in this chapter).

TECHNIQUE ■ Figure 7–6A shows a short oblique fracture of the tibia. The proximal aspect of the left tibia shows the menisci and limits of the articular surface (Fig. 7–6B). It is usually advantageous to have the stifle flexed at a right angle. The pin is then inserted through the skin and along the medial border of the patellar ligament, entering the proximal end of the tibia approximately ¼″ caudal to the cranial surface of the tibial tubercle (Fig. 7–6B, C). Entering the pin too far caudally will not allow full extension of the stifle joint. After entering the marrow cavity, the pin should glide along the medial cortical surface.

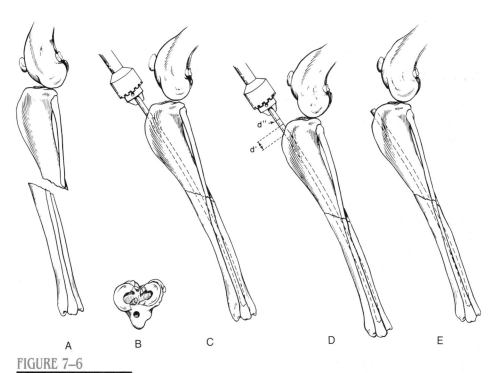

A   B   C   D   E

FIGURE 7–6

Intramedullary pinning technique for the tibia. (A) Serrated short oblique fracture of the tibia. (B) Proximal aspect of the left tibia showing menisci and limits of articular surface. Circle depicts the approximate location for insertion of an intramedullary pin. The stifle should be flexed at a right angle. The pin is inserted through the skin along the medial border of the patellar ligament, entering the proximal end of the tibia approximately ¼″ caudal to the tibial tubercle. (C) Reduced fracture and intramedullary pin, lateral view. The pin should be inserted well into the distal end. (D) Pin retracted about ¼″ (d′); pin cut (d″). (E) With a countersink and mallet, the pin is returned to the original depth. Sufficient pin is left protruding for removal at the time of clinical union.

The reduced fracture and intramedullary pin are shown in Figure 7–6C. The pin should be inserted well into the distal end, and this should be confirmed radiographically. The pin is retracted about ¼″ (d′), then cut (d″). With a countersink and mallet, the pin is returned to the original depth. This seats the pin so that the proximal end does not interfere with movement of the stifle joint and still keeps the pin protruding sufficiently for removal (Fig. 7–6D, E). The fracture site should be compressed while the pin is redriven with the countersink and mallet.

SUPPLEMENTAL FIXATION

INTRAMEDULLARY PIN AND UNILATERAL EXTERNAL FIXATOR ■ In unstable fractures, the addition of a unilateral external fixator, 1/1 pin (half Kirschner) splint, adds markedly to stability and guards against rotation. This combination can be used for a wide range of fractures. The splint is placed on the medial surface of the leg (Fig. 7–7). One fixation pin is placed in each of the upper and lower segments. Each pin is inserted through both cortices at an angle of about 70° to the long axis of the bone and is connected by outside clamps and a bar. The splint is removed after a good primary callus has formed (approximately 4 weeks), and the intramedullary pin is removed at clinical union. If the

FIGURE 7–7   FIGURE 7–8

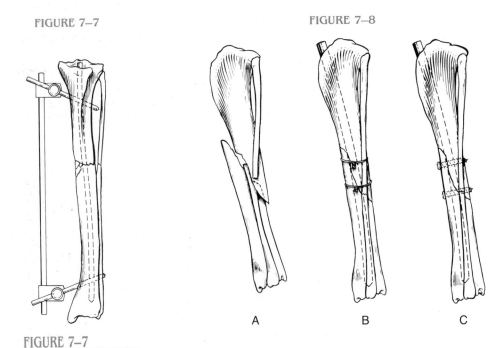

A   B   C

FIGURE 7–7

Intramedullary pin and external fixator, 1/1 pin (half Kirschner) splint, for unstable fractures. If this does not accomplish stability, use a 2/2 pin external fixator.

FIGURE 7–8

(A) Long oblique fracture of the tibia. *(B)* An open approach exposes the fracture, which is held in reduction by self-holding bone forceps. An intramedullary pin is inserted from the proximal end of the tibia, followed by placement of cerclage wires. *(C)* Same fracture immobilized by intramedullary pin and lag screws inserted off center to avoid pin. If the fixation shown in *(B)* and *(C)* does not appear to give sufficient stability, do not hesitate to add an external fixator at the time of the original surgery.

fracture is more comminuted than shown in Figure 7–7 or is in a large dog, a 2/2 pin external fixator may be indicated to accomplish rigid stability.

INTRAMEDULLARY PIN AND CERCLAGE WIRES OR BONE SCREWS ■ The use of cerclage wires or lag screws in addition to an intramedullary pin works well on long oblique or spiral fractures and certain butterfly segment fractures. This same group of fractures is also amenable to the use of lag screws and bone plates or external fixator fixation. Figure 7–8 presents an example of this pinning method.

In Figure 7–8, an open approach is performed to reduce a long oblique tibial fracture, which is held in reduction by use of self-holding bone forceps. The intramedullary pin is then inserted from the proximal end of the tibia, followed by placement of cerclage wires. Figure 7–8C shows the same fracture, immobilized with the use of an intramedullary pin and lag screws inserted off center to avoid the intramedullary pin. This procedure is more amenable to larger dogs. Lag screws of relatively small diameter are used. In both cases, no additional external fixation is used. The pin is removed at clinical union, and the cerclage wires and lag screws are usually left in place.

EXTERNAL FIXATOR

This splint (Fig. 7–9) may be used on practically all fractures of the tibial shaft, including delayed unions and nonunions, and on corrective osteotomies. The splint is placed on the *medial surface* of the leg. In this position, it does not interfere with walking, and it is less subject to being bumped or becoming hooked on objects.

Whenever possible, the pins are placed in the same plane and connected by a common connecting bar. The external fixator is particularly adaptable to open fractures because the segments can be immobilized without invading or placing metallic fixation in the contaminated open area. The external fixator

FIGURE 7–9

Unilateral external fixator, 3/3 pins. *(A)* Open multiple fracture of the tibia. *(B)* Splinting offers rigid uninterrupted fixation of fracture segments without invading the contaminated area. The use of 3/3 pins helps to further distribute the forces to which the pins are subjected, thus reducing the possibility of pin loosening before clinical union.

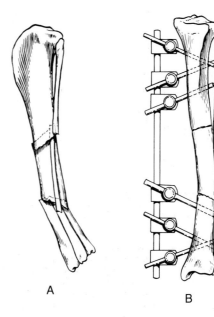

A   B

can also be used in combination with other supplemental fixation (e.g., cerclage wires, lag screws, and intramedullary pins).

Figure 7–9A shows an open multiple fracture of the tibia of 3 days' duration, with suppurative discharge. The patient's temperature was 104.5° F, and the animal was markedly depressed. One of the basic fundamentals of treating fractures of this type is rigid uninterrupted fixation of the fracture segments (Fig. 7–9B). By use of the external fixator, 3/3 pins, this can be accomplished in minimal operating time without invasion of the infected area. The open area is also accessible for local treatment. Some accuracy of reduction can be sacrificed, but the bone should be straight and not rotated. We proceeded with fixation immediately in this situation. The animal was also treated systemically and locally with antibiotics.

BONE PLATES

Plates can be used on most fractures of the tibial shaft, including nonunions, or corrective osteotomies.[2, 3] Bone plates are the first method of choice for fixation in multiple and complex fractures and are particularly useful in larger dogs and semidomesticated animals. Plates are usually placed on the medial surface of the bone. Whenever possible, it is best to apply them so that compression is exerted at the fracture site.

Case Studies

CASE 1 ▪ Figure 7–10 shows a multiple fracture of the tibia. This animal also had a multiple fracture of the radius and ulna. When an animal has fractures involving two or more legs, rigid uninterrupted fixation is indicated. If at all possible, the fixation should make return to function possible during the healing period. Bone plate fixation, in most cases, is the best means of accomplishing this objective.

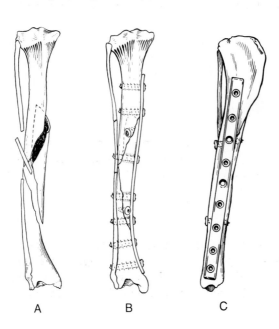

A   B   C

FIGURE 7–10

(A) Multiple fracture of the tibia. (B, C) Shaft has been anatomically reconstructed using two lag screws. Neutralization plate applied on medial surface of tibia.

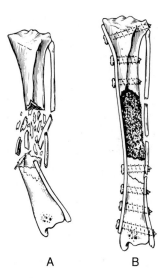

FIGURE 7–11

Multiple fracture of the tibia in a 10-year-old dog. *(A)* Entire center portion markedly comminuted. *(B)* Following application of a buttress plate, the small fracture fragments were left in place and the imperfections were filled in with autogenous cancellous bone. Fracture of this type may also be treated by use of frozen cylindrical allograft and a DCP plate.

A　　　　B

The shaft was anatomically reconstructed using two lag screws (Fig. 7–10B, C). A neutralization plate was then applied on the medial surface of the tibia. The radius was also plated.

CASE 2 ■ Figure 7–11A illustrates a multiple fracture of the tibia in a 10-year-old dog. The entire central portion was markedly comminuted, and anatomical reconstruction of the cylinder of bone appeared impossible. A buttress plate was applied and remaining deficits were filled in with autogenous cancellous bone (Fig. 7–11B). The use of bone graft material speeds healing and filling in of the imperfections. When this type of fracture is treated, healing in older patients is very slow and may not continue to a satisfactory completion without the aid of bone graft material. The basic objectives are to restore length, supply rigid uninterrupted fixation, and supplement imperfections in the area with bone graft material.

DISTAL TIBIAL FRACTURES

Fracture of the Distal Tibial Epiphysis

This fracture is observed primarily in the immature animal.[1,2] In some animals, it may constitute a separation at the epiphyseal line. In other animals, it may be a combination of fracture and separation (Fig. 7–12A, B).

CLOSED FIXATION

Reduction and fixation vary with the individual case. Sometimes reduction may be accomplished closed by a combination of traction, countertraction, and manipulation. If any degree of stability is obtained following reduction, fixation may be accomplished by use of a combined plaster of Paris or fiberglass

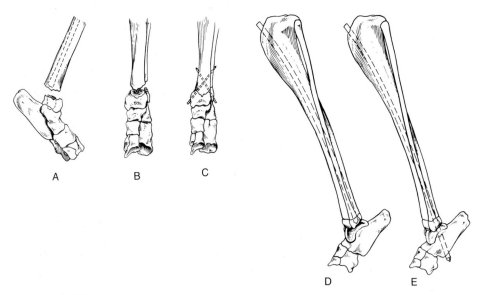

FIGURE 7-12

Fixation of a distal tibial physeal fracture. *(A, B)* Salter-Harris I fracture of the distal tibia and fibula. *(C)* Diagonally placed pins or Kirschner wires are started at the medial and lateral malleoli. Supplemental coaptation fixation is also needed. *(D)* Intramedullary Steinmann pin fixation is adequate to maintain reduction when well supported by external coaptation fixation. *(E)* Intramedullary Steinmann pin fixation crosses the talocrural joint. External coaptation fixation is required to minimize damage to the joint and to prevent bending or breaking of the pin. This is the least desirable method of fixation.

cast and a modified Thomas splint. With the hock flexed just a little more acutely than the angle of the standing position, the plaster cast is applied to cover the foot and extends upward to about the stifle joint. Flexing the hock joint increases the stability. The modified Thomas splint is attached with adhesive tape to the plaster cast. When the combination is used, the plaster cast serves to immobilize the local area, and the modified Thomas splint further immobilizes the entire leg. This will also prevent soft tissue damage around the proximal end of the cast. A long-leg (above the stifle) cast could also be used.

OPEN APPROACH AND FIXATION

An open approach may be mandatory for satisfactory reduction in some cases. In this situation, the longitudinal incision is usually made on the medial side. Suturing the soft tissues over the reduced fracture and adding a cast and modified Thomas splint may also afford good immobilization.

In some cases, more rigid fixation is indicated. One way of accomplishing this is by the insertion of two small diagonally placed pins starting at either the medial or lateral malleolus. Supplemental fixation using a plaster cast is also indicated (Fig. 7–12C).

Another method of internal fixation is use of an intramedullary pin. The pin inserted from the proximal end traverses the entire length of the tibial shaft and is anchored into the distal tibial epiphysis (Fig. 7–12D). The amount of anchorage gained is small but adequate if well supported by external fixation—usually a plaster or fiberglass cast.

An alternative method is use of an intramedullary pin that traverses the entire length of the shaft and hock joint. The hock should be in the angulation of the standing position. This technique, however, has the disadvantage of causing injury to the articular surface. The hock should also be supported by supplemental external fixation until the pin is removed (Fig. 7–12E). Even though the pin traverses the joint, most animals have a good recovery of function and range of movement.

AFTERCARE

Whichever form of immobilization is used, activity is restricted during the healing period. The intramedullary pin or diagonally inserted pins can be removed when adequate primary callus has formed (within approximately 3 weeks). The external fixation is usually continued until clinical union has been reached.

SHEARING INJURY AS A COMPLICATION

This topic is addressed in Chapter 20.

FRACTURES OF THE MEDIAL OR LATERAL MALLEOLUS

Fractures of either or both of the malleoli give rise to instability of the tarsocrural joint, resulting in subluxation or dislocation.[1-3] The two most important factors in the treatment of fractures in the hock are:

1. Maintenance of integrity of the hock mortise.
2. Complete re-establishment of the weight-bearing surfaces of the tibia and tibial tarsal bone.

The hock is functionally a hinge with motion in one plane, flexion and extension. The bony structure is designed as a mortise and tenon with considerable inherent stability. The mortise is formed by the lateral malleolus (at the distal end of the fibula), the distal articular surface of the tibia, and the medial malleolus. The tenon is the trochlea and body of the tibial tarsal bone, which is shaped to fit snugly into the mortise. The tibia and fibula and tibial tarsal bone are bound together by numerous ligaments.

TREATMENT

Intraperiosteal fractures of the malleolus without displacement usually respond to cast or coaptation splinting. In fractures with displacement, it is virtually impossible to obtain and maintain accurate repositioning without internal fixation. Failure to stabilize properly will result in movement at the fracture site and a loose-fitting joint with subsequent degenerative joint disease.

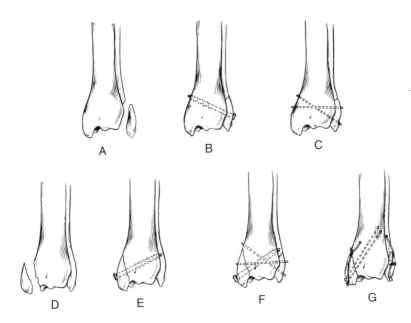

FIGURE 7–13

Malleolar fractures. *(A)* Fracture of the lateral malleolus (distal end of fibula). *(B)* Immobilization using a cancellous screw or *(C)* two threaded Kirschner wires. *(D)* Fracture of the medial malleolus. *(E)* Immobilization using a cancellous bone screw. *(F)* Fractures of both malleoli with fixation. *(G)* Fixation with two Kirschner wires and a figure-8 tension band wire.

In most cases, rigid fixation can be best instituted by the use of bone screws, tension band wire, or threaded pins. Screws are usually used in medium- and large-size dogs, and threaded Kirschner pins are used in the small dogs and cats. The screws or pins should pass in a proximal direction and anchor completely through the cortex on the opposite side of the tibia. Ligaments that have been ruptured should be repaired by suturing. Supplemental fixation is usually indicated in the form of a cast until healing has reached the stage of clinical union.

CASE STUDY ■ A fracture of the lateral malleolus (at the distal end of the fibula) is shown in Figure 7–13A. Anatomical reconstruction of the joint is of first importance. Immobilization is accomplished using a cancellous screw or two threaded Kirschner wires (Fig. 7–13B, C). In the fracture of the medial malleolus (Fig. 7–13D), immobilization is accomplished by use of a cancellous bone screw (Fig. 7–13E).

Figure 7–13F shows fractures of both malleoli with fixation. Supplemental external fixation should also be applied with the hock in slightly overflexed position. In large dogs, fractures of one or both malleoli may be fixed using two Kirschner wires and a figure-8 tension band wire (Fig. 7–13G). With this fixation and restricted activity, no additional external fixation is usually needed.

REFERENCES

1. Brinker WO: Fractures in Canine Surgery, 2nd Archibald ed. Santa Barbara, American Veterinary Publications, Inc, 1974, pp 949–1048.
2. Brinker WO: Small Animal Fractures. East Lansing, MI, Depart Cont Ed Press, Michigan State University, 1978.
3. Brinker WO, Hohn RB, Prieur WD: Manual of Internal Fixation in Small Animals. New York, Springer-Verlag, 1984, pp 180–190.
4. Dingwall JS, Sumner-Smith G: A technique for repair of avulsion of the tibial tubercle in the dog. J Sm Anim Pract 12:665, 1971.
5. Pettit GD, Slattet DH: Tension-band wires for fixation of an avulsed canine tibial tuberosity. J Am Vet Med Assoc 163:242, 1973.
6. Ramadam RO, Vaughan LC: Disturbances in the growth of the tibia and femur in dogs. Vet Rec 104:433, 1979.
7. Hunt JM, Aitken ML, Denny HR, et al: The complications of diaphyseal fractures in dogs: a review of 100 cases. J Sm Anim Pract 21:103–119, 1980.
8. Goodship AE, Kenwright J: The influence of induced micromovement upon the healing of experimental tibial fractures. J Bone Joint Surg 67B:650–655, 1985.
9. Piermattei DL: An Atlas of Surgical Approaches to the Bones of the Dog and Cat, 3rd ed. Philadelphia, WB Saunders Company, in preparation.
10. Boone EG, Johnson AL, Montavon P, et al: Fractures of the tibial diaphysis in dogs and cats. J Am Vet Med Assoc 188:41–45, 1986.

8

Fractures of the Tarsus, Metatarsus, and Phalanges

THE TARSUS

Injuries to the tarsus generally involve fracture of one or more bones, impairment of ligaments, or, occasionally, a combination of these. Ligamentous injuries are most commonly seen in athletic animals, whereas fractures are common in a variety of animals. Only fractures will be covered in this chapter; the other injuries are discussed in Chapter 20.

The bony anatomy of the hindfoot is complicated and must be well understood before any repairs are attempted. Figure 8–1 reviews these bones and provides a comprehensive resource for interpreting radiographs. Ligaments of the hock and tarsus are shown in Figure 20–32. Beginning at the hock joint and continuing distally, the terms *cranial* and *caudal* are replaced by the terms *dorsal* and *plantar*.

Generally, approaches to the various bones are made directly over the injured bone because there are no muscles of any size covering them. Nerves, vessels, and tendons are retracted as necessary to a low exposure. A tourniquet is invaluable for decreasing oozing hemorrhage. VETRAP* bandage material has proved very satisfactory for this purpose (Fig. 8–2). Although the bandage is best sterilized in ethylene oxide, it can be sterilized in the autoclave at minimal time and temperature settings, much like the process of preparing rubber gloves (250° F for 12 minutes).

Use of the tourniquet has the disadvantage of producing more postoperative swelling. Application of a cast or splint should be delayed for 48 to 72 hours, with the foot supported in a Robert Jones bandage during this time.

Fractures of the Calcaneus

A calcaneal fracture is a very disabling injury because it destroys the ability of the gastrocnemius muscle and the rest of the common calcanean tendon

---

*Animal Care Products, 3M Company, St. Paul, Minnesota.

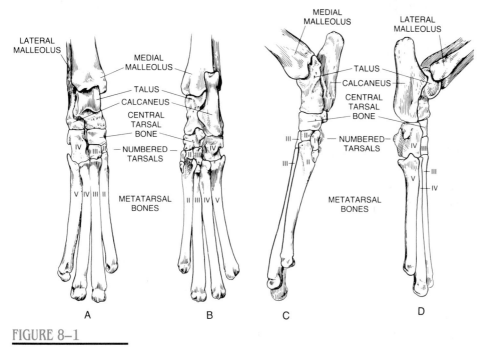

FIGURE 8–1

Bones of the tarsus, metatarsus, and phalanges. *(A)* Dorsal view. *(B)* Plantar view. *(C)* Medial view. *(D)* Lateral view.

apparatus to prevent hyperflexion of the hock joint, resulting in a plantigrade stance. As a result of muscle tension on the tendons, there is considerable pull on the free fragment and, therefore, marked displacement of the fragment. Fractures occur most commonly at the tuber or in the shaft (Figs. 8–3*A* and 8–4*A*) and less commonly near the base (Fig. 8–5*A*). Because the plantar ligament of the calcaneo-quartile part of the proximal intertarsal joint originates at the base of the calcaneus, fractures in this region cause subluxation and hyperextension of this joint. (For further discussion of tarsal hyperextension, see Chapter 20.)

Calcaneal fractures are not uncommon injuries of the racing Greyhound and are usually associated with central tarsal (Tc) bone fractures. When there is no accompanying Tc bone fracture there is invariably a plantar proximal intertarsal subluxation.[1]

The bending loads on the free fragment make conservative treatment with an external cast impossible. Fixation by a Steinmann pin or a screw is very questionable as well because both will usually bend, even with the limb in a splint. Tension band wiring with Kirschner wires is an ideal fixation method in most cases because it allows the bending loads to be converted to compression forces, is applicable to any size animal, is inexpensive, and requires no special equipment. (For further explanation of the tension band technique, see Figure 1–27.) Occasionally, a comminuted fracture requires application of a bone plate, which is best placed laterally. When possible the plate should be supplemented with a tension band wire, placed as shown in Figure 8–4*B, C*.

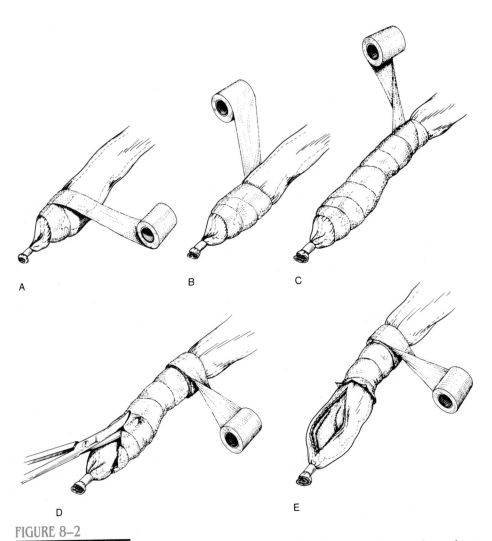

FIGURE 8–2

Application of a VETRAP tourniquet. *(A)* After the foot has been draped in sterile stockinet bandage, a roll of 2″ sterile VETRAP is secured around the toes. *(B)* The VETRAP is wrapped very tightly as it is being wound proximally. *(C)* When well proximal to the surgical field, the elastic bandage is wrapped several times in one area while the bandage is twisted 180°. This forms the tourniquet. *(D, E)* The stockinet and VETRAP are cut to expose the surgical field, in this case the phalanges.

FIGURE 8–3

(A) Fracture of the tuber calcanei. (B, C) Two Kirschner wires, 0.045″ or 0.062″ in diameter, placed side by side, as far medially and laterally as possible. Note that the tendon of the superficial digital flexor has been retracted medially. The exact position of the transverse hole for the wire is not critical and is usually at midshaft or slightly distal as shown here.

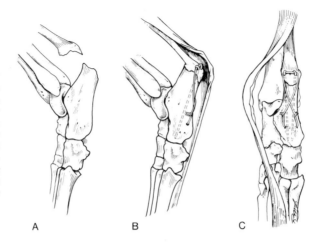

A   B   C

TENSION BAND WIRE FIXATION ■ Surgical approach by means of a plantarolateral incision to the calcaneus is not complicated.[2] Reduction of the fracture and application of fixation are simplified if the tendon of the superficial digital flexor is freed from the tuber by incision of the lateral retinaculum and retracted laterally. The tension band wires must be applied between the tendon and the bone, not superficial to the tendon (Fig. 8–3B, C).

Two methods of application of the tension band are shown. The method shown in Figure 8–3 is the conventional one and is used for fractures of the tuber. It has the disadvantage of creating some irritation of the tendon of the superficial digital flexor as it glides over the tuber. This is minimized by

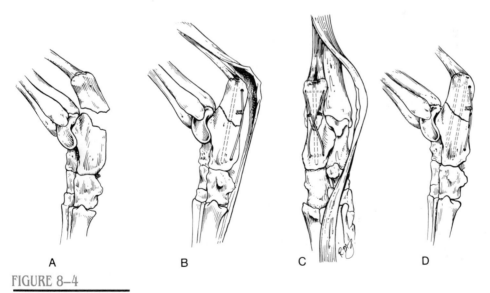

A   B   C   D

FIGURE 8–4

(A) Fracture of the shaft of the calcaneus. (B, C) A single Steinmann pin, $\frac{5}{64}″$ to $\frac{1}{8}″$ in diameter, has been countersunk in the tuber. This pin position allows the wire to be placed through a drill hole in the tuber, which minimizes irritation of the tendon of the superficial digital flexor. A single pin is used when the fracture reduces well and is stable relative to rotation in the reduced position. (D) If the fracture line is smooth or slightly comminuted, two smaller countersunk pins or Kirschner wires in the sagittal plane are used because they provide more rotational stability.

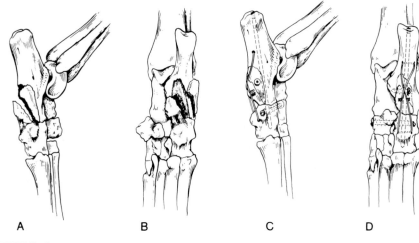

A   B   C   D

FIGURE 8–5

(A, B) Comminuted fracture of the base of the calcaneus. The tarsus hyperextends at this level. Further instability is created by a dorsomedial luxation of the central tarsal bone, a fairly common complication of this type of calcaneal fracture. *(C, D)* The central tarsal bone is reduced first to establish some stability at the proximal intertarsal joint. Fixation is done with a 3.5-mm bone screw through the central tarsal bone into the fourth tarsal bone. This screw is not lagged, but threaded into both bones with the central tarsal held in a reduced position with vulsellum forceps. (For more details, see Figure 20–59). The slab fracture on the lateral side of the calcaneus is lag screwed with a 2.0- or 2.7-mm screw. A 5/64″ Steinmann pin is placed in the calcaneus and seated in the fourth tarsal bone. The tension band wire is placed from midshaft in the calcaneus to the plantar tubercle of the fourth tarsal bone, dorsal to the tendon of the superficial digital flexor tendon. The tension band wire holds the second fragment in place. An additional lag screw may be useful in some cases.

placing the pins as plantarolateral and medial as possible and seating the bent end of the pin close to the bone. Following bone healing, these pins and the wire occasionally must be removed because of soft tissue irritation.

The method shown in Figure 8–4 eliminates these problems by countersinking the pin, but it is applicable only to fractures of the shaft or base. The stainless steel wire must be adequate in size. The following sizes are recommended: up to 15 to 20 pounds—22 gauge (0.635 mm); 20 to 40 pounds—20 gauge (0.812 mm); and over 40 pounds—18 gauge (1.02 mm).

TENSION BAND WIRE AND LAG SCREW FIXATION ■ Comminuted fractures involving the base of the calcaneus (Fig. 8–5A, B) usually require small lag screws for fixation of the slab-like bone fragments from the distolateral region of the bone. This type of fixation is illustrated in Figure 8–5C, D.

AFTERCARE ■ Generally, external casts are not necessary postoperatively except for severely comminuted fractures. In such cases, a short lateral splint (see Fig. 19–13) is applied for approximately 4 weeks or until some radiographic signs of bone healing are seen. A Robert Jones bandage may be useful for a few days to minimize soft tissue swelling. Exercise is restricted until clinical union occurs. Prognosis is generally good.

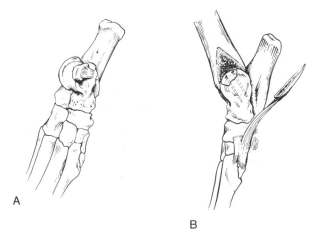

FIGURE 8–6

(A) Fracture of the medial ridge of the talus. (B) Medial malleolus osteotomized and reflected to allow placement of two Kirschner wires, which are countersunk beneath the surface of the articular cartilage. Alternatively, 1.5- or 2-mm screws could be used. The malleolus is replaced by the pin and tension band wire technique (see Figure 1–27).

Fractures of the Talus

Fractures of this bone may be intra-articular, involving either the medial or the lateral ridge of the trochlea (Figs. 8–6 and 8–7), or may be extra-articular in the neck (Fig. 8–8), the body, or the base (Fig. 8–9). Fractures of the ridges, especially the lateral, are difficult to visualize radiographically. Dorsolateral

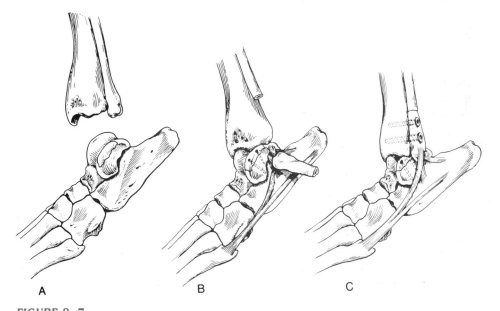

FIGURE 8–7

(A) Fracture of the lateral ridge of the talus. (B) The fibula is osteotomized 1.5 to 2 cm from the tip of the malleolus, dissected free from the tibia, and rotated caudally or distally on the intact short part of the collateral ligament. (See Figure 20–43 for more detail.) It is necessary to cut a short ligament between the tibia and fibula to reflect the fibula. When the foot is supinated (rolled inward), the fracture can be visualized. It is fixed by two or three Kirschner wires countersunk beneath the articular cartilage. Alternatively, 1.5- or 2-mm screws could be used. (C) The fibula is attached by two lag screws, small pins, or Kirschner wires. The small cut ligament is not sutured. Note: If exposure of the caudal portion of the condyle is essential, the short collateral ligament is cut close to the fibula. It is reattached with a suture that engages the ligament and is then passed medial to lateral through two drill holes in the malleolus and tied on the lateral side.

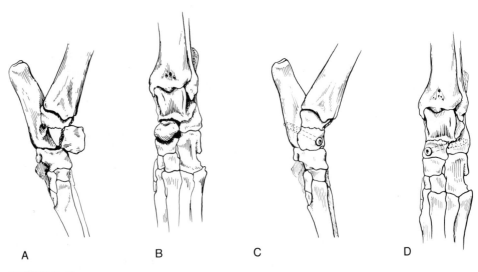

FIGURE 8–8

(A, B) Fracture of neck of talus with typical luxation of body and base. (C, D) Reduction is obtained by flexion and lateral bending at the proximal intertarsal joint and is maintained with vulsellum forceps. A 3.5- or 4.0-mm screw (shown here) is used in average- to large-size breeds. It is not essential that this screw be lagged if the bone is properly reduced and held in place with forceps.

oblique views in both flexion and extension are most useful. Lameness is severe, and there is generally some effusion in the joint. Severely comminuted fractures may require arthrodesis (see Chapter 20). The etiology is usually obscure but may involve a fall or jump. Prognosis for intra-articular fractures is variable, depending on the accuracy of reduction of the fracture. The prognosis is good for neck and body fractures.

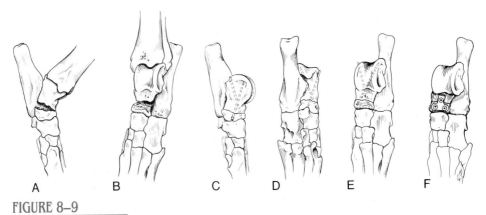

FIGURE 8–9

(A, B) Fracture through the body of the talus. (C–E) Kirschner wires are crossed in the bone. The proximal pin must be cut close to the bone to avoid irritation of the deep digital flexor tendon. (F) T-plates of the 1.5-, 2-, and 2.7-mm series can be used in some cases. Here, a 2.7-mm plate has been cut to fit the bone. Because only one screw is placed in the proximal fragment, external support is essential.

FRACTURE OF THE TROCHLEAR RIDGES

These fractures are generally stabilized by 0.035″ or 0.045″ Kirschner wires that are countersunk beneath the articular surface. Lag screw fixation is preferable, but the fragments are often too small. When fragment size permits, 1.5- and 2.0-mm screws can be used. The screw heads may be countersunk beneath the cartilage surface when used in an articulating area. Fractures of the medial ridge (see Fig. 8–6) are approached by osteotomizing the medial malleolus of the tibia.[2] In the same way, the lateral ridge is approached by osteotomy of the distal fibula (see Fig. 8–7) to allow maximum exposure of the lateral side.[3]

Aftercare ■ A lateral splint (see Fig. 19–13) or short cast (see Fig. 19–10) is placed on the lower limb for 4 weeks, followed by a support bandage for 2 weeks. Exercise is restricted for 6 to 8 weeks. Prognosis ranges from poor to good, depending on the exactness of reduction and stability achieved. Degenerative joint disease is the sequela when this joint fracture does not heal perfectly.

FRACTURE OF THE TALAR NECK

A fracture of the talar neck (Fig. 8–8A, B is usually accompanied by luxation of the body of the bone. In cats and small dogs seen soon after injury, it may be possible to do a closed reduction and to maintain fixation by a snug-fitting short-leg cylinder cast (see Fig. 19–10), but in most animals it will not be possible to maintain position of the fragments with a cast. These animals require internal fixation, best supplied in the form of a lag screw between the body of the talus and the calcaneus. A neck fracture is exposed by proximal extension of the approach to the central tarsal bone.[2]

Aftercare ■ Because the lag screw crosses the tarsal sinus (a gap between the calcaneus and talus), it is somewhat subject to bending with early weight-bearing; the screw is thus best protected by a short lateral splint (see Fig. 19–13) for 4 weeks. Exercise is restricted for 6 to 8 weeks. The 3.5-mm cortical

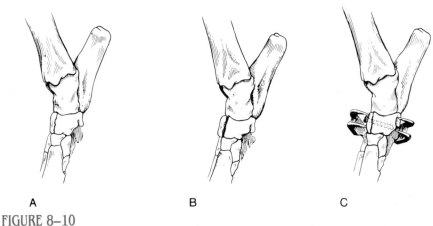

A   B   C

FIGURE 8–10

(A) Dorsal slab fracture of the central tarsal bone with minimal displacement (type 1). *(B)* Dorsal slab fracture of the central tarsal bone, slightly displaced (type 2). *(C)* A 2.7-mm lag screw is placed in the center of the fragment. The fragment is held in the reduced position with vulsellum forceps and the screw is placed between the teeth of the forceps.

screw is considerably stronger in bending than the 4.0-mm cancellous screw shown here and may be a better choice in this application. Prognosis is good in this injury.

FRACTURE OF THE TALAR BODY

In these cases (Fig. 8–9A, B), the base of the talus does not luxate, but there is a slight subluxation of the talocalcaneal joint. Fixation is usually by means of multiple Kirschner wires because the neck of the bone is often too small to accommodate a lag screw. Ideally, two wires are crossed in the bone (Fig. 8–9C, D, E). In some cases, bone plates can be used for fixation. T-plates of the 1.5-, 2.0-, and 2.7-mm series can be adapted to this fracture and provide relatively good stability (Fig. 8–9F). The bone is approached by a combination of the approaches to the medial malleolus and the central tarsal bone.[2]

Aftercare ■ Neither fixation is very rigid and both should be protected for 4 to 6 weeks postoperatively by a short lateral splint (see Fig. 19–13). The prognosis is generally good.

Fractures of the Central Tarsal Bone

These fractures[4] (Figs. 8–10 through 8–13) rarely occur except in the racing Greyhound. They are usually seen in the right foot. This is the "off" foot—toward the outside of the track—and the bone is subject to tremendous compression forces during turns. These forces literally explode the bone out of its position in the midst of the other six tarsal bones, producing a variety of fractures and subluxations of the bone. The fracture types are explained in detail below. Type 4 fractures are most common (68 percent) and most often, are accompanied by associated fractures of the fourth tarsal bone (T4), calcaneus, or T4 and the lateral aspect of the base of metatarsal V.[5] In nonracing animals, the simpler fracture types can be seen; more commonly, however, the bone is luxated intact except for a portion of the plantar process (see Chapter 20).

Fixation is by one or two lag screws, followed by coaptation in a lateral splint or short cast. The bone is approached by a dorsomedial incision.[2] The details of fixation for each fracture type follow.

TYPE 1 FRACTURE ■ A small slab is seen on the dorsal surface of the bone, with minimal displacement (Fig. 8–10A). In the past, these fractures have been treated primarily with a short lateral splint (see Fig. 19–13). Generally, they heal well with 4 to 6 weeks of immobilization, but occasionally they displace a little more during healing and thus create a slight incongruity at the proximal intertarsal joint space. For this reason, type 1 fractures are best treated with a lag screw, as are type 2 fractures.

TYPE 2 FRACTURE ■ Slightly more displacement of the dorsal slab differentiates a type 2 fracture from a type 1 fracture (Fig. 8–10B). A single 2.7- or 3.5-mm lag screw centered in the middle of the fragment is placed in a dorsoplantar direction (Fig. 8–10C).

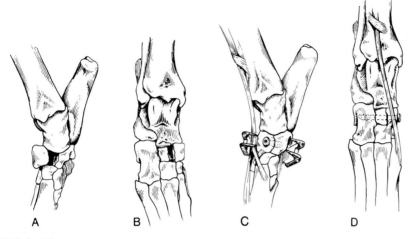

FIGURE 8–11

(A, B) Dorsomedial displacement of the medial portion of the central tarsal bone (type 3). *(C, D)* The 3.5- or 4.0-mm lag screw has been inserted in a mediolateral direction. The tendon of insertion of the tibialis cranialis muscle and the ligament between the central and third tarsal bones are shown for orientation. Reduction is accomplished by laterally displacing and flexing the metatarsus to allow the fragment to be wedged back into the joint space. It is held by vulsellum forceps while the screw is inserted.

TYPE 3 FRACTURE ■ Approximately one third to one half of the bone is fractured in the median plane and is displaced medially or dorsally (Fig. 8–11A, B). A single 3.5- or 4.0-mm lag screw is placed in a mediolateral and slightly plantar direction and seats in the fourth tarsal bone. The screw is placed just proximal to the origin of the ligament between the central and third tarsal bones (Fig. 8–11C, D).

TYPE 4 FRACTURE ■ This injury is a combination of fracture types 2 and 3 (Fig. 8–12A, B). The joint space may be narrowed if the lateral undisplaced half of the bone is comminuted. This will lead to slight hyperextension and varus deformity (toes displaced medially) of the foot. Because of the severe instability of the tarsus induced by this injury, fractures of other tarsal bones, especially the base of the calcaneus and T3 and T4, should be suspected. Fixation is a combination of the two lag screws used for type 2 and 3 fractures. Exact placement of the screws is critical to ensure that both of them will be able to be placed in this small bone (Fig. 8–12C, D). The mediolateral screw must be placed first at the junction of the middle and distal third of the bone. The dorsoplantar screw is placed at the junction of the proximal and middle third of the bone. The angle of the drill bit is important because it must pass proximal to the first screw and also avoid entering the proximal intertarsal joint. If other fractures are present, they are often reduced spontaneously during reduction of the central tarsal bone. Fixation of these fractures is illustrated in Figures 8–5, 8–14, and 8–15.

TYPE 5 FRACTURE ■ Severely comminuted and displaced (Fig. 8–13A, B), these injuries carry the poorest prognosis for racing. If soundness of the animal for kennel activity is the only consideration, closed reduction and immobilization

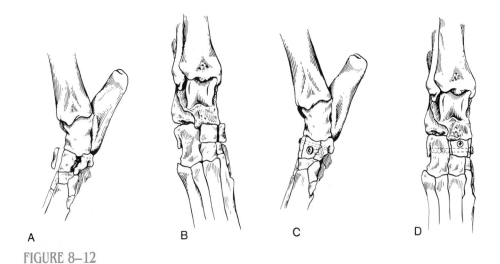

FIGURE 8–12

(A, B) Dorsal and medial displacement of two fracture fragments of the central tarsal bone (type 4). There may be comminution of the central part of the bone with slight varus deformity of the foot. *(C, D)* The medial fragment is reduced first and the 4.0-mm lag screw is placed mediolaterally as far distally in the bone as possible. The 2.7-mm lag screw is placed next in a dorsoplantar direction. Because this screw must not enter the proximal intertarsal joint, the exact angle of the drill hole is critical. Using partially threaded 4.0-mm screws for the mediolateral lag screw gives an extra millimeter of clearance between the two screws over the fully threaded 3.5-mm screw.

in a short cylinder cast for 6 weeks are sufficient. These animals will have slight hyperextension and varus deformity of the foot. If optimal results are desired, a buttress plate and cancellous bone graft (see Chapter 3) are utilized (Fig. 8–13C, D). The objective is to restore and maintain the normal joint

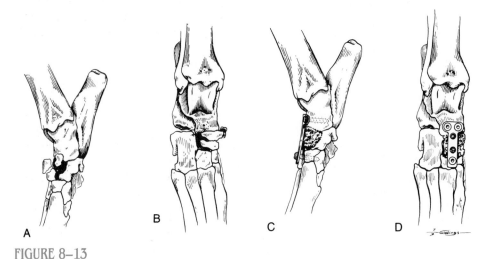

FIGURE 8–13

(A, B) Comminuted fracture of the central tarsal bone (type 5). Note the varus deformity of the tarsus and metatarsus. *(C, D)* A finger plate (2.7-mm screws) has been used as a buttress plate to restore the joint space occupied by the central tarsal bone. No fixation of the fragments is possible because of their small size. The fragments are placed loosely back into the space, and the entire area is packed with autogenous cancellous bone graft obtained from the proximal tibia.

space and thereby prevent deformity of the foot. Fragments of the bone are left in place, and cancellous graft is packed into the spaces. Ligamentous injury on the lateral side of the joint may accompany these fractures and may be difficult to evaluate until the fracture is stabilized. Repair of the ligament or arthrodesis of the unstable joint should be performed for optimum function (see Chapter 20).

Aftercare ■ Lag screw fixation in these cases is not sufficiently rigid to allow early weight-bearing, especially in the Greyhound. These animals are very tolerant of pain and will use the limb excessively, even in kennel confinement. A short lateral splint or short cast (see Figs. 19–13 and 19–10) is applied for 4 weeks. Close confinement is maintained for 8 weeks, at which point radiographs are made. If fracture healing is satisfactory, gradually increasing exercise is allowed; at 12 weeks postoperatively, regular training is allowed.

Bone screws do not need to be removed unless the screw enters the proximal intertarsal joint, as may happen with the dorsoplantar screw in type 4 fractures (Fig. 8–12C, D). These animals remain slightly lame until the screw is removed. A screw in the joint may also loosen and back out, again requiring removal. The plate used in type 5 injuries should be removed in most cases at 3 to 6 months postoperatively, especially if any attempt will be made to race the dog. Motion in the tarsus will cause the screws to loosen, which causes pain and prevents return to racing form.

PROGNOSIS ■ With anatomic reduction and rigid fixation, good healing and return to competitive racing can be anticipated in 71 percent of dogs with fracture types 1 through 4.[6] Type 5 injuries carry a more guarded prognosis for racing, although most patients will become sound for breeding or pet purposes. Some type 4 and 5 injuries also have fractures of the base of the calcaneus (see Fig. 8–5) or proximal intertarsal plantar ligament injuries with subluxation and hyperextension of that joint (see Chapter 20). Again, the prognosis for racing is poor, but soundness of condition for kennel activity can be expected. Treatment is a combination of the methods described above with the methods for a fracture of the calcaneus and for hyperextension at the proximal intertarsal joint.

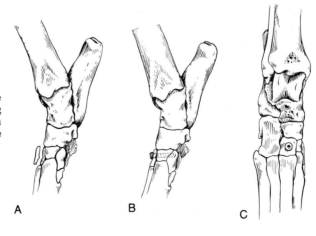

FIGURE 8–14

(A) Dorsal slab fracture of the third tarsal bone. (B, C) Lag screw fixation with 2.7-mm screw placed in the center of the fragment.

A   B   C

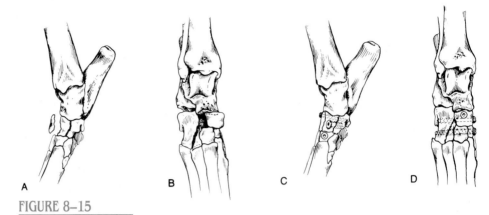

FIGURE 8–15

(A, B) Type 4 fracture of the central tarsal bone with fracture of the head of the fourth tarsal bone. *(C, D)* Double lag screw (4.0 and 2.7 mm) fixation of the central tarsal bone is accomplished first, followed by placement of a 3.5-mm lag screw that is started in the second tarsal bone and passes through the third and into the fourth tarsal bone.

Fractures of Numbered Tarsal Bones

In our experience, we have not seen fractures of the first and second tarsal bones, nor have they been reported. Occasionally, the third tarsal bone may be fractured on the dorsal surface in racing Greyhounds (Fig. 8–14A). A slab fracture similar to the central tarsal type 1 and 2 fractures, it may be treated either by a closed reduction and casting or, preferably, by lag screw fixation (Fig. 8–14B, C).

Fractures of the fourth tarsal bone seen in nonracing animals are usually nondisplaced and respond well to casting. More serious injuries are seen in Greyhounds, usually in conjunction with fractures of the central tarsal bone (Fig. 8–15A). Some of these require internal fixation, whereas others heal well with a cast following internal fixation of the central tarsal bone. The decision is based primarily on the amount of displacement, always bearing in mind that the fracture will probably displace farther while in the cast. If internal fixation of the central tarsal bone is indicated, it is very little additional work to place a screw or Kirschner wire in the fourth tarsal bone (Fig. 8–15C, D).

The third and fourth tarsal bones are exposed by incision directly over the bones. The third tarsal incision is simply a distal continuation of the approach to the central tarsal bone.[2]

Aftercare ■ A short lateral splint or short cast (see Figs. 19–13 and 19–10) is applied for 4 weeks. Exercise restrictions for racing animals are the same as for animals with central tarsal fractures. For nonracing animals, close confinement is maintained for 6 weeks, followed by 4 weeks of gradual return to normal activity.

THE METATARSUS, PHALANGES, AND SESAMOIDS

Fractures of these bones are virtually identical to fractures of the corresponding bones of the metacarpus and forefoot and are covered in Chapter 12.

REFERENCES

1. Ost PC, Dee JF, Dee LG: Fractures of the calcaneus in racing Greyhounds. Vet Surg 16:53, 1987.
2. Piermattei DL: An Atlas of Surgical Approaches to the Bones of the Dog and Cat, 3rd ed. Philadelphia, WB Saunders Co, in preparation.
3. Earley TD: Fractures of the Tarsus. Presented at Canine Carpus and Tarsus Short Course, University of Tennessee, Nov. 21–22, 1981.
4. Dee JF, Dee J, Piermattei DL: Classification, management, and repair of central tarsal fractures in the racing Greyhound. J Am Anim Hosp Assoc 12:398–405, 1976.
5. Boudrieau RJ, Dee JF, Dee LG: Central tarsal bone fractures in racing Greyhounds: a review of 114 cases. J Am Vet Med Assoc 184:1486, 1984.
6. Boudrieau RJ, Dee JF, Dee LG: Treatment of central tarsal bone fractures in the racing Greyhound. J Amer Vet Med Assoc 184:1492, 1984.

Fractures of the Scapula

CLASSIFICATION

Fractures of the scapula are relatively uncommon and may be classified on the basis of the following anatomical locations.[1-3]

1. The body.
2. The spine and acromion process.
3. The neck (including the supraglenoid tuberosity and coracoid process) and glenoid cavity.

The most frequently encountered complications are pulmonary contusions, rib fractures, pneumothorax, pleural effusions, foreleg paralysis, and injury to the suprascapular nerve.[4] Long-standing complications include limitation of range of movement and osteoarthrosis in unreduced fractures of the neck or articular surface.

TREATMENT

Conservative Treatment

Most scapular body fractures are not grossly displaced because of the protection of the surrounding muscle mass and rib cage. A fracture can be treated closed unless there is loss of congruity of the articular surface or a distinct change in the angulation of the shoulder joint articulation. Many fractures respond well to simple limitation of the animal's activity. In some instances, a modified Velpeau bandage adds greatly to the animal's comfort. The leg is flexed along the chest wall, padded, and bound to the body (see Fig. 19–16).

Open Approach to the Scapula and Shoulder Joint

The approach varies considerably, depending on the area of involvement (Fig. 9–1).[1-3, 5]

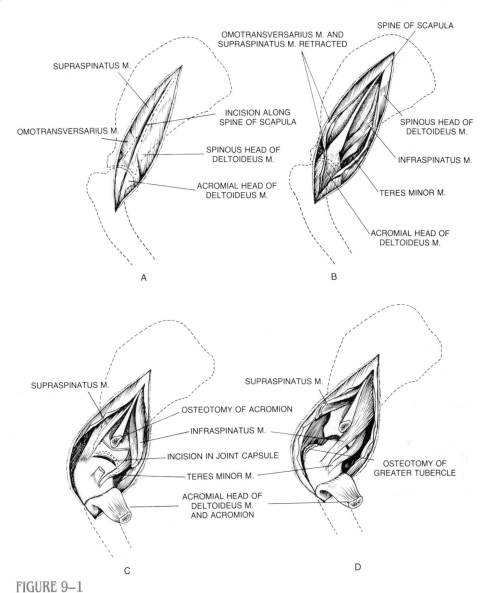

FIGURE 9–1

Open approach to the scapula and shoulder joint. *(A)* A longitudinal skin incision over spine of scapula extends distally over shoulder joint. The omotransversarius muscle is severed from its insertion on the fascia and spine of the scapula and is reflected cranially. *(B)* Fractures of body and spine; the infraspinatus and supraspinatus muscles are reflected caudally and cranially, respectively, from the spine. *(C)* Fractures of neck; the acromion process is osteotomized so that the acromial head of the deltoid muscle can be reflected distally. The infraspinatus and supraspinatus muscles are reflected caudally and cranially, respectively. Their tendons of insertion may be severed for more exposure. The suprascapular nerve is located as it crosses the lateral surface of the neck just distal to the acromion process. In fractures involving the articular surface, the joint capsule is incised between the scapula and humerus for exposure. *(D)* In avulsion fractures of the coracoid process or supraglenoid tuberosity or in multiple neck fractures, the belly of the brachiocephalicus muscle is reflected cranially. The greater tuberosity of the humerus is osteotomized and insertion of the supraspinatus muscle is reflected proximally for exposure and working room.

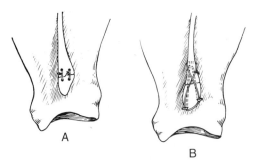

FIGURE 9–2

(A) Reattachment of the osteotomized or fractured acromion process by use of two stainless steel wires. *(B)* Kirschner wire and a figure-8 tension band wire.

Reduction and Fixation

Surgical treatment is indicated primarily for those cases in which there is gross displacement of the fracture segments, loss of congruity, or change in angulation of the articular surface, and avulsion fractures.[1–3, 5]

METHODS OF FIXATION ■ The following implants may be used:

1. Stainless steel wire sutures.
2. Cancellous or cortical bone screws.
3. Steinmann pins or Kirschner wires.
4. Semitubular plates or small bone plates.

Figure 9–2A shows the reattachment of a fracture or osteotomized acromion process by use of two stainless steel wires. A Kirschner wire and a figure-8 tension band wire may be used in larger dogs (Fig. 9–2B).

Figure 9–3 depicts an avulsion fracture of the supraglenoid tuberosity and transverse fracture of the body and spine. Immobilization of the supraglenoid tuberosity is accomplished by use of a cancellous bone screw. A small inverted semitubular plate with screws anchored at the junction of the spine

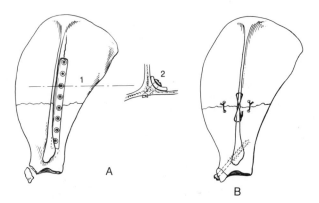

FIGURE 9–3

(A) Avulsion fracture of supraglenoid tuberosity and fracture of the scapular body. (1) A small inverted semitubular plate with screws anchored at the junction of the spine and blade can immobilize fractures of the spine and body. (2) Cross-sectional view of semitubular plate and scapula. *(B)* Supraglenoid tuberosity immobilization by use of a cancellous bone screw. Some fractures of the body and spine are amenable to interfragmentary wiring and a tension band wire.

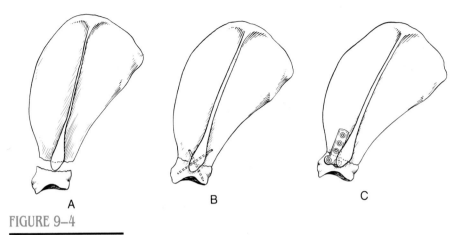

FIGURE 9–4

(A) Transverse fracture at the junction of the scapular body and neck. (B) Immobilization by insertion of two Kirschner wires. (C) Immobilization by a small bone plate; the suprascapular nerve is elevated to insert the bone plate.

and blade may be used to immobilize fractures of the spine and body, particularly in larger dogs.

In Figure 9–4, a transverse fracture at the junction of the body and neck is immobilized by the insertion of two Kirschner wires. When the fracture is being reduced, the suprascapular nerve must not be trapped between the fracture segments. Figure 9–4C shows immobilization by a small plate. The suprascapular nerve is elevated to insert the plate.

A T-fracture of the scapular neck and glenoid is shown in Figure 9–5A.

Immobilization is accomplished by a cancellous screw and two diagonally inserted Kirschner wires. Figure 9–5C shows multiple fractures of the scapular neck and glenoid with immobilization by the use of Kirschner wires and bone screw. Fractures of this type require the pattern of open approach indicated in Figure 9–1D. The surgeon must visualize the articular surface of the glenoid during the reduction and fixation procedure. The fracture is usually reduced

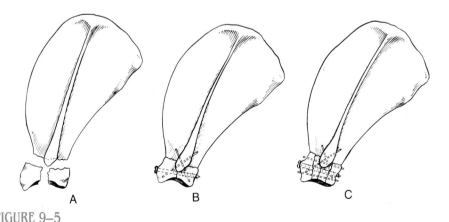

FIGURE 9–5

(A) T fracture of scapular neck and glenoid. (B) Immobilization by a cancellous screw and two diagonally inserted Kirschner wires. (C) Multiple fracture of the scapular neck and glenoid; immobilization by Kirschner wires and a lag screw.

and held by self-holding bone forceps and Kirschner wires prior to insertion of the bone screw. Two or more screws are preferable if there is room. The Kirschner wires and screws are left in place and are not removed unless indicated.

REFERENCES

1. Brinker WO: Fractures in canine surgery, 2nd Archibald ed. Santa Barbara, American Veterinary Publications, Inc, 1974, pp 949–1048.
2. Brinker WO: Small Animal Fractures. East Lansing, MI, Depart Cont Ed Press, Michigan State University, 1978.
3. Brinker WO, Hohn RB, Prieur WD: Manual of Internal Fixation in Small Animals. New York, Springer-Verlag, 1984, pp 127–133.
4. Tomes PM, Paddleford RR, Krahwinkel DJ. Thoracic trauma in dogs and cats presented for limb fractures. J Am Vet Med Assoc 21:161–166, 1985.
5. Piermattei DL: An Atlas of Surgical Approaches to the Bones of the Dog and Cat, 3rd ed. Philadelphia, WB Saunders Co, in preparation.

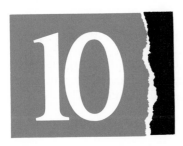

Fractures of the Humerus

The majority of fractures involving the humerus are in the middle and distal thirds.[1] Occasionally, fractures of this bone may be accompanied by foreleg paresis or paralysis resulting from nerve injury. In most cases, a patient with a humeral fracture carries the affected leg with the elbow dropped and with the paw resting on its dorsal surface because of a weakening of the extension musculature. Nerve injury may occur at the fracture site or in the brachial plexus, or it may be due to avulsion of spinal nerves from the cord. Nerve impairment may be temporary or permanent; fortunately in most cases it is the former. Establishing the presence of intact pain sensation by toe pinch may be helpful in differentiation. Nerve conduction studies can be used to establish whether nerves are intact, but results are not reliable until about 7 days postoperatively.

CLASSIFICATION

Fractures of the humerus may be classified anatomically.[2–5]

1. The proximal end.
2. The shaft.
3. The supracondylar region.
4. The medial or lateral aspect of the humeral condyle.
5. The intercondylar region.

PROXIMAL FRACTURES
Fracture of the Proximal Humeral Epiphysis

This is an uncommon injury that occurs in young animals prior to physeal closure. It may be a result of direct or indirect force (avulsion).

TREATMENT
Reduction

Usually closed reduction can be accomplished, particularly in cases of recent origin. Immobilization may be accomplished by use of a modified Velpeau bandage encircling the chest and the affected leg with the joints flexed (see Fig. 19–16).

An open (craniolateral) approach and reduction can be performed. A longitudinal incision is made along the craniolateral surface of the humerus. The belly of the brachiocephalicus muscle is reflected cranially. The dislocation is reduced by levering.

Immobilization

Immobilization may be accomplished by one of the following techniques:

1. Suturing of the ruptured soft tissues and application of a Velpeau bandage.

2. Internal fixation, which is necessary in most cases, carried out by the insertion of one or more Steinmann pins, Kirschner wires, Rush pins, or cancellous bone screws on the crest of the greater tuberosity extending down the shaft of the bone (Figs. 10–1 and 10–2).

Case Studies

CASE 1 ■ Figure 10–1 shows a Salter-Harris Type I fracture of the proximal humeral epiphysis. Fixation is accomplished using Kirschner wires. This method is preferred in relatively young animals because it is less apt to bring about premature closure of the epiphyseal line. Ordinarily, reduction is easy to maintain, and two or more relatively small Kirschner wires are used. In Figure 10–1C, fixation is performed by use of a cancellous bone screw. The bone screw enters on the ridge of the greater tuberosity and anchors in the cancellous bone in the proximal end of the humeral shaft. This procedure is reserved for use on animals that are close to maturity, because it may bring about premature closure and cessation of growth in the area.

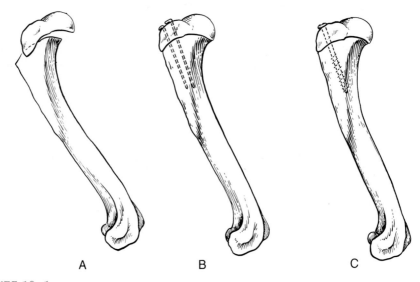

A   B   C

FIGURE 10–1

(A) Salter-Harris I fracture-separation of the proximal humeral physis. *(B)* Fixation using Kirschner wires and *(C)* a cancellous bone screw. This method is reserved for animals that are close to maturity.

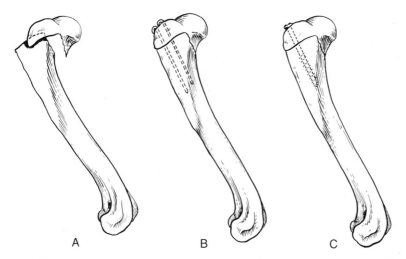

FIGURE 10–2

(A) Salter-Harris II fracture-separation of the proximal humeral physis. (B) Fixation using Kirschner wires and (C) a cancellous bone screw. This method is reserved for animals that are close to maturity.

CASE 2 ■ In the Salter-Harris Type II fracture shown in Figure 10–2, fixation is accomplished using Kirschner wires or a cancellous bone screw. Again, use of a lag screw is reserved for use in animals nearing maturity.

Proximal Metaphyseal Fractures

If displacement is present, reduction is necessary because the bone segment or callus may encroach on the joint or brachial plexus or change the functional angle of the shoulder joint and thus limit range of movement or alter function. Reduction and immobilization are the same as for physeal fractures; however, most cases respond best with internal fixation.

For the impacted fracture shown in Figure 10–3, reduction is usually satisfactory and only immobilization is indicated. The intramedullary pin is inserted closed, starting on the ridge of the greater tuberosity and proceeding distally.

SHAFT FRACTURES

Considerable overriding resulting from spastic contraction of the brachial muscles is usually seen with these fractures.[2-6] The distal segment is usually tilted cranially.

Treatment

CLOSED REDUCTION AND FIXATION

Closed reduction is occasionally possible, particularly in cats and small dogs, when the fracture is of the transverse or short oblique type and can be readily palpated. Immobilization may be done by these methods:

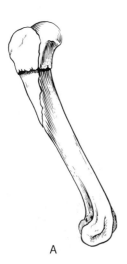
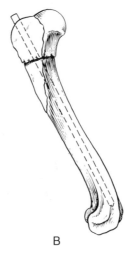

FIGURE 10–3

(A) Impacted fracture of the proximal humeral metaphysis. (B) The intramedullary pin is inserted closed, starting on the ridge of the greater tuberosity and proceeding distally.

A   B

INTRAMEDULLARY PINNING ■ The pin is inserted through the skin and bone just lateral to the ridge of the greater humeral tuberosity and then is inserted distally into the shaft. A half Kirschner splint may be added for supplemental fixation (see Figs. 10–6 and 10–7F).

EXTERNAL FIXATOR ■ This splint is illustrated in Figures 10–8A, B and 1–14C.

OPEN REDUCTION

A lateral approach is usually preferred. Figure 10–4 shows the craniolateral open approach to the shaft of the humerus.[2, 6] This approach may be used to expose the proximal three fourths of the humerus.

Figure 10–5 shows a medial open approach to the shaft of the humerus.[2, 6] This approach may be used to expose the distal half of the shaft of the humerus.

INTERNAL FIXATION

The more common methods of internal fixation are:

1. Intramedullary pin alone or with supplemental fixation (see Fig. 10–7).
2. Unilateral external fixator alone or with supplemental fixation.
3. Plate alone or with supplemental fixation.

Rarely is the modified Thomas splint or a coaptation splint used as the sole method of fixation or as auxiliary fixation. With a modified Thomas splint, the ring acts as a fulcrum at the fracture site.

INTRAMEDULLARY PIN ■ The chief indication for using an intramedullary pin as the sole method of fixation is for transverse or short oblique fractures in small dogs and cats. The Steinmann pin is usually inserted from the proximal end by entering the skin and bone just lateral to the ridge of the lateral tuberosity

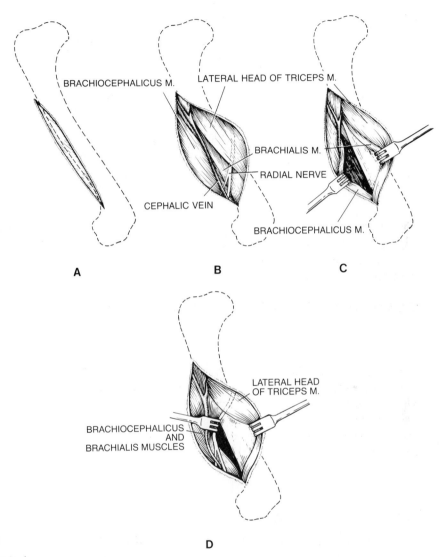

FIGURE 10–4

Craniolateral open approach to the shaft of the humerus. (A) Longitudinal skin incision over craniolateral surface of the humerus. (B) The radial nerve obliquely circles the lower third of the humerus between the lateral head of the triceps and brachialis muscles; the nerve is located and avoided. (C) The brachiocephalicus muscle is reflected cranially and the brachialis muscle is reflected caudally. (D) For fractures located a little further distally, the brachialis muscle and radial nerve are reflected cranially. On closure, the fascia is sutured and a second row of sutures is placed in the subcutaneous tissue and skin.

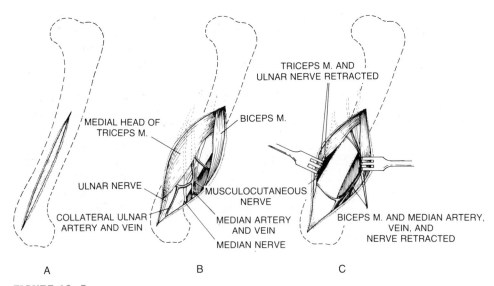

FIGURE 10–5

Medial open approach to shaft of humerus. (A) Longitudinal skin incision over distomedial surface of humerus. (B, C) By careful blunt dissection, the triceps muscles are reflected caudally and the biceps muscle is reflected cranially. Vessels and nerves are usually retracted with the muscles.

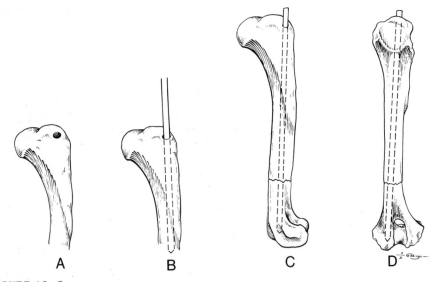

FIGURE 10–6

Internal fixation with an intramedullary pin. (A, B) The Steinmann pin is inserted from the proximal end by entering the skin and bone in an oblique fashion just lateral to the ridge of the greater tuberosity of the humerus. (C) After the bony anchorage is secured in the outer cortex, the pin is directed distally in the marrow cavity. (D, E) The pin is directed to pass along the medial cortex of the shaft and anchors well down in the medial condyle. Care must be taken that the pin is not too large to pass through the medial epicondylar area. If too large, it will break through into the elbow joint.

near its base (Fig. 10–6A, B). (Note that the pin enters near the base of the curve.) After bony anchorage is secured in the outer cortex, the pin is directed distally in the marrow cavity to pass along the medial cortex of the shaft and anchors well down in the medial condyle (Fig. 10–6C, D).

INTRAMEDULLARY PIN AND AUXILIARY FIXATION ■ The intramedullary pin may be used in combination with other methods of fixation in unstable fractures. Following an open approach, the fracture is first reduced, and the intramedullary pin is inserted in the proximal segment. During insertion of the pin into the distal segment, the two segments are held firmly in the reduced position with one or two self-locking bone forceps. Allowing one segment to rotate on the other during insertion results in a loose-fitting pin. In order to ensure passage of the pin down into the medial condyle, the bone fragments are bowed slightly medially at the fracture site. The auxiliary fixation is applied next.

The methods of auxiliary fixation are as follows:

1. Cerclage wires (Fig. 10–7A).
2. Hemicerclage wires (Fig. 10–7B).
3. Orthopedic stainless steel wire inserted to secure the cortical fragments to each other and the intramedullary pin at the fracture site (interfragmentary wire) (Fig. 10–7C).
4. Lag screw fixation (Fig. 10–7D).
5. Two or more intramedullary pins (Fig. 10–7E).
6. External fixator, 1/1 pins for stable fractures (Fig. 10–7F). The 2/2 pins configuration is used on unstable fractures.

UNILATERAL EXTERNAL FIXATOR ■ This splint may be used on most types of fractures; however, it is most commonly used on multiple and open fractures. The splint is placed on the craniolateral surface of the bone. If the distal segment is too

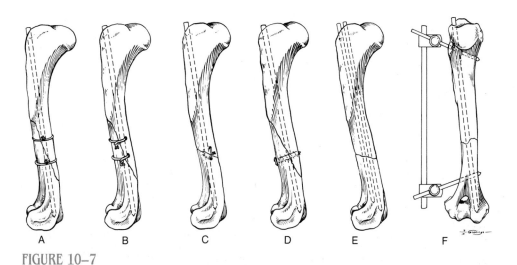

A   B   C   D   E   F

FIGURE 10–7

Intramedullary pin and auxiliary fixation. (A) Cerclage wires. (B) Hemicerclage wires. (C) An orthopedic wire secures cortical fragments to each other and the intramedullary pin at fracture site. (D) Lag screw fixation. (E) Use of two pins. (F) Unilateral external fixator, 1/1 pins.

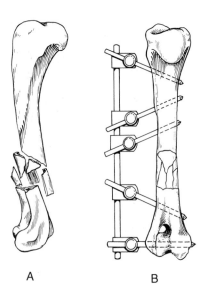

A   B

FIGURE 10–8

(A) Multiple fracture of the distal third of the humeral shaft. (B) External fixator, 3/2 pins. The distal pin is usually inserted first in the transcondylar position. The proximal pin is inserted next, followed by application of connecting bar and clamps, then the three center pins.

short to allow the placement of two fixation pins proximal to the supratrochlear foramen (see Fig. 1–14C), the distal pin may be inserted in a transcondylar position (Fig. 10–8B).

Figure 10–8 shows a multiple fracture of the distal third of the humeral shaft. In Figure 10–8B, the external fixator is shown in place. The distal (threaded or smooth) pin is usually inserted first in the transcondylar position, immediately distal to the most prominent protuberance of the lateral and medial surface of the condyle. The proximal pin is inserted, followed next by application of the connecting bar and clamps, then by insertion of the three center pins. This placement of pins may be used when the distal segment is too short to accommodate two pins placed above the condyle; this technique also allows full range of movement of the elbow joint during the healing period.

BONE PLATE (COMPRESSION TYPE) ■ Bone plates are applicable to most types of shaft fractures, particularly in large dogs. In many cases, the plate may be applied on the cranial surface to advantage. The lateral surface has two disadvantages: marked curvature of the bone and location of the radial nerve and brachialis muscle. The plate must be placed under these structures.

A multiple fracture of the proximal humeral shaft is shown in Figure 10–9. Fixation is by application of a bone plate to the cranial surface. Screws that cross the fracture line are inserted with a lag effect through the plate.

Figure 10–10 shows a midshaft humeral fracture with a caudal butterfly segment. The butterfly segment is first reduced with the proximal segment and fixed with a lag screw (Fig. 10–10B). The distal segment is next reduced and attached with a second lag screw. A neutralization plate is applied to the cranial surface (Fig. 10–10C). A neutralization plate may be applied to the lateral surface (Fig. 10–10D), although the surgical exposure and application are more difficult because they must be placed under the brachialis muscle and radial nerve.

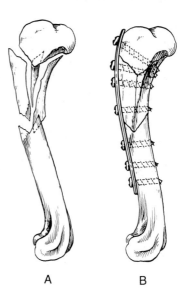

FIGURE 10-9

(A) Multiple fracture of the proximal humeral shaft. (B) Fixation by application of bone plate to cranial surface. Screws crossing the fracture line are inserted with a lag effect through the plate.

SUPRACONDYLAR FRACTURES

In supracondylar humeral fractures,[2-5] the fracture line may vary somewhat; however, it usually passes through the supratrochlear foramen. In young animals, the injury may be a combination fracture and physeal separation (a Salter-Harris Type II injury). Even though the fracture may be reduced closed, an open approach is usually indicated for the application of internal fixation.

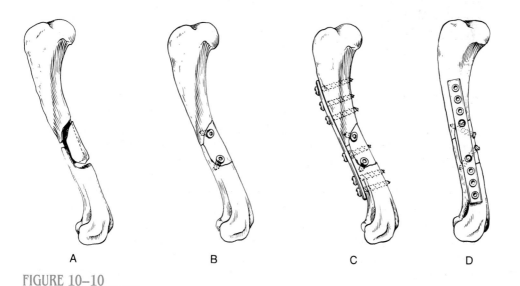

FIGURE 10-10

(A) Midshaft humeral fracture with a caudal butterfly segment. (B) The butterfly segment was first reduced with the proximal segment and fixed with a lag screw. The distal segment was next reduced and attached with a second lag screw. (C) Neutralization plate applied to cranial surface. (D) A neutralization plate may be applied to the lateral surface, although surgical exposure and contouring the plate may be more difficult.

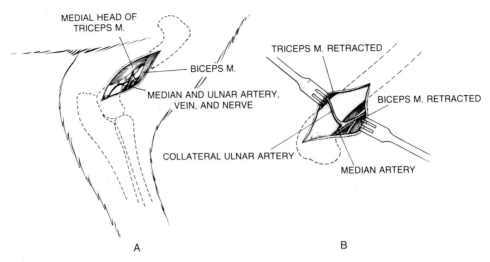

FIGURE 10–11

Open reduction of a supracondylar fracture, medial approach. (A) Longitudinal incision through skin and fascia over medial surface of distal end of humerus. (B) Fracture site exposed by blunt dissection between biceps and triceps muscles.

Best results are obtained by using rigid internal fixation, which allows movement of the joint during the convalescent period.

Treatment

OPEN REDUCTION

The skin incision may be medial (Fig. 10–11), lateral (Fig. 10–12), or both, or a near-midline longitudinal incision on the caudal surface may be used. In

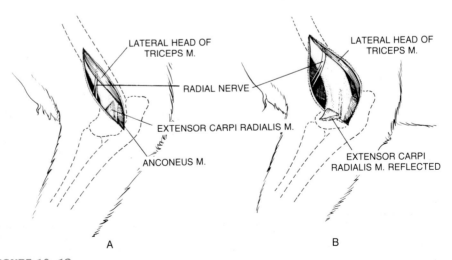

FIGURE 10–12

Open reduction of a supracondylar fracture, lateral approach. (A) Skin incision along lateral epicondyloid crest. (B) The lateral head of the triceps muscle is elevated caudally and the fracture site is exposed through separation of the extensor carpi radialis muscles.

most instances, both the medial and lateral incisions are used. In some multiple fractures in this area, the transolecranon (caudal) approach may give the best visualization and working area (see Fig. 10–20).

The exact method of fixation may be dictated by the individual fracture. Following are five suggestions:

1. Insert a double-pointed Steinmann pin retrograde through the shaft of the humerus along the medial cortex, reduce the fracture, and run the pin well into the medial aspect of the condyle. This type of fixation will allow rotation at the fracture site unless the fracture is serrated and interlocking on reduction (Fig. 10–13).

2. Insert a double-pointed Steinmann pin into the medial aspect of the condyle as just described. In addition, insert another pin (usually of a smaller diameter) from the lateral epicondyle across the fracture to anchor in the medial cortex of the humeral shaft proximal to the fracture line (Fig. 10–14A).

3. Insert a double-pointed Steinmann pin into the medial side of the

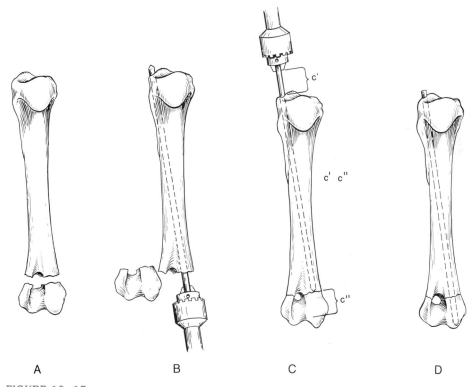

| A | B | C | D |

FIGURE 10–13

Placement of an intramedullary pin for a supracondylar fracture. *(A)* Fracture of the supracondylar type. *(B)* The fracture site is exposed from the medial side, and a double-pointed pin, started near the medial cortex, is inserted retrograde. *(C)* A pin chuck is attached at the proximal end at a distance (c′) that corresponds to the length of the condyle (c″). The fracture is reduced, and the elbow joint is extended prior to insertion. *(D)* Final position; if fracture segments do not interlock, rotation is possible at fracture site and supplemental fixation is indicated.

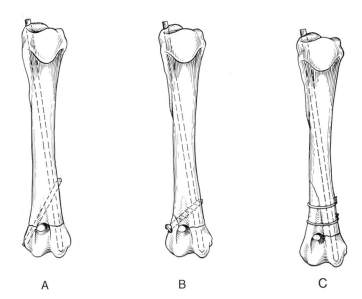

A   B   C

FIGURE 10–14

Intramedullary pin and auxiliary fixation for a supracondylar fracture. *(A)* An additional pin is inserted up the lateral epicondyle and penetrates the medial cortex. *(B)* A lag screw is inserted in addition to the pin. *(C)* Two cerclage wires are added for supplemental fixation.

condyle as in number 1, above. In addition, insert a bone screw with a lag effect starting on the lateral side and anchoring in the medial cortex of the humeral shaft. This will bring about compression at the fracture site. When applicable, this is the preferred method (Fig. 10–14B).

4. Insert a double-pointed Steinmann pin down into the medial condyle as described. In addition, insert one or more cerclage wires if the fracture is of the oblique type (Fig. 10–14C).

5. Insert Rush pins at the medial and lateral epicondyles and drive them simultaneously into the shaft of the humerus (Fig. 10–15).

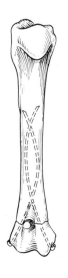

FIGURE 10–15

Two Rush pins give good stabilization.

Note: All methods of fixation allow movement of the joint during the convalescent period. Intramedullary pins are removed after the fracture reaches the stage of clinical union.

Aftercare ■ The incision area is usually covered with a well-padded dressing until the skin sutures are removed. In most cases, no additional fixation is required; however, it is best to limit activity during the healing period.

FRACTURES OF MEDIAL OR LATERAL ASPECT OF THE HUMERAL CONDYLE (UNICONDYLAR)

Fractures of the lateral portion occur much more frequently than fractures of the medial portion.[1-5] The lateral portion is the major weight-bearing part, and its smaller lateral supracondylar ridge makes it biomechanically weaker. The procedure for reduction and fixation will vary, depending on the length of time since injury, the amount of swelling and edema, and the ease with which the fragments can be palpated.

As a result of muscular pull, the prereduction radiograph will usually show the fractured lateral portion to be dislocated proximally and rotated laterally and cranially. The fractured medial epicondyle is usually rotated medially and caudally. Subluxation is present in the elbow joint.

Recent fractures of the lateral and medial aspect of the humeral condyle are shown in Figures 10–16*A* and 10–17*A*. Within the first 36 to 48 hours after injury, there is usually minimal swelling, and the fragment can be palpated.

Treatment

REDUCTION AND FIXATION

The fractured leg is placed in the Gordon extender (see Fig. 1–7) for 10 to 15 minutes to fatigue the muscles and overcome spastic contraction. While still in the Gordon extender, the leg is prepared and draped for surgery. By use of

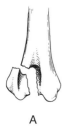
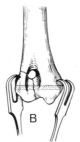
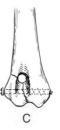
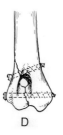

FIGURE 10–16

(A) Recent fracture of the lateral aspect of the humeral condyle. *(B)* In place of a condyle clamp, reduction may be maintained by use of a vulcellum or similar forceps. Area to accommodate transcondylar bone screw. *(C)* Bone screw insertion with lag effect. *(D)* Insertion of additional bone screw proximal to the supratrochlear foramen adds to stability.

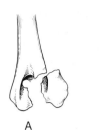
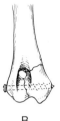
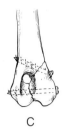

A   B   C

FIGURE 10–17

(A) Recent fracture of the medial aspect of the humeral condyle. *(B)* Bone screw insertion with lag effect. *(C)* Insertion of additional bone screw proximal to the supratrochlear foramen adds to stability.

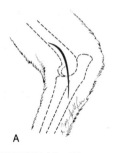
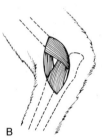
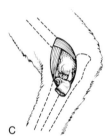
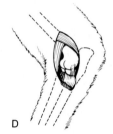

A   B   C   D

FIGURE 10–18

Craniolateral approach to the canine elbow. *(A)* Skin incision over the lateral aspect of the humeral condyle. *(B)* Reflection of skin exposes the lateral head of the triceps, extensor carpi radialis, and brachialis muscles. *(C)* The lateral head of the triceps muscle retracted caudally and the distal aspect of the extensor carpi radialis is incised and retracted distally, exposing the joint capsule and lateral collateral ligament. *(D)* The joint capsule (not shown) is incised, exposing the humeral condyle.

FIGURE 10–19

Condyle clamp maintains reduction during fixation procedure. The holes in the clamp are centered approximately on the palpable points of the medial and lateral epicondyles.

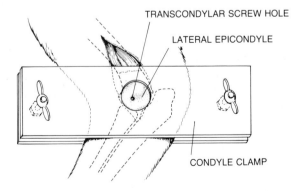

TRANSCONDYLAR SCREW HOLE

LATERAL EPICONDYLE

CONDYLE CLAMP

a lateral or medial approach (see Figs. 10–11 and 10–12), the fracture area is exposed. A craniolateral approach has also been described and reported as giving good visualization and excellent clinical results[7] (Fig. 10–18). The fracture is reduced, and a condyle clamp or vulsellum-type forceps (self-retaining type) is applied (Figs. 10–19 and 10–16B). A condyle clamp or similar instrument is essential to maintain reduction during the fixation procedure. The holes in the clamp are centered approximately on the palpable points of the medial and lateral epicondyles. The points of entry and exit of the transcondylar hole to be drilled are immediately below these two points.

The screw hole is started by a trocar-pointed pin, then enlarged with a drill of the appropriate size to accommodate the bone screw. The bone screw is inserted. Compression at the fracture site may be obtained by using a cancellous bone screw or a cortical bone screw inserted with a lag effect (Figs. 10–16C and 10–17B). In the very immature dog, minimal or no compression is advisable because of crushing of soft bone and possible physeal compression.

For longer-standing fractures of the lateral or medial epicondyle, if the fragments cannot be accurately palpated or reduced or if the fracture is more than 48 hours old, this procedure is modified by performing a transolecranon approach[6, 8] (Fig. 10–20) or a craniolateral approach[7] (Fig. 10–18) to expose the fracture site. When the patient is very young, a triceps tenotomy is advisable in preference to an osteotomy of the olecranon process.[9] Blood clots or soft tissue between the fracture segments is removed. Following reduction, a vulsellum or similar self-retaining forceps is applied, and a transcondylar lag screw is inserted.

The insertion of an additional bone screw proximal to the supratrochlear foramen is highly advisable because it adds to stability, particularly in large dogs (see Figs. 10–16D and 10–17C). Small threaded pins may be used on the toy breeds that are too small for bone screws. Small vulsellum forceps is used to obtain compression during the insertion procedure.

Aftercare ■ Additional stabilization, when indicated, may be accomplished by the application of a Robert Jones dressing. During the healing period, exercise should be allowed, but limited. The bone screw may be removed in the young growing animal (up to approximately 4 months of age), but it is usually left in place in those over this age unless otherwise indicated.

BICONDYLAR (INTERCONDYLAR) FRACTURES— T OR Y FRACTURES OF THE CONDYLE

This type of fracture occurs most frequently in mature animals and usually results from trauma exerting torsional stress.[1–5, 11] The spaniel breeds are particularly prone to this fracture. Spastic contractions of the muscles of the foreleg pull the ulna and radius proximally between the fractured medial and lateral portions of the condyle.

Treatment

Perfect anatomical reduction of the fractured articular surfaces with uninterrupted rigid fixation and movement of the elbow is mandatory for the best

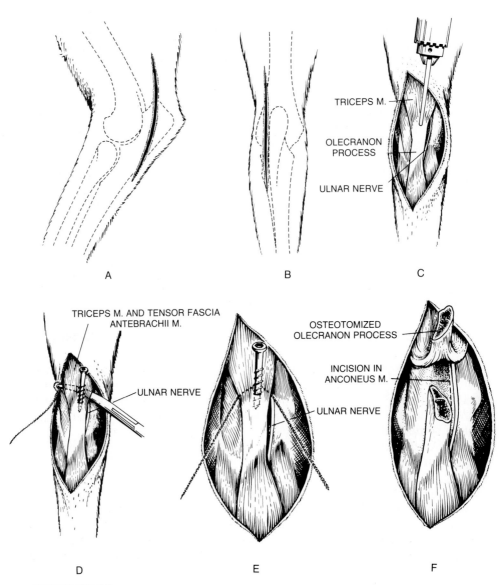

FIGURE 10–20

Transolecranon (caudal) approach for supracondylar, unicondylar, or bicondylar fractures. *(A, B)* Longitudinal skin incision on caudolateral aspect of elbow. *(C)* The skin and fascia are reflected both medially and laterally to expose olecranon process, insertion of the triceps muscle, and condyle of the humerus. A hole is drilled through the olecranon process and into the marrow cavity of the ulna to a depth sufficient for insertion of a bone screw. The ulnar nerve (medial side) is located and isolated. *(D)* Starting from the medial surface, the separation between the triceps and tensor fasciae antebrachii muscles and the anconeus muscle is developed. *(E)* Olecranon process transected with a Gigli wire or bone saw. *(F)* The transected olecranon process and its muscle attachments are reflected proximally as a unit.

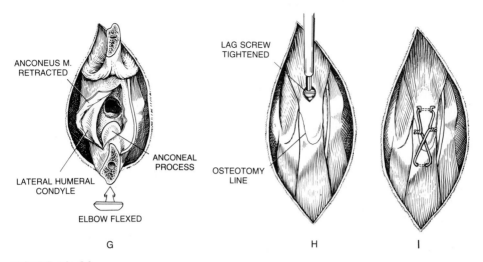

LAG SCREW
TIGHTENED

ANCONEUS M.
RETRACTED

ANCONEAL
PROCESS

OSTEOTOMY
LINE

LATERAL HUMERAL
CONDYLE

ELBOW FLEXED

G   H   I

FIGURE 10–20

Continued (G) Attachment of anconeus muscle and joint capsule severed from the medial supracondylar ridge and reflected laterally. *(H)* Closure by reattachment of the anconeus muscle and replacement of the osteotomized olecranon process. The lag screw may be further supported by a tension band wire. *(I)* The olecranon process may also be attached by use of two Kirschner wires and a tension band wire.

functional results. This type of fracture is one of the most challenging to repair in veterinary medicine; any errors in reduction and fixation lead to decreased range of movement, abnormal wear, and joint degenerative changes. More conservative methods, such as the application of a modified Thomas splint or cast, result in an unreduced fracture, marked decrease in range of movement following healing, and abnormal wear, giving rise to secondary osteoarthritis changes.

OPEN REDUCTION

The transolecranon (caudal) approach usually gives the best visualization of the fracture area.[6, 8] This approach gives good exposure of the caudal surface of the distal end of the humerus, including the condyle, trochlea, and anconeal process. This technique may also be used to expose the area for corrective surgery on complicated fractures of the humeral condyle or for a dislocated elbow.

Two other approaches that may be used are (1) proximal ulnar osteotomy[11] and (2) triceps tenotomy.[10] The latter is usually reserved for use in small dogs and cats.

In cats, two anatomical differences are to be noted when making surgical approaches in this area:

1. The median nerve passes through the supratrochlear foramen.
2. The ulnar nerve lies under the short portion of the medial head of the triceps muscle.

REDUCTION AND FIXATION

The transolecranon approach is performed as described previously. Following removal of the organizing clot and fibrin, the epicondyles are reduced and temporarily held by one or two vulsellum or similar forceps (Fig. 10–21A). The addition of one or two transverse Kirschner wires dorsally or cranially increases stability for drilling. The hole is drilled for insertion of the transcondylar bone screw. This hole may be drilled directly from the lateral or medial surface (Fig. 10–21A) or from the fracture surface (Fig. 10–21B).

Before the transcondylar hole is drilled, there should be perfect anatomical reduction of the articular cartilages of the humeral condyle along the fracture lines. The humeral condylar and humeral shaft should be checked for good approximation of the fracture site. Less than anatomical reduction may impinge the anconeal process, limit range of movement, or result in abnormal wear. The transcondylar bone screw is inserted with a lag effect (Fig. 10–21B, C).

Various methods may be used to reattach the condyle to the humeral shaft. The method is dictated to a certain extent by the fracture pattern, size of the animal, and the equipment available. The objective is rigid uninterrupted fixation that is capable of withstanding considerable abuse during the healing period. Documentation studies on T and Y fractures of the humerus indicate that less than adequate fixation in this area is the most frequent cause of failure.[1] Bone plate fixation gives the highest percentage of successful results.[1]

In most cases, it is advantageous to carry out the reduction and fixation as described. In some cases, however, it may be advantageous to first reduce and fix one of the epicondyles to the humeral shaft and to then reduce the remaining epicondyle and insert the transcondylar bone screw.

Figure 10–21 presents some suggested methods of fixation. The condyles are secured by vulsellum forceps, and a lag screw is inserted (Fig. 10–21A, B). An intramedullary pin is inserted in retrograde fashion at the fracture site

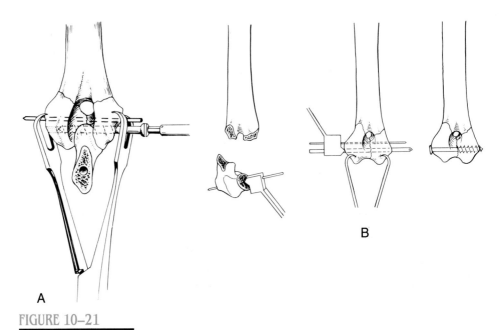

FIGURE 10–21

Methods of fixation for bicondylar fracture. Reduction is usually maintained during the fixation procedure by use of a vulsellum forceps and transcondylar Kirschner wire. (A) The hole may be drilled and the screw inserted directly from the medial or lateral surface or (B) from the fracture surface. The Kirschner wire is usually removed after lag screw insertion.

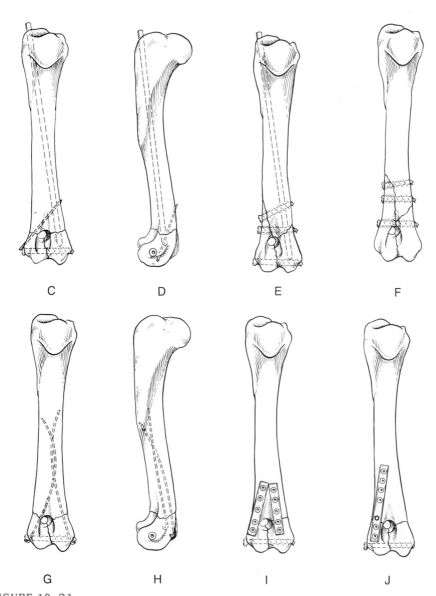

FIGURE 10–21

Continued (C, D) Intramedullary pin inserted retrograde fashion at fracture site and driven into medial aspect of the condyle. An additional pin, inserted just distal to the lateral epicondylar ridge and directed obliquely across fracture through medial cortex of the shaft, gives good two-point fixation in stable type fractures. *(E)* An intramedullary pin in combination with lag screws gives interfragmentary compression. *(F)* If the arms of the Y fracture are relatively long, they may be attached using lag screws. *(G, H)* Fixation using two Rush pins. *(I)* Fixation using two small bone plates in large dogs for comminuted (unstable) fractures. *(J)* Fixation using one bone plate inserted along the medial epicondylar ridge and shaft.

and is then driven into the medial epicondyle (Fig. 10–21C, D). An additional pin is inserted just distal to the lateral epicondylar ridge and directed diagonally across the fracture and through the medial cortex of the shaft. This gives good two-point fixation if the fracture is of the stable type.

An intramedullary pin can also be used in combination with one or more lag screws (Fig. 10–21E). This gives interfragmentary compression and is preferable to the use of a diagonal pin when applicable. If the arms of the Y fracture are relatively long, they may be attached using several lag screws (Fig. 10–21F). Fixation can also be accomplished using two Rush pins (Fig. 10–21G, H), two small bone plates (Fig. 10–21I), or one larger bone plate inserted along the medial epicondylar ridge and shaft (Fig. 10–21J). The last is usually the method of choice.

Aftercare ■ A modified Robert Jones dressing is applied with the leg in the angulation of the standing position. This is left in place for 3 to 7 days. Exercise is limited during the healing period, and the intramedullary pin is removed after healing. Concomitant fixation is left in place unless indicated otherwise.

REFERENCES

1. Brinker WO: Fracture Documentation Studies at Michigan State University. Unpublished data, 1971–1978.
2. Brinker WO: Fractures in Canine Surgery, 2nd Archibald ed. Santa Barbara, American Veterinary Publications, Inc, 1974, pp 949–1048.
3. Brinker WO: Small Animal Fractures. East Lansing, MI, Depart Cont Ed Press, Michigan State University, 1978.
4. Brinker WO, Hohn RB, Prieur WD: Manual of Internal Fixation in Small Animals. New York, Springer-Verlag, 1984, pp 134–144.
5. Bardet JF, Hohn RB, Olmstead ML: Fractures of the humerus in dogs and cats: a retrospective study of 130 cases. Vet Surg 12:73–77, 1983.
6. Piermattei DL: An Atlas of Surgical Approaches to the Bones of the Dog and Cat, 3rd ed. Philadelphia, WB Saunders Co, in preparation.
7. Turner TN, Hohn RB: Craniolateral approach to the canine elbow for repair of condylar fractures or joint exploration. J Am Vet Med Assoc 176:1264–1266, 1980.
8. Mostosky UV, Cholvin NR, Brinker WO: Transolecranon approach to the elbow joint. Vet Med 54:560, 1959.
9. Dueland R: Triceps tenotomy approach for distal fractures of the canine humerus. J Am Vet Med Assoc 167:82–86, 1974.
10. Lenehan TM, Nunamaker DM: Lateral approach to the canine elbow by proximal diaphyseal osteotomy. J Am Vet Med Assoc 180:523–530, 1982.
11. Matthiesen DT, Walter M: Surgical management of distal humeral fractures. Comp Cont Ed 6:1027–1036, 1984.

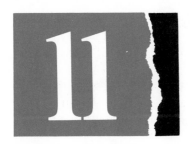

Fractures of the Radius and Ulna

All types of fractures can be seen involving either or both the radius and ulna. The development of angulation and rotation at the fracture site, delayed union, and nonunion are not uncommon sequelae, and measures to prevent them should be kept in mind constantly.

CLASSIFICATION

Fractures of the radius and ulna may be classified as follows:[1, 2]

1. Fracture of the proximal ulna, involving the trochlear notch or olecranon.
2. Fracture of the proximal radial epiphysis.
3. Fracture of the proximal ulna and dislocation of the radius.
   a. Fracture of the proximal ulna with dislocation of the radial head and remaining ulna.
   b. Fracture of the proximal ulna with dislocation of the radial head and separation of the radius and ulna (Monteggia fracture).
4. Shaft fractures.
5. Fractures of the distal radius and ulna.
   a. Fracture of the distal articular region or styloid processes.
   b. Fracture at the distal epiphysis of the radius.

FRACTURE OF THE PROXIMAL ULNA INVOLVING THE TROCHLEAR NOTCH OR OLECRANON

Following a fracture, the pull of the triceps muscles lifts the fracture segments proximally and bends the ulna toward the shaft of the humerus (Fig. 11–1A). For best results, this pull should be equalized by use of the tension band principle. In general, the tension band wire is used on stable fractures, and a plate is used for unstable fractures.[1–4]

Surgical Procedure

A longitudinal skin incision is made just off the midline along the caudal surface of the proximal ulna. By blunt dissection or subperiosteal reflection,

195

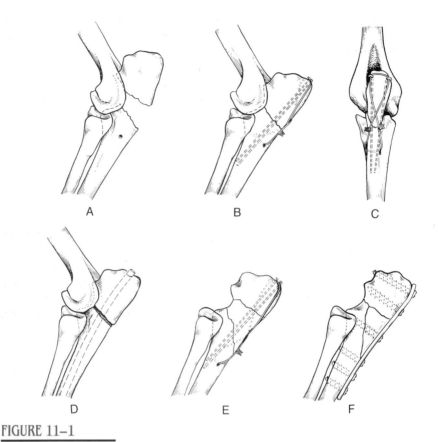

FIGURE 11–1

(A) Transverse fracture of the olecranon process. *(B, C)* Fixation using two Kirschner wires and a figure-8 tension band wire works very well on stable fractures involving the articular surface. *(D)* Fixation with a smooth intramedullary pin alone is inadequate; as the proximal segment slides proximally, a gap develops at the fracture site and delayed union or nonunion results. With a fracture in this location, pins or screws used alone are subject to bending or fatigue fracture. *(E)* Fractures involving the articular surface must be anatomically reduced and may be stabilized using the tension band wire if they are stable on reduction. *(F)* In large dogs or in comminuted fractures (unstable fractures), the semitubular or dynamic compression plate (DCP) may be used as a tension band. In some comminuted fractures, it may be advantageous to place the plate on the lateral surface of the ulna.

the fracture site and the shaft of the ulna about 1″ distal to it are exposed. The fracture is reduced. If the articular surface is involved, anatomic reduction is mandatory for restoration of good joint function.

Two Kirschner drill wires are started in the proximal end near the caudal edge of the olecranon process and are driven distally into the shaft of the ulna. They are directed to engage the cranial cortex of the ulna distal to the trochlear notch in preference to going directly down the marrow cavity because this may not adequately prevent rotation (Fig. 11–1B). A transverse hole is drilled through the distal ulna below the fracture line.

A figure-8 wire connects the protruding pins on the proximal end with the hole that was drilled transversely in the distal segment. It is important to place the wire through the triceps tendon, directly on the bone rather than over the surface of the tendon. The top protruding portions of the pins are bent over caudally in hook fashion, cut off, and rotated 180° cranially into the triceps insertion. With this type of fixation, the Kirschner wires guard against rotation and shear forces at the fracture line, and the figure-8 wire transforms tension force into compression. Small plates can function as tension bands in larger breeds and are especially useful in comminuted fractures (Fig. 11–1F).

Aftercare ■ In most cases, no additional fixation is required. Activity should be limited during the healing period. The pins and wire should be removed if there is any indication of irritation or loosening after the fracture is healed.

FRACTURE OF THE PROXIMAL RADIAL EPIPHYSIS

The radial head is rarely fractured. It may or may not be accompanied by dislocation of the elbow joint.[1–3] There is usually history of trauma. Separation at the physeal plate always threatens to disturb growth. Anatomic reduction and fixation are indicated.

Figure 11–2 shows an epiphyseal fracture-separation of the radial head. Simple Kirschner wire fixation is used. If closed reduction cannot be accomplished, opening is indicated. Healing is rapid, and the wire is removed in 2 to 3 weeks. A light Robert Jones dressing may be indicated for temporary additional support. Premature closure of the physis and shortening of the radius are not uncommon sequelae (Chapter 14).

FRACTURE OF THE PROXIMAL ULNA AND DISLOCATION OF THE RADIUS

Fracture of the Proximal Ulna and Dislocation of the Radial Head and Remaining Portion of the Ulna

In this type of fracture, the dislocated portion is usually cranial and proximal in relation to the joint. If the fracture is relatively recent in origin, a closed reduction often can be accomplished by a combination of traction and countertraction along with caudal pressure on the radius to manipulate the radial head back into the reduced position. Internal fixation may be accomplished by inserting a pin from the proximal end of the olecranon process into the shaft of the ulna.

In some cases, it may be necessary to perform an open approach to

FIGURE 11–2

(A) Epiphyseal fracture of the radial head. (B) Simple Kirschner wire fixation. The wires enter the bone near the joint surface and proceed distally and diagonally.

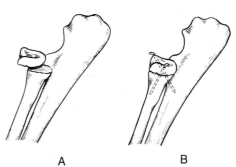

A   B

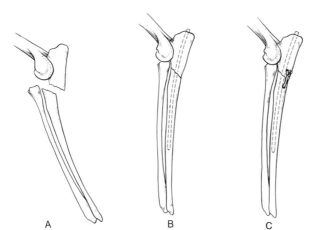

FIGURE 11–3

(A) Fracture of ulna with dislocation of the radial head. (B) Immobilization by use of an intramedullary pin in the ulna and a coaptation splint. (C) The addition of a hemicerclage wire improves stability at the fracture site.

accomplish accurate reduction. The pin in the ulna may be inserted either from the proximal end or by use of the retrograde technique. If indicated, a hemicerclage wire may be inserted in the ulna for additional stabilization and compression (Fig. 11–3). If temporary additional external support is indicated, it may be in the form of a modified Robert Jones dressing. Exercise is restricted during the healing period.

Fracture of the Proximal Ulna with Dislocation of the Radial Head and Separation of the Radius and Ulna (Monteggia Fracture)

The radius and ulna are separated as a result of rupture of the radial annular ligament.[1–5] Frequently, there is soft tissue (usually one or more of the extensor muscles) interposed between the two bones. An open approach may be necessary to accomplish reduction.

The usual procedure is to repair the ulnar fracture (with a bone plate or intramedullary pin) and to then suture the annular ligament to restore and maintain apposition of the radius and ulna (Fig. 11–4A, B). If suturing the annular ligament is not possible, apposition between the radius and ulna can be accomplished by the use of several bone screws (Fig. 11–4C). Ordinarily, this procedure should not be used in the young growing animal because it interferes with normal shifting of the ulna on the radius in the growing process and may result in incongruency of the elbow joint and/or radius curvus. It should also not be used on members of the feline family because supination and pronation are a part of the normal function of the foreleg. If it is used out of necessity, the screws should be removed 3 to 4 weeks postoperatively to allow return of normal motion between the radius and ulna.

FRACTURES OF THE RADIAL AND ULNAR SHAFTS

A high percentage of the fractures involving the shaft of the radius and ulna occur in the middle and distal thirds with both bones involved.[1–3] However,

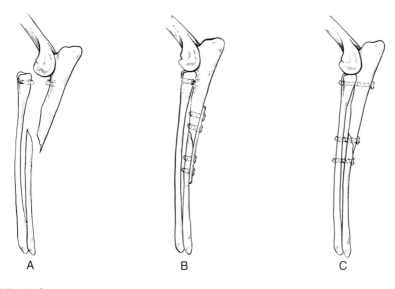

FIGURE 11–4

(A) Monteggia fracture. (B) Repair by immobilizing the ulna with a bone plate and suturing the annular ligament. (C) Fixation by use of bone screws. The ulna is fixed to the radius.

these fractures occur at all levels and include all types; in a few cases, they may involve only the radius or ulna.

The development of angulation, rotation, delayed union, and nonunion at the fracture site are not uncommon sequelae when the bones are handled improperly. Two of the more common mistakes are using fixation methods that allow rotation at the fracture site and removing the fixation device before the callus becomes sufficiently mature for weight-bearing. Shaft fractures that are unstable or those involving the proximal third of the radius and ulna should be immobilized with rigid internal fixation because a coaptation splint or cast does not satisfactorily eliminate internal movement or rotation.

The most frequently used methods of stabilization for diaphyseal fractures of the radius and ulna are:[1-7]

1. External coaptation splint or cast. This is usually limited to green-stick and stable fractures of the young animal.
2. External fixator with or without supplemental internal fixation.
3. Plates with or without supplemental internal fixation.

Treatment

CLOSED REDUCTION AND EXTERNAL FIXATION

Green-stick and stable fractures in the young and intraperiosteal fractures respond well to external fixation, usually in the form of a plaster of Paris or fiberglass cast, coaptation splint, or Thomas splint. Any time an external splint is applied, it should be checked periodically, and the animal's activity should be limited. With unlimited activity, external splints may become loose or cause development of ulcerated areas.

Stable fractures usually respond to external fixation. Reduction may be accomplished closed by a combination of traction, countertraction, and digital manipulation. In many instances, open reduction is preferable to closed manipulation, which may cause an undue amount of trauma to tissue in the fracture site.

There is a tendency for the carpus to hyperextend, develop valgus deviation, and rotate outward postoperatively (owing to loss of tone in the flexor muscle group). The position of the foot on standing and walking while favoring the leg is also a factor. To prevent this unfavorable development when an external splint is used, the foot should be placed in a position of slight varus, flexion, and inward rotation. Ordinarily, this can be accomplished best with a plaster of Paris or similar molded cast.

SPLINTING ■ As the sole method of fixation, the use of a Thomas splint, Mason metasplint, or similar coaptation splint is limited to the more stable and more distal fractures (e.g., green-stick and certain intraperiosteal fractures). Many splints have a tendency to loosen and need constant rechecking to make sure they are accomplishing the intended objective. For complete fractures, the position of slight varus, flexion, and inward rotation is difficult or impossible to obtain and maintain when these splints are used. It is also difficult and may be impossible to immobilize the joint adequately above and below the fracture.

CASTS ■ In stable fractures, a plaster of Paris or similar molded cast may be used as the sole method of fixation. If a cast is used on an unstable fracture, overriding frequently develops at the fracture site. Overpadding inside the cast allows for torsional movement at the fracture site and may result in delayed union, nonunion, or malunion.

If the cast is applied when the leg is swollen, looseness and instability may result if the cast is not readjusted. Casts are frequently used as supplemental fixation along with various internal fixation devices. Figure 11–5 illustrates the principle of location of fracture vs. length of cast for applying a plaster of Paris or fiberglass cast.

OPEN APPROACH

The main indications for the open approach[1, 2, 8] are as follows:

1. When reduction by closed methods is difficult or impossible.

2. When there is difficulty in maintaining reduction in the process of applying fixation. (Viewing the fracture site during this process is most helpful.)

3. When internal fixation is applied. The choice of approach may vary, depending on the location of the fracture and the objective to be accomplished.

CRANIOMEDIAL APPROACH TO THE RADIUS [1, 2, 8] ■ In most instances, this is the preferred approach because the radius is subcutaneous in this area and can be exposed with a minimum of hemorrhage. Figure 11–6 illustrates this technique.

CRANIOLATERAL APPROACH TO THE RADIUS AND ULNA [1, 2, 8] ■ (See Figure 11–7.)

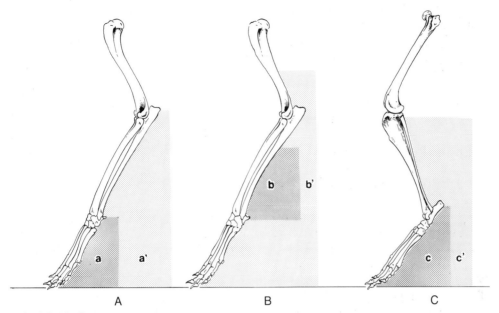

FIGURE 11–5

Application of a plaster of Paris or fiberglass cast. (A) Stable fractures of the carpus or foot (a) may be immobilized with a cast extending to the top of the olecranon process caudally and slightly below the elbow joint cranially to allow use of the elbow joint (a'). (B) Stable fractures of the ulna and radius (b) may be immobilized with a cast extending to the midhumeral region (b'). (C) Stable fractures of the tarsus (c) may be immobilized with a cast extending to the proximal tibial region (c').

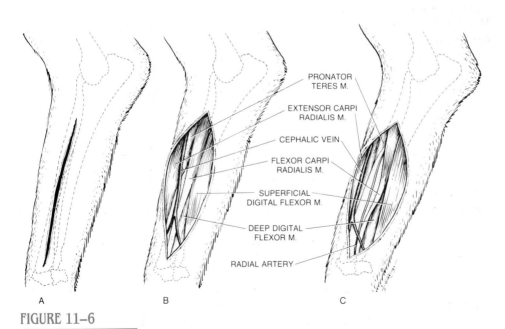

PRONATOR
TERES M.

EXTENSOR CARPI
RADIALIS M.

CEPHALIC VEIN

FLEXOR CARPI
RADIALIS M.

SUPERFICIAL
DIGITAL FLEXOR M.

DEEP DIGITAL
FLEXOR M.

RADIAL ARTERY

FIGURE 11–6

Craniomedial approach to the shaft of the radius. (A) The skin is incised longitudinally along the craniomedial border of the radius; right leg shown. (B, C) The large cephalic vein along the cranial border and the small radial artery and vein along the caudal border of the radius should be avoided. The extensor carpi radialis muscle is located cranially, and the pronator teres and flexor carpi radialis muscles are located caudally.

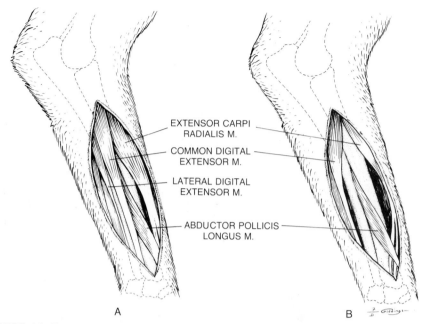

EXTENSOR CARPI
RADIALIS M.

COMMON DIGITAL
EXTENSOR M.

LATERAL DIGITAL
EXTENSOR M.

ABDUCTOR POLLICIS
LONGUS M.

A   B

FIGURE 11-7

Craniolateral approach to the shaft of the radius and ulna. (A) Longitudinal incision is made through the skin and fascia along the craniolateral border of the radius; right leg shown. (B) The common and lateral digital extensor muscles are separated, exposing the radius and portions of the ulna. In comparison to the craniomedial approach, more hemorrhage is encountered in this approach as there are usually many small vessels traversing the area.

CAUDAL APPROACH TO THE ULNA ■ The caudal border of the ulna can be palpated subcutaneously. The skin and fascia are incised longitudinally along the shaft. The flexor carpi ulnaris and deep digital flexor muscles are separated to expose the fracture site. Subperiosteal reflection of the origin of the flexor carpi ulnaris muscle can be used to expose the trochlear notch.

INTERNAL FIXATION

Following open reduction, some stable fractures may be immobilized by external methods. All unstable fractures and most of the stable fractures respond best to internal fixation.

EXTERNAL FIXATOR ■ This splint is adaptable to most shaft fractures of the radius and ulna. It is particularly indicated in open fractures, delayed unions, nonunions, and corrective osteotomies. The splint works particularly well with small dogs. In most instances, the pins are inserted on the medial or craniomedial border of the radius because the bone is more superficial in this location and the splint is in the position of least interference from cages, fences, and so forth.

All of the various configurations (unilateral, bilateral, biplanar) may be used. In the author's experience, however, the unilateral is adequate in almost all cases, is the simplest to apply, and has the fewest complications. This

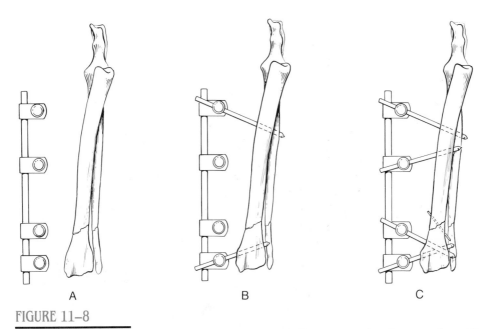

FIGURE 11-8

Applying an external fixator with one connecting bar and all pins inserted in the same plane. *(A)* The fracture is openly reduced and held with locking forceps; a connecting bar with four single clamps is prepared. *(B)* The proximal and distal pins are inserted in the same plane; the connecting bar and outer clamps are attached. *(C)* Middle clamps are positioned; the two inside pins are inserted through holes in the middle clamps. The nuts on the clamps are securely tightened. In some cases, an additional obliquely directed Kirschner wire is inserted to give more stability at the fracture site. If the fracture pattern is a longer oblique, insertion of a lag screw is indicated.

method requires the placement of all pins in the same plane (Fig. 11–8). A comminuted fracture of radius and ulna with single-bar, external fixator, 3/3 pins is shown in Figure 11–9. Depending on the size of the animal and complexity of the fracture, 2/2, 3/3, or 4/4 pins may be used. On some of the very comminuted fractures, a biplanar configuration (one unilateral splint on medial surface and one on the cranial) may be indicated.

INTRAMEDULLARY PIN ■ Because the radius is relatively straight and both ends are completely covered with articular cartilage, the shaft is not as amenable to intramedullary pin fixation as are the other long bones. In small dogs, the pin may be used to assist in holding end-to-end alignment in stable fractures. In general, the pin that is inserted is too small to approximate the marrow cavity in size. There are better methods of fixation available.

These are several methods of insertion:

1. The pin is started at the styloid process, then continues up through the marrow cavity, Rush pin style (Fig. 11–10A).

2. The pin is inserted obliquely through the cranial cortex and marrow cavity of one segment into the marrow cavity of the other segment, Rush pin style (Fig. 11–10B).

3. The pin is inserted in the proximal segment and protrudes distally by ¼″. The distal segment is then telescoped over the protruding segment of the pin. This procedure is usually restricted for use in small dogs (Fig. 11–10C).

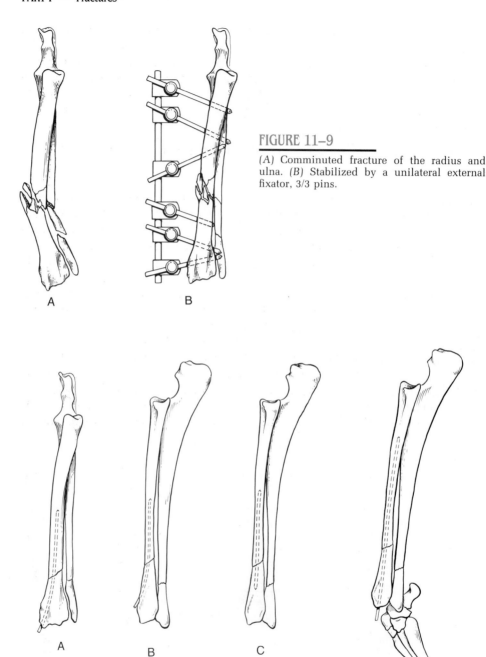

FIGURE 11–9

(A) Comminuted fracture of the radius and ulna. (B) Stabilized by a unilateral external fixator, 3/3 pins.

FIGURE 11–10

Insertion of intramedullary pins. (A) A pin is started at the styloid process, continuing up through the marrow cavity in a Rush pin style. (B) The pin is inserted obliquely through the cranial cortex and marrow cavity of one segment into the marrow cavity of the other segment in a Rush pin style. (C) Insertion of a pin in proximal segment with ¼" of pin protruding distally. The distal segment is then telescoped over the protruding segment of the pin. (D) With the antebrachiocarpal joint flexed, the pin entered from the distal end of the radius (not recommended). A, B, and C above need additional stability (e.g. external fixator, coaptation splint), since the intramedullary pins fit loosely in the marrow cavity.

A disadvantage of this method is that removal, if necessary, is difficult (e.g., in the presence of infection).

4. The antebrachiocarpal joint is flexed, and the pin is entered from the distal end of the radius (Fig. 11–10D). We do not recommend this method because the pin must enter at the articular border, and this may give rise to secondary joint complication at a later date (e.g., there may be loss of full extension and osteoarthritis.

In all cases, supplemental external fixation is essential during the healing period.

BONE SCREWS ■ Long oblique or spiral fractures of the radius and ulna may be stabilized with lag screws for holding alignment and exerting interfragmentary compression at the fracture site (Fig. 11–11A). This fixation must be supplemented with either external (coaptation splint) or internal fixation. Internal fixation may consist of a bone plate (Fig. 11–11B), an intramedullary pin in the ulna (Fig. 11–11C), or an external fixator (Fig. 11–11D). The latter may still need external splint support. Figure 11–11E illustrates a short distal fracture of the radius and ulna stabilized by applying a dynamic compression plate (DCP) on the medial surface of the radius.[7]

BONE PLATES ■ Plates are adaptable to most radial and ulnar shaft fractures.[1-7] The usual procedure is to plate the radius. If the radius is well stabilized, fixation of the ulna is usually unnecessary. In large dogs, it is generally recommended that small plates be placed on both the radius and ulna in preference to one large plate placed on the radius. The large plate may be too

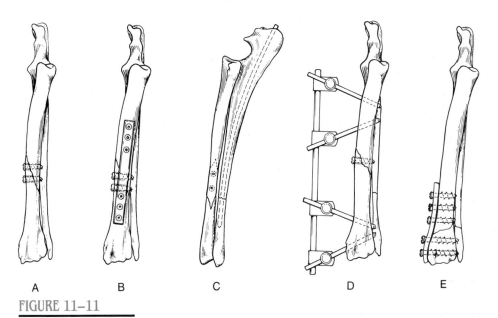

A   B   C   D   E

FIGURE 11–11

Bone screws. (A) Long oblique or spiral fractures of the radius and ulna may be stabilized by lag screws to hold alignment and to exert interfragmentary compression at the fracture site. Additional stabilization may consist of a coaptation splint, a plate (B), an intramedullary pin in the ulna (C), or an external fixator (D). Application of the plate on the medial surface of the radius serves very well on short distal fractures (E).

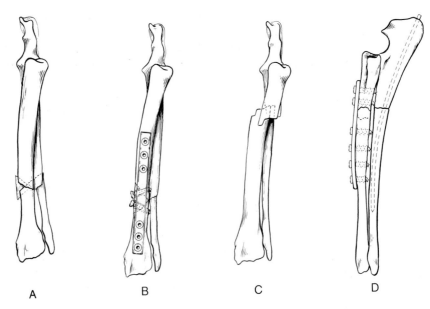

A   B   C   D

FIGURE 11–12

(A) Butterfly segment fracture of the radius with a fracture of the ulna. *(B)* Fixation with two lag screws and a neutralization plate on the radius. *(C)* Short oblique fracture near the proximal end of the radius and ulna in a German shepherd dog. *(D)* Fixation using a compression plate on the radius. Because the proximal segment is short and only two screws were used, additional fixation is possible by inserting an intramedullary pin in the ulna.

large to accomplish adequate soft tissue closure at the time of implantation, or it may interfere with movement of the extensor tendons.

Regular plates, DCPs, or semitubular plates may be used. The plate most frequently used is the DCP because it has the built-in potential of compression at the fracture site. A semitubular plate must be of sufficient size, and bending

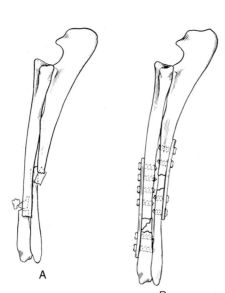

A   B

FIGURE 11–13

(A) Comminuted fracture of the radius and ulna in a large St. Bernard dog. *(B)* Fixation using two neutralization plates.

must be minimal in contouring it to fit the bone surface. See Chapter 1 for suggested plate size.

Figure 11–12A, B illustrates a butterfly segment fracture of the radius with a transverse fracture of the ulna. Figure 11–12C, D illustrates a short oblique fracture at the proximal third of the radius and ulna stabilized by a DCP on the radius and an intramedullary pin in the ulna. In Figure 11–13, a comminuted fracture of the radius and ulna is shown. Two neutralization plates are used. In large dogs, this procedure appears preferable to using one large plate on the radius.

FRACTURES OF THE DISTAL RADIUS AND ULNA

Fractures of the Styloid Process of the Radius

Fractures involving the styloid process give rise to instability of the antebrachiocarpal joint. Open reduction and internal fixation are indicated. In most cases, additional external support is indicated during the healing period (4 to 6 weeks).

Figure 11–14 presents examples of some of the various methods of fixation. In this oblique fracture of the radial styloid process, fixation may be done with two Kirschner wires, a tension band wire, or a lag screw.

Fracture of the Articular Surface of the Radius

Occasionally, fractures involve a central area of the distal radial articular surface. The principles of treating articular fractures dictate perfect anatomic reduction by means of an open approach and rigid internal fixation. Lag screws are used whenever possible, and Kirschner wires are used for fragments that are too small for lag screws.

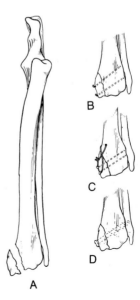

FIGURE 11–14

(A) Oblique fracture of the styloid process of the radius. Fixation by (B) two Kirschner wires, (C) a tension band wire, or (D) a lag screw.

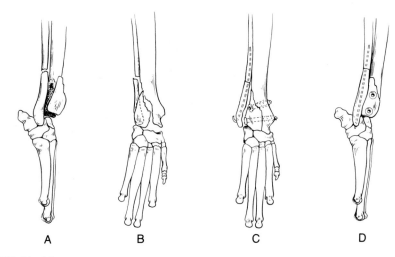

FIGURE 11–15

(A, B) Fracture of the lateral portion of the distal radius and distal ulna. *(C, D)* Lag screw fixation of the distal radius with 4.0-mm cancellous screws and Kirschner wire intramedullary fixation of the ulna. A coaptation splint is usually indicated for additional stability (4 to 6 weeks).

Figure 11–15 shows a fracture of the lateral portion of the distal radius and distal ulna. Lag screw and Kirschner wire intramedullary fixation is used, plus coaptation splinting for 4 to 6 weeks.

Fracture of the Ulnar Styloid

These fractures may occur in association with luxation or subluxation of the antebrachiocarpal joint (Fig. 11–16) or in isolation (Fig. 11–17). Because the

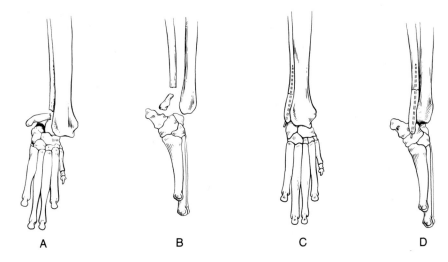

FIGURE 11–16

(A, B) Fracture of the ulnar styloid with palmar luxation of the antebrachiocarpal joint. *(C, D)* Intramedullary fixation of the styloid. If any ligaments and the joint capsule are ruptured, they are repaired and a coaptation splint is added.

FIGURE 11–17

(A) Fracture of the ulnar styloid. *(B, C)* Fixation with a Kirschner wire and tension band wire. Add a coaptation splint for stability, if indicated.

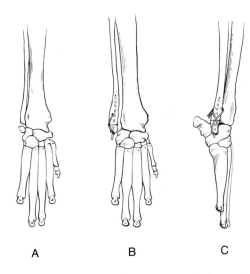

A   B   C

ulnar collateral ligaments originate on the styloid process, it is essential to fix these fractures to help stabilize the joint, especially in large, active animals. Supplemental external fixation is necessary.

REFERENCES

1. Brinker WO: Fractures in Canine Surgery, 2nd Archibald ed. Santa Barbara, American Veterinary Publications, Inc, 1974.
2. Brinker WO: Small Animal Fractures. East Lansing, MI, Depart Cont Ed Serv, Michigan State University, 1978.
3. Brinker WO, Hohn RB, Prieur WD: Manual of Internal Fixation in Small Animals. New York, Springer-Verlag, 1984.
4. Schwarz PD, Schrader SC: Ulnar fracture and dislocation of the proximal radial epiphysis (Monteggia lesion) in the dog and cat: a review of 28 cases. J Am Vet Med Assoc 185:190–194, 1984.
5. DeAngelus M, Olds RB, Stoll SE, et al: Repair of fractures of the radius and ulna in small dogs. J Am Anim Hosp Assoc 9:436–441, 1973.
6. Phillips IR: A survey of bone fractures in the dog and cat. J Small Anim Pract 20:661, 1979.
7. Tearse L: Fractures of distal radius and ulna. Breckenridge, CO, 15th Annual Conference of Veterinary Orthopedic Society, 1988.
8. Piermattei DL: An Atlas of Surgical Approaches to the Bones of the Dog and Cat, 3rd ed. Philadelphia, WB Saunders Co, in preparation.

12

Fractures of the Carpus, Metacarpus, and Phalanges

THE CARPUS

As with injuries to the tarsus, carpal injuries may consist of fractures, ligamentous injuries, and various combinations.[1] Fractures are covered in this chapter and ligamentous injuries are detailed in Chapter 21.

There are six carpal bones arranged in two rows, with three major joints. The bony anatomy of the forefoot is depicted in Figure 12–1, and the ligamentous structures are shown in Figure 21–34. Distal to the radius, the terms *cranial* and *caudal* are replaced by *dorsal* and *palmar*.

Fracture of the Radial Carpal Bone

Fractures of this bone, which, with the radius, forms the antebrachiocarpal joint—the major joint of the carpus—are usually manifested as chips or slabs off the articular surfaces[1] (Figs. 12–2, 12–3A, and 12–4). They are most often seen after injuries resulting from jumps or falls and in dogs undergoing heavy exertion such as sled dogs, field trial dogs, and other working breeds.

Fragments are apparently created by a compressive force combined with shear. There is little tendency for these fragments to heal spontaneously, and the bony or cartilaginous fragments usually become joint mice, creating an acute inflammatory reaction in the joint, leading to synovitis and degenerative joint disease. Lameness is severe but subsides somewhat in a few weeks. The dog may be sound when rested but becomes lame when exercised. Soft tissue thickening around the joint may become obvious after a few more weeks as a result of synovitis and arthritis.

Diagnosis requires a high index of suspicion because radiographs (non-screen film or high-detail screens) must be made in oblique planes and in flexion and extension to verify the fracture. Sometimes, only a unilateral arthrosis is seen, but if the history supports a traumatic cause, this is sufficient

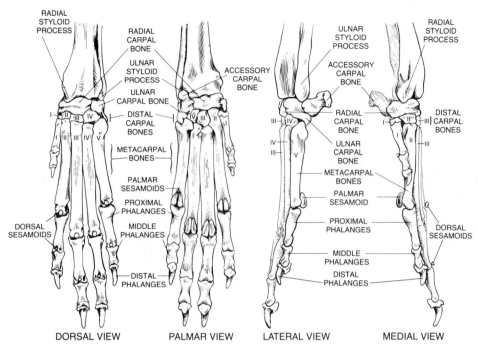

FIGURE 12–1

Bones of the carpus, metacarpus, and phalanges.

FIGURE 12–2

Comminuted dorsal slab fracture of the radial carpal bone. The fragments are excised in this type of injury.

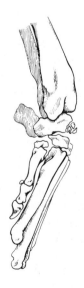

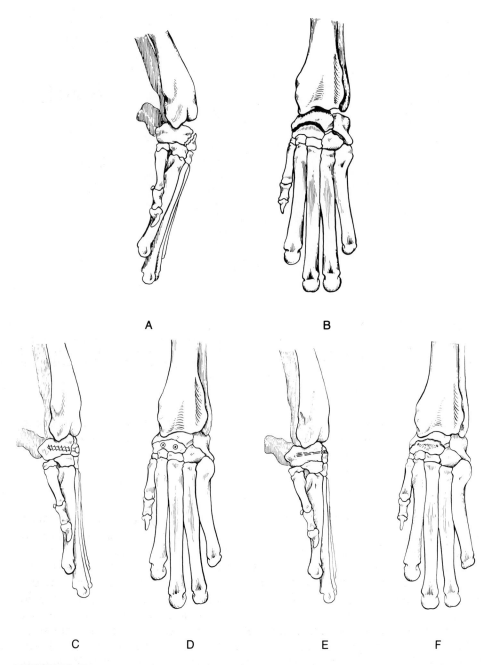

A   B

C   D   E   F

FIGURE 12–3

(A, B) Dorsal slab fracture of the radial carpal bone. (C, D) Two lag screws of 1.5- or 2-mm diameter are countersunk beneath the articular surface when the fragment is large enough. (E, F) Smaller fragments may be secured by two or more Kirschner wires countersunk beneath the surface of the articular cartilage or bone.

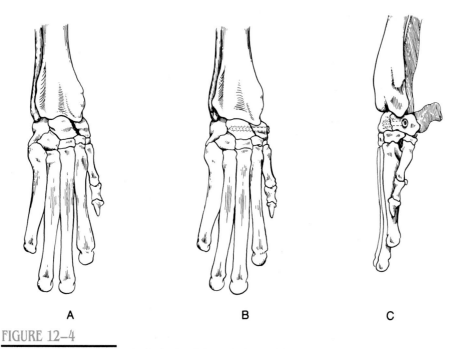

A   B   C

FIGURE 12–4

(A) Oblique fracture through the body of the radial carpal bone. (B, C) Lag screw fixation with a 2.7-, 3.5-, or 4.0-mm lag screw inserted from the medial surface of the bone. The screw is placed through the insertions of the radial collateral ligaments (see Figure 21–34). In this position, the screw head will not interfere with joint motion.

justification for exploration of the joint. Undisplaced fragments may reattach if the joint is splinted for 4 weeks. The prognosis is uncertain, however, and many patients require surgery later.

SURGICAL TECHNIQUE

Surgery may be performed with a tourniquet (see Figure 8–2), and most fractures can be exposed from a cranial approach.[2] Considerable synovial proliferation and inflammation may complicate the exposure. When the fragment is located, a decision is made to reattach or remove the fragment. To be reattached, the fragment must be large enough to handle; moreover, the fracture surfaces should not be severely eburnated, as may happen in a chronic fracture. If small screws are used, their heads must not interfere with any other structures (Figs. 12–3C, D and 12–4B, C). Kirschner wires countersunk below the level of the cartilage or bone are a most useful method (Fig. 12–3E, F). Stainless steel wire is occasionally useful in opposing fragments. Fragments are often excised because they cannot be reattached (Fig. 12–5). In this situation, the desired result is an adequate fibrocartilage scar to fill in the defect. Prognosis is usually good unless the bone is comminuted; this situation then usually calls for arthrodesis (see Figure 21–44).

Aftercare ■ A short molded palmar splint or short cast (see Figures 19–14 and 19–10) is applied for 3 to 4 weeks following fixation of the fragments. Exercise is limited for 6 to 8 weeks, until there is radiographic evidence of healing. If

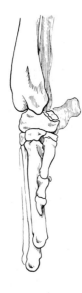

FIGURE 12-5

Fracture of the palmaromedial portion of the radial carpal bone (mediolateral view). Such fragments are simply excised because they are not on the main weight-bearing area of the bone.

the fragments are excised, the joint is rested in a similar splint for 10 days, after which light exercise is advisable through the fourth postoperative week.

Fracture of the Accessory Carpal Bone

Fractures of the accessory carpal bone are seen most commonly in the racing Greyhound but may be seen occasionally in most of the large breeds. Most fractures are self-induced avulsions (grade III sprains or strains; see Chapter 22), rather than caused by outside trauma. Johnson[3, 4] has described these fractures and proposed the following classification system:

CLASSIFICATION

INTRA-ARTICULAR FRACTURES

TYPE I, DISTAL BASILAR ■ Avulsion fracture of the distal margin of the articular surface at the origin of the accessoroulnar carpal ligaments (Fig. 12–6A).

TYPE II, PROXIMAL BASILAR ■ Avulsion fracture of the proximal margin at the insertion of the ligaments to the radius, ulna, and radial carpal bone (Fig. 12–6C).

EXTRA-ARTICULAR FRACTURES

TYPE III, DISTAL APICAL ■ Avulsion fracture of the distal margin of the palmar end of the bone at the origin of the two palmar accessorometacarpal ligaments.

TYPE IV, PROXIMAL APICAL ■ Avulsion fracture of the tendon of insertion of the flexor carpi ulnaris muscle at the proximal surface of the palmar end of the bone (see Figure 12–8).

COMBINED INTRA-ARTICULAR AND EXTRA-ARTICULAR FRACTURES

TYPE V, COMMINUTED FRACTURE OF THE BODY ■ May extend into the articular surface (see Figure 12–9).

Type I fractures comprise 67 percent of the injuries in the racing Greyhound and occur almost exclusively in the right limb, whereas type III injuries are the least common and occur mainly in the left limb.[4] Type II injuries rarely occur alone; they are usually seen concurrently with type I fractures. In other breeds, type IV and V fractures predominate.

CLINICAL SIGNS

In track injuries, the dog usually comes off the track mildly lame, but clinical signs may not be noted until the day following the injury when slight lameness and swelling are observed in the region of the accessory carpal bone. Clinical signs include swelling of the carpus, pain on digital pressure lateral to the accessory carpal bone, and pain on carpal flexion. Rest will lead to diminution of these signs, but a chronic low-grade lameness persists when exercise is resumed. There is very little tendency for complete healing to occur with conservative treatment such as external splinting or casting of the limb.

TREATMENT

Although simple excision of the fragment in type I injuries has been advocated,[5] less than 50 percent of our animals so treated have ever won a race.

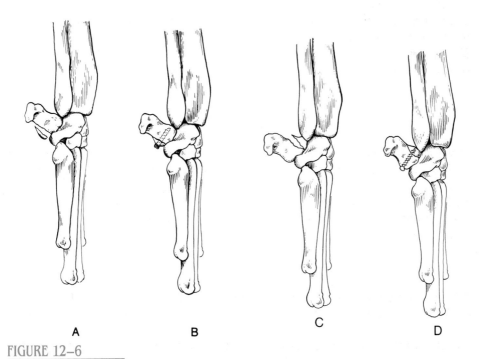

A   B   C   D

FIGURE 12–6

(A) Typical distal-basilar (type I) fracture of the accessory carpal bone. (B) Fixation of the fracture with a 2-mm screw. (C) Proximal basilar (type II) fracture of the accessory carpal bone. (D) Fixation with a 2-mm screw.

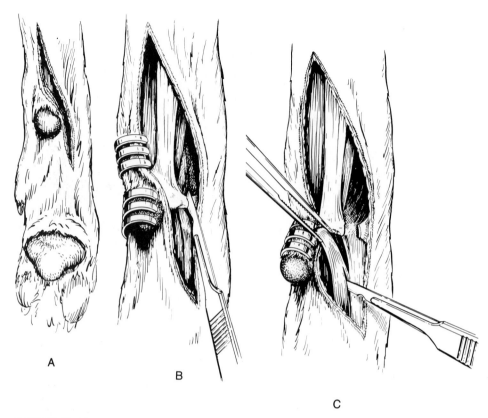

A

B

C

FIGURE 12–7

Approach and screw fixation of a fracture of the accessory carpal bone. *(A)* Right carpus, palmar view. Skin incision extends from the base of the metacarpus to the distal third of the radius. *(B)* Incision of antebrachial fascia reveals a tendinous slip from the ulnaris lateralis tendon to the free end of the accessory carpal bone, which is incised. *(C)* The abductor digiti quinti muscle is sharply dissected from the bone and from between the two accessorometacarpal ligaments (see Figure 21–34).

With this technique, successful healing seems to depend on scar tissue reattachment of the ligaments to the bone. Failure to achieve this results in instability of the accessory carpal bone, leading to inflammation and degenerative joint disease. Because scar tissue does not have nearly the tensile strength of ligamentous tissue, it does not adequately replace the ligament in areas of high tensile stress.

In our practice, screw fixation of type I, II, and III injuries has resulted in approximately 90 percent of these dogs returning and winning a race. Although the case numbers are too small yet to allow any valid conclusions, these results are encouraging, and this approach is our preferred treatment (Figs. 12–6 and 12–7).

A palmarolateral approach is made[2] (Fig. 12–7A). The fragment is reduced and clamped with small, pointed reduction forceps,* or Lewin forceps (Fig. 12–7D). Fixation is accomplished by a 2.0-mm screw that is not placed as a lag screw (Fig. 12–7D, E). The bone clamp is used to supply compression

*Synthes LTD (USA), Wayne, Pa.

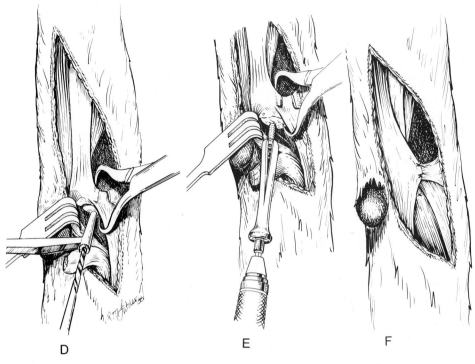

D   E   F

FIGURE 12-7

Continued (D) The accessorometacarpal IV ligament is retracted medially. The fragment is reduced and clamped with small, pointed, reduction forceps or Lewin forceps. A 1.5-mm drill is used to place a drill hole in the center of the fragment. If the drill is held parallel to the metacarpus, the angle will be correct to prevent entering the joint space. *(E)* The hole is measured and tapped, and a 2-mm screw driven with the clamp in place. This is not a lag screw; the clamp supplies compression. *(F)* The tendinous slip from the ulnaris lateralis tendon is sutured, followed by the antebrachial fascia, and then the skin.

because drilling with a 2-mm bit to produce a glide hole probably poses an unnecessary risk of splitting the fragment. Additionally, it is very difficult to judge the depth needed for a gliding hole in such a small bone fragment. Closure of the approach includes suturing of the abductor digiti quinti muscle and the tendinous slip from the ulnaris lateralis tendon to the accessory carpal bone (Fig. 12–7F).

Fractures seen more commonly in nonracing animals include an avulsion fracture of the free end of the bone (Fig. 12–8A) and varying degrees of comminution of the bone (Fig. 12–9). The avulsion is in the insertion of the flexor carpi ulnaris muscle and causes mild but persistent irritation until the fragment is removed (Fig. 12–8B–D). Internal fixation of comminuted fractures is probably not feasible very often, and most limbs treated for this injury are cast in 20 degrees of flexion with surprisingly good healing and function if the fracture is entirely extra-articular. If there is an intra-articular component, an attempt should be made to do an internal fixation of that part of the fracture.

Aftercare ■ Following screw fixation, a molded palmar splint or short cast (see Figs. 19–14 and 19–10) is applied with the carpus flexed 20 degrees. The splint is maintained for 4 weeks. Complete confinement is enforced through

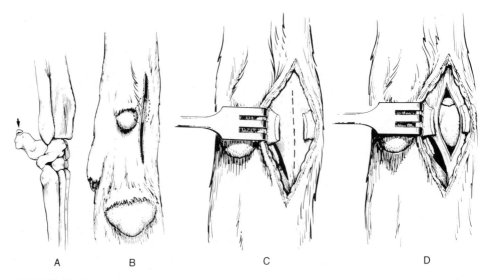

A   B   C   D

FIGURE 12-8

(A) Avulsion of part of the insertion of the flexor carpi ulnaris muscle on the free end of the right accessory carpal bone (type IV fracture). (B) Skin and antebrachial fascia incisions for removal of the fragment are slightly lateral to the bone. (C) The tendinous slip from the ulnaris lateralis muscle is incised over the free end of the bone and a midsagittal incision is made in the tendon of the flexor carpi ulnaris. (D) Careful dissection through the tendon will reveal the fracture fragment, which is then dissected free; care must be taken to avoid unnecessary trauma to the tendon. The tendon incision is closed with interrupted sutures, followed by the tendinous slip over the free end of the bone, the antebrachial fascia, and the skin.

FIGURE 12-9   FIGURE 12-10

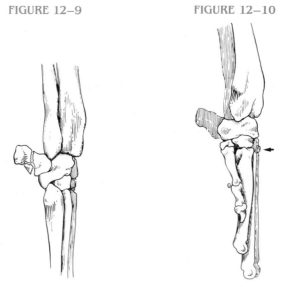

FIGURE 12-9

Comminuted type V fracture of the accessory carpal bone. This fracture was splinted in 20 degrees of flexion and healed well.

FIGURE 12-10

A small fracture on the dorsal surface of the third carpal bone. This fragment was excised.

the eighth postoperative week, followed by 4 weeks of gradually increasing activity. Regular training is started by the 12th week.

Following excision of fragments, the splint is maintained for 2 weeks, followed by an elastic bandage for 2 more weeks. Exercise is restricted for 4 more weeks. Splinting of a comminuted fracture is maintained until radiographic signs of healing are obvious, usually in about 6 weeks. Full exercise should not be started until 3 or 4 weeks after splint removal.

Fracture of the Ulnar and Numbered Carpal Bones

We have not observed fractures of the ulnar carpal bone. Fracture of the distal row of numbered bones is rare and usually is manifested as a small chip or slab on the dorsal surface (Fig. 12–10). Clinical signs of intermittent mild lameness and joint effusion are noted. Because these bones are smaller, radiographic diagnosis and reattachment of fragments are more difficult. Multiple oblique views are often necessary for visualization.

Because these bones are all directly in contact with the synovium, adhesions form early between the fragments, or the damaged articular surface, and the synovial membrane. Most of these fractures are treated by excision of fragments and curettage of the damaged articular surface to ensure fibrocartilaginous scar formation. Small nondisplaced fragments may reattach and heal following 3 to 4 weeks of splinting of the carpus.

THE METACARPUS

Fractures of the metacarpal bones occur in all three anatomic regions of the bone—the base (proximal end), the shaft, and the head (distal end).

Fracture of the Base

The medial (second) and lateral (fifth) bones are most commonly involved (Figs. 12–11A and 12–12A). Because these areas are points of ligamentous insertion, varying degrees of valgus (lateral) displacement of the foot are seen with fractures of the second metacarpal, and varus (medial) displacement with fifth metacarpal fractures. Some injury of the carpometacarpal ligaments may be noted, which may also result in hyperextension at the carpometacarpal level (see also Chapter 21).

Fixation of displaced fractures is usually done by the tension band wire technique (Fig. 12–11B and Fig. 12–12B, C). Lag screws are also useful in some cases (Fig. 12–11C). Undisplaced fractures may be treated by external fixation, but there is usually some displacement of the fragment during healing. A very secure splint or short leg cast (see Figs. 19–14 and 19–10) must be used.

Comminuted fractures in larger breeds may be handled with small plates, combined with lag screws and/or cerclage wires (Fig. 12–13). Racing Greyhounds are subject to stress fractures of the second metacarpal (and third metatarsal) of the right foot. These fractures are undisplaced and often show

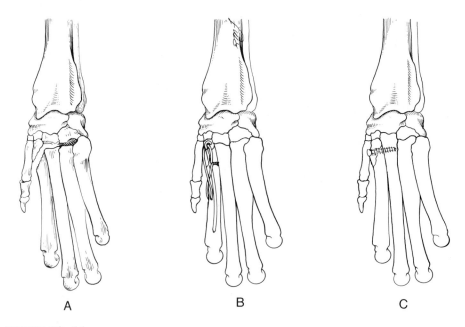

A   B   C

FIGURE 12–11

(A) Fracture of the base of the second metacarpal bone is usually associated with valgus (lateral) deviation of the foot. (B) Fixation with Kirschner wire and tension band wire. (C) Fixation with lag screw.

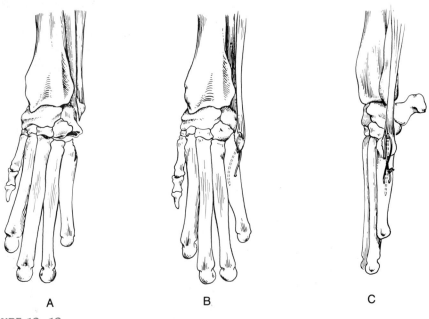

A   B   C

FIGURE 12–12

(A) Fracture of the base of the fifth metacarpal bone. The tendon of insertion of the ulnaris lateralis muscle causes the fragment to be displaced proximally. Some varus (medial) deviation of the foot may be present. (B, C) Fixation is by the tension band wire technique. The Kirschner wire is 0.045″ in diameter, and the stainless steel wire is 22 gauge. This fracture could also be repaired with a lag screw.

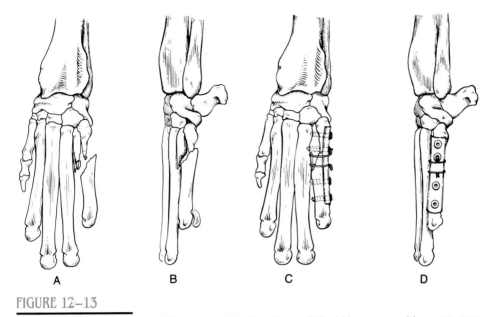

FIGURE 12–13

(A, B) Comminuted fracture of the proximal shaft and base of the fifth metacarpal bone. *(C, D)* A one-third tubular plate, 2.7-mm screws, and 22-gauge cerclage wire fixation. The two proximal screws were applied in lag fashion.

some callus formation (Fig. 12–14). Fixation is by a palmar splint, maintained for 4 weeks. Lag screw fixation is indicated when there is no response to immobilization.

Aftercare ■ Primary fixation by casting or splinting will require the device to be worn for about 6 weeks, except in the case of the stress fracture, which requires only 4 weeks. If internal fixation is used, a molded palmar splint or

FIGURE 12–14

(A, B) Stress fracture of the second metacarpal bone, right forefoot. This fracture is specific in the racing Greyhound. The fracture is usually incomplete and undisplaced and may extend into the articular surface of the base; unless it is seen very early, it will have some periosteal callus formation, which is usually palpable.

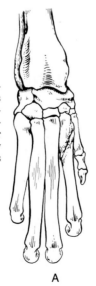

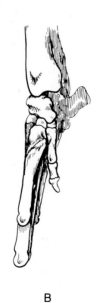

short cast (see Figs. 19–14 and 19–10) is maintained for 3 to 4 weeks. Exercise is restricted for 3 to 4 weeks after splint removal.

Fracture of the Shaft

Fracture of one or even two metacarpals is not a serious injury, especially if the two middle bones are not involved. They heal quite readily in a simple palmar splint as a result of the splinting effect of the remaining bones. When three or all four bones (Fig. 12–15A) are broken, the situation is quite different, however, especially in the large and giant breeds. Here, simple splints often create a delayed union or malunion at best, with nonunion often resulting. This is a problem particularly when preformed spoon splints are used. Additionally, a valgus deformity and palmar bowing of the bones may occur because they are not adequately supported in the spoon splint (Fig. 12–15B, C). When closed reduction and external fixation are used, a molded splint or cast of plaster of Paris, thermomoldable plastic, or fiberglass is advisable (see Chapter 19). Because the device is molded to the foot, the bony support is improved. The splint or cast should be maintained until radiographic signs of healing are well advanced, which typically occurs within 4 to 8 weeks, varying with the age of the animal.

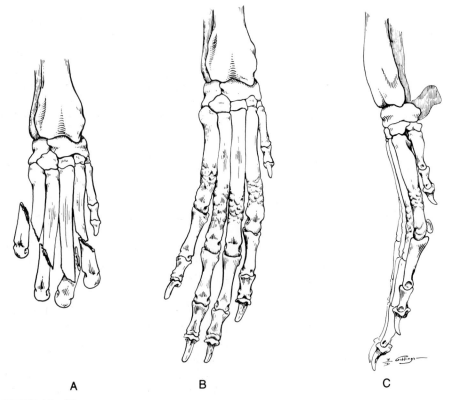

A   B   C

FIGURE 12–15

(A) Multiple metacarpal shaft fractures. (B, C) Closed reduction and inadequate external fixation resulted in valgus deformity and palmar bowing of the metacarpus.

Internal fixation is indicated when two or more bones are involved, especially if they are the middle bones. Other indications for internal fixation include severely comminuted or displaced fractures, nonunion, and malunion. Even simple single bone fractures may warrant internal fixation for optimal functional results in large athletic breeds.

INTERNAL FIXATION

INTRAMEDULLARY PINS ■ Kirschner wires, Steinmann pins, and Rush pins are all applicable to the metacarpal/metatarsal bones. They are indicated in transverse and oblique fractures that are not highly comminuted. They can be combined with cerclage wires in long oblique fractures. The pin should not fill the medullary canal too tightly because it will interfere with medullary blood supply and delay healing. In most cases it is best to think of the pin as merely an internal splint to maintain reduction of the bone and to rely on an external cast/splint to furnish a good deal of the immobilization needed for fracture healing. A method of introducing the pins that does not damage or interfere with motion of the metacarpophalangeal joint will produce the best functional results and allow the external fixation to be removed as soon as there is sufficient callus to support the pin.

One acceptable method is to introduce the pin from the distal end of the bone at the dorsal edge of the articular cartilage. Although this causes the pin to enter the bone at a slight angle, nevertheless, if the pin is not too large and stiff to bend slightly it should glide proximally in the medullary canal. The fracture is reduced and the pin driven into the proximal fragment until it is well seated in the base of the bone. The pin is then retracted 5 mm, a hook is bent and the end cut, and then the pin is driven back into the bone until the hook is close to the bone surface. In this manner, there is very little pin protruding from the bone to irritate the joint, yet the pin is easily removed (Fig. 12–16). Retrograde insertion (from the fracture site) is advocated by some, but it is difficult to avoid penetrating the distal articular surface with this method.

The metacarpophalangeal joint is kept in flexion in a splint or cast (see below), and the pins are removed after healing. If the pins do penetrate articular cartilage, the splint should be maintained until healing is complete and the pins removed, before allowing active weight-bearing.

If the bone is large enough to accept a ¹⁄₁₆″ (1.5 mm) Rush pin, the hook will not have to be bent by the surgeon, and the pin can be inserted at some distance from the articular surface (Fig. 12–17C). Generally, a Rush pin will provide more rigid fixation than a straight intramedullary pin.

CERCLAGE WIRES ■ The general rules given in Chapter 1 apply to application of wires in the metacarpus or metatarsus. Useful wire sizes vary from 20 gauge to 24 gauge (0.8 to 0.4 mm). Of primary importance is that the cerclage wire must be tight or it will devascularize the underlying bone because of movement of the wire. An important difference in the metacarpus/metatarsus from their application in long bones is that on occasion cerclage wires are used as primary fixation. This is possible because external casts/splints are always used to support the internal fixation. More commonly, however, cerclage wires are combined with intramedullary pins (Fig. 12–17C).

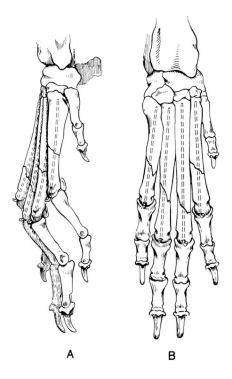

FIGURE 12–16

(A, B) Intramedullary fixation of multiple metacarpal fractures. Kirschner wires are inserted in the distal segment, staying as close as possible to the dorsoproximal edge of the metacarpophalangeal joint capsule. The fracture is reduced and the pins are driven into the base of the bone. The pins are then bent to a hook shape and driven as close to the bone as possible to allow more extension of the toes and easier removal of the pins.

A   B

FIGURE 12–17

(A) Oblique shaft fracture of the fifth metacarpal in a racing Greyhound. (B) Fixation by 2.7-mm lag screws. This method was chosen over pinning or cerclage wiring because there is less joint and soft tissue irritation. Primary bone union was achieved. (C) Cerclage wires and ¹⁄₁₆″ diameter Rush pin. The articular surface is not invaded.

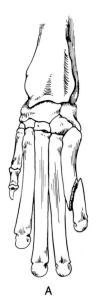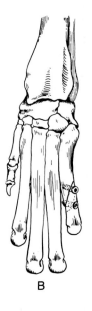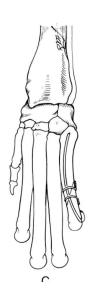

A   B   C

LAG SCREWS ■ Interfragmentary fixation with lag screws, as with cerclage wire, is occasionally used as primary fixation in the metacarpus/metatarsus when supported with an external cast or splint. The advent of 1.5- and 2.0-mm screws has increased the usefulness of this method in long oblique or spiral fractures. It is rarely possible to combine intramedullary pinning with lag screws because of the small size of the bones; thus screws are generally used alone (Fig. 12–17B) or in conjunction with bone plates (Fig. 12–13C, D). The same general guidelines as discussed in Chapter 1 apply to the application of lag screws here.

BONE PLATES ■ Small plates are valuable in larger breeds for fixation of very unstable fractures (Fig. 12–13) and for nonunion fractures (Fig. 12–18). Because of their stability, external support does not have to be maintained as long as with other methods. Four weeks is typically sufficient to allow limited active use of the limb. Plate and screw sizes typically range from 1.5 to 2.7 mm; both flat and semitubular style plates are useful. See Chapter 1 for a discussion of plating techniques.

Aftercare ■ In all cases of internal fixation, the foot should be supported in a molded splint or cast until radiographic signs of bone healing are obvious. This typically ranges from 3 to 6 weeks.

Bone plates are usually removed in 3 to 4 months, especially in athletic animals. Bone screws and cerclage wires can usually be left with no harmful effects. Intramedullary pins inserted from the distal joint area should be removed as soon as callus formation is well established. Rush pins can usually be left in place if desired.

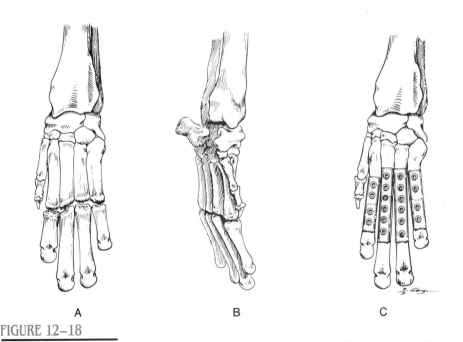

A   B   C

FIGURE 12–18

(A, B) Nonunion fracture of all metacarpals, 9 months' duration. (C) Multiple bone plate fixation. Size of plate will vary from a 1.5- to 2.7-mm screw size. Good healing was achieved using 2.7-mm plates and screws in this 80-pound (36 kg) dog.

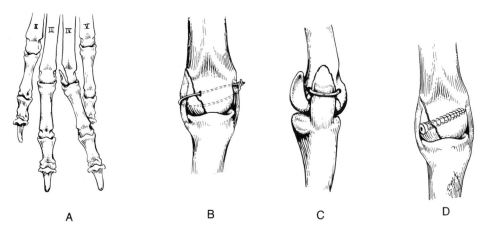

FIGURE 12–19

(A) Fracture of the medial condyle of the head of the fourth metacarpal bone. Valgus deformity of the toe results. *(B, C)* Wire fixation of fragments. To avoid having to drill a hole through the small fragment, two holes are drilled in the metacarpal bone and the wire (22 gauge in a 60-pound animal) passed through the holes and around the fragment. If the wire can be passed through the ligamentous tissue, it will have less tendency to slip off the fragment. *(D)* Lag screw fixation with 1.5- or 2.0-mm screws is ideal if the fragment is large enough.

Fracture of the Head

One of the most common injuries in this region is a fracture of the condyle. Such a fracture results in instability and luxation/subluxation of the metacarpophalangeal joint (Fig. 12–19) because the collateral ligaments of the joint originate on the condyle. The condylar fragment may be quite small (Fig. 12–19A), or it may involve half the head.

Internal fixation offers the best chance for return to normal function, especially in the athletic animal. Closed reduction and external casting usually result in an unstable joint, or the intra-articular alignment of the fragments may be poor, resulting in degenerative joint disease. Internal fixation may be done with wire (Fig. 12–19B, C) or by lag screws (Fig. 12–19D). Failure to repair these injuries may necessitate amputation at the metacarpophalangeal joint to restore function in the athletic animal, especially if the third or fourth bone is involved. For further discussion of amputation, see Chapter 21.

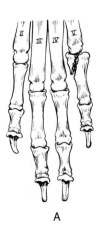
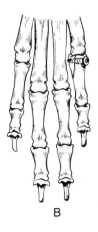

FIGURE 12–20

(A) Fracture of the base of the first phalanx. *(B)* Lag screw fixation using a 2.0- or 1.5-mm screw.

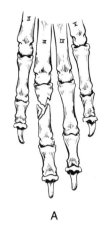

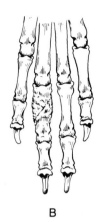

A

B

FIGURE 12–21

(A) Comminuted fracture of the first phalanx. (B) Four weeks after coaptation splintage. Although there is considerable callus at this stage, good alignment of the bone has been maintained.

Aftercare ■ A molded palmar splint or cast is applied for 4 weeks, and exercise is limited for 6 to 8 weeks.

PHALANGES

Fractures of the head and base are handled in much the same way as described for metacarpal fractures, except that the fragments are often smaller and more difficult to secure (Fig. 12–20). As a result, amputation may need to be considered more often. Fractures of the shaft are most commonly treated by closed reduction and external fixation (Fig. 12–21), although internal fixation should be considered for a performance animal (Figs. 12–22 and 12–23). Surgical exposure is quite simple because the bone is immediately beneath the skin.[2] As in the case of metacarpal fractures, both cerclage wires and lag screws are suitable as primary fixation when supplemented with external support.

Aftercare ■ A molded plastic bivalve splint (see Figure 19–15) is applied either as primary fixation or as support for internal fixation. Three to 6 weeks of splinting are usually needed for primary fixation, and 3 to 4 weeks are sufficient for support of internal fixation.

FIGURE 12–22

(A) Oblique fracture of the first phalanx in a racing Greyhound. (B) Because of the need for rapid return to function, internal fixation with a 2.7-mm lag screw was chosen. Use of two smaller screws would provide more stability.

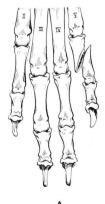

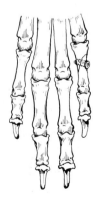

A

B

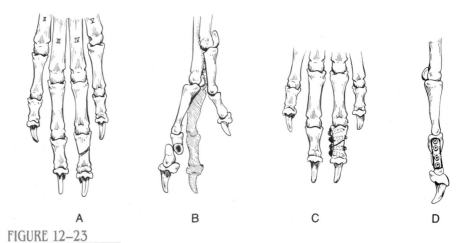

FIGURE 12–23

(A, B) Short oblique fracture of the second phalanx in a racing Greyhound. *(C, D)* Because the fracture line was too short for a lag screw, a miniplate was used with 2.0-mm screws. An excellent functional result was obtained. The plate was left in place because it had not affected the dog's performance.

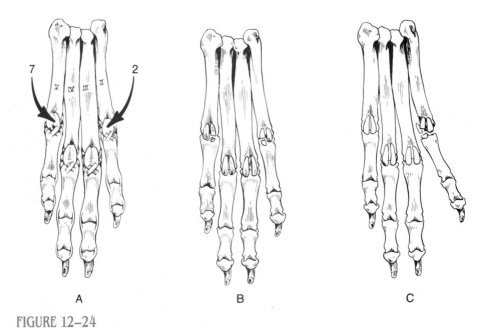

FIGURE 12–24

(A) Ligaments of the palmar sesamoids of the metacarpophalangeal joints. The sesamoids are numbered from medial to lateral, 1 to 8, with 2 and 7 being the most commonly injured. *(B)* Fractures of the distal third of sesamoid 7 and midportion of sesamoid 2. Only the small fragment of 7 is removed, whereas all of 2 is removed. *(C)* Fracture of sesamoid 2 with fracture of the base of the second metacarpal bone. The sesamoid is excised and the metacarpal fracture wired or lag-screwed as in Figure 12–19.

THE PROXIMAL SESAMOIDS

Large-breed dogs are the primary victims of fractures of the proximal sesamoids of the metacarpophalangeal joint.[5] Excessive tension on the digital flexor tendons can cause the sesamoid bone, which is quite long and banana-shaped, to fracture near its midportion. Sesamoids are numbered from medial to lateral; because there are two sesamoids at each metacarpophalangeal joint, they are numbered from 1 to 8 (Fig. 12–24A). The sesamoids that are most commonly injured are the second and seventh (Fig. 12–24B, C). Either the forelimbs or hindlimbs can be involved. Sudden lameness occurs, accompanied by swelling, pain on palpation, and crepitus. This lameness rapidly subsides, and the animal shows lameness only on exercise. Tenderness on deep palpation over the bones remains. Bilateral injuries are not uncommon.

High-detail screens or nonscreen radiographic techniques are helpful in diagnosing these fractures. Treatment in the acute stage consists of splinting. Some fractures will heal sufficiently, but many will later require surgery for excision of the bone fragments. All chronic cases should undergo operation.

The bone is exposed by an incision just medial or lateral to the large central pad, directly over the joint.[2] The fragments are sharply dissected free of their ligamentous attachments. On occasion, only a small portion of the bone is fractured. If this piece is less than one third of the total bone, it is usual to leave the larger fragment and remove the smaller. When the fracture is in the midportion, both fragments are removed. A snug bandage is maintained for 7 to 10 days postoperatively. Activity is restricted until 6 weeks postoperatively. A good prognosis can be given for surgically treated cases.

THE DORSAL SESAMOIDS

The dorsal sesamoid bones of the metacarpophalangeal bones (Fig. 12–1) are attached proximally to the common digital extensor and interosseous muscles, and distally via a ligament to the proximal phalanx. These small bones are rarely involved with any injury or pathological process, although they are commonly mistaken for chip fractures of the joint when seen radiographically. However, one dog has been seen in our practice that had a chronic lameness and exhibited pain and crepitus on flexion of the digits. Radiographic signs of degenerative joint disease of the metacarpophalangeal joint were present. The lameness and clinical signs were relieved by surgical excision of the affected dorsal sesamoid.

REFERENCES

1. Piermattei DL, Wind A: Orthopedic problems of the lower limbs. Proc Am Anim Hosp Assoc 341–350, 1977.
2. Piermattei DL: An Atlas of Surgical Approaches to the Bones of the Dog and Cat, 3rd ed. Philadelphia, WB Saunders Co, in preparation.
3. Johnson KA: Accessory carpal bone fractures in the racing Greyhound: classification and pathology. Vet Surg 16:60, 1987.
4. Johnson KA, Piermattei DL, Davis PE, et al: Characteristics of accessory carpal bone fractures in 50 racing Greyhounds. Vet Comp Orth Traum 2:104, 1988.
5. Berg JA: Fractures of the palmar and plantar sesamoid bones as a cause of lameness in the dog. J Am Vet Med Assoc 163:968, 1973.

13

Fractures and Dislocations of the Upper and Lower Jaw

Fractures of the jaws[1, 2] are characterized by swelling, deviation of the segments, malocclusion of the teeth, and blood-stained saliva. With few exceptions, all jaw fractures are open and contaminated or infected. These fractures may be unilateral or bilateral with single or multiple fracture lines. In general, healing is rapid (3 to 5 weeks), requiring less time than do the long bones. The exception to this general statement on healing is fractures through infected sockets and symphyseal fractures in the elderly toy breeds where considerable osteoporosis precedes the fracture.

DIAGNOSIS AND GENERAL TREATMENT

Diagnosis is usually based on a history of trauma, sudden onset, appearance, and a palpable fracture. Radiography is also helpful in discerning fracture lines and displacement but is supplemental to a thorough physical examination under anesthesia or sedation.

The objective of treatment should be the implantation of fixation so that the animal can have restricted use of the mouth to eat and drink following reduction and fixation. With few exceptions, this goal can be achieved.

Surgical treatment varies considerably, and in practically all cases, some type of fixation is indicated. The tension band side is the alveolar border, and fixation should be applied on this side when possible.

With a few exceptions, bone fragments are replaced in the reduction process and are not discarded. Realignment is usually best checked with the jaw closed and the teeth occluding. Following reduction and fixation, the torn gingiva is sutured to keep food and contaminants out of the wound. Suturing also aids in stabilizing the fracture segments and in converting the area to a closed fracture.

Even though the tissues in the mouth are very effective in eliminating infection, systemic antibiotics are advisable. Chronic osteomyelitis in connection with primary jaw fractures is rare.

In performing the fixation procedure in many cases, particularly the more

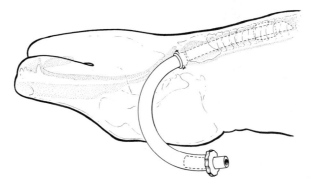

FIGURE 13–1

Pharyngostomy tube. After the animal is stabilized on gas anesthesia, the tracheal tube is changed to pass through a pharyngostomy opening and down the trachea. This allows fixation to be applied with the mouth closed and the teeth occluding.

complicated ones, a tracheostomy—or, preferably, a pharyngostomy—is done to maintain anesthesia. This technique assures an open airway while the animal's mouth is closed and the teeth are occluded during the procedure.

After the animal is stabilized on gas anesthesia, the tracheal tube is changed to pass through the pharyngostomy opening. This allows the surgeon to apply fixation with the animal's mouth closed and the teeth occluding (Fig. 13–1). Good occlusion of the teeth is mandatory following the application of fixation. After the surgery is completed, the tracheal tube is removed, and the pharyngostomy opening is allowed to heal by granulation.

FRACTURES OF THE MANDIBLE

Fixation of the Mandibular Symphysis

The method of immobilization depends on the presence or absence of teeth and the stability of the reduced fragments.[1–3, 7] If the incisor teeth are present and the fracture-separation is stable, a simple, interrupted stainless steel wire suture may be adequate (Fig. 13–2A). If the bases of the third incisor and canine teeth fit close together, a hand chuck may be used to force a Kirschner drill wire between them, thus allowing easy placement of the wire suture (Fig. 13–2B).

Stability may be improved by the insertion of a transmandibular pin (smooth or threaded) or a bone screw (Fig. 13–2C, D). Figure 13–2E suggests the location from the lateral surface for insertion, which is usually just rostral to the mental foramen. In many cases, a combination of fixation methods is used.

Another method consists of using an encircling wire (Fig. 13–2F). The wire is inserted to hug the bone under the skin and gums and penetrates the soft tissue to be tightened.[2, 7] Fractures in this area usually heal rapidly, and fixation can be removed in 3 to 5 weeks.

Fixation of Mandibular Body Fractures

A wide variety of fractures may be encountered; ingenuity is required to devise the best type of fixation. The various methods of fixation[1–5] include the use of:

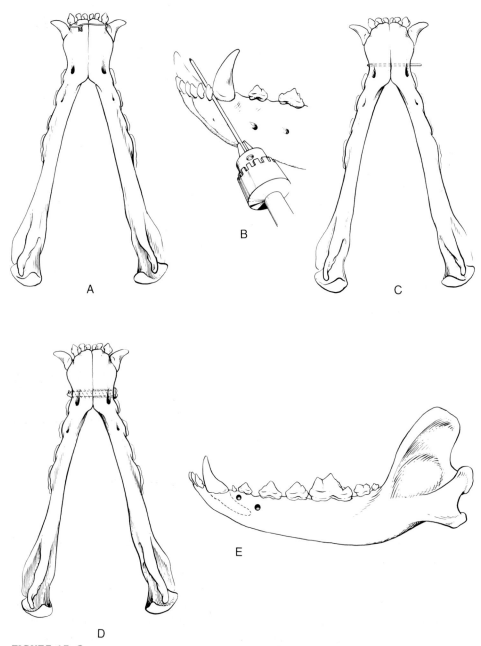

FIGURE 13–2

Fixation of the mandibular symphysis. *(A)* Simple, interrupted stainless steel wire suture. *(B)* A hand chuck forces a Kirschner drill wire between the base of the third incisor and canine teeth, allowing easy placement of wire sutures. *(C)* Insertion of a transmandibular pin, smooth or threaded, or a bone screw *(D)* to improve stability. *(E)* Suggested location from the lateral surface for insertion, which is usually just rostral to the mental foramen.

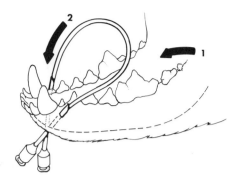

FIGURE 13–2

Continued (F) Immobilization by use of an encircling wire. The wire (usually 20 gauge) is inserted by using two 16-gauge needles and twisted outside the skin on the ventral surface. The mouth is closed with the teeth occluding when the final twisting is done.

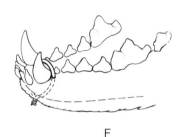

F

1. Interfragmentary stainless steel wire (18 to 24 gauge) around the base of the teeth on each side of the fracture. This places it on the tension band side.

2. Interfragmentary stainless steel wire inserted through bone fragments of the mandible.

3. Intramedullary pins.

4. External fixator.

5. Acrylic prosthesis or acrylic pin external fixation splint.

6. Bone plates.

7. Combinations of the above.

A method or combination of methods must be used that gives stability at the fracture site.

INTERDENTAL STAINLESS STEEL WIRE AROUND THE BASES OF THE TEETH ■ This method works best when there is a solid tooth on each side of the fracture line and when the fracture is stable in nature (Figs. 13–3A, B and 13–4F). Occasionally, this is modified so that the wire is passed between the roots of the adjacent teeth (Fig. 13–3B). The guide hole is made with a small Kirschner wire and a pin chuck.

INTERFRAGMENTARY STAINLESS STEEL WIRE ■ Some oblique, multiple, and noncomminuted unstable fractures lend themselves to simple interrupted wire fixation. A longitudinal incision is made over the ventral surface of the mandible, and the soft tissue is reflected to expose the fracture area. The fragments are drilled, usually with a Kirschner drill wire, so that the inserted wire crosses

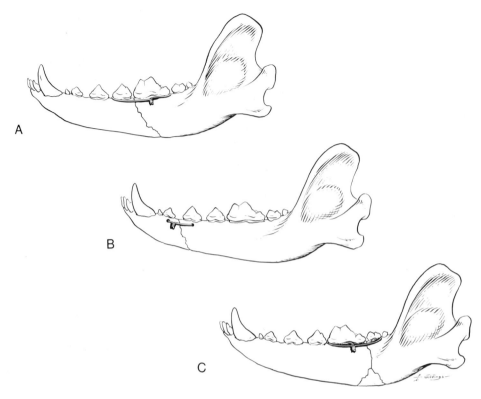

FIGURE 13-3

Fixation of a fracture of the body of the mandible. (A) Interdental wire around the bases of the fourth premolar and the first molar. (C) Interdental wire around the bases of the first and second molars. (B) Modified method, with wire through drill holes between the roots of the adjacent teeth.

the fracture line at a right angle (Fig. 13–4). These are left in place unless removal is indicated. Stability must be accomplished at the fracture site; if not, some modification or another fixation method is in order.

INTRAMEDULLARY PINNING [1-3] ■ The diameter of the pin will vary with the size of the mandible, ranging from 0.035, 0.045, and 0.062 or $\frac{1}{16}$″. The point of entry varies, usually starting retrograde with the shorter segment. The pin is kept near the ventral border to interfere less with the roots of the teeth and structures in the mandibular canal (Fig. 13–5). The pins are removed following clinical union. The mandible is very dense, and intramedullary pins are difficult to pass, except in the mandibular canal, which causes some damage to the vessels and nerves. However, from clinical observations, this sequela appears to be of minor significance.

EXTERNAL FIXATOR ■ This device[1-4] is useful for:

1. Nonunion fractures; bone grafting is indicated in many cases (see Chapter 3).
2. Multiple fractures (Fig. 13–6A, B).

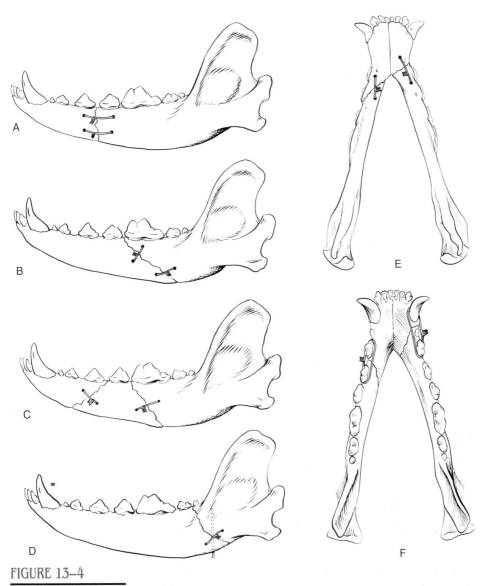

FIGURE 13-4

(A–C) Examples of interfragmentary wire in various areas. *(D)* Interfragmentary wire supplemented with a short intramedullary pin or Kirschner wire. *(E, F)* Two views of a rostral stable bilateral body fracture treated with both interfragmentary and interdental wires.

3. Bilateral fractures (Fig. 13–6C).

4. Unstable or gunshot fractures where bone is missing. The gums are sutured following reduction and fixation. In the healing process, the missing segment may fill in if bone chips and periosteum are still present. In others, a bone graft is indicated (Fig. 13–6D).

SURGICAL PROCEDURE ■ Two pins are usually inserted in each fragment, but one pin in the rostral fragment may be sufficient if it passes transversely through

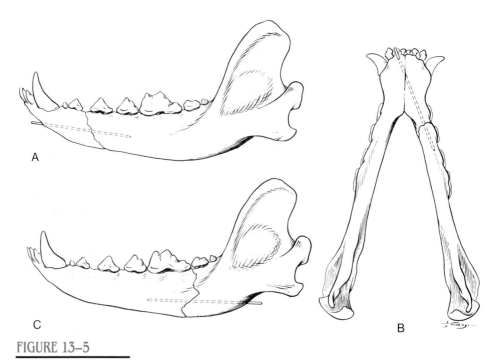

FIGURE 13–5

(A, B) An intramedullary pin for a cranial body fracture crosses the symphysis rostrally. *(C)* Intramedullary pin for caudal body fracture; the pin penetrates the cortex rostral and ventral to the angular process.

both halves of the mandible (Fig. 13–6*B–D*). The procedure is usually as follows:

    1. Close the animal's mouth with the fracture reduced and the teeth occluding.

    2. Insert the rostral and caudal pins through the skin and soft tissues into the bone.

    3. Attach the bar with single clamps and an empty center clamp.

    4. Insert the third pin through the center clamp and tighten. This essentially lines up the three pins in a common plane and attaches them with three single clamps and a common connecting bar.

In some patients, wire around the base of the teeth is indicated to improve stability (Fig. 13–6*C*). In general, the splint is well tolerated.

Aftercare ■ Postoperative treatment consists primarily of restricting the animal's jaw activity by feeding soft, small pieces of food. Toys or play that would stress the jaws should be eliminated until healing is evident.

ACRYLIC PIN EXTERNAL FIXATION SPLINT[5] ■ Because the external fixator splint has some inherent limitations in pin placement and connective bar attachment, polymethyl methacrylate (nonsterile dental acrylic) may be substituted as the connecting bar.

Surgical Procedure ■ A tracheal tube is inserted through a pharyngostomy incision to ensure an open airway. The mouth is closed, and reduction includes occlusion of the teeth. At least two or more pins should be placed in each

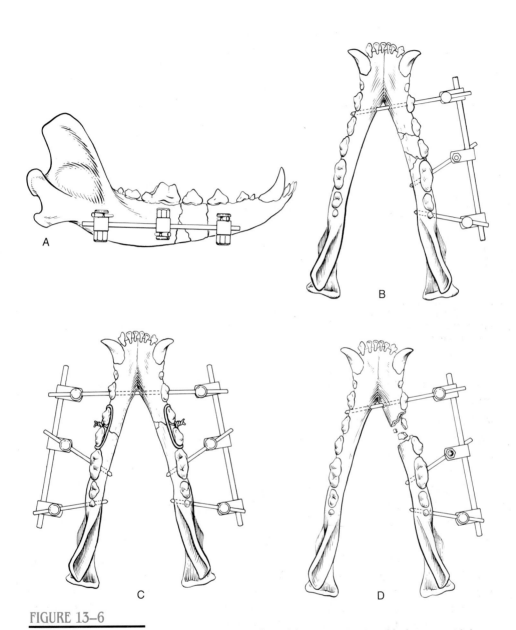

FIGURE 13–6

External fixator. *(A, B)* Multiple fractures. *(C)* Bilateral fractures. *(D)* Unstable fracture with bone missing. In most cases, the splint can be applied so that it does not extend beyond the length of the mandible, thus it does not interfere with eating or drinking. If the bone chips are left in place and the gums closed, in most cases the bone deficit will bridge over without the addition of a bone graft.

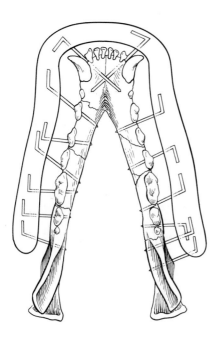

FIGURE 13–7

Modified acrylic external fixator. With the mouth closed, the fracture reduced, and the teeth occluding, two or more Kirschner wires are inserted into each major segment. The wires are bent and included in an acrylic mold. This apparatus has the disadvantage of protruding beyond the length of the jaw, thus making it more vulnerable to bumping and cumbersome when eating. In many cases, the same configuration can be applied by first bending the connecting bar of the external fixator, then inserting the Kirschner pins through the holes in the clamps and through the skin and soft tissue and into the bone.

major bone segment. Small fragments may be skewered with divergent Kirschner wires. The protruding pins are bent to better hold the molded acrylic connecting bar (Fig. 13–7). The acrylic usually takes about 8 to 10 minutes to set. Following healing, the pins can be cut between the acrylic and jaw and removed with a hand chuck. Because this fixation extends beyond the lower jaw, it may interfere with eating, and hand feeding may be necessary.

BONE PLATES[2, 4] ■ These are particularly useful for the more complex fractures and bilateral fractures. They afford good rigidity and almost unrestricted use of the jaws immediately after surgery.

Surgical Procedure ■ A pharyngostomy incision is made (see Figure 13–1), with insertion of a tracheal tube to ensure an open airway. The jaw is exposed with a ventral incision (see Figure 13–9D). Compression forceps are applied to compress the fracture segments and hold them in the reduced position while the bone plate is contoured to fit the surface perfectly. The plate is then attached with bone screws. Contouring the plate is a most important step in ensuring proper occlusion of the teeth. The plate is usually placed laterally near the ventral border to avoid placing the screws in the mandibular canal. In some cases, it is advisable to add a wire around the base of the teeth (tension side) for additional stability.

Figures 13–8A and B show a fractured mandible immobilized with a mini dynamic compression plate (DCP). In Figure 13–8C, a bilateral fracture is immobilized with two small reconstruction plates. A ventral approach to the body of the mandible is also shown (Fig. 13–8D).

Fixation of the Mandibular Vertical Ramus

Various methods of fixation may be used, including Kirschner wires, stainless steel wire, and mini bone plates. Figure 13–9 illustrates a lateral approach to

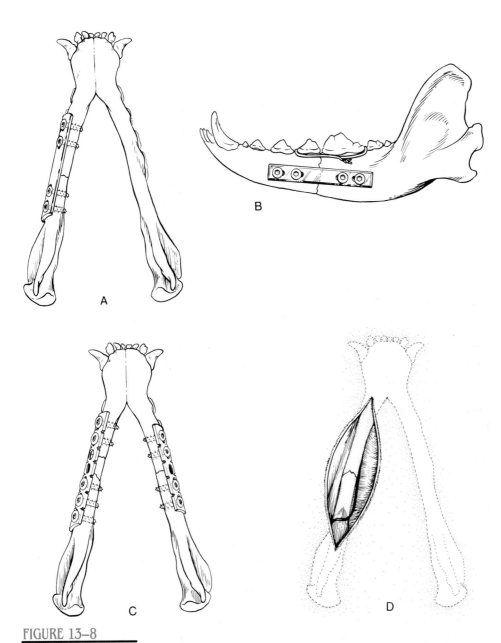

FIGURE 13-8

(A) Fractured mandible immobilized with a mini dynamic compression plate (DCP) and tension wire, ventral view; (B) Lateral view. (C) Bilateral fracture immobilized with two reconstruction plates, ventral and lateral views. The reconstruction plate is very adaptable to contouring to fit the bone surface. (D) Ventral approach to the body of the mandible showing the digastricus muscle (caudal), platysma muscle (lateral), and mylohyoid muscle (medial). A branch of the facial vein crosses the digastricus muscle.

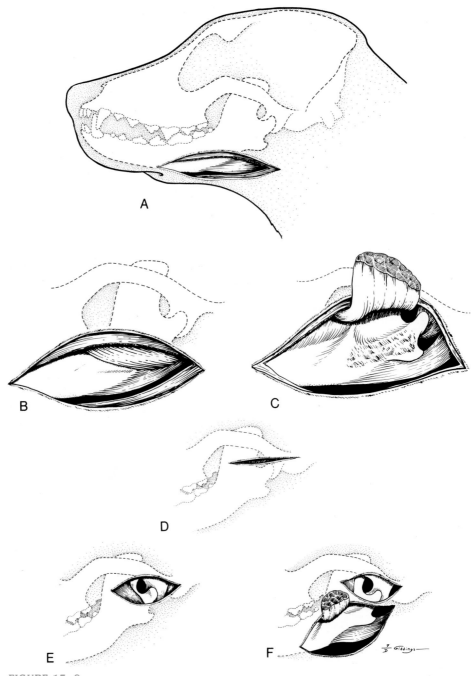

FIGURE 13-9

Surgical approach to the ramus and temporomandibular joint. (A) Ventrolateral approach to the caudal angular portion of the ramus. Skin incision along the ventrolateral border; separation of the platysma muscle exposes the digastricus muscle. (B) Further separation of the soft tissue exposes portion of the mandible, masseter muscle, and digastric muscle. (C) Subperiosteal reflection of the masseter muscle exposes angular and condyloid processes and masseteric fossa. (D) Longitudinal skin incision along ventral border of zygomatic arch and temporomandibular joint. (E) Platysma muscle and fascia incised along same line. This tissue is reflected ventrally, exposing the lateral surface of the joint and the upper portion of the condyloid process. (F) The tissue between the two incisions is tunneled beneath for visualization, reduction, and fixation.

the ramus and temporomandibular joint. Fixation methods for fractures of the ramus are shown in Figure 13–10.

FRACTURES OF THE UPPER JAW

Fractures of the incisive and maxillary bones[2, 4, 5] are usually readily diagnosed by observation and palpation. They are accompanied by bleeding from the nose and mouth, and disfigurement with some loss of dental malocclusion.

The primary objective is reestablishment of dental occlusion. Accomplishing this goal usually returns approximately normal appearance to the nose, upper jaw, and face.

Fixation

Fixation can usually be accomplished by placing a stainless steel wire around the base of the teeth on each side of the fracture line. The torn gingiva and palate are sutured (Fig. 13–11A, B). If the hard palate is split, a wire suture inserted underneath the mucosal covering of the hard palate and anchored to

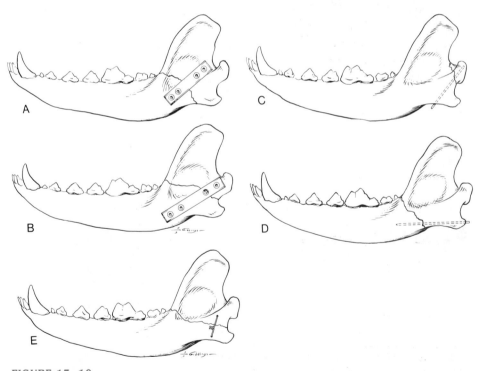

FIGURE 13–10

Fixation methods for fractures of the ramus. (A) Fracture just rostral to the angular process immobilized by a bone plate. (B) Fracture between the angular and condyloid processes immobilized by use of a bone plate. (C) Condyloid process fracture immobilized by an intramedullary pin placed from the ventral border of the mandible. (D) Fracture rostral to the angular process immobilized with an intramedullary pin placed through the angular process. (E) Fracture between the angular and condyloid processes immobilized by an interfragmentary wire.

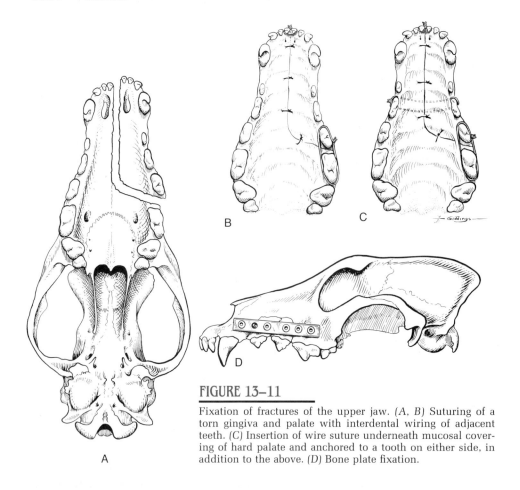

FIGURE 13–11

Fixation of fractures of the upper jaw. *(A, B)* Suturing of a torn gingiva and palate with interdental wiring of adjacent teeth. *(C)* Insertion of wire suture underneath mucosal covering of hard palate and anchored to a tooth on either side, in addition to the above. *(D)* Bone plate fixation.

a tooth on either side may be indicated in addition to wiring the teeth and suturing the palate and gingiva (Fig. 13–11C).

Some fractures of the incisive bone or maxilla are amenable to bone plate fixation (Fig. 13–11D). Exposure is gained by incising the gums along the base of the teeth and reflecting the soft tissue to expose the fracture area. Occasionally, massive bilateral fractures of the nasal and maxillary bones and mandible are encountered. Reconstruction and immobilization may include using an acrylic pin external fixator[5] or wiring the jaws together using the eyelet method of wiring[6] to maintain occlusion during the healing period. Food and liquids may have to be given by use of an implanted pharyngostomy tube.

Surgical Procedure for Combined Bilateral Fractures of the Upper and Lower Jaws If They Cannot Be Stabilized Separately

The animal is maintained on gas anesthesia through a pharyngostomy tube. The bones are realigned where possible and wired. The torn palate and gingiva are sutured. Next, a pharyngostomy tube (see Figure 13–1) is inserted for feeding and supplying water through a new opening on the other side. The

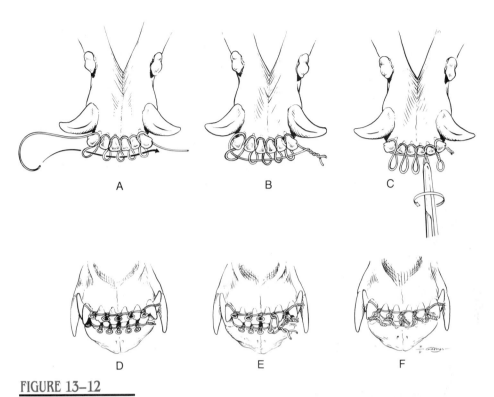

FIGURE 13–12

Surgical procedure for bilateral fractures of both upper and lower jaws if they cannot be stabilized separately. (A–F) Procedure for wiring the jaws together using the eyelet method.

jaws are wired together using the eyelet method of wiring (Fig. 13–12).[6, 7] Postoperative care consists of maintaining the animal with food and water through the pharyngostomy tube. Healing is usually rapid, and the jaws are wired together for 3 to 6 weeks.

Note: Occasionally, this style of wiring can be used to advantage on certain fractures of the mandible to provide immobilization of the entire lower jaw.

REFERENCES

1. Brinker WO: Fractures in Canine Surgery, 2nd Archibald ed. Santa Barbara, American Veterinary Publications, Inc, 1974, pp 949–1048.
2. Brinker WO: Small Animal Fractures. East Lansing, MI, Depart Cont Ed Serv, Michigan State University, 1978.
3. Rudy RL: Internal fixation of jaw fractures. 19th Annual AO/ASIF Course on Surgical Fixation of Fractures. Ohio State University, Columbus, OH, March 9–12, 1988.
4. Brinker WO, Hohn RB, Prieur WD: Manual of Internal Fixation in Small Animals. New York, Springer-Verlag, 1984, 210–218.
5. Egger EL: Management of mandibular fractures with acrylic-pin external fixation splints. 15th Annual Conference of the Veterinary Orthopedic Society. Breckenridge, CO, Feb. 20–27, 1988.
6. Merkley DF, Brinker WO: Facial reconstruction following massive bilateral maxillary fracture in the dog. J Am Anim Hosp Assoc 12:831–833, 1976.
7. Lantz GC: Interarcade wiring as a method for fixation in selected mandibular injuries. J Am Anim Hosp Assoc 17:599–603, 1981.

14

Fractures and Corrective Surgery in Young Growing Animals

OSTEOTOMY

An osteotomy is the surgical division of the bone and is usually indicated to correct bony deformities that may include both angular and rotational changes.[1,2] These may occur in one plane; however, most involve two or more planes. The surgeon must keep this in mind in planning and carrying out the corrective surgical procedure.

Surgical Procedure ■ After the leg is prepared for surgery, an elastic bandage or Vet Wrap* is applied as an Esmarch bandage with a tourniquet above. An open approach is carried out to expose the operative bone area. A longitudinal incision is made through the periosteum, which is peeled back as a layer using the osteotome or periosteal elevator. The bone is osteotomized using a bone saw, Gigli wire, osteotome, or double-action bone cutter. The double-action bone cutter is preferred if the bone is soft enough because healing takes place in a shorter period of time since less heat is generated in the cutting process. If bone graft is added at the osteotomy site, it is placed between the bone and periosteum. Fixation is applied, and the surgical area is closed in layers.

Osteotomy Methods

TRANSVERSE OSTEOTOMY ■ This technique is used for correction of rotational deformity, angulation deformity, or a combination of both. Kirschner wires may be inserted in each section of bone before the osteotomy is done so that the amount of derotation can be determined. Figure 14–1 illustrates the corrective procedure, and Figure 14–2 is a case illustration of its use.

---

*Vet-Wrap 3M Animal Care Products, St. Paul, MN.

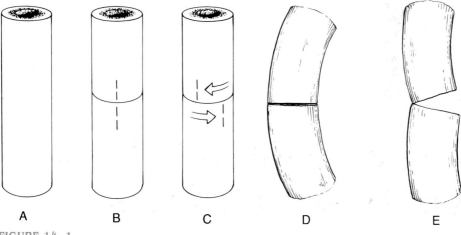

FIGURE 14-1

Transverse osteotomy. *(A–C)* Correction of a predetermined rotational deformity. *(D–E)* Open wedge type. A single transverse cut is made, rotational and angular deformities are corrected, stabilization is applied, and the deficit is filled with a bone graft.

CUNEIFORM OSTEOTOMY ■ In the closed wedge procedure, a predetermined size wedge of bone is removed from the point of maximal deformity (Fig. 14–3). Figure 14–4 is a case illustration of its use.

OBLIQUE OSTEOTOMY ■ An oblique cut is usually made parallel with the distal articular surface. The proximal point is inserted into the medullary cavity of the distal fragment. This procedure usually increases length slightly and can be used to correct rotation and varus or valgus deformity. It is most frequently used in corrective surgery for radius curvus (Fig. 14–5).

FRACTURES IN YOUNG BONE

This chapter describes separations and fractures involving the physis before closure and diaphyseal fractures in animals up to 4 or 5 months of age.[1, 2] Beyond this period of time, treatment is the same as for the adult animal.

FIGURE 14-2

Intertrochanteric osteotomy for varization and retroversion of the femoral neck. In malformation and osteoarthritis of the hip, the joint mechanics will be improved and the pain reduced by this procedure. *(A)* The transverse osteotomy line is made just proximal to the tip of the lesser trochanter. *(B)* The second osteotomy line is made about 3–6 mm from the lateral border and on an osteotomy angle determined by using the goniometer. *(C)* After rotation to correct anteversion, a 3.5 DCP or special hook plate is used for fixation.

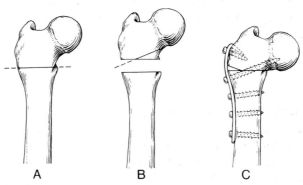

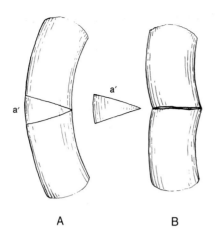

FIGURE 14-3

Cuneiform osteotomy. *(A, B)* Closed wedge type. A predetermined size wedge of bone (a′) is removed from the point of maximal deformity.

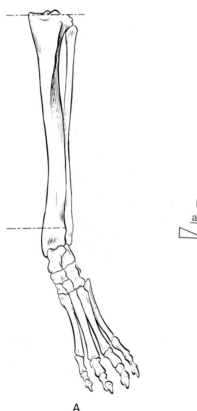

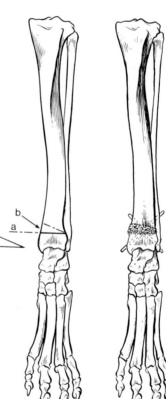

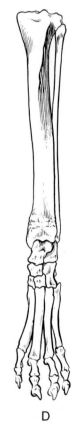

A   B   C   D

FIGURE 14-4

Cuneiform osteotomy used for correction of an angular deformity caused by partial premature closure of the distal tibial physis. *(A)* Preoperative craniocaudal view. Line (a) indicates the planned location of the osteotomy cut. *(B)* To arrive at the size wedge to remove, a paper tracing is made off the AP radiogram and cut out. A transverse cut is made near the tip of the area of greatest curvature (a). The distal portion is then moved so that it is in a straight line with the proximal portion of the tibia. The wedge indicated by the overlap of paper (b) is the size to remove. Because angular deformities and rotation encompass more than one plane, final adjustments will need to be made before application of fixation. *(C)* Because the segment was relatively short, cross pins were used for fixation at the osteotomy site. The removed wedge of bone was cut in small pieces and laid in the area as a bone graft. The fixation was further stabilized with a coaptation splint. *(D)* Clinical union was present at 7 weeks, and the splint and pins were removed.

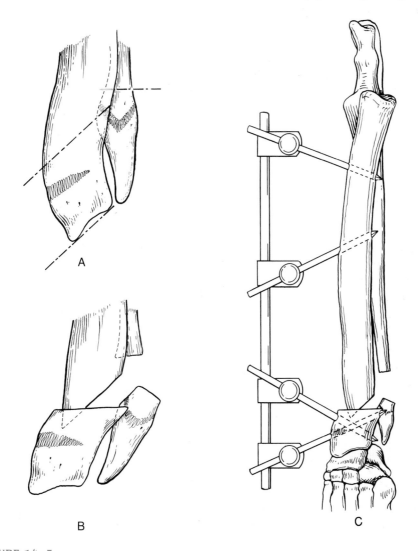

FIGURE 14–5

Oblique osteotomy. (A) The oblique line is drawn parallel with the radiocarpal joint surface at the area of greatest curvature. (B) Transverse osteotomy of the ulna, then oblique osteotomy of the radius. The pointed proximal segment of the radius is placed in the center of the distal segment. (C) The foot is derotated and held so that it is in a straight line with the proximal portion of the radius and ulna while the external fixator is applied medially.

Young bones are more resilient and elastic than older bones and thus withstand greater deflection before incomplete or complete fracture. The periosteum is attached loosely to the diaphysis and strips easily when subjected to trauma. Blood collects beneath it, and the resulting subperiosteal hematoma is soon converted to callus.

Healing is rapid (2 to 4 weeks, depending on age), and most animals produce an abundant callus regardless of the method of stabilization. Remodeling is very active and is completed quickly, with all evidence of the fracture obliterated. Nonunion is very unusual.

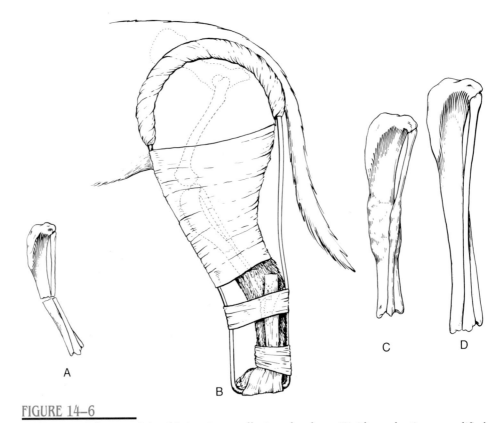

FIGURE 14–6

(A) Transverse fracture of the tibia in a toy poodle 8 weeks of age. (B) After reduction, a modified Thomas splint was applied. (C) Splint removed 2 weeks after treatment. (D) Fracture remodeled 4 weeks after treatment.

In articular fractures, anatomic reduction and rigid fixation are necessary to restore a functional joint. Fractures or trauma in the physeal area may arrest or alter growth, resulting in shortening or distortion of the limb. Because changes occur so quickly following trauma, it is fundamental that reduction and fixation be carried out as soon as possible.

Fixation

Some fractures may be treated by closed means—limb splintage (Thomas splints, coaptation splints, and so forth) (Fig. 14–6). If limb splintage is used, it must be properly applied and kept in good repair; otherwise hazards may be encountered, including valgus deformity, rotation, ligamentous laxity, and others. Internal fixation is used primarily for these types of acute fractures:

1. Fractures causing rotational deformity or excessive shortening.
2. Fractures resulting in incongruency of an articular surface.
3. Fractures affecting the physeal plate and thus future bone growth.

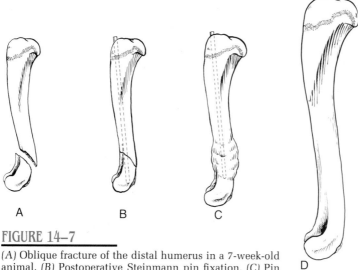

FIGURE 14-7

(A) Oblique fracture of the distal humerus in a 7-week-old animal. *(B)* Postoperative Steinmann pin fixation. *(C)* Pin removed 2 weeks postoperatively. *(D)* Fracture remodeled 4 months postoperatively.

Diaphyseal Fractures Resulting in Rotational Deformity or Excessive Shortening

The following types of fixation are used:

INTRAMEDULLARY PIN (FIG. 14–7)[1, 2] ■ In proportion, pins used in the young are relatively smaller in diameter than those used in the adult. Because cancellous

FIGURE 14-8

(A) Comminuted open fracture of the tibia in a 9-week-old animal. *(B)* Clinical union at 2½ weeks; external fixator removed at this time.

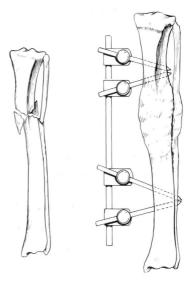

A   B

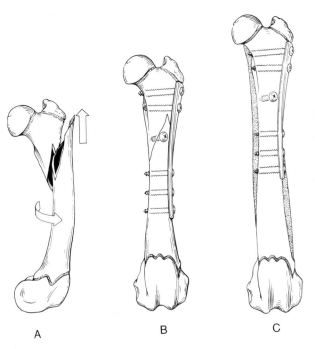

FIGURE 14-9

(A) Spiral femoral fracture with marked shortening and rotation in a Doberman 11 weeks of age. *(B)* Postoperative fixation with 3.5 bone plate and lag screw. *(C)* The fracture line had totally disappeared, and the plate was removed 4 weeks postoperatively. Another method of fixation, in this case, may have been to use two cerclage wires and an intramedullary pin.

bone is present in a high percentage of the marrow cavity, the pin stabilizes the fracture better in young animals.

EXTERNAL FIXATOR (FIG. 14-8) ■ The fundamentals of using the splint are the same in the young as in adult animals; however, healing is rapid, less fixator stiffness is required, and 2/2 pins are usually sufficient. The pins should not traverse the physis or penetrate paired bones such as the radius and ulna.[7]

BONE PLATE (FIG. 14-9) ■ When used, bone plates should be minimal in size and removed early (after approximately 3 to 5 weeks, depending on age and circumstances).

Fractures Resulting in Change in Angulation or Incongruency of the Articular Surface: Salter-Harris Classification[3]

Longitudinal growth of bone is the result of enchondral ossification occurring in the epiphyseal and metaphyseal areas. The process is a sequence of coordinated events; multiplication, growth, and degeneration of the cartilage cell, followed by calcification and vascularization of the cartilage matrix, then production of primary spongiosa, which is followed by bony trabeculae of the metaphysis.

Excess load applied to the immature bone may result in dislocation, fracture, or a crushing type injury. Because the strength of the fibrous joint capsule and ligaments is two to five times greater than that of the metaphyseal-physeal junction, the latter is more prone to injury (e.g., separation, dislocation, fracture).

Growth plates can be classified on the basis of their locations. There are two types:

Pressure growth plates are located at the ends of the long bones and transmit forces through the adjacent joint. Pressure growth plates produce the majority of the longitudinal growth.

Traction growth plates are located where muscles originate or insert. A traction growth plate contributes little to bone length (e.g., the tibial tubercle).

Salter and Harris (Table 14–1) (Fig. 14–10) have anatomically classified epiphyseal injuries in man into five types to give prognostic evaluation.[3, 4] The various types of injuries are the result of different types of forces being applied to various areas of the leg at different stages of maturity of the growth plate. The younger the animal, the greater the chance for growth deformity even with early reduction and fixation.

CONSIDERATIONS IN THE TREATMENT OF SALTER-HARRIS TYPE I–IV INJURIES[1, 2]

Open reduction and internal fixation of fractures involving joints are indicated if congruent articular surfaces cannot be obtained and maintained by conservative means. The majority of fractures in small animals need open reduction and rigid internal fixation.[1, 2] Kirschner wire fixation of bone fragments is an excellent method; healing is rapid, and the wires can be removed in 2 to 4 weeks. If more stability is needed, threaded Kirschner wires or screws may be indicated.

With meticulous surgery, early reduction, and rigid fixation, the response

TABLE 14–1

Salter-Harris Classification of Separations or Fracture-Separations Involving a Growth Plate and the Adjacent Metaphysis and Epiphysis

TYPE OF FRACTURE	RADIOGRAPHIC FINDINGS	PRINCIPAL ANATOMIC REGION INVOLVED
Type 1 (Fig. 14–10A)	Physeal separation; displacement of the epiphysis from the metaphysis at the growth plate	Proximal humerus and femur, distal femur
Type 2 (Fig. 14–10B)	Small corner of the metaphyseal bone fractured, with displacement of the epiphysis from the metaphysis at the growth plate	Distal femur and humerus, proximal humerus, proximal tibia
Type 3 (Fig. 14–10C)	Fracture through the epiphysis and part of the growth plate, but the metaphysis unaffected	Distal humerus
Type 4 (Fig. 14–10D)	Fracture through the epiphysis, growth plate, and metaphysis; several fracture lines may be seen	Distal femur, distal humerus
Type 5 (Fig. 14–10E)	Soft tissue swelling, but no bony abnormalities seen following the injury	Distal ulna, distal radius, distal femur
Type 5 (Fig. 14–10F)	Two months after trauma, shortening of ulna and partial closure with angular deformity of radius	

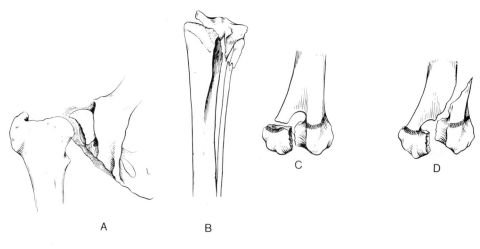

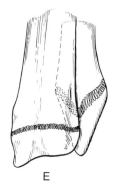

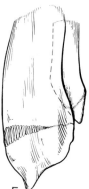

FIGURE 14–10

Salter-Harris classification of epiphyseal fractures involving the growth plate, adjacent metaphysis, and epiphysis. *(A)* Type 1 physeal fracture; displacement of the epiphysis from the metaphysis at the growth plate. *(B)* Type 2 small corner of the metaphyseal bone fractured with displacement of the epiphysis from the metaphysis at the growth plate. *(C)* Type 3 fracture through the epiphysis and part of the growth plate. Metaphysis unaffected. *(D)* Type 4 fracture through the epiphysis, growth plate, and metaphysis. *(E)* Type 5 soft tissue swelling but no bony abnormalities seen immediately following the injury. *(F)* Type 5 2 months after the trauma; closure and shortening of the ulna and partial closure with an angular deformity of the radius are evident.

to Type I–IV injuries is very encouraging for healing and return to normal or at least satisfactory function. The surgical approach and fixation methods are similar to those described for the corresponding areas in the adult animal. Figures 14–11 and 14–12 depict most of fracture-separations that occur in the region of the physis and suggest methods of stabilization.

CONSIDERATIONS IN THE TREATMENT OF SALTER-HARRIS TYPE V INJURY [1–19]

Type 5 injury to the growth plate can result in temporary delay in growth, altered growth, or premature closure and cessation of growth. The entire growth plate or a localized region within the growth plate may close prematurely. In paired bones, the premature closure may involve one or both bones, resulting in partial or complete growth impairment.[1, 2] The degree of alteration of growth is proportional to the growth potential remaining at the time of injury.

Frequently, the immediate resultant pathology may be too insignificant for clinical observation, but with time (one to several weeks) signs and alterations begin to appear.

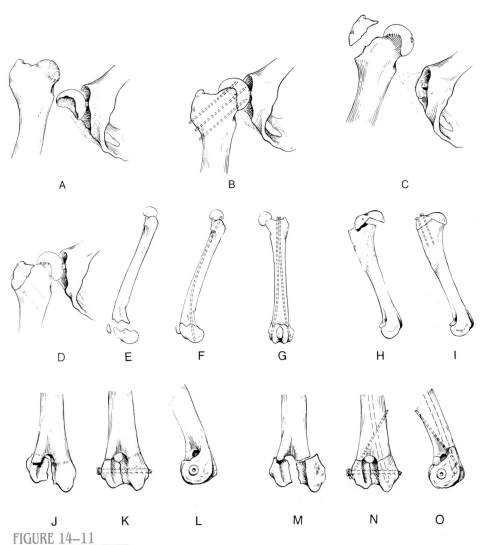

FIGURE 14-11

Physeal fractures of the femur and humerus. *(A)* Type 1 injury to the pressure physis; separation of the proximal femoral physis. *(B)* Fixation with three smooth Kirschner wires. *(C, D)* Type 1 injury to the traction physis; avulsion or fracture of the trochanter major and dislocation of the coxofemoral joint. After reduction of the femoral head, the trochanter is relocated and fixed in place with two Kirschner wires. *(E–G)* Type 1 injury to the pressure physis; separation of the distal femoral physis. Reduction and fixation using two small intramedullary pins. *(H, I)* Type 1 injury to the pressure physis; fracture of proximal humeral epiphysis. Fixation by insertion of two Kirschner wires entering on the ridge of the greater tuberosity. *(J–L)* Type 3 injury to the pressure physis; fracture between the medial and lateral aspects of the humeral condyle with separation at the lateral part of the epiphyseal line. Fixation with a transcondylar lag screw. *(M–O)* Type 3 bicondylar fracture of the humeral condyles with separation along the entire epiphyseal line. Fixation with a transcondylar screw and two pins.

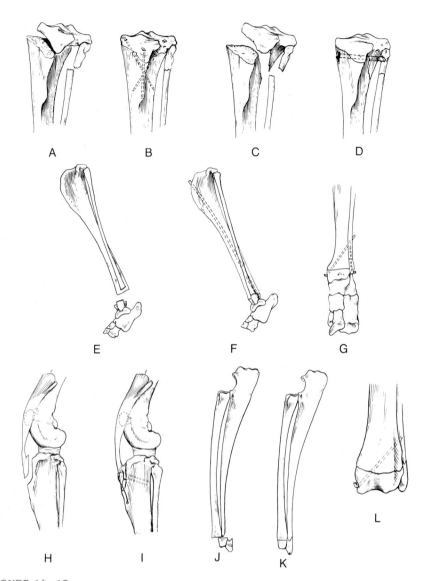

FIGURE 14–12

Physeal fractures of the tibia and radius and ulna. (A, B) Type 1 injury to the pressure physis. Fracture of the proximal tibial physis with a fracture of the fibula. Fixation with three obliquely inserted Kirschner wires. (C, D) Type 2 injury to the pressure physis; fracture of the proximal tibial physis and a small portion of the metaphysis. Fixation with a cancellous screw under the physis. (E–G) Type 1 injury to the pressure physis. Fracture of the distal tibial and fibular physis. If the parts are stable on reduction, the hock is flexed to a right angle and fixed in this position for 2 to 3 weeks with a cast. The right angle places the bone segments in the most stable position. If this fracture is unstable on reduction, a small intramedullary pin is inserted from the proximal end of the tibia down into the epiphysis, or two small pins are inserted through the malleoli. A cast is applied for additional stabilization. (H, I) Type 1 injury to the traction physis. Avulsion of the tibial tubercle. Fixation by a tension band wire. (J, L) Type 1 separation of the distal physis of the radius and fracture of ulna. The segments are usually stable on reduction (K) but require external stabilization with a coaptation splint. If segments appear unstable after reduction, a Kirschner wire (L) should be inserted diagonally through the radial styloid process into the diaphysis.

Clinical characteristics of premature partial or complete closure of the physis include lameness, shortened limb, angular deformity (valgus or varus), rotation, discomfort, crepitation, and restricted range of movement. Radiography should include both limbs, with special attention to the physis, the adjacent metaphysis, and the joints above and below the growth arrest. This study should determine (1) length of bone or bones, (2) width of the joint space at either end of the shortened bone, (3) direction of diaphyseal bowing, (4) angulation of the foot, (5) range of movement, and (6) extent of pathological changes in the joints above and below the physeal injury.

The treatment of pathological changes in Salter-Harris Type V injury presents more complex problems when paired bones (e.g., radius and ulna) are involved. The radius and ulna must grow in a synchronous manner to promote normal growth and maintain congruency of their common articular surfaces. The ulna grows from two growth plates. The proximal physis, which closes between approximately 187 and 222 days, contributes only to olecranon length and is usually not significant to premature physeal closure anomalies. The distal ulnar physis is responsible for 100 percent of the longitudinal growth distal to the elbow joint and equals the combined growth of the proximal and distal radial physis. The radius grows from both the proximal physis (40 percent) and distal physis (60 percent) and provides the major weight-bearing surface of the elbow joint (75 to 80 percent). Closure of these physes ranges from about 220 to 250 days.

Abnormal development from asynchronous growth between the radius and ulna can result from retarded growth of the distal ulnar physis, distal radial physis, or proximal radial physis. Resultant dysplasias are common orthopedic problems and vary depending on the physis or physes involved, the age of the animal at time of involvement, and the span of time since injury.

Two cardinal considerations in planning corrective surgery are (1) the operative procedure should increase or at least maintain length because closure of the physis always results in a shorter bone (limb), and (2) corrective surgery should be carried out early to avoid or to at least minimize irreversible pathological changes.

TYPE V—DISTAL ULNAR PHYSIS CLOSURE

Premature closure of the distal ulnar physis and subsequent deformities are the most common complications of physeal injury (Fig. 14–13A). The conical shape of the distal ulnar physis is unique to the dog. In all other animals, the radial and ulnar physes are flat and predisposed to shearing fractures, and after reduction, the prognosis for uninterrupted growth is usually good. The canine distal ulnar physis is unable to shear because of the conical configuration, and thus shear forces are transformed to compressive forces and injury. Significant retardation in growth of the distal ulnar physis results in a shortened ulna, which acts as a bowstring to restrict longitudinal growth of the radius. This retardation produces various degrees of cranial and/or lateral bowing of the distal radius, radial shortening, valgus deformation, and external rotation of the foot, elbow subluxation, and degenerative joint disease in the carpal and elbow joints. With cessation of growth of the ulnar diaphysis and

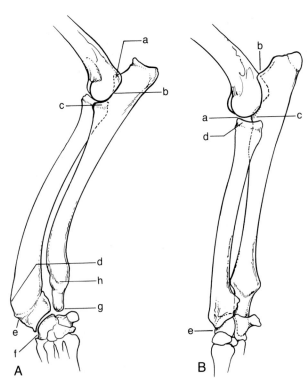

FIGURE 14–13

(A) Radiographic changes characteristic of premature closure of the distal ulnar physis. With a cessation of growth of the ulna and continued growth of the radius, there is remodeling of the anconeal process with sclerosis (a), elbow subluxation with flattening of the trochlear notch (b) and distal displacement of the styloid process (c), anterior bowing of the radius (d), opening of distal radial physis (e) with increased angulation of the radiocarpal joint (f), and secondary arthritic changes. There is proximal relocation of the ulnar styloid (g) because of the shortened ulna. The distal ulnar physis is closed (h). *(B)* Radiographic changes characteristic of premature closure of the distal or proximal radial physis. With a cessation of growth of the radius, there is increased width of the humeroradial joint space (a), proximal displacement of the anconeal process (b), remodeling of the trochlear notch and coronoid process (c), and development of secondary osteoarthritis. There is posterior and lateral displacement of the radial head (d). Angular deformity may or may not be present; however, there is usually some increase in radiocarpal joint space (e) and evidence of radial physis closure.

continued growth of the radius, the humeral condyle is forced proximally and can result in subluxation and damage to the anconeal process. The most severe lesion occurs in the distal half of the trochlear notch, resulting in degenerative cartilage changes, fracture of trabeculae in the subchondral bone, and alteration in joint morphology.

Lameness is usually the first sign of premature closure of the distal ulnar growth plate. Beginning radiographic changes are usually visible at this time, and corrective surgery is indicated to avoid or to at least minimize subsequent changes. Removal of a 1 to 3″ section of the distal ulna (including periosteum) is required to remove the bowstring effect. Corrective osteotomy of the radius to realign the foot is performed at the same time. Use of the external fixator is usually the preferred method of fixation (Fig. 14–14).

Figure 14–14 shows a healed fracture of the radius with premature closure of the distal ulnar physis in a 5-month-old Afghan hound. Treatment originally consisted of application of a Mason metasplint. The radiographs taken 3 weeks after the injury revealed a clinically healed radius, leg shortening of 10 mm, premature closure of the distal ulnar growth plate, moderate valgus deformity of foot, and early signs of incongruency of the elbow joint.

The primary objectives were to restore congruency of the elbow joint and to correct the cranial bowing of the radius and valgus deformity of the foot.

Removal of a 1½″ section of the ulna (including periosteum) corrects the bowstring effect, and, in most instances (with minor deformity), the proximal ulna will readjust in position and make the correction needed for congruency at the elbow joint. An oblique osteotomy of the radius at the fracture site was used to derotate the foot and straighten the radius.

In Figure 14–14C, the external fixator is in place, following removal of a section of the ulna and corrective osteotomy of the radius. At 4½ weeks postoperatively, the radius was healed and the elbow joint was congruent and had a full range of movement (Fig. 14–14D). The external fixator was removed at this time.

Note: If the periosteum is removed with the section of ulna, the ends of the ulna will not heal back together. This is desirable because healing together of the ulnar ends in the growing animal re-establishes the bowstring effect. Operating by use of an Esmarch bandage gives good visualization, and with care the periosteum can be removed; it also reduces surgical operating time.

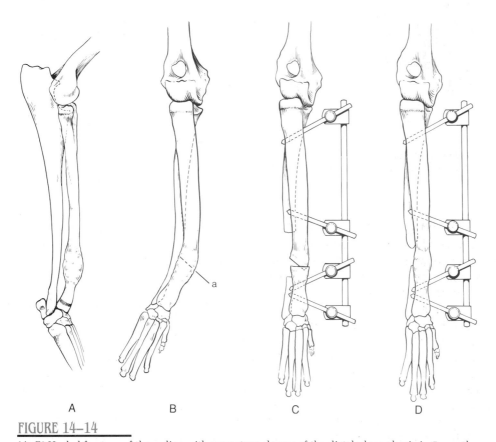

A   B   C   D

FIGURE 14–14

(A, B) Healed fracture of the radius with premature closure of the distal ulnar physis in 5-month-old Afghan hound. Preoperative lateral and craniocaudal views. *(C)* A 1½″ section of the ulna (including periosteum) was removed, the oblique cut (a) in the radius was made at the point of greatest curvature, the point of the radius was inserted into the medullary cavity of the distal radial segment, the foot and distal section of radius was held so that it was in line with the proximal end of the leg, and the external fixator was applied on the medial surface. *(D)* At 4½ weeks postoperatively, healing of the radius has occurred and the elbow joint is congruent with a good range of motion; the external fixator was removed at this point.

If there is marked incongruency of the elbow with or without distal changes, a proximal ulnar osteotomy (Fig. 14–17) allows the proximal end to shift proximally and re-establish congruency as well as possible with the deformed articulating surfaces. A small Steinmann pin is used for stabilization.

TYPE V PROXIMAL OR DISTAL RADIAL PHYSIS CLOSURE

Less common than premature closure of the distal ulnar physis is premature closure of either the proximal or distal radial physis (Fig. 14–13B). Premature closure of either physis results in shortening of the radius, although the leg may remain straight. Asymmetric closure alters growth and usually results in some degree of angular deformity. As the ulna grows, the shortened radius is pulled distally by the radioulnar ligament, bringing about an increase in joint space between the radial head and humeral condyle. As discrepancy of growth between the radius and ulna continues, the medial and lateral collateral ligaments of the elbow impinge the humeral condyle on the coronoid process with subsequent displacement and an increase of humeroulnar joint space, elongation of the articular notch, and sometimes fragmentation of the coronoid process and degenerative joint disease. There are also changes in the radio-carpal joint, which may include angular deformity and an increase in joint space. The first clinical sign of closure is a gradual onset of lameness. Beginning radiographic changes are present at this time, and surgery is indicated to check or minimize joint changes.

Corrective osteotomy of the radius is needed to restore length and congruency of the elbow joint. Bone lengthening with plate fixation is usually the method of choice. For animals over 5½ months of age, one lengthening will usually be sufficient. For those under this age, the procedure may need to be repeated in 6 to 8 weeks to restore length and congruency. If the closure is accompanied by angular deformity, corrective osteotomy for this defect may be delayed until the lengthening osteotomy is about healed (Fig. 14–15).

Figure 14–15 shows premature closure of the distal growth plate of the radius, with shortening and early secondary incongruency of the articular surfaces in the elbow joint in a 4-month-old large dog. The animal had started to favor the leg 2 weeks before presentation. The leg appeared to be straight from both lateral and cranial views.

The objective was to restore approximately normal length to the radius and thus restore congruency to the articular surfaces of the elbow joint. Because the animal had approximately 4 months of growth left, the operative procedure was expected to be repeated to maintain a good elbow joint.

A transverse midshaft osteotomy of the radius was performed (Fig. 14–15B). The bone segments were wedged apart 15 mm with a bone spreader, and a semitubular plate was inserted for fixation. Congruency of the elbow joint was restored. At the 3-month re-examination, the osteotomy area was filled with bone. Shortening of the radius and incongruency of the elbow were again evident. Lameness returned about 3 weeks prior to this re-examination. Discrepancy between the coronoid process of the ulna and the articular surface of the radius was evident (Fig. 14–15C).

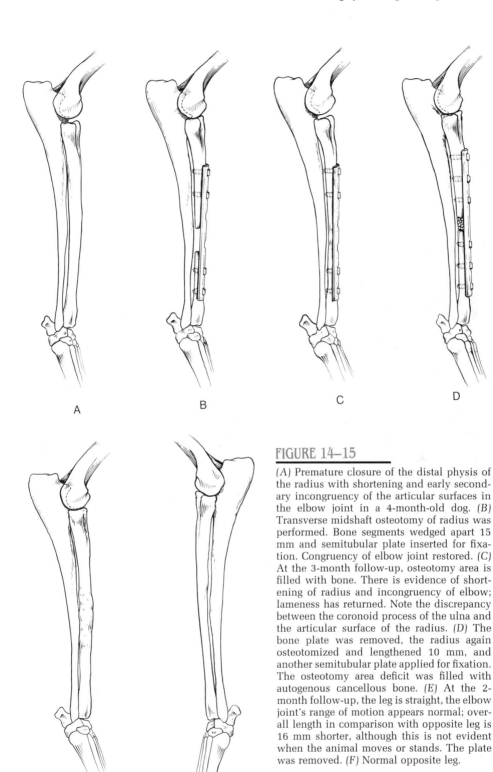

A

B

C

D

E

F

FIGURE 14–15

(A) Premature closure of the distal physis of the radius with shortening and early secondary incongruency of the articular surfaces in the elbow joint in a 4-month-old dog. *(B)* Transverse midshaft osteotomy of radius was performed. Bone segments wedged apart 15 mm and semitubular plate inserted for fixation. Congruency of elbow joint restored. *(C)* At the 3-month follow-up, osteotomy area is filled with bone. There is evidence of shortening of radius and incongruency of elbow; lameness has returned. Note the discrepancy between the coronoid process of the ulna and the articular surface of the radius. *(D)* The bone plate was removed, the radius again osteotomized and lengthened 10 mm, and another semitubular plate applied for fixation. The osteotomy area deficit was filled with autogenous cancellous bone. *(E)* At the 2-month follow-up, the leg is straight, the elbow joint's range of motion appears normal; overall length in comparison with opposite leg is 16 mm shorter, although this is not evident when the animal moves or stands. The plate was removed. *(F)* Normal opposite leg.

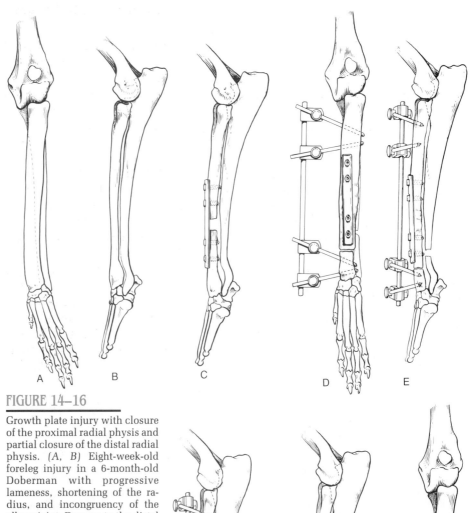

FIGURE 14–16

Growth plate injury with closure of the proximal radial physis and partial closure of the distal radial physis. *(A, B)* Eight-week-old foreleg injury in a 6-month-old Doberman with progressive lameness, shortening of the radius, and incongruency of the elbow joint. Damage to the distal radial physis with partial closure resulted in some progressive valgus deformity and outward rotation of the foot. *(C)* Lateral view following transverse osteotomy. The segments were slowly wedged apart 11 mm by exerting constant pressure with a bone spreader, restoring length to the radius and congruency to the elbow joint. A semitubular buttress plate was applied. In 1 month, healing at the osteotomy site was nearly complete, the elbow joint appeared congruent, leg function had markedly improved. *(D, E)* The ulna and radius were osteotomized, derotation and straightening of the foot were carried out, and an external fixator was applied to the medial surface of the radius. *(F)* After 7 weeks, both osteotomy sites were

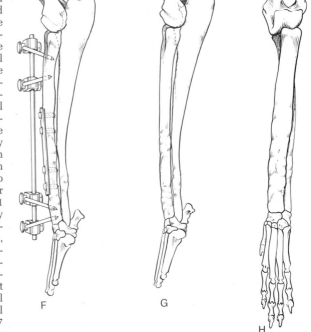

well healed and the plate and external fixator were removed. *(G, H)* At 1 year, the leg was straight when viewed laterally and cranially; there was a 10° loss of flexion at the elbow joint, the elbow joint appeared congruent, the affected leg was slightly shorter than the opposite normal leg, function was good.

The bone plate was removed, and the radius was again osteotomized and lengthened by 10 mm. A semitubular plate was applied for fixation (Fig. 14–15D). At the 2-month follow-up, the leg was straight, the elbow joint range of motion appeared normal, and function was good (Fig. 14–15E). The overall length in comparison to the opposite leg was 16 mm shorter; however, this was not evident on standing or moving. The normal opposite leg is shown in Figure 14–15F.

PARTIAL OR COMPLETE PREMATURE CLOSURE OF THE DISTAL AND PROXIMAL RADIAL PHYSES IN THE SAME LIMB ■ For this condition, the objectives of corrective osteotomy are to restore congruency of the elbow joint and realign the foot. Treatment varies with the individual set of circumstances. Because the leg is already shorter than the opposite leg, it is advisable to plan the surgical procedure so that the leg is lengthened or, at least, not shortened further (Fig. 14–16).

A 6½-month-old Doberman had suffered a foreleg injury approximately 8 weeks previous to being treated (Fig. 14–16). Lameness was intermittent at first but became continuous and progressive during the preceding 3 weeks. Radiographs revealed premature closure of the proximal radial physis, shortening of the radius, and incongruency of the elbow joint. There was also evidence of damage to the distal radial physis along with altered growth,

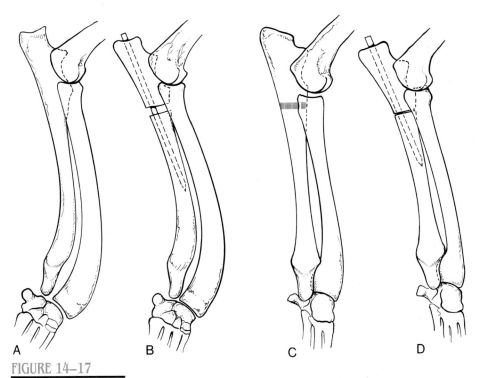

A   B   C   D

FIGURE 14–17

(A) Another approach for improving congruency of the elbow joint in connection with ulnar shortening is to do a proximal ulnar osteotomy to allow the proximal end to move upward. *(B)* An intramedullary pin is used for stabilization. *(C, D)* For cases in which the radial shortening is minimal and the animal is about mature, removal of a short section of the ulnar diaphysis to restore congruency of the radial head and humeral condyle is another solution. A small Steinmann pin is used for stabilization.

resulting in some valgus deformity and outward rotation of the foot, which—the owner had stated—was becoming more pronounced.

The first objective was to restore radial length and elbow congruency; the second objective was to correct the angular deformity and external rotation of the foot at a later date.

A transverse osteotomy was performed and the segments were wedged apart by 11 mm using a bone spreader; this restored length to the radius and congruency to the articulating surfaces of the elbow joint. A semitubular plate (buttress plate) was applied for fixation (Fig. 14–16C). In 1 month, healing at the osteotomy site was well under way, and the elbow appeared stable. Leg function had improved markedly. At this time, the ulna and radius were osteotomized, angulation and rotation were corrected, and an external fixator was applied for fixation on the medial surface of the radius.

In 7 weeks, the osteotomy sites were well healed. The bone plate and external fixator were removed. When the animal was rechecked at 1 year of age, good functional use of the leg was evident (Fig. 14–16G, H). The leg appeared straight from both lateral and cranial views. There was a 10° loss of flexion at the elbow joint; however, it was not discernible on walking or running. The affected radius was slightly shorter than the opposite normal radius. The animal adjusted by slightly increasing extension at the shoulder and elbow joints; this was not evident on standing or moving.

For cases in which the ulna shortening is minimal and the animal is about mature, a short section of the ulna can be removed (Fig. 14–17A, B). This allows the proximal segment of ulna to move upward, thus reestablishing congruency of the elbow joint. A small Steinmann pin is used for stabilization.

For cases in which the radial shortening is minimal and the animal is about mature, one can remove a short section (ostectomy) of the ulna to restore congruency of the radial head with the humeral condyle. A small Steinmann pin is used for stabilization (Fig. 14–17C, D).

REFERENCES

1. Brinker WO: Small Animal Fractures. East Lansing, MI. Depart Cont Ed Serv, Michigan State University, 1978.
2. Brinker WO, Hohn RB, Prieur WD: Manual of Internal Fixation in Small Animals. New York, Springer-Verlag, 1984, pp 255–264, 225–238.
3. Salter RB, Harris WR: Injuries involving the epiphyseal plate. J Bone Joint Surg 45-A:587, 1953.
4. O'Brien T, Morga JP, Suter PF: A radiographic study of growth disturbances in the forelimb. J Small Anim Pract 12:19, 1961.
5. Clayton-Jones DA, Vaughan LC: Disturbance in the growth of the radius in dogs. J Small Anim Pract 11:453–468, 1970.
6. Newton CD, Nunamaker DM, Dickinson CR: Surgical management of radial physeal growth disturbance of dogs. J Am Vet Med Assoc 167:1011–1018, 1975.
7. Noser GA, Carrig CB, Brinker WO, et al: Asynchronous growth of the canine radius and ulna: effects of cross pinning the radius to the ulna. Am J Vet Res 38:601–610, 1977.
8. Olsen N, Brinker WD, Carrig C: Asynchronous growth of canine radius and ulna: Effect of longitudinal growth of radius. Am J Vet Res 40:3, 1979.
9. Noser G, Carrig CB, Merkley D, et al: Asynchronous growth of the canine radius and ulna: effects of cross-pinning the radius to the ulna. Am J Vet Res 38:601, 1977.
10. Kleine LJ: Radiographic diagnosis of epiphyseal plate trauma. J Am Anim Hosp Assoc 7:250–255, 1971.
11. Carrig CB, Morgan JP: Asynchronous growth of the canine radius and ulna: early radiographic changes following experimental retardation of longitudinal growth of the ulna. J Am Vet Radial Soc 16:121, 1975.
12. Skaggs S, DeAngelis MP, Rosen H: Deformities due to premature closure of the distal

ulna in fourteen dogs: a radiographic evaluation. J Am Anim Hosp Assoc 9:496–500, 1973.

13. Dieterich HF: Repair of radius curvus in a two-stage surgical procedure: a case report. J Am Anim Hosp Assoc 10:48–52, 1974.

14. Newton CDE: Surgical management of distal ulna physeal growth disturbances in dogs. J Am Vet Med Assoc 164:479–487, 1974.

15. Vaughan LC: Growth plate defects in dogs. Vet Rec 98:185–189, 1976.

16. Olson NC, Carrig CB, Brinker WO: Asynchronous growth of the canine radius and ulna: effect of retardation of longitudinal growth of the radius. Am J Vet Res 40:351, 1979.

17. Olson NC, Brinker WO, Carrig CB: Premature closure of the distal radial physis in two dogs. J Am Anim Hosp Assoc 176:906, 1980.

18. Olson NC, Brinker WO, Carrig CB, et al: Asynchronous growth of the canine radius and ulna: surgical correction following experimental premature closure of the distal radial physis. J Vet Surg 10:3, 1981.

19. Fox, SM: Premature closure of the distal, radial and ulnar physes in the dog, Part I. Pathogenesis and Diagnosis. Comp Cont Ed 6:128–139, 1984. Part II. Treatment. Comp Cont Ed 6:212–220, 1984.

20. Gilson SD, Piermattei DL, Schwarz AD: Treatment of humeroulnar ulnar subluxation using a dynamic ulnar osteotomy. A review of 13 cases. Veterinary Orthopedic Society Meeting, Feb 20–27, 1988, Breckenridge, CO.

PART II

Lameness and Joint Surgery

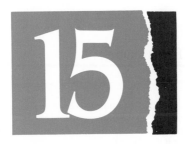

Physical Examination for Lameness

Veterinary diagnosticians frequently encounter patients with a history of lameness or pain of obscure origin. In a veterinary hospital environment, excitement and apprehension often seem to cause a chronic lameness to disappear or painful maneuvers to go unnoticed by the animal. Historical information, careful observation and palpation, and proper radiography are paramount in assessing the patient and in advising appropriate therapy. Not every case deserves the comprehensive examination as described in this chapter. The intended use of the animal, the economics of the case, and the animal's cooperation are also factors that guide the veterinarian. When undue pain is elicited or when further damage is caused by manipulations, the examination is purposefully left incomplete or is done under anesthesia at a later time.

History

In general, certain historical information should be obtained, such as age, breed, gender, identification of the lame limb, the degree of pain or lameness, its duration, other limb involvement, known trauma, changes with weather, exercise, time of day, or rest, and treatments that have been tried. Other information such as anorexia, depression, fever, multiple-limb involvement, and so forth may be important to know. With severe progressive lameness (without history of trauma), neoplasia should be considered. Owners often report sudden onset of lameness in the animal that later proves to be chronic in origin. This is usually not an attempt to deceive but a failure of the owner to note the slow development of lameness. At some point the animal can no longer withstand the discomfort, and the lameness becomes apparent even to the untrained eye (Table 15–1).

TABLE 15–1

Causes of Lameness in the Dog (Excluding Fractures and Minor Soft Tissue Injuries)

REAR LIMB	FORELIMB
Growing Dog	**Growing Dog**
1. hip dysplasia	1. osteochondritis dissecans (OCD)*—shoulder
2. avascular necrosis (Legg-Calvé-Perthes)	2. luxation/subluxation shoulder—congenital
3. avulsion of long digital extensor	3. avulsion supraglenoid tubercle
4. osteochondritis dissecans (OCD)*—stifle	4. osteochondritis dissecans (OCD)*—elbow
5. osteochondritis dissecans (OCD)*—hock	5. UAP (ununited anconeal process)
6. luxating patella complex	6. FCP (fragmented coronoid process)
7. genu valgum	7. UME (ununited medial epicondyle)
8. eosinophilic panosteitis	8. elbow incongruity
Medium—Large breeds = 1, 3–8	a. congenital
Toy—Small breeds = 2, 6	b. physeal injury
Chondrodystrophied breeds = 1, 2, 6, 8	9. radius curvus
	10. retained cartilaginous cores (ulna)
Adult Dog	11. eosinophilic panosteitis
A. arthritis (or continuum) 1–7	Medium—Large breeds = 1, 4–7, 8b, 9–11
B. luxating patella complex	Toy—Small breeds = 2, 8, 9
C. eosinophilic panosteitis	Chondrodystrophied breeds = 2?, 5, 8a, 8b, 9, 11
D. cruciate/meniscal syndrome	
E. inflammatory joint disease	**Adult Dog**
F. neoplasia	A. arthritis (or continuum) 1–6, 8, 9
Medium—Large breeds = A$_1$, A 3–7, B, F	B. UME (ununited medial epicondyle)
Toy—Small breeds = A$_2$, B, D–F	C. eosinophilic panosteitis
Chondrodystrophied breeds = A$_1$, A$_2$, B, D–F	D. bicipital tenosynovitis
	E. calcification of supraspinatus tendon
	F. contracture of infraspinatus or supraspinatus
	G. bone/soft tissue neoplasia
	H. luxation/subluxation—shoulder
	I. inflammatory joint disease
	Medium—Giant breeds = A, 7, 11, I
	Toy—Small breeds = 2, G, H, I
	Chondrodystrophied breeds = 2?, A–5, A–8, A–9, C, H, I

*OCD = osteochondritis dissecans.

The animal should then be observed standing for such conditions as weakness, asymmetrical limb trembling, spasms, asymmetry of the head, neck, or limb carriage, unequal weight-bearing, bowleg or knock-knee, muscle atrophy, and favoring a limb. After a routine general examination of the heart, lungs, lymph nodes, and abdomen, examination for the lameness should be undertaken.

Observation of Gait

One of the first tasks for the diagnostician is to observe the animal's gait, both at a walk and at a trot. Running is usually not as helpful. If lameness is still not apparent, having the animal gait in tight clockwise and counterclockwise circles or go up and down stairs may elucidate abnormalities. Besides obvious limping, the following signs should be noted if present: shortened strides, dragging of the toenails, "toeing-in" or "toeing-out," hypermetria, "bunny-hopping," stumbling, ataxia, criss-crossing of the rear legs, asymmetry of gait or stance, or abnormal sounds upon ambulation. A bobbing motion of the head will often be observed with forelimb lameness. In its attempt to remove weight from the leg, the animal lifts its head as the lame limb is placed.

NEUROLOGICAL EXAMINATION

With the animal standing, conscious proprioception should be tested in the forelimbs and rear limbs. The animal's limbs should be under the body in a normal fashion (Fig. 15–1) and not abducted. With the examiner supporting the animal's chest or groin area with one hand, the other hand gently and slowly turns the patient's toes over so that weight-bearing occurs on the dorsum of the paw. The animal should quickly right the paw. Delay of more than one second or an absence of perception and reaction to this proprioceptive reflex may mean involvement of the nervous system rather than the musculoskeletal system. This test is extremely important in the situation of the older German shepherd dog with known or suspected hip dysplasia that is described as "worsening." More times than not, in our experience, it is a spinal problem, and the abnormal proprioceptive response can help determine this. Severe hip dysplasia will not result in neurological deficits. Non-neurological causes of an apparent neurological deficit include mental depression or extreme acute pain (i.e., a recent fracture).

In recumbent traumatized patients, the paw pinch, knee jerk, and anal reflexes are important in assessment of neurological status. *Voluntary* movement should be observed. Limb withdrawal after paw pinching does not mean it is conscious and voluntary. When the cause of pain is obscure, especially in breeds susceptible to disc disease, the animal's neck and back should be flexed, extended, and palpated.

PALPATION FOR ASYMMETRY

Before an individual limb is examined, the diagnostician's hands should be placed simultaneously over each side of the animal's shoulders, back, and legs in an attempt to detect asymmetry of size, shape, heat, and sensitivity. This is extremely helpful for detecting tumors, abscesses, or atrophy in long-haired breeds.

The diagnostician examines the rear limbs for asymmetry by observing the standing animal from behind. The following areas are quickly palpated

FIGURE 15–1

Conscious proprioceptive response is elicited while the dog is standing with the limbs in a normal position. The dog is supported while the toes are turned over and released. A delay or absence of the dog's quickly returning the toes to a normal position may mean neurological rather than orthopedic problems.

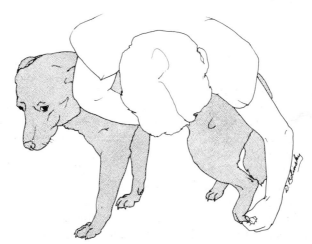

and compared with the opposite side: the gluteal area, trochanter major area, cranial thigh, patellar region, patellar ligament, tibial tubercle, cranial tibia (shin), and cranial tarsometatarsal regions. The caudal and plantar structures, such as the caudal thigh, stifle, popliteal lymph nodes, gastrocnemius muscle, calcaneal tendon, and caudal hock region are palpated in the same way. With each hand simultaneously palpating contralateral limb areas, subtleties of abnormality can be detected, leading to such diagnoses as coxofemoral luxation, fracture, stifle swellings, and gastrocnemius muscle rupture.

Similar methods are used to examine the foreleg. Muscle atrophy in the shoulder region is best detected by comparing the prominences of the spines of the scapulae. Abnormal distance from the acromion to the greater tubercle of the humerus may indicate dislocation. Palpation from the distal lateral epicondyle toward the olecranon (over the anconeus muscle) may help to detect swelling of the elbow. Normally, the anconeus muscle is flat; a bulge under the muscle could indicate increased synovial fluid.

Closer examination of the limb is then performed in total lateral, not sternal, recumbency. This allows easy restraint and patient relaxation and avoids abnormal muscular tension that may obscure instabilities.

SEDATION

In general, it is best to avoid administering a sedative upon initial examination so that areas of sensitivity or unusual crepitation may be detected. If the animal is too tense or unmanageable, sedation may be used; it should be realized, however, that sedation may interfere with accurate assessment of reflexes and pain (as in eosinophilic panosteitis) and the detection of some types of crepitation (meniscal click). The suspected area of involvement should be investigated last, if possible, to avoid causing pain early in the investigation and to avoid missing other areas of involvement. In most instances, it is better to examine the normal limb first in order to allow relaxation for the animal and to assess "normal" reactions from maneuvers.

JOINT MANIPULATION

Manipulations of the joints are used to detect instability, incongruency, luxation or subluxation, pain, abnormal range of motion, and abnormal sounds. It must be remembered that palpation of the involved area may not elicit a pain response. Likewise, when a painful reaction or crepitation is detected, it may originate some distance away from the part being examined.

Forelimb

DISTAL JOINTS

To be thorough, the diagnostician should examine the forelimb from the toe to the shoulder. The toes are spread apart, and the nails, webbing, and pads are inspected and manipulated. The phalangeal and metacarpophalangeal joints are palpated for stability, which is best done with the joints in extension. The palmar sesamoids of metacarpophalangeal joints 2 and 5 are subjected to digital pressure to check for pain. The joints are directly medial and lateral to the large metacarpal pad. The carpus is flexed, extended, and palpated closely for swelling, laxity, or instability; the elbow is examined in the same way. A bulge between the lateral epicondyle and proximal elbow could mean increased joint fluid from several diseases of the elbow. Hyperextension of the elbow may cause pain in association with an ununited anconeal process.

SHOULDER

The shoulder is examined by gentle flexion, extension, and rotation, followed by hyperextension and hyperflexion while the opposite hand stabilizes the scapula. When osteochondritis dissecans of the shoulder is present, the patient may flinch or yelp, especially on hyperextension. While holding the acromion with one hand, the examiner may push, pull, adduct, or abduct the shaft of the humerus in order to detect luxation or subluxation. Sedation may be necessary for accurate evaluation. When these procedures are used, many normal shoulder joints "pop" or "click" without any significance. Inflammation and sensitivity of the biceps tendon origin may be tested by extending the elbow and bringing the entire limb caudally alongside the thoracic wall while applying digital pressure to the tendon region.

BONE PALPATION

Bone or periosteal pain (from eosinophilic panosteitis, traumatic periostitis, tumors, and so on) is elicited by gentle pressure directly over the distal, middle, and proximal ends of the long bones. Because squeezing the muscle may cause pain, the muscles should be pushed aside if possible before the bone is palpated. The radius, ulna, and humerus of the normal leg are palpated first. When an area affected by eosinophilic panosteitis is touched, a sudden wincing, limb withdrawal, yelping, or, rarely, biting is usually elicited in even the most stoic patient. Limb withdrawal is also seen when the patient becomes bored or irritated by the examination. Therefore, the maneuver should be repeated and the reaction should be reproduced to yield a positive finding.

Rear Limb

The procedure for examining the rear limb is similar and the toe examination is identical to those for the forelimb. The hock is given a valgus (inward) and varus (outward) stress, especially when trauma has occurred recently. Many partial instabilities are concurrent with other more apparent pathology.

STIFLE

Stifle swelling can be detected by comparing the rear limbs while the dog or cat is standing and, hopefully, bearing weight equally. With stifle swelling, the patellar ligament is less distinct because effusion or fibrosis pushes outward and "buries" the ligament. The medial/lateral width of the femoral condyles just caudal to the patella often increases as a result of the production of osteophytes or capsular thickening. Either this thickness or the indistinct patellar ligament should alert the clinician that the stifle is involved. More thorough examination is carried out in lateral recumbency.

The stifle is gently flexed and extended several times with the palm of one hand over the cranial aspect of the joint to detect crepitation, grating, clicking, or snapping. This maneuver is not painful even in a pathological joint (except fracture), and the examiner can feel the animal relax. The craniolateral aspect of the joint is palpated for a "lump" in young large-breed dogs. If present, a lump may represent an avulsion of the long digital extensor tendon. The area just lateral to the patella and trochlear ridges is palpated for thickness and smoothness.

PATELLAR LUXATION ■ Because the examination is relatively painless, patellar luxation should be checked for before cruciate instability. To check for medial patellar instability, the animal's knee is extended, the toes are internally rotated, and thumb pressure is placed on the lateral aspect of the patella (Fig. 15–2). Conversely, for lateral luxations, the stifle is slightly flexed, the toes are externally rotated, and pressure is applied on the medial aspect of the patella with the index and middle fingers (Fig. 15–3). The patella normally moves slightly medially and laterally, but it is pathological when it hops out of the trochlear groove. Sometimes the patella may be luxated by just rotating the paw with the stifle extended. Whether this abnormality is the cause of lameness depends on severity of the lameness, the presence of a permanently

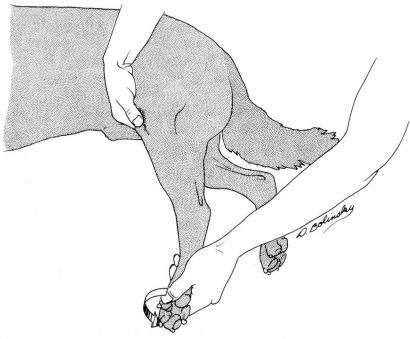

FIGURE 15–2

For the patella to be luxated medially, the stifle is extended and the toes are rotated medially while the patella is pushed medially.

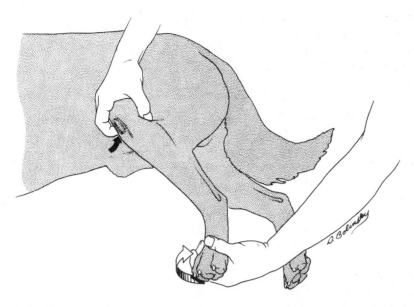

FIGURE 15-3

For the patella to be luxated laterally, the stifle is partially flexed and the toes are rotated laterally while the patella is pulled laterally.

luxated patella (patellar ectopia), erosion of the patella or femoral condyle, and the absence of any other problem being detected in the animal's limb or spine.

In tiny puppies with patellar ectopia or severely swollen stifles, the patella may be difficult to find. However, the tibial tubercle is usually prominent and identifiable. Its cranial, medial, or lateral position is noted. As the patellar ligament is palpated proximally, a pea-size hardness can be detected one to two inches (depending on animal size) from the ligament's insertion.

COLLATERAL LIGAMENT INSTABILITY ■ Medial joint instability is diagnosed when the joint line "opens" upon proper stress. This is accomplished by holding the stifle slightly extended, while the index and middle fingers of one hand are placed parallel to the medial joint line and the distal tibia is angulated laterally (abducted) with the other hand. Normally, the taut medial collateral and cruciate ligaments and joint capsule allow no distraction of the tibia and femur. In the same way, lateral collateral ligament injury is detected by placing the thumb perpendicular to the lateral joint line at the level of the fibular head. With the limb moderately extended, an outward stress of the stifle is accomplished by adducting the distal tibia.

CRUCIATE LIGAMENT ABNORMALITIES ■ Finally, the animal is examined for craniocaudal instability of the stifle, indicative of cruciate ligament abnormalities. In the normal animal, this is not a painful maneuver; however, where there has been a rupture, some pain may be elicited, causing tenseness. Usually, some degree of drawer movement is detected by gentle, patient manipulation. If the animal is too tense, however, some sedation may be indicated.

The presence and amount of drawer movement vary with the tenseness and size of the animal, the duration of pathology, and the kind of cruciate pathology present. Except in young puppies, there is no craniocaudal drawer movement in normal dogs and cats. If there is the slightest amount, then some form of cruciate pathology exists. Some internal rotation of the tibia as the joint is flexed is normal but this will increase with cranial cruciate rupture. If surgery is to be performed, accurate assessment of drawer movement should be undertaken after anesthesia is administered.

Drawer movement is due to the tibia's sliding cranially or caudally in relation to the femur. Theoretically, cranial drawer occurs with anterior cruciate ligament rupture, and caudal drawer occurs with caudal cruciate ligament rupture. Indirect cranial drawer movement (tibia compression test[1]) can be elicited by holding the leg in standing position while hyperextending (dorsiflexing) the hock. This tenses the gastrocnemius muscle, which compresses the femur and tibia together. In the anterior cruciate ligament–deficient stifle, the tibia will slide forward. This motion is detected by the palm and index finger of the opposite hand. This maneuver is not particularly painful. Direct drawer is the use of the hands directly around the stifle, which may elicit pain and reflexive tightening of the knee. With the examiner standing caudal to the animal, the hands are positioned as close to bone as possible to prevent other tissues (such as muscle and skin) from moving. The index finger of one hand is placed on the proximal end of the patella while the thumb is placed over the lateral fabellar region. The index finger of the other hand is placed on the tibial crest, and the thumb is positioned caudal to the fibular head (Fig. 15–4). The wrist should be straight. Frequently, the novice bends the wrist, resulting in inability to "drawer" the unstable stifle. With the stifle slightly flexed and held at that angle, the tibia is pushed gently forward and then is pushed caudally.

Rotation should be prevented. The maneuver should be done quickly because if it is performed more slowly, the examiner loses a sense of quantitating the amount of drawer movement present. Sometimes the stifle is already in a cranial drawer position and needs to be reduced caudally before cranial drawer motion can be detected. If there is concurrent patellar luxation,

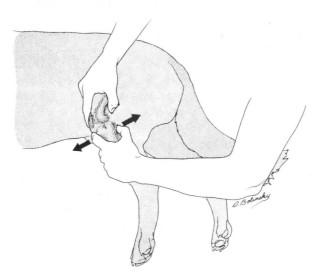

FIGURE 15–4

For stifle drawer movement to be palpated, the thumb and index finger surround the caudal distal gfemur (*fabellar region*) and proximal patella while the other thumb and index finger surround the tibial crest and caudal fibular head. The leg is flexed slightly and the femur is held steady while the tibia is pushed directly cranially and caudally, swiftly and gently. The manipulation is repeated in extension and flexion.

the patella should be relocated in the trochlea and held there while drawer movement is attempted. The drawer maneuver is repeated in 80 to 90 degrees of flexion and full extension. In most animals, the greatest amount of drawer movement occurs when the stifle is in slight flexion.

Partial drawer movement (less than that expected with a full fresh tear of the cranial cruciate ligament in the relaxed patient) may mean any of the following:

1. A partial tear or stretching of the cranial cruciate ligament. Drawer motion in these cases is usually only detected in flexion.

2. A full tear of the cranial cruciate with a displaced torn meniscus wedged between the tibia and femur.

3. A chronically ruptured cranial cruciate ligament with joint capsule fibrosis.

4. A torn caudal cruciate ligament.

An exception worth mentioning is cruciate disease of large breeds of dogs. Often, they will have relatively and absolutely less drawer movement than small dogs. There is also more of a tendency for abnormal internal rotation rather than cranial drawer movement.

Isolated tears of the caudal cruciate ligament are rare (a 2 percent occurrence). They may be suspected in any of the following situations:

1. Grade II drawer movement is detected, especially in flexion. (Grade IV drawer movement is that perceived in an acute full tear of the cranial cruciate ligament. Grades I to III are subjective estimates of less than full drawer.)

2. Caudal drawer movement is detected. (However, it may be difficult to determine the direction of the drawer movement if the tibia at rest is luxated caudally. "Cranial" drawer actually reduces the luxation and may be mistaken as true anterior drawer.)

3. A sudden cessation of cranial drawer movement occurs as the cranial cruciate becomes taut. With cranial cruciate ruptures, this cessation is not abrupt.

A pathological meniscus may be suspected if a definite click is palpated or heard during flexion or extension or during drawer movement manipulations or while gaiting the animal. Sedation often causes the disappearance of these findings.

PELVIS AND COXOFEMORAL JOINT

Next, the pelvis and coxofemoral joint are examined. A rectal examination may be indicated to detect pelvic fracture or a painful prostrate, which can lead to weakness or mimic rear-limb lameness. In trauma cases, the tuber ischii and wing of the ilium are pushed, pulled, or rotated while the examiner checks for instability, crepitation, or elicitation of pain.

The relationship of the trochanter major of the femur to the wing of the ilium and ischium is noted. According to procedure, its relative position to the opposite limb should have been noted earlier in the standing animal. If imaginary points and lines connecting them are placed on the dorsal wing of the ilium, ischium, and trochanter major, a triangle is formed (Fig. 15–5). This triangle appears altered from the one formed on the normal opposite side

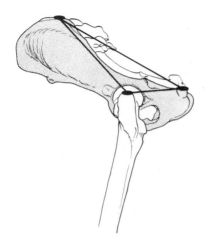

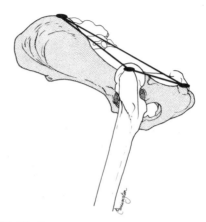

FIGURE 15-5

Areas are palpated on the wing of the ilium, tuber ischii, and trochanter major. If imaginary lines are drawn between these points in a normally conformed hip joint, a triangle is formed.

FIGURE 15-6

With hip dislocation, the triangular shape becomes altered when compared with the other normal hip of the dog (compared with Figure 15-5).

when there is muscle atrophy, coxofemoral luxation (Fig. 15-6), subluxation or luxation with or without osteoarthrosis as a result of hip dysplasia, fractures of the femoral neck, slipped capital femoral epiphyses, Legg-Calvé-Perthes disease, and so forth. The distance from the trochanter major to the ischium should be compared. This distance is greater with craniodorsal coxofemoral luxation.

The hip joint is manipulated by grasping the stifle with one hand while the palm of the other hand rests on the trochanter major region. The hip is flexed, extended, and rotated. Some clicks that are normal may be detected as muscles jump over prominences. Crepitation from severe cartilage erosion may be detected. Crepitation from the stifle, however, may resound in the hip (and vice versa), giving a false interpretation.

Ortolani's sign, elicited in humans to detect hip laxity, may be used in the dog for the same purpose.[2] This test can be performed in the unsedated (or sedated) dog by grasping the stifle in one hand while using the other hand to stabilize the pelvis and identify the trochanter major. As the stifle is pushed slowly upward (parallel to the femoral shaft axis), it subluxates the hip. The stifle is then abducted, which causes the unstable femoral head to slide back into the socket, eliciting a click that can be detected by the opposite hand on the trochanter major (Fig. 15-7).

Hip joint laxity may be detected in the following manner: One hand grasps the midfemoral region with the thumb lateral, the rest of the fingers medial. The index finger of the other hand rests on the trochanter major with the palm stabilizing the dorsal acetabular area. The distal femur is elevated so that the femur lies parallel to the examining table. The femur is lifted quickly and laterally and then relaxed as the opposite index finger pushes the trochanter medially toward the socket.

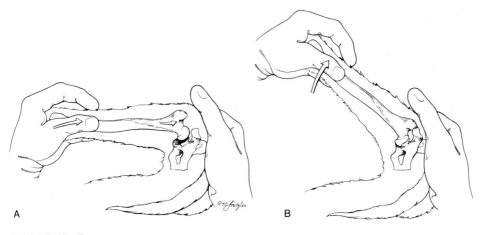

FIGURE 15–7

Ortolani's sign: Subluxation due to hip dysplasia may be created by pushing the stifle proximally and parallel to the femur (A). Reduction of the subluxation results in a "thud" that is detected by the other hand on the trochanter major region when the stifle is abducted (B).

In many breeds of nondysplastic puppies, there is no lateral movement or subluxation; in others, some looseness is normal. Many investigators have disputed this technique in diagnosing hip dysplasia in pups 8 to 10 weeks old. In young adult dogs (6 to 9 months old), however, laxity of ¼ inch or more is probably indicative of hip dysplasia and may mean more than the pathology seen on the radiograph. The older dysplastic dog seldom has this instability. This last maneuver may be painful for many dogs with either normal or abnormal hips and may result in tenseness. This tenseness is probably due to the digital pressure on the medial aspect of the thigh. Sedation is frequently needed for meaningful evaluation if instability is not detected.

BONE PALPATION

The tibia and femur are palpated for periosteal pain in the same manner as described for the forelimb.

REFERENCES

1. Henderson RA, Milton JL: The tibial compression mechanism: A diagnostic aid in stifle injuries. J Am Anim Hosp Assoc 14:474–479, 1978.

2. Chalman JA, Butler HC: Coxofemoral joint laxity and the Ortolani sign. J Am Anim Hosp Assoc 21:671–676, 1985.

Structure and Function of Joints

The purpose of joints is to afford the greatest stability to the body during weight-bearing and motion. Proper diagnosis and management of joint disease depend on understanding the basic anatomy and physiology of the musculoskeletal system. With recent advances using the scanning electron microscope and histochemical and biochemical techniques, articular cartilaginous diseases are beginning to be understood. Cures for stopping or reversing osteoarthrosis are on the horizon. The material presented in this chapter should guide clinicians in arriving at rational treatments and stimulate researchers in pursuing clinical problems.

CONNECTIVE TISSUES

The work horse of the musculoskeletal system is connective tissue. Its components are outlined in Table 16–1 and are mentioned throughout the next two chapters. It is extremely important that their relationships be understood.

CLASSIFICATION OF JOINTS

Joint classification[1, 2] is summarized in the following way. Joint diseases of animals ordinarily involve the diarthrodial joints.

FIBROUS JOINTS (SYNARTHROSES) ■ These joints have little motion.

    1. Syndesmoses. These have considerable intervening connective tissue (for example, the temporohyoid joint).
    2. Sutures (for example, the skull).
    3. Gomphosis (for example, the tooth socket).

CARTILAGINOUS JOINTS ■ These joints have limited motion, which permits compression and stretching.

    1. Hyaline cartilage (synchondrosis) (for example, the costochondral junction, epiphyseal plate of the long bones of growing animals).

TABLE 16–1

Components of Connective Tissue in Joints

CELL TYPES	FIBERS (PROTEINS)	MATRIX (GROUND SUBSTANCE)
Fibroblast	Elastin	Proteins
Chondrocyte	Reticulin	Mucopolysaccharides (proteoglycans),
Osteocyte	Collagen (hydroxyproline)	hyaluronic acid, chondroitin
Synoviocyte		sulfate, keratosulfate
Myocyte		Water

2. Fibrocartilage (amphiarthrosis) (for example, the mandibular symphysis).

SYNOVIAL JOINTS (DIARTHROSES) ▪ These joints allow the greatest amount of movement.

COMPONENTS OF SYNOVIAL JOINTS

All synovial joints have a joint cavity, joint capsule, synovial fluid, and articular cartilage (Fig. 16–1). Some joints, in addition, have intra-articular ligaments, menisci, and fat pads.

The articular surface of bone is covered by hyaline cartilage. The bones are united by a joint capsule and ligaments. The joint capsule is composed of an inner synovial membrane that produces synovial fluid and an outer fibrous layer that aids joint stability. The range of motion in joints is limited by muscles, ligaments, joint capsule, and bone shapes.

Any mechanical system wears out with time, and animal joints are no exception. Wear and tear occur with aging but may be hastened or exaggerated by trauma, disease, and structural and biochemical changes in the articular cartilage.[2] Lubrication—which decreases friction—is vital in keeping the "machine" in proper working condition. This lubrication can be affected by the nature and geometry of the articulating surfaces, the synovial membrane,

FIGURE 16–1

Schematic drawing of joint components. (*A*) Joint cavity with joint fluid. (*B*) Articular cartilage. (*C*) Subchondral bone. (*D*) Synovial lining. (*E*) Fibrous joint capsule.

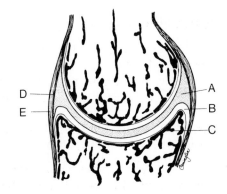

the physical and chemical properties of the synovial fluid, the load on the joint, and the type of joint movement.[2]

Synovial Membrane

The synovial membrane is highly vascular, blends with the periosteum as it reflects onto bone, and covers all structures within the joint except articular cartilage and menisci. The synovial lining may extend beyond the fibrous layer and may act as bursae under tendons and ligaments. Basically, the synoviocytes have two functions: phagocytosis and synovial fluid production.

Synovial Fluid

Synovial fluid is a dialysate of blood to which mucoprotein has been added by the synoviocytes.[2] Its chief function is lubrication, which decreases friction, thereby decreasing wear and tear to articular cartilage. The synovial fluid also provides nutrition to the articular cartilage and maintains electrolyte and metabolite balance.

The chief mucoprotein of synovial fluid is hyaluronic acid, which is highly polymerized and prevents serum proteins of high molecular weight from entering the fluid. Joint fluid proteins increase with inflammatory conditions either because of a decrease in this polymerized state of hyaluronic acid or as a result of an increase in the capillary permeability of the subsynovium. Both situations cause joint effusion. Corticosteroids are thought to interfere with production of hyaluronic acid.[3]

Inflammatory joint conditions may be distinguished from noninflammatory conditions by analysis of joint fluid (see Table 17–2). In inflammatory conditions, the protein electrophoretic pattern of synovial fluid is altered, sugars are decreased, the cell population increases, and cell type ratios change. The polymerized state of hyaluronic acid can be estimated using the glacial acetic acid precipitate test.[3–5] The quality of mucin decreases rapidly in the presence of some infections and can slowly decrease in chronic osteoarthritis.

The viscosity of the synovial fluid is related to this mucoprotein; it is higher in small joints and at low rates of shear and use (walking, standing). A decrease in viscosity during more rapid joint movement causes less drag and, therefore, less friction of the joint surfaces. Cold temperatures may cause increased viscosity and, therefore, drag to joint surfaces. This partly explains the necessity for "warming up" prior to athletic pursuits.

Articular Cartilage

Joint cartilage is the recipient of most blows and jolts to the skeleton.[6] Its resilience buffers these blows, preventing erosion and shortening of bones. This surface also allows gliding action of joints.

Grossly, normal adult articular cartilage is white, smooth, glistening, and translucent. It lacks blood vessels, lymphatic vessels, and nerve endings.[7] Nutrients must pass the synovial barrier and the cartilage matrix barrier before reaching the chondrocytes. Thus, a mechanical or chemical joint injury is not recognized by the animal until a synovial reaction occurs. Some agents used to treat synovial disease may be deleterious to the articular cartilage (for example, corticosteroids in rheumatoid arthritis) but are not detected by cartilage cells owing to this lack of nerve endings in the cartilage. Because cartilage lacks blood vessels, the inflammatory repair process following trauma is impossible until deep lesions invade subchondral bone.[8]

The thickness of the articular cartilage is generally greater when:

1. The joints are larger.
2. The joints are under considerable functional pressure.
3. Friction is increased.
4. The joints are not very congruent.
5. The joints are greatly used.
6. The animals are younger.
7. The joints are exercised.[7]

Histologically, articular cartilage is composed of chondrocytes, fibers, and ground substance. Eighty percent of cartilage is water, 10 percent is collagen, and 10 percent is proteoglycan.[8]

There are four layers of articular cartilage, not including a surface membrane (lamina splendens), based on fiber orientation and shape of chondrocytes:

1. Tangential (surface layer).
2. Transitional (intermediate layer).
3. Radial (deep layer).
4. Calcified[7, 10, 11] (Fig. 16–2).

The chief nourishment for the cartilage comes from the synovial fluid, with 7 to 10 percent coming from the blood vessels of the subchondral bone.[9]

CELLS ■ Chondrocytes in mature cartilage are sparse but are metabolically quite active despite their appearance on light microscopy. The intermediate-zone cells are active in synthesizing protein and other components of matrix, as well as collagen. In immature cartilage, mitoses occur in the surface zone (resulting in growth of the cartilaginous mass during adolescence) and in the basilar layers (accounting for growth of the bony epiphysis). At skeletal maturity, however, mitoses are absent under normal conditions and cartilage cells are incapable of division. There is recent evidence that under certain situations, such as cartilage laceration and osteoarthritis, the chondrocyte can reinitiate cell synthesis and multiple division of a single cell (clone).[8]

FIBERS ■ Collagen fibers are imbedded in matrix. They are not normally visible by light microscopy because the refractive index is the same as that of the ground substance.[2] They may be seen by phase-contrast microscopy or electron microscopy.[7] Freyberg has postulated that the fibers form hoops or wickets[6] (Fig. 16–2). The surface arrangement of the cartilage fibrils provides a slightly irregular surface that prevents adhesions of opposing articular surfaces when

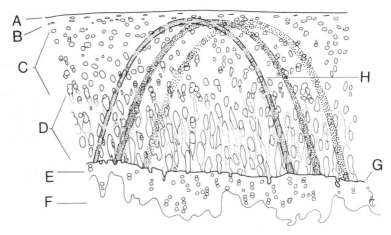

FIGURE 16–2

Schematic drawing of articular cartilage histology showing its layers and fibril arrangement. (*A*) Surface membrane. (*B*) Tangential zones. (*C*) Intermediate zones. (*D*) Radial zone. (*E*) Calcified zone. (*F*) Subchondral zone. (*G*) Tide mark. (*H*) Fibrils or "wickets."

lubricated by synovial fluid.[2] This superficial layer of tightly packed fibers resists shear forces during joint movement.[12] When pressure is applied at the surface, the fibrils expand laterally while the thickness decreases. When the pressure is released, the fibrils rebound as a result of their elasticity.[6] This elasticity decreases with continuous compression or with age. The resiliency of cartilage also depends on the fibrils being "buoyed" by matrix proteoglycans.[12] The intermediate layer has the greatest shock-absorbing capacity because of the high content of bound water.[12]

If the superficial layers of fibers are lost through erosion (trauma), the matrix comes into closer contact with joint enzymes, leading to further degradation. This layer can then be considered like the integument as a first line of defense for the rest of the cartilage.

MATRIX ■ The matrix or ground substance of articular cartilage is composed of bound water and proteoglycans. Subunits of proteoglycans are called glycosaminoglycans, such as chondroitin 6-sulfate, chondroitin 4-sulfate, and keratosulfate. These macromolecules are stiffly extended in space as a result of their strong negative charges, repelling one another. They are hydrophilic and bind to the collagen fibers, thereby creating a barrier to absorption of substances from synovial fluid. Only substances having a small molecular weight permeate normal articular cartilage. The barrier to outward flow of organic components is thought to be the factor for its resiliency and resistance to deformation of the articular cartilage.[8]

The health of cartilage matrix may be measured by using metachromatic histochemical stains such as toluidine blue O or safranin-O. Loss of metachromasia (and thus chondroitin sulfate) is characteristic of degenerating cartilage[13] and is directly proportional to the severity of the disease.[14] Staining is thus an excellent research tool.

Significant softening of the articular cartilage has been seen in dogs undergoing experimental stifle immobilization for 11 weeks.[15] Rabbit knees immobilized for 6 days underwent extensive loss of metachromatic staining.[16] Mobilization, therefore, is critical to the health of articular cartilage.

Diseases, injuries, or toxic agents affecting matrix or fibers result in changes that can be permanent, painful, and crippling. Understanding these mechanisms may elucidate a cure or reversal of these changes.

HEALING OF THE ARTICULAR CARTILAGE

In normal situations, mitotic figures are not seen in the articular cartilage of adult animals. However, in lacerations to the articular cartilage or in osteoarthrosis, the chondrocyte can reinitiate DNA synthesis and cell division possibly by release of biological suppression of the replicatory apparatus.[8]

If lacerations in adult animals are confined to the upper layers of the avascular articular cartilage, no inflammation or effective healing can occur. Mitotic activity does occur but ceases one week after initial injury. In rabbits, these superficial lacerations neither healed nor progressed to more serious disorders within one year of injury. When lesions were deep and invaded the subchondral vascular bone, reparative granulation tissue invaded the defect, which then changed to fibrocartilage by metaplasia. The end result, years after injury, is a discolored, roughened pit surrounded by smooth hyaline cartilage.[8] Allowing this vascularity to reach the surface is the theoretical reason for curetting or drilling a defect that results from osteochondritis dissecans. Continuous passive motion[17, 18] (where the animal is placed in a confining apparatus with the affected limb attached to a machine that moves the leg at preselected rates and ranges of motion for 2 to 4 weeks) has shed new light on articular cartilage healing. However, it remains to be seen if there are practical applications in veterinary medicine.

REFERENCES

1. Evans HE, Christensen GC: Miller's Anatomy of the Dog. Philadelphia, W. B. Saunders Company, 1979, p 95.
2. Gardner E: Structure and function of joints. In Hollander JL (ed): Arthritis and Allied Conditions. Philadelphia, Lea & Febiger, 1972, pp 32–50.
3. Van Pelt RW, Connor GH: Anatomy and physiology of articular structures. Vet Med 57:135–143, 1962.
4. Van Pelt RW: Arthrology Lecture Course. East Lansing, Mich., Michigan State University, 1967.
5. Hollander JL: The Arthritis Handbook. West Point, Pa., Merck, Sharp, & Dohme, Inc., 1974.
6. Freyberg RW: The joints. In Sodeman WA, Sodeman WA, Jr. (eds): Pathologic Physiology: Mechanisms of Disease. Philadelphia, W. B. Saunders Company, 1967, Chapter 32.
7. Jaffee HL: Structure of joints, bursal mucosae, tendon sheaths. In Metabolic Degenerative and Inflammatory Diseases of Bones and Joints. Philadelphia, Lea & Febiger, 1972, pp 80–104.
8. Mankin HJ: The reaction of articular cartilage to injury and osteoarthritis. N Engl J Med 291:1285–1292, 1974.
9. Moroudas A: Transport through articular cartilage and some physiological implications. In Ali SG, Elves MW, Leaback DH (eds): Proceedings of the Symposium on Normal and Osteoarthrotic Articular Cartilage. Middlesex, England, Institute of Orthopaedics, 1974, pp 33–40.
10. Wittberger H: Ultrastructure of canine articular cartilage: Comparison of normal and degenerative (osteoarthritic) hip joints. Am J Vet Res 36:727–739, 1975.
11. Van Pelt RW: Pathologic findings associated with idiopathic arthritides in cattle. J Am Vet Med Assoc 149:1283–1290, 1966.
12. Johnson LC: Joint remodeling as a basis for osteoarthritis. J Am Vet Med Assoc 141:1237–1241, 1962.
13. Collins DH, McElligott JF: Sulfate ($S^{35}O_4$) uptake by chondrocytes in relation to his-

tological changes in osteoarthritic human articular cartilage. Ann Rheum Dis 19:318–330, 1960.

14. Mankin HJ, Dorfman H, Lippiello L: Biochemical and metabolic abnormalities in articular cartilage from osteo-arthritic human hips. II. Correlation of morphology with biochemical and metabolic data. J Bone Joint Surg 53:523–537, 1971.

15. Jurvelin J, Kiviranta I, Tammi M, Helminen JH: Softening of articular cartilage after immobilization of the knee joint. Clin Orthop Rel Res 207:246–252, 1986.

16. Troyer H: The effect of short term immo-bilization on the rabbit knee joint cartilage. Clin Orthop Rel Res 107:249–257, 1975.

17. Salter RB, Simmonds DF, Malcolm BW, et al: The biological effect of continuous passive motion on the healing of full-thickness defects in articular cartilage. J Bone Joint Surg 62-A:1232–1250, 1980.

18. Driscoll SW, Salter RB: The repair of major osteochondral defects in joint surfaces by neochondrogenesis with autogenous osteoperiosteal grafts stimulated by continuous passive motion. Clin Orthop Rel Res 206:131–140, 1986.

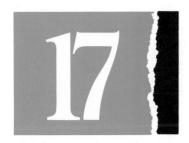

Cartilage and Joint Abnormalities

Pain, deformity, and limb malfunction can result from improper joint physiology. Many acute joint conditions progress to chronic osteoarthrosis. The aim of the orthopedist is to minimize or stop these changes. In chronic osteoarthrosis, the objective is to minimize patient discomfort and improve limb function.

DEFINITIONS

ARTHRITIS ■ The simple definition of arthritis is inflammation of a joint. Many orthopedic conditions in veterinary medicine do not cause any long-lasting appreciable inflammation of the synovial lining and are therefore best termed "arthrosis."

ARTHROSIS ■ The term arthrosis refers to a noninflammatory degenerative joint condition characterized by a lack of inflammation in the synovial lining and the presence of normal or near-normal synovial fluid.

OSTEOARTHRITIS (OSTEOARTHROSIS) ■ The common arthritis seen in veterinary medicine is a slowly progressive cartilage degeneration with osteophyte production usually caused by trauma or microtrauma (abnormal wear). There is very little inflammation of the synovial lining (and therefore few changes in the synovial fluid) compared with the more inflammatory disease conditions of joints. The synovial response is the basis for classifying joint disease. Because it is degenerative and not inflammatory, a more proper term is osteoarthrosis, or degenerative joint disease (DJD).

CLASSIFICATION OF JOINT DISEASE

Joint diseases are classified in the following way[1]:

Noninflammatory Joint Disease
1. Degenerative joint disease (DJD), osteoarthritis, osteoarthrosis
   a. Primary
   b. Secondary

2. Traumatic
3. Neoplastic
Inflammatory Joint Disease
1. Infectious
2. Noninfectious
   a. Immunological
      (1) Erosive
      (2) Nonerosive

NONINFLAMMATORY JOINT DISEASE

Osteoarthrosis

PRIMARY DEGENERATIVE JOINT DISEASE ■ Primary DJD is a degeneration of cartilage in elderly individuals occurring for no known reason other than the wear and tear that comes with aging. Mankin, however, points out that aged cartilage does not show the same changes as osteoarthrotic cartilage.[2] Consequently, contradictions in various histochemical and biochemical data exist because of the types of abnormal cartilage that are analyzed and not identified as to source.

Most people older than 40 years of age have some degree of degeneration in the hip, knee, or interphalangeal joints of the fingers (Heberden's nodes). Much interest in this phenomenon has been generated in human medicine. Animals are useful as research models for osteoarthrosis. Bentley has stated that a suitable model is valuable in facilitating further study of the pathogenesis of the disease and the effects of various treatments upon it.[3] The ideal model for DJD should start with the loss of matrix and should progress to fissuring, fibrillation, erosion of cartilage, subchondral sclerosis, osteophyte production, and mild synovial inflammation.

TABLE 17-1

Conditions Predisposing to Secondary Degenerative Joint Disease*

CONGENITAL
1. Achondroplasia (generalized conformational defects of the limbs).
2. Localized conformational or postural defects (for example, bowleggedness, straight hocks).
3. Chronic hemarthrosis with hemophilia.

DEVELOPMENTAL
1. Osteochondritis dissecans.
2. Failure of ossification centers to fuse (for example, ununited anconeal or possibly coronoid processes).
3. Abnormal development of joints (for example, hip dysplasia, congenital elbow luxations).
4. Premature epiphyseal closure (for example, radius curvus) resulting in carpal DJD from angular deformity and elbow DJD from joint incongruity, owing to asynchronous growth of the radius and ulna.
5. Miscellaneous conditions (patellar luxations).

ACQUIRED
1. Damage to articular surfaces.
   a. Post-traumatic (for example, fractures of articular surfaces, unusual shoulder stress seen in sled-pulling huskies).
   b. Sequelae to inflammatory joint disease (for example, osteophytes seen secondary to instability from rheumatoid arthritis).
2. Damage to supporting structures of joints (for example, tendons, ligaments, menisci).
3. Aseptic necrosis (for example, Legg-Calvé-Perthes disease of the femoral head).
4. Neuropathies (for example, abnormal range of motion resulting from abnormal pain and proprioception sense).

*Printed by permission of Pederson NC: Canine joint disease. In 1978 Scientific Proceedings, 45th Annual Meeting of the American Animal Hospital Association, 1978, pp 359–366.

SECONDARY DEGENERATIVE JOINT DISEASE ■ Secondary DJD develops secondarily from known conditions that affect the joint and supporting structures. This is perhaps the most common type observed in small animals. Those conditions predisposing animals to secondary DJD are outlined by Pedersen[1] and appear in Table 17–1.

DEGENERATION OF THE ARTICULAR CARTILAGE

Bentley[3] states that the cartilage breakdown starts when compression or shear stresses cause cell damage, releasing cathepsin, which in turn induces loss of proteoglycans and water. This decreases cartilage resiliency and leaves collagen exposed so that fissuring (fibrillation) occurs. Additional chondrocyte damage then occurs, and additional cathepsin is released ad infinitum.

Other investigators hypothesize that excessive wear occurs in this damaged cartilage with normal physical stresses and that the degradation products released into the joint space produce secondary synovitis and sometimes inflammation[4] (hence, pain and effusion in acute flare-ups of a chronic situation[5]). There are attempts at repair in the forms of granulation tissue, chondrocyte proliferation, clones, increased mucopolysaccharide production, and osteophytes. However, with degradative enzymes, lack of orientation in regenerating tissue, and abnormal stress caused by these unstable joints, physiological repair attempts are usually negligible. Two instances, however, have been reported that may show some reversibility of osteoarthrosis.[6]

In a case of hip osteoarthrosis, devitalized tissue was removed and a metal device interposed between the acetabulum and femoral head. Imperfect hyaline articular cartilage formed under the prosthesis. The implication is that the prosthesis protected the reparative granulation tissue from mechanical abrasion.

In another case of osteoarthrosis of the hip, wedge osteotomies of the femur with reangulation of the femoral head were done. Subsequently, radiographs showed regression of the osteoarthrosis.[6] Wilson stated that there was an increase in the joint space and more reformation of cartilage.[7]

Changes in Bone

Two changes in bone occur in the presence of osteoarthrosis: the production of marginal osteophytes and the appearance of subchondral sclerosis.

OSTEOPHYTES ■ Marginal osteophytes may protrude into the joint or may develop within capsular structures or ligamentous attachments to joint margins. Their shape is determined by mechanical forces and the surface contour from which they protrude.[2] McDevitt and colleagues showed this to begin histologically seven days after experimental rupture of the cranial cruciate ligament in dogs.[8] At first, there was an accumulation of fibroblast-like cells at the synovial membrane–articular cartilage junction, which by four weeks had changed to woven bone with a few chondrocytes. By eight weeks, trabecular patterns were seen in the early osteophyte along with resorption of the femoral cortex underneath, allowing some communication of bone marrow from each area. By 16 weeks after the rupture, the osteophytes consisted of trabecular bone covered by thick cartilage. By 48 weeks, the trabeculae and marrow of the osteophyte and distal femur were confluent. Some investigators have proposed that hyperplasia of the cartilage margin is invaded by vascular granulation tissue with subsequent bone formation.[9] The reason for these osteophytes is unclear, and the theories are contradictory.[9–11]

SCLEROSIS ■ Under areas of cartilage erosion, sclerosis (eburnation) occurs. The denuded bone becomes polished and grossly resembles ivory or marble and represents advanced cartilage destruction. Turek believes that an early stage of this condition results from endochondral ossification of the lower layers of cartilage, which histologically are detected by double "tidemarks" (wavy hematoxylin-staining lines demarcating the interface between calcified and noncalcified hyaline cartilage).[11]

Changes in Synovial Membrane

The synovial membrane in degenerative joint disease generally appears normal. The surface may show some hyperplasia, but very little inflammatory response, except in certain forms of hip osteoarthritis in humans and large animals.

Changes in Cartilage

Early gross changes in articular cartilage consist of a localized soft or velvety area that changes to a yellow-to-dull-white color with pits, and with depressions and linear grooves becoming apparent. In advanced disease, the cartilage may be soft and spongy. In areas where subchondral bone is exposed and subjected to wear, a highly polished eburnated surface may be present.[12] In joints with apposing articular surfaces, "kissing" or mirror-image lesions develop.[12, 13] Osteophytes develop at joint margins where the synovium reflects off the chondral-perichondral junction. Osteophytes sometimes form in an area not covered by synovium.

HISTOLOGICAL ■ Collins has defined the histological progression of osteoarthrosis as follows[14]:

1. Loss of surface cartilage layers.
2. Diffuse increase in numbers of cells.
3. Moderate decrease in metachromatic staining, indicating loss of proteoglycans. In experimental sectioning of the cranial cruciate ligament in dogs, McDevitt[8] and associates found this loss 16 weeks after the rupture.
4. Ingrowth of subchondral vessels through the tidemark (the wavy hematoxylin-stained line demarcating the interface between calcified and noncalcified hyaline cartilage).
5. Vertical clefts beginning at the surface (flaking).
6. "Fibrillation" when clefts extend to the calcified zone.
7. Further loss of metachromatic staining.
8. Cloning or clumping of chondrocytes.
9. Focal areas of erosion down to the subchondral bone, leaving exposed sclerotic bone.
10. Subchondral cyst formation.
11. Patches of new cartilage seen over eroded areas and osteophytes.

The stages just enumerated are not always present and do not always occur in the order given. Sokoloff[6] states that in some cases extensive erosions and eburnation occur without marginal osteophytes, whereas in other cases many osteophytes may be seen without appreciable change in the articular cartilage—such as in many naturally occurring cruciate ligament ruptures in dogs.

BIOCHEMICAL ■ In osteoarthrotic cartilage, collagen is renewed with a different type of collagen that is larger in diameter than the type found in skin and bone. The synthesis of protein and glycosaminoglycans is markedly increased—although the total quantity found is decreased—and is proportional to the disease severity in mild or moderate cases. In severe cases, there is a failure of this reparative process. This irreversibility suggests that treatment should be instituted at a relatively early stage of the disorder while there is still a capability of providing cells and matrix for repair of minimal to moderate defects.[15] Lacerations and chemical lesions do not show this reparative reaction. It may be feasible to treat lesions of cartilage with agents that decrease enzymatic degradation or with materials that could enhance repair (salicylates, uridine diphosphates).[15]

CLINICAL SIGNS

Osteoarthrosis in Humans

Because subjective patient descriptions are lacking in veterinary medicine, the clinical signs and symptoms of osteoarthrosis in people will be reviewed.[16]

PAIN

The prominent sign is pain that occurs upon use of the part and that is relieved by rest. The pain is usually described as aching and is poorly localized. With more advanced cases, pain may occur with minimal activity or even at rest. At times, it may awaken a person after tossing and turning during sleep owing to loss of joint "splinting," which limits painful motion during the waking hours. Pain may be exacerbated by changes in the weather, such as temperature, humidity, and barometric pressure.

The origin of this pain may arise from several areas:

1. Elevation of normally sensitive periosteum due to marginal osteophytes.
2. Pressure on exposed subchondral bone.
3. Trabecular microfracture.
4. Pinching or abrasion of synovial villi.
5. Mild synovitis.
6. Capsular inflammation.

According to Gardner, pain in capsules and ligaments is stimulated by twisting or stretching.[17] There are pain fibers in the capsule and ligaments but few in the synovium. However, there are pain fibers in the adventitia of blood vessels supplying these areas. Gardner theorizes that increased sensitivity during weather changes is due to reflex blood flow to the area of the joints; in addition, the pain may be referred from one area of the limb to another as a result of reflex spasms of the flexor muscles.

Pain is often nonexistent in osteoarthrosis. In one study, only 30 percent of people with radiographic or pathological evidence of osteoarthrosis had any symptoms.[16] Generally, when there were symptoms, there was little correlation between degree of pathology and severity of pain.

STIFFNESS ■ Stiffness upon arising from a resting position is common and usually lasts less than 15 minutes. The stiffness is due to a change in the elasticity of periarticular structures. Loss of joint range of motion (ROM) may be due to joint surface incongruity, muscle spasm and contracture, capsular contraction, or mechanical block from osteophytes or joint mice.

CREPITATION ■ Upon palpation, the human joint may show localized tenderness. Pain elicited by passive motion may be prominent. Joint crepitation (grating, crackling) from erosion or incongruity may be palpated; however, normal joint cracking or snapping is believed to be a slipping of tendons or ligaments over a bony prominence when the joint is flexed.[18] The examiner may note loss of ROM. Bony ankylosis (fusion) of joints is very uncommon with osteoarthrosis. The joint may be swollen because of synovial reaction, increased joint fluid, or the presence of osteophytes.

OBESITY ■ It is still unresolved whether obesity is a contributing factor in osteoarthrosis.[16] Logically, it appears that a heavier weight would mechanically abrade a damaged joint more quickly. In mice with a genetic predisposition for primary degenerative joint disease, obesity did not alter the course of the disease. Epidemiological studies in humans, however, indicate that osteoarthrosis is more common in obese, rather than nonobese, individuals.

Osteoarthrosis in Dogs

Most of our experience with osteoarthrosis deals with the dog; the cat rarely has osteoarthrosis except after obvious injury. Hip dysplasia has been diagnosed sporadically in cats.[19]

PAIN ■ A discussion of pain is noteworthy, since our clients usually complain that their pet is in pain, or they may ask whether the animal is in pain when known osteoarthrosis exists. First of all, many dogs, as with some people, are stoic and do not let their pain bother them. Since they cannot tell us they are in pain and even though they may not cry or yelp, it is difficult to advise an owner whether an osteoarthrotic animal is experiencing pain, especially since we know that human patients with osteoarthrosis are commonly without pain.

An example of stoicism in a dog may occur in the event of fresh fractures. Many times, a dog will allow gentle palpation, radiographic positioning, and body movement without wincing, cringing, gasping, crying, yelping, or biting. Is this dog in pain? The answer is believed to be yes.

Another finding is that excitement or nervousness may override the dog's sensitivity to pain. For example, a client may say, "He limps all day except when he goes out chasing rabbits"; or lameness may disappear as the pet approaches the veterinary environment.

The most prominent sign of limb pain with osteoarthrosis is lameness. Limping or unusual gait can occur with other conditions, such as shortened limb (without pain), mechanical dysfunction (that is, patellar ectopia, contracture of the infraspinatus muscle), a stiff leg (usually from previous fracture), neurological problems, or neuromuscular weakness. After examination of the limb, shortening or mechanical problems can be eliminated. Limping, then, is usually caused by pain. This is contradictory to a client's comment that the limping dog "doesn't seem to be in any pain." Clients fail to understand that dogs are more tolerant and less vocal than humans.

Other signs of pain—besides crying out, yelping, sensitivity upon palpation, and favoring a limb—include loss of tolerance to exercise and reluctance to play, jump on furniture, or go up and down stairs. When rear legs are involved, the dog may "bunny hop," take short, mincing steps, sit with the painful leg cocked to the side rather than underneath the body, or show pacing, irritability (especially with children), and personality change. When viewing a dog with obvious lameness, the owner or another veterinarian may have judged that the dog has a "shoulder" or "hip" lameness. Identifying the location of pain may be difficult based on gait observation. The astute clinician should not make preconceived diagnoses based upon other opinions.

Pain elicited upon palpation is variable. Many dogs with known osteoarthrosis of a joint will not react to palpation. Identifying the area where pain has been elicited can be challenging at times. It is difficult to isolate and move one joint without moving other tissues or without pressing on a sensitive area during the manipulation. If a young dog has eosinophilic panosteitis of the radius or ulna, the area may be grasped tightly while the shoulder joint is examined. When the dog cringes, the examiner is thinking about the shoulder joint and forgets that the elbow is extended and the forearm tissues are compressed.

The osteoarthrotic dog is similar to humans in regard to the pain worsening with cold, damp weather and a change in physical activity. This physical activity may include taking longer walks or runs than usual; slipping on ice and stretching contracted tendons, capsules, and other parts; or climbing stairs that have not been part of the routine. Although pain may be increased, it usually does not persist for more than a week or two. If it does, the clinician should be alerted to further problems (for example, a ruptured cranial cruciate ligament with hip dysplasia, fracture of osteophytes, further progression of pathology—such as meniscal damage occurring with chronic cruciate ligament disease). However, some chronically osteoarthrotic dogs progress to the stage where lameness or pain is continual.

The fact that in humans the radiographic signs may not correlate with the severity of the symptoms may help the veterinary clinician understand why a dog with severe osteoarthrosis of the hips may act totally normal without clinical signs, or why the dog may be more lame on the less arthritic hip, as shown by radiography.

A few comments concerning the theorized origin of pain from osteoarthrosis are in order. If osteophytes stretch sensitive periosteum, does debridement of these proliferations alone help the patient? Experimental data are lacking. If reflex muscle spasms from osteoarthrosis accentuate pain in people, can this be one of the benefits of pectinotomy for hip dysplasia in dogs? In cranial cruciate ligament rupture or partial rupture, the synovium is frequently reddened and corrugated. Can synovectomy in dogs relieve pain by eliminating hypertrophied synovial villi that can become pinched?

STIFFNESS ■ Upon arising from a resting state, an arthritic dog experiences stiffness. As with people, in earlier stages, this stiffness disappears as dogs "warm out of it." As time goes by, this stiffness may become continual as fibrosis and decreased ROM about the joint occur. The decreased ROM is not as common or as great as in people, probably because of the degree of use a dog would have compared with a person, whose pain threshold is probably lower.

CREPITATION ■ Crepitation is palpated on dogs with severe osteoarthrosis. The examiner must be careful at times in determining the source of crepitation since, if great, it can resound throughout the limb. If the stifle is palpated and crepitation originates from the hip, the examiner may get the impression that the stifle is the origin of the crepitation. Sutures beneath the skin from previous surgery may also give a feeling of crepitation; however, this sensation will be of a quality different from the kind that comes from bone rubbing on bone.

OBESITY ■ The question of whether obesity contributes to the development of osteoarthrosis is pertinent in veterinary medicine. Most arthritic dogs that we see are overweight. Common sense tells us that extra stress on the joint contributes to abrading and degenerating cartilage more quickly. For instance, hypernourished puppies with hip dysplasia potential have shown more degenerative joint disease than those whose diets were restricted;[20] however, this does not indicate that the diet was the cause of hip dysplasia. In cases of ruptured cruciate ligaments, our clinical impression is that larger dogs develop osteophytes more quickly than smaller dogs. This may also be related to the fact that smaller dogs may "carry" or favor the leg, thus resulting in less damage from weight-bearing. In some cases, dogs with chronic pain from osteoarthrosis seemed to improve with weight reduction alone.

AGE ■ Osteoarthrosis rarely is seen (radiographically or pathologically) in very immature animals, as compared with older dogs, except for cartilage diseases such as Legg-Perthes or osteochondrosis. For example, a mature, large dog with cruciate disease would begin to develop osteophytes within seven to ten days after the rupture. Although the literature is sparse concerning natural rupture in young dogs, a few cases have been seen in which young dogs with chronic lameness (that is, two months or more) associated with cruciate disease do not have remarkable cartilage change.

TREATMENT

The best treatment for osteoarthrosis is prevention. When a known disease condition is present in which a potential for osteoarthrosis exists, the clinician should advise corrective measures or environmental changes to lessen the problem (for example, surgery for cruciate ligament rupture, diet for over-weight dogs with hip dysplasia, and slinging for early Legg-Calvé-Perthes disease of the femoral head). It is interesting to note that Murray states that excessive athletic activity in children is likely an important cause (especially in males) of subsequent degenerative joint disease of the hip.[21] This contradicts those veterinarians and owners who believe that young dogs with hip dysplasia or with a potential for hip dysplasia should be heavily exercised to develop muscle mass and prevent or minimize osteoarthrosis.

Objectives

The objectives of treatment for osteoarthrosis in animals are to relieve pain, to maintain function and range of motion (unless undertaking arthrodesis), and to maintain or regain normal activity.

Nonsurgical Methods

REST ■ During flare-ups of osteoarthrosis, mild inflammation exists as debris is being absorbed and removed by the synovium. Weight-bearing activities tend to aggravate and prolong this inflammation.[22] Total disuse, however, may lead to excessive muscle atrophy and joint stiffness. In most animals, total limb inactivity is unusual. If inactivity seems to be a problem, gentle passive range of motion exercises may be warranted. When the animal is overusing a joint affected by early osteoarthrosis or in cases of early traumatic arthroses, coaptation splints, casts, or slings for two to three weeks may be useful.

HEAT ■ Heat is very beneficial in relieving muscle spasm and pain. This may be accomplished by soaking a facecloth or towel in fairly warm water and applying it around the joint for ten minutes, two to three times per day. Therapeutic ultrasound is an effective method of applying heat in animals. The dose range depends on the depth of penetration desired and ranges from 5 to 10 watts (total dose) twice daily for 5 to 10 days. In acute joint injuries, however, cold rather than heat is indicated to decrease pain, swelling, and hematoma formation.

EXERCISE ■ Our usual recommendation concerning degree of exercise is rest during acute flare-ups and moderate self-regulated activity during remission. Encouraging an animal to overexert behind a bike or car or on an exercise treadmill is not advised. A dog will often not "feel" its limitations when excited (until later) to please an owner, chase a rabbit, or follow another dog in a race. Swimming is an excellent exercise for osteoarthrosis of joints since non–weight-bearing range of motion exercise decreases joint capsule adhesions.

MEDICATION ■ Most medications do nothing to reverse osteoarthrosis. By eliminating the animal's own defense mechanism (pain), overexertion and aggravation of joint degeneration are possible. Therefore, any pain-killing drugs administered should be accompanied by rest. Medication should be used only if needed as determined by the animal's discomfort or decreased function, not by radiographs. The use of medication may also eliminate the owner's concern about pain and may thus delay diagnosis and proper management of some orthopedic conditions (for example, osteochondritis dissecans of the elbow and shoulder and cruciate ligament instability). Aspirin or buffered aspirin (5 grains twice a day for a 25- to 40-pound dog) is the first drug of choice since it is effective, free from most side-effects, readily available in the home, and inexpensive. If vomiting occurs, feeding prior to aspirin administration is often helpful.

The mechanisms of aspirin and aspirin-like drugs (acetaminophen, phenylbutazone, meclofenamic acid) are not totally known. The most recent tenable theory is that these agents inhibit the synthesis of prostaglandins, which are important mediators of inflammation. Aspirin itself has been shown to have a protective effect against the degeneration of articular cartilage.[23] Other substances such as phenylbutazone, selenium, vitamin E, orgotein, and meclofenamic acid have been used with varying success.

Corticosteroids are frequently used by clinical veterinarians to treat lameness. Although short-term use is tolerated, long-term systemic use has undesirable systemic mineralocorticoid effects. Intra-articular corticosteroids repeatedly given to rabbits have been shown to decrease synthesis of proteoglycans and therefore hasten a type of cartilage destruction resembling chondromalacia.[24] This condition may lead to a Charcot-like joint[23] (see **Neurectomy**). Corticosteroids, if used, should be given only occasionally and accompanied by rest for two to three weeks. In general, a continuing regimen of corticosteroids for arthritis should be used only as a last resort. Fortunately, cats infrequently need chronic pain medication. They are, however, more resistant to the various side effects of exogenous corticosteroids than are dogs and humans.[25] As with other animals, the reduction in pain caused by medications should be accompanied by rest.

Newer medications for osteoarthrosis in people aim to decrease joint stiffness. Stiffness is due to new collagen formation in joint capsules that has unstable intermolecular covalent bonds. In normal mature collagen, these bonds are not reducible biochemically, but new or pathological collagen can lose its strength completely when broken down by drugs such as penicillamine.[26] Its practical use in animals is unknown. Other medications are aimed at increasing proteoglycans (for example, uridine diphosphate in rabbits[15]), decreasing its degradation, replacing proteoglycans with synthetic analogs, or increasing the limited healing properties of articular cartilage.[5] These drugs are on the horizon.

DIET ■ Although it has not been proved that obesity aggravates osteoarthrosis in genetically prone mice, common sense and positive clinical results lead us to recommend weight loss in overweight animals. Weight reduction alone has been very effective for animals that were two to three times their normal weight.

Surgical Methods

Surgery for osteoarthrosis should be considered where pain or function is not helped by reasonable conservative measures. Operations include debridement of osteophytes and joint surfaces, soft tissue or muscle release, arthrodesis (bony fusion of a joint), arthroplasty, osteotomy, pseudoarthrosis, neurectomy, and limb amputation.[27]

DEBRIDEMENT ■ The removal of osteophytes may decrease the "tugging" on the joint capsule and therefore prevent pain, although the real efficacy is unknown.

Regrowth of osteophytes may occur, especially if the inciting cause (e.g., instability) is not corrected. Debridement of joint mice, cartilage flaps, proliferative synovium, or degenerative ligaments is also performed. Debridement is often used in conjunction with other procedures. Smoothing joint surfaces may enhance joint congruency and improve stability and joint fluid lubrication.

MUSCLE RELEASE ■ A prime example of helping pain and function involves cutting the pectineus muscle or tendon in canine hip dysplasia. The exact effect is uncertain, but improvement may be due to destroying a painful spastic muscle, decreasing the forces between the painful femoral head and acetabulum, or reangulating an eroded area in the coxofemoral joint to allow weight-bearing on a less damaged area of cartilage.

ARTHRODESIS ■ Fusion of the carpal and tarsal regions is a fairly common procedure in dogs and is effective in relieving instability and pain. The canine limb functions satisfactorily with these fusions. Shoulder, elbow, and stifle fusions are attempted less often; they have a slightly greater chance of fusion failure, and greater gait impairment results than with fusions in the more distal areas. When arthrodesis is performed properly, however, a remarkable degree of function is obtained.

ARTHROPLASTY ■ Arthroplasty means any plastic or surgical reconstruction of a joint. A synovectomy may fall into this category.[28] Total hip replacement is another example of an arthroplastic procedure. This is now a fairly common procedure in small animal referral centers. Other prosthetic joints are not commercially available at present.

OSTEOTOMY ■ In humans, wedge osteotomy on the proximal femur is an older, accepted treatment for coxofemoral arthritis. The reangulated femoral head is nailed or plated in a more varus precalculated position (see Fig. 14–2), which brings immediate relief of pain and can increase the joint space radiographically as some reformation of surface cartilage occurs.[7] Wilson stated that simply breaking the bones is what brings relief, possibly owing to a decongestive effect by altered venous drainage; mere trochanteric osteotomy without altering the femoral angle also gave immediate pain relief.[7] It was not clear whether reformation of cartilage is possible.

Bentley produced osteoarthrosis in rabbits by injecting papain into coxofemoral joints.[3] He then studied the effects three and six months after osteotomy. Results showed an increased blood supply to the femoral head and acetabulum, increased bone formation in the femoral head, and increased marrow activity. These changes can cause the clearance of bone cysts and subchondral sclerosis. The subchondral marrow cells produce fibrocartilage, and, coupled with a more favorable redistribution of forces in the hip, a continuous surface layer is reformed.

Wedge osteotomy of the proximal femur has been performed in North America after having been used with encouraging results in Switzerland.[29] Our experience is that, although dogs are helped clinically, osteoarthrosis is still progressive.[30] Pelvic osteotomy (see Chapter 20) is another example of an osteotomy usually used to prevent osteoarthrosis rather than to treat osteoarthrosis.

PSEUDOARTHROSIS ■ A good example of pseudoarthrosis is resection of the femoral head and neck in dogs and cats. It is a simple, effective technique for relieving pain in dogs and cats. Pseudoarthrosis can be useful for treating problems with the digits, if necessary.

NEURECTOMY ■ Sectioning a sensory nerve to relieve pain has been used in large animals but not in companion animals. The diffuse nerve supply to an area is one reason why neurectomy may fail in dogs. In humans lacking nerve supply to a joint (Charcot's joint, often caused by syphilis or diabetes), joint destruction is massive as a result of the absence of normal body responses in protecting a painful area.[11] Pursuing therapies along this line seems unwarranted.

AMPUTATION ■ A final treatment that should be avoided is amputation of a limb or toe. In a few instances, however, such as a chronically infected, destroyed joint caused by a resistant organism, this treatment may be in the patient's best interest.

In conclusion, treatment of osteoarthrosis should include a proper balance of client instruction, moderate medication, and surgery if applicable.

Traumatic Joint Disease

Obvious traumatic joint conditions involve dislocation (luxation), instability from ligamentous disruption, and fracture. They may be categorized under acquired degenerative joint disease. However, there are some general guidelines for selecting a rational treatment.

DISLOCATION (LUXATION)

Dislocations result in obvious mechanical dysfunction. Normal nourishment and lubrication of the articular cartilage are lacking, and weight-bearing on incongruent surfaces leads to further traumatic injury to the cartilage surfaces. In some instances, open reduction is less traumatic than prolonged abortive attempts at closed reduction (for example, an elbow that has been dislocated five or more days). Therefore, gentle closed reduction should be attempted as soon as possible before muscle spasticity prevents easy relocation or before the animal tries to bear weight too soon on an unstable joint. Most joints should be immobilized from one to four weeks after reduction, depending on the degree of instability remaining after reduction. A relocated elbow may not need any support, whereas a relocated hock may require four weeks of support. When the joint is so unstable that immobilization will not maintain reduction, then some form of internal stabilization may be needed, such as capsular or ligament repair, pinning across joints, and other techniques.

FRACTURE

A fracture through a joint is obviously serious when it affects a major movable joint. The hip and elbow joints are most frequently involved. The aim of repair is to reduce the fracture line perfectly in order to decrease incongruency and subsequent degree of osteoarthrosis. Another objective in surgery is to stabilize fractures well enough to allow early weight-bearing, which helps decrease joint stiffness and maintain range of motion. In general, pins, wires, and screws should not be placed through articular cartilage unless absolutely necessary. If so, non–weight-bearing areas of cartilage should be selected if a choice is possible.

INSTABILITY

Instability from ligament rupture often involves the stifle joint. The ligament or its function should be repaired as soon as possible so that instability does not cause osteophytes, erosion, or possible discomfort from the resulting arthritis. Instability seen with congenital laxity, such as in hip dysplasia, causes microtrauma of articular surfaces, deformity of bony contours, eventual erosion of cartilage surfaces, and osteoarthrosis. Simple "reefing" or imbrication of the joint capsule does not result in a permanent stability in these hips, in luxating patellas, or in cruciate rupture instability.

Thus, early repair of joint injuries is indicated to minimize the irreversible changes that may occur. Usually some osteoarthritis will form, and the surgeon attempts to minimize these changes so that the animal may lead a comfortable life. The client should be advised, however, that the joint will never be as normal as it was prior to injury, in spite of the best effort made. This may change the performance of a working dog. When performance has to be maximum (for example, in police, tracking, or sled dogs), the dog's function in life may have to be changed. There have been cases, however, in which strenuous activities were resumed and the animal performed well.

Neoplastic Joint Disease

Neoplasms in joints are rare. From 1952 to 1978, there were only 29 cases in dogs and three in cats reported in the literature.[31] Primary tumors are termed synoviomas, synovial sarcomas, and giant cell tumors. These tumors are characterized by slow-growing swellings about a joint that occasionally cause pain upon joint movement. Initially upon radiography, only a soft tissue mass may be seen. There may be calcium deposits within the soft tissue. Later there is destruction of the adjacent cortical bone followed by cancellous bone destruction. The tumor may appear encapsulated, but often there are extensions into fascial planes and surrounding tissues, resulting in a high rate of recurrence following extirpation.[31]

Wide surgical resection is advisable. Postoperative radiation therapy results in the dog are unknown. In humans, there is a decreased frequency of local recurrence following postoperative radiation. If recurrences appear, amputation may be the best course to follow.

INFLAMMATORY JOINT DISEASE

Inflammatory joint diseases caused by infection or immunological factors are not rare in pet practice, but they occur infrequently. These conditions are characterized by inflammation of the synovial membrane with resultant

TABLE 17–2
Synovial Fluid Changes in Various Types of Canine Arthritis*

| CONDITION | NUCLEATED CELLS/CU MM | DIFFERENTIAL | |
		Mononuclear	Neutrophils
Normal	250–3000	94–100	0–6
Degenerative joint disease	1000–5000	88–100	0–12
Erosive arthritis (rheumatoid-like)	8000–38,000	20–80	20–80
Nonerosive arthritis (all types)	4400–371,000	5–85	15–95
Septic arthritis	40,000–267,000	1–10	90–99

*Printed by permission of Niels Pedersen, Proceedings of the American Animal Hospital Association, 1978, p 365.

changes in the synovial fluid (Table 17–2).[1] Lameness and gait impairment are the signs seen most frequently. Systemic signs may include fever, lethargy, anorexia, and leukocytosis.

Infectious Disease

ARTHRITIS

Joint infections are usually caused by bacteria that enter the joint either by way of penetrating wounds or by way of the bloodstream. Fortunately, these instances are rare, but when an infection occurs, it can be devastating to the joint. Our experience with pets (other than neonates) differs from that of other investigators,[1] in that joint infections usually have been caused by external wounds (e.g., surgery, gunshot, abrasions, lacerations). The severity of joint destruction depends on the type of bacteria and the duration of infection. *Corynebacterium pyogenes* infection causes severe pannus formation (granulation) over cartilaginous surfaces, whereas *Clostridium* species can elaborate collagenase. *Streptococcus* and *Staphylococcus* produce kinases that activate plasminogen and result in plasmin, which removes chondroprotein from cartilage matrix.[32] All these infections result in severe and widespread cartilage damage.

SIGNS ■ Pain and lameness are consistent findings. The joint is swollen, warm, and tender upon palpation. If the soft tissue trauma is extensive, the former signs may be present without infection.

DIAGNOSIS ■ It is expedient to perform synovial fluid analysis and Wright's staining of the centrifuged exudate. This staining technique is more helpful than a Gram's stain in picking up the presence of bacteria. Culture and sensitivity of this fluid are mandatory, although synovial biopsy culture is better.[33] Early radiographs may show capsular distention, and subchondral lysis may appear later. Bacteria readily attach to the synovium. Therefore, it may be well to massage and "pump" the joint prior to joint tap so that the bacteria may break off into the fluid.

TREATMENT ■ In acute cases, treatment should be undertaken immediately. The exudate should be evacuated (by aspiration or by arthrotomy), the synovium cultured, the fluid smeared on a slide, and Wright's stain applied. High levels of appropriate antibiotics, depending on the results of the smear, are given systemically. However, antibiotics given before the culture is taken may prevent bacterial growth of the culture. Antibiotics should be given before the culture and sensitivity results are received because of the disaster that may result if protection had been withheld for the few days during which test results are being anticipated. Choice of antibiotics may be changed when the sensitivity results are known. Penicillin G in high doses (30,000 IU/pound twice a day) is good to start with. Ampicillin and the cephalosporins are also useful. These antibiotics should be continued from two to four weeks.

Early infections (within the first 24 to 48 hrs) may respond to joint aspiration alone without arthrotomy. Arthrotomy, however, allows debridement of necrotic material, removal of fibrin clots, which may serve as a nidus for infection, and subtotal synovectomy if joint motion is restricted by the thickened joint capsule encroaching on the articular cartilage.[33] Local instillation of antibiotics is contraindicated for two reasons: Systemic antibiotics achieve adequate levels in the joint; chemical synovitis may be created, thereby enhancing the inflammation.[34]

Initially, the joint should be supported by a soft splint or bandage to reduce pain and inflammation. When clinical signs regress, gentle range of motion exercise and minimal weight-bearing may be allowed. If the joint is destroyed, arthrodesis may be indicated after the infection clears.

Noninfectious Diseases

IMMUNOLOGICAL JOINT DISEASE

Joint conditions believed to be the result of the immune mechanism can be divided into those that erode cartilage (rheumatoid arthritis) and those that do not (systemic lupus erythematosus).[1] These conditions are becoming better known in veterinary medicine as the literature describing clinical cases and our diagnostic tools expand. Most of our knowledge comes from human medicine, where these diseases are common and potentially crippling or life threatening.

Erosive Inflammatory Disease

RHEUMATOID ARTHRITIS

Rheumatoid arthritis is defined as a severe, often progressive, polyarthritis of unknown etiology.[35] It was first described in the dog in 1969,[36] and other cases have been described since.[37-39]

PATHOGENESIS ■ The exact pathogenesis is unknown but has been summarized as follows.[40] Endogenous IgG protein becomes altered for some unknown reason and stimulates IgG and IgM antibodies (called rheumatoid factors), which then combine to form immune complexes in the joint. These complexes activate the complement sequence, resulting in leukotaxis. Leukocytes phagocytize the immune complexes, thereby releasing lysosomal enzymes that alter the components of the joint. These enzymes contain collagenase; cathepsins, which disrupt basement membranes; and proteases, which can cleave glyco-proteins.[41] The more prolonged the synovitis, the more prominent the joint damage.[42] This succession of events is the basis for using anti-inflammatory drugs. Surgical synovectomy[43] removes the immune complexes and can be effective in humans if it is performed early.

SIGNS AND SYMPTOMS ■ The clinical signs and course of the disease may vary, as they do in humans. Depression, fever, and anorexia may occur with or without lameness. Joint swelling may be subtle or obvious. Often, more than one joint may be affected. With severe involvement, cartilage erosion may be detected by palpating crepitation. Erosions may be explained by the proliferative granulation tissue arising from the synovium, which crosses the articular surface (pannus) or invades the subchondral bone at the synovial attachments. Erosions in cartilage not covered by pannus may be caused by granulation tissue arising from the epiphyseal marrow, which erodes the subchondral bone.[44] Joint instability of the carpus and tarsus may be apparent while the dog is ambulatory. Drawer movement from stretching or tearing the cruciate ligaments may be palpated. Toes may dislocate. Spontaneous exacerbations and remissions occur.

DIAGNOSIS ■ The diagnosis of rheumatoid arthritis is not provable. In humans, there is no pathognomonic characteristic or test. The American Rheumatism Association has established 11 criteria (Table 17–3),[45] and a definitive diagnosis is made if a patient shows at least seven of 11 characteristics. Subcutaneous nodules (criterion 6) have not been reported in the dog.[39]

The rheumatoid factor test in humans yields false positive and false negative results. The latex particle rheumatoid factor test using human IgG as performed in clinical laboratories has given poor results in the dog.[46] In institutions using canine antigen, if the titer is high and other clinical signs are compatible with rheumatoid arthritis, a presumptive diagnosis of rheumatoid arthritis can be made because there are not too many diseases that can cross react. A negative rheumatoid factor test, however, does not exclude the diagnosis. Synovial histopathology reveals lymphoid and plasma infiltrates and is very nonspecific.

Radiographic changes[47] occurring in this disease include soft tissue swelling, increased joint fluid, decreased joint space, and lytic areas in the subchondral bone and juxta-articular bone. Disuse osteoporosis appears at a

TABLE 17–3

Diagnostic Criteria for Rheumatoid Arthritis*

1. Morning stiffness
2. Pain or tenderness on joint motion
3. Soft tissue or fluid swelling in one or more joints
4. Swelling of another joint
5. Symmetrical onset of joint swelling and symptoms
6. Subcutaneous nodules (para-articular)
7. Radiographic changes typical of rheumatoid arthritis
8. Positive rheumatoid factor test
9. Poor mucin precipitate of synovial fluid
10. Characteristic histological changes of synovial membrane
11. Characteristic histological changes in nodules

*From Primer of the Rheumatic Diseases, 7th ed. New York, American Rheumatism Association, The Arthritis Foundation, 1973.

later stage, and osteophytes form when instability occurs. The joint space decreases as cartilage becomes thinner, and it is seen especially in the carpal and tarsal joints.

In one report,[37] four of ten cases of rheumatoid arthritis occurred in the Shetland sheepdog. In our experience, the Shetland sheepdog and collie have been prone to this condition. Often, the presenting signs are breakdown of the ligaments and tendinous support of the carpus or tarsus. Minimal trauma (for example, fighting or jumping out of a truck) may have made the owner suddenly aware of the lameness or joint angulation. Similar presenting signs have been noted elsewhere.[39] The cartilage change seen on radiographs (that is, lysis) or arthrotomy may be minimal. The inflammatory response may cause necrosis within bundles of collagen, leading to weakening and rupture of tendons and ligaments.[48]

Joint infections may be difficult to differentiate from rheumatoid arthritis. History and clinical course help to distinguish the two.

Other diseases that may mimic clinical signs of rheumatoid arthritis include traumatic arthritis and degenerative joint disease. History of sudden onset and the fact that only one joint may be involved help to distinguish these from rheumatoid arthritis. Usually, synovial fluid analysis is valuable. Shifting leg lameness is seen with hypertrophic pulmonary osteopathy (HPO); however, careful limb palpation for swelling and radiography can usually elucidate this disease.

Other inflammatory diseases have joint fluid analyses as well as systemic signs similar to those characteristic of rheumatoid arthritis. In bacterial endocarditis, there may be a heart murmur, electrocardiographic changes, and little erosion of the cartilage. Systemic lupus erythematosus (SLE) may be difficult to distinguish from rheumatoid arthritis in the early stages. SLE does not tend to cause erosions of cartilage, and it can have a high antinuclear antibody (ANA) titer.

TREATMENT ■ Anti-inflammatory agents are used to block the production or action of the local mediators of the inflammatory response. Immunosuppressant drugs may be tried.[44] In general, it is wise to start treatment with the least toxic drug and to change therapy only when the maximum tolerated dose is ineffective.[49] In veterinary medicine, economics may play a considerable role. Salicylates (for example, aspirin) are considered to be very effective in their anti-inflammatory and analgesic effects and are still considered the first form of therapy for humans.

The most common cause of failing to achieve therapeutic results in humans is administration of an inadequate dose.[48] The dose in dogs for rheumatoid arthritis is 25 to 35 mg/kg (5 grains/20 pounds body weight) every eight hours.[39] Aspirin should be buffered and given with food to decrease gastric irritation. It has been shown that salicylates retard the disappearance of cartilage whereas corticosteroids hasten it.[50] Corticosteroids (such as prednisolone, 0.5 mg/pound twice a day) can be used as necessary if aspirin fails to decrease the active inflammation. Intra-articular injections of corticosteroids are seldom indicated. If the patient is not responsive to high levels of aspirin and is nonambulatory, the clinician may be forced to consider joint injections. However, multiple joint injections cause cartilage degeneration and cyst formation and thus should be used as a last resort.[24, 51]

Other aspects of treatment consist of weight reduction, rest during flare-ups, mild exercise (swimming is excellent), synovectomy, and arthrodesis. Synovectomy and arthrodesis are practical only if one or two joints are involved.

LYME ARTHRITIS

We are just beginning to see this relatively new disease, most prevalently on the East and West Coasts and in the Midwest. The condition can have an acute onset of severe joint pain (polyarticular or monarticular) and may result in erosive cartilage lesions as well as degeneration of intra-articular structures (cruciate ligaments and menisci). The condition is caused by *Borrelia burgdorferi*, a spirochete transmitted by ticks (or other vectors). The joint reaction may well be an autoimmune phenomenon. The disease is diagnosed by analyzing of serum for titer and treated with tetracyclines for 10 to 21 days. The joint inflammation is treated with salicylates for several months at tapering doses.

Nonerosive Inflammatory Disease

These joint conditions involve three categories of disease: SLE, those associated with chronic infectious processes, and idiopathic conditions. The symptoms can mimic rheumatoid arthritis, but erosions are rare and systemic involvement occurs. Lameness and weakness are common.

SYSTEMIC LUPUS ERYTHEMATOSUS

The distinguishing feature of SLE is its serological abnormalities (LE cell or antinuclear antibody positive). In humans, glomerulonephritis caused by aggregation of immune complexes in the kidney may cause death. Aspirin may control the joint aspects of this disease, but not the kidney changes.[49] Therefore, prednisolone is recommended and may be combined with cytotoxic drugs such as cyclophosphamide or azathioprine.[52] Polymyositis has been reported in the dog.[53]

ARTHRITIDES WITH CONCOMITANT CHRONIC INFECTIOUS DISEASE

The presenting picture was reported as being the same as SLE, except that a disease process (dirofilariasis—chronic fungal or bacterial infections of the heart, ears, or genitourinary system) was concurrent. Reversal of joint changes occurred when there was a resolution of the primary problem.[52] Rheumatic fever in humans (preceded by *Streptococcus* pharyngitis) may result in polyarthritis that is sterile, probably owing to circulating immune complexes.

REFERENCES

1. Pedersen NC: Canine joint disease. In 1978 Scientific Proceedings, 45th Annual Meeting of the American Animal Hospital Association, South Bend, Ind., 1978, pp 359–366.

2. Mankin HJ: Discussion of pathogenesis of osteoarthrosis. In Ali SG, Elves MW, Leaback DH (eds): Proceedings of the Symposium on Normal and Osteoarthrotic Articular Cartilage. Middlesex, England,

Institute of Orthopaedics, 1974, pp 301–317.

3. Bentley G: Experimental osteoarthrosis. In Ali SG, Elves MN, Leaback DH (eds): Proceedings of the Symposium on Normal and Osteoarthrotic Articular Cartilage. Middlesex, England, Institute of Orthopaedics, 1974, pp 259–284.

4. Ali SY: Discussion of pathogenesis of osteoarthrosis. In Ali SG, Elves MN, Leaback DH (eds): Proceedings of the Symposium on Normal and Osteoarthrotic Articular Cartilage. Middlesex, England, Institute of Orthopaedics, 1974, pp 301–317.

5. Sokoloff L: The general pathology of osteoarthritis. In Ali SG, Elves MN, Leaback DH (eds): Proceedings of the Symposium on Normal and Osteoarthrotic Articular Cartilage. Middlesex, England, Institute of Orthopaedics, 1974, pp 111–124.

6. Sokoloff L: The pathology and pathogenesis of osteoarthritis. In Hollander JL (ed): Arthritis and Allied Conditions. Philadelphia, Lea & Febiger, 1972, pp 1009–1029.

7. Wilson JN: The place of surgery in the treatment of osteoarthritis. In Ali SG, Elves MN, Leaback DH (eds): Proceedings of the Symposium on Normal and Osteoarthrotic Articular Cartilage. Middlesex, England, Institute of Orthopaedics, pp 227–232.

8. McDevitt C, Gilbertson E, Muir H: An experimental model of osteoarthritis: Early morphological and biochemical changes. J Bone Joint Surg 59:24–35, 1977.

9. Marshall JL: Periarticular osteophytes. Initiation and formation in the knee of the dog. Clin Orthop 62:37–47, 1969.

10. Freyberg RH: The joints. In Sodeman WA, Sodeman WA Jr (eds): Pathologic Physiology: Mechanisms of Disease. Philadelphia, W. B. Saunders Company, 1967.

11. Turek SL: Orthopaedics—Principles and Their Application. Philadelphia, J. B. Lippincott, 1967.

12. Van Pelt RW: Comparative arthrology in man and domestic animals. J Am Vet Med Assoc 147:958–967, 1965.

13. Riddle WE: Healing of articular cartilage in the horse. J Am Vet Med Assoc 157:1471–1479, 1970.

14. Collins DH: The Pathology of Articular and Spinal Diseases. London, Edward Arnold and Company, 1949.

15. Mankin HJ: The reaction of articular cartilage to injury and osteoarthritis. N Engl J Med 291:1335–1340, 1974.

16. Moskowitz RW: Symptoms and laboratory findings in osteoarthritis. In Hollander JL (ed): Arthritis and Allied Conditions. Philadelphia, Lea & Febiger, 1972, pp 1032–1053.

17. Gardner E: Structure and function of joints. In Hollander JL (ed): Arthritis and Allied Conditions. Philadelphia, Lea & Febiger, 1972, pp 32–50.

18. Lockie LM: Examinations of the arthritic patient. In Hollander JL (ed): Arthritis and Allied Conditions. Philadelphia, Lea & Febiger, 1972, pp 15–26.

19. Hayes HM, Wilson GP, Burt JK: Feline hip dysplasia. J Am Anim Hosp Assoc 15:447–449, 1979.

20. Olsson S, Hedhammer A, Kasstrom H: Hip dysplasia and osteochondrosis in the dog. In Proceedings of Voojaarsdagen 1978 (The Netherlands Small Animal Veterinary Association). Amsterdam, Royal Netherlands Veterinary Association, 1978, pp 70–72.

21. Murray RO: Aetiology of degenerative joint disease. A radiological re-assessment. In Ali SG, Elves MW, Leaback DH (eds): Normal and Osteoarthrotic Articular Cartilage. Middlesex, England, Institute of Orthopaedics, 1974, pp 125–130.

22. Hollander JL: The Arthritis Handbook. West Point, Pa., Merck, Sharp & Dohme, 1974.

23. Short CR, Beadle RE: Pharmacology of antiarthritic drugs. Vet Clin North Am 8:401–418, 1978.

24. Mankin HJ: The reaction of articular cartilage to injury and osteoarthritis. N Engl J Med 291:1285–1292, 1974.

25. Scott DW: Feline dermatology, therapeutics. J Am Anim Hosp Assoc 16:434–456, 1980.

26. Jayson MIV, Herbert CM, Bailey AJ: Studies on collagen crosslinks in osteoarthritis. In Ali SG, Elves MW, Leaback DH (eds): Proceedings of the Symposium on Normal and Osteoarthrotic Articular Cartilage. Middlesex, England, Institute of Orthopaedics, 1974, pp 219–220.

27. Moskowitz RW: Treatment of osteoarthritis. In Hollander JL (ed): Arthritis and Allied Conditions. Philadelphia, Lea & Febiger, 1972, pp 1054–1070.

28. Bradney IW: Treatment of osteoarthritis of the femoro-tibial joint in the dog by synovectomy and debridement and repair of the anterior cruciate ligament. J Small Anim Pract 20:197, 1979.

29. Walker T, Prieur WD: Intertrochanter femoral osteotomy. Sem Vet Surg Med 2:117–130, 1987.

30. Braden TD: Personal communication. Unpublished data. Michigan State University, 1988.

31. Madewell MR, Pool R: Neoplasms of joints and related structures. Vet Clin North Am 20:511–521, 1978.

32. Van Pelt RW, Langham RF, Shight SD: Lesions of infectious arthritis in calves. J Am Vet Med Assoc 149:303–311, 1966.

33. Brown SG: Infectious arthritis and wounds of the joints. Vet Clin North Am 8:501–510, 1978.

34. Van Pelt RW, Langham RF: Nonspecific polyarthritis secondary to primary systemic infection in calves. J Am Vet Med Assoc 149:505–511, 1966.

35. Schultz RD: Immunological diseases of the

dog and cat. Vet Clin North Am 4:153–174, 1974.

36. Tiu SK, Suter PF, Fischer CA, Dorfman HD: Rheumatoid arthritis in a dog. J Am Vet Med Assoc 154:495–502, 1969.

37. Newton CD, Lipowitz AJ, Halliwell RE, et al: Rheumatoid arthritis in dogs. J Am Vet Med Assoc 168:113–121, 1976.

38. Newton CD, Lipowitz AJ: Canine rheumatoid arthritis: A brief review. J Am Anim Hosp Assoc 11:595–599, 1975.

39. Alexander JW, Begg S, Dueland R, et al: Rheumatoid arthritis in the dog: Clinical diagnosis and management. J Am Anim Hosp Assoc 12:727–734, 1976.

40. Ward PA, Zvaifler NJ: Complement-derived leukotactic factors in inflammatory synovial fluids of humans. J Clin Invest 50:606–616, 1971.

41. Robinson WD: The etiology of rheumatoid arthritis. In Hollander JL (ed): Arthritis and Allied Conditions. Philadelphia, Lea & Febiger, 1972, pp 297–301.

42. Anderson RJ: The diagnosis and management of rheumatoid synovitis. Orthop Clin North Am 6:629–639, 1975.

43. Sbarbaro J: Synovectomy in rheumatoid arthritis. In Hollander JL (ed): Arthritis and Allied Conditions. Philadelphia, Lea & Febiger, 1972, pp 623–629.

44. Pedersen NC, Pool RC, Castles JJ, Weisner K: Noninfectious canine arthritis: Rheumatoid arthritis. J Am Vet Med Assoc 169:295–303, 1976.

45. Rodnan G, McEwen C, Wallis SL: The primer of rheumatic disease. JAMA 224(Suppl)662–804, 1973.

46. Lipowitz AJ, Newton CD: Laboratory parameters of rheumatoid arthritis of the dog: A review. J Am Anim Hosp Assoc 11:600–606, 1975.

47. Biery DN, Newton CD: Radiographic appearance of rheumatoid arthritis in the dog. J Am Anim Hosp Assoc 11:607–612, 1975.

48. Sokoloff L: The pathology of rheumatoid arthritis and allied disorders. In Hollander JL (ed): Arthritis and Allied Conditions. Philadelphia, Lea & Febiger, 1972, pp 1054–1070.

49. Mills JA: Nonsteroidal anti-inflammatory drugs. N Engl J Med 290:781–784, 1974.

50. Roach JE, Tomblin W, Eysing EJ: Comparison of the effects of steroid, aspirin and sodium salicylate on articular cartilage. Clin Orthop 106:350–356, 1975.

51. Moskowitz RW, Davis W, Sammarco J, et al: Experimentally induced corticosteroid arthropathy. Arthritis Rheum 13:236–243, 1970.

52. Pederson WC, Weisner K, Castles JJ, et al: Noninfectious canine arthritis: the inflammatory nonerosive arthritides. J Am Vet Med Assoc 169:304–310, 1976.

53. Krum SH, Cardinet GH, Anderson BC, Holliday TA: Polymyositis and polyarthritis associated with systemic lupus erythematosus in the dog. J Am Vet Med Assoc 170:61–64, 1977.

18

Osteochondrosis

Osteochondrosis is a disturbance of cell differentiation in metaphyseal growth plates and joint cartilage. If this condition results in a dissecting flap of articular cartilage with some inflammatory joint changes, it may then be termed *osteochondritis dissecans*. This condition is very common in many species.[1–12] By understanding the origins of these lesions, the veterinarian can devise a rational treatment for this condition at various stages and degrees of severity.

PATHOLOGY

Olsson[1] has characterized osteochondrosis as a generalized skeletal disturbance of endochondral ossification in which either parts of the physis (epiphyseal plate) or lower layers of the articular surface fail to mature into bone at a symmetrical rate. This results in focal areas of thickened cartilage that are prone to injury.

Bone growth (osteogenesis) in the metaphyseal area of the long bones occurs at the physis (growth plate) through endochondral ossification (bone formation following a cartilage precursor). The end of the bone—the epiphysis—must also grow. This occurs by endochondral ossification of the deeper layers of the surface articular cartilage. Osteochondrosis in the physeal area can result in an ununited anconeal process, retained cartilaginous cores at the distal ulna, and genu valgum (knock-knee). Osteochondrosis of the articular surface can lead to osteochondritis dissecans in several joints (shoulder, stifle, hock, elbow, and vertebral articular facets[12]) and, possibly, to a fragmented coronoid process and ununited medial epicondyle of the elbow.[1]

The form of osteochondrosis seen most frequently in the United States is osteochondritis dissecans of the scapulohumeral joint.

Histopathology

Cordy and Wind[2] give a histological sequence for the various stages of osteochondrosis. They studied the "normal" histology of the humeral heads from 14 dogs of large breeds 3 to 18 months of age. The predilective site for osteochondritis dissecans had thicker-than-normal subchondral trabeculae that contained calcified cartilage until the dogs were eight months of age. Nonpredilective sites of the humeral head showed ossified cartilage remnants in the trabeculae, which remained only until the animal reached 5 months of age. In three of these "normal" control animals, however, there were tongues of unossified cartilage that extended into the subchondral bone region (Fig. 18–1A). The cartilage in the oldest of these three dogs contained necrotic chondrocytes. These three dogs probably had osteochondrosis, which might have progressed to the clinical lesions of osteochondritis dissecans had they been allowed to live.

In the control animals, the "tidemark" (a wavy hematoxylin-stained line demarcating the junction of the calcified and noncalcified layers of cartilage) was faint in younger animals but dark-stained in those animals 6 to 7 months of age. In the predilective site, however, the tidemark was not prominent until the animals were 9 months old. This tidemark can be likened to a cementing

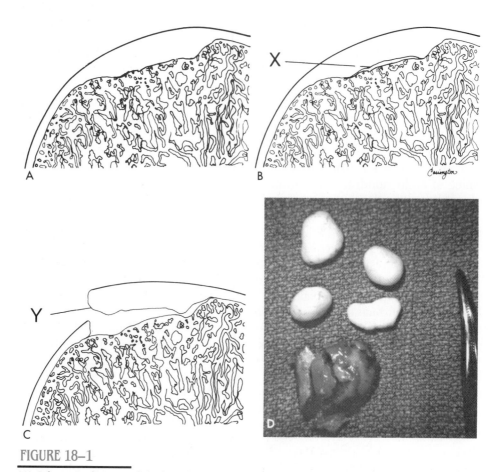

FIGURE 18–1

(A) Schematic diagram of thickened cartilage representative of osteochondrosis. (B) Osteochondrosis with a horizontal cleft that may heal or turn into osteochondritis dissecans. (X represents a crack in the calcified cartilage zone.) (C) Osteochondritis dissecans with flap formation. (Y represents the flap.) (D) Specimens from the radiograph shown in Figure 18–2E. Note the color difference between the fractured osteophyte and the four white joint mice.

substance. It may be that the predilective site has a weaker attachment (until the animal is 9 months of age) to the calcified cartilage zone than other areas of the humeral head.

A greater degree of asymptomatic pathology was seen in two other dogs.[2] Upon gross visualization of the smooth humeral head, a yellowish discoloration was seen bilaterally at the predilective sites. Histologically, there were debris-filled horizontal clefts along the tidemark region with thickened cartilage above it (Fig. 18–1B). This thickened cartilage superficial to the horizontal cleft contained some unorganized and necrotic chondrocytes.

When osteochondrosis progresses so that a vertical cleft breaks through the surface, the disease can then be termed osteochondritis dissecans. It is at this point that lameness may occur. According to Pedersen and Pool,[11] if the subchondral capillary bed is able to surround, bridge over, and bypass this area of chondromalacia, then endochondral ossification can occur without a clinical lesion developing. If the vertical cleft radiates and becomes more extensive than in one linear spot, the cartilage can then form a movable flap (Fig. 18–1C). These flaps, at this stage, are twice the normal cartilage thickness. Histologically, the surface appears normal, whereas the deep layers contain disorganized chondrocytes with some necrosis and calcification.[2] Bone was not found in these flaps except in two of 31 instances. In these cases, vascularized connective tissue extended to the flap from the underlying bone marrow of the bed. This vascularized cartilage then underwent endochondral ossification, thereby allowing bone to form within the flap.

The bed of the defect formed a saucer-shaped depression covered by a granular, grayish-white material that histologically represented the calcified cartilage zone. Beneath this zone, there was a thin layer of new fibrous tissue or fibrocartilage. Deeper to this, trabecular bone was normal, and no necrosis, comminution, or eburnation was present, at least in the early stages of this condition.

After the flap forms (at 6 to 7 months of age), it cannot heal back to the humeral head. It undergoes further calcification and may stay in place or become detached. Since there is not much room, these joint mice fall into the cul-de-sac of the joint capsule just caudal to the humeral head, or they may collect in the tendon sheath of the bicipital tendon. If the flap detaches early (when the animal is 6 to 7 months old), the joint mouse may not be radiographically visible. With time and greater calcification, however, the joint mouse may then be seen.

These joint mice may be engulfed by the synovium, or they may remain free within the joint. They may grow in size, since they are being nourished by synovial fluid. Often they become rounded (Fig. 18–1D).

PATHOGENESIS

The pathogenesis of osteochondritis dissecans can be considered as a thickened area of articular cartilage that is not cemented down well to the underlying subchondral bone. Some chondrocytes may die. A tangential force, such as the scapula hitting the humerus during running and jumping, can crack this weakened area horizontally; if the trauma is continued, it may crack vertically through the articular surface allowing synovial fluid to bathe the deep layers of degenerating cartilage, which in turn causes a synovitis. If there is no further stress (e.g., the stress of walking or running), the lesion may have a chance to heal. With further stress, the crack becomes circumferential, forming a nonhealing flap. The flap will continue to stimulate synovitis until removed. The cause of the thickened cartilage is unknown; however, a hereditary predilection is suspected. Feeding three times the recommended calcium intake has also produced osteochondrosis.[13]

RADIOGRAPHIC APPEARANCE

Since the bulk of normal cartilage is uncalcified, the early radiographic lesions (at 4 to 6 months of age) of osteochondrosis are represented by a flattening of the subchondral bone (Fig. 18–2A). With further growth of the epiphysis (not the defect), the lesion becomes saucer-shaped (when the animal reaches 6 to 7 months of age) (Fig. 18–2B). If the lesion progresses to osteochondritis dissecans, the flap starts to calcify; the flap that remains in the bed of the defect thus is made visible at 7 to 8 months of age or older (Fig. 18–2C). In advanced cases, this calcified flap may then be elevated from the contour of the humeral head (Fig. 18–2D), or it may fall off and lay caudoventral to the humeral head as joint mice (Fig. 18–2E). Occasionally, a cartilage flap is not apparent. In such cases contrast arthrography is very useful in demonstrating the presence of a flap. Any of the intravenous contrast media can be used, following a dilution to a 20 percent solution. For a large breed dog, 3 ml is sufficient.

TREATMENT

In the early stages of radiographically diagnosed osteochondrosis, when there is no clinical evidence of pain or lameness, rest and restricted diet (decreased calories if overweight, and cessation of any calcium supplementation) are indicated. Less weight-bearing and less stress, such as vigorous play, may eliminate the tangential stresses that may cleave the thicker cartilage horizontally. If the dog is lame and young (5 to 7 months of age), rest and restricted diet may work. Rest can include confinement with leash walks or slinging the leg so that no weight-bearing is possible. However, surgery is indicated if lameness has persisted past six weeks, if the dog is 8 months of age or older, or if a flap or mouse is seen upon radiography. These latter signs mean a nonhealing flap has appeared.

The first objective of surgery is to remove the flap or joint mouse that is irritating the synovium and gouging the opposite cartilaginous surfaces. A second objective is to remove any cartilage in the periphery of the bed that is not adherent to the underlying tissue. A third concern is whether the bed should be curetted. Curettage is sometimes recommended because granulation tissue from the bleeding subchondral bone invades the defect and fills it more quickly with fibrocartilage. (On the other hand, curettage may be unnecessary because the calcified cartilage layer remaining may proliferate and may make

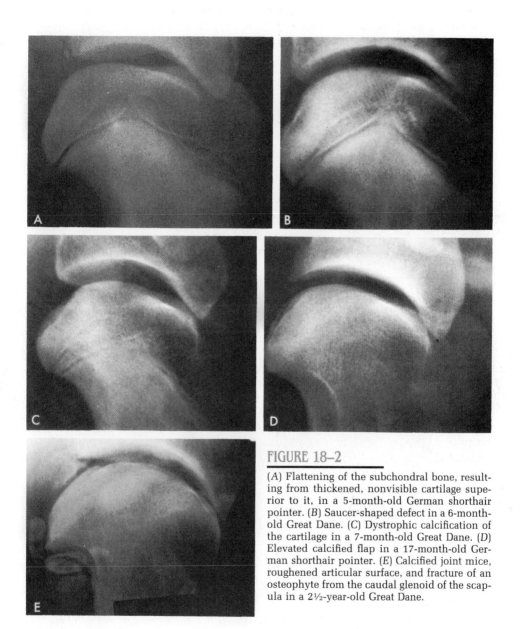

FIGURE 18–2

(A) Flattening of the subchondral bone, resulting from thickened, nonvisible cartilage superior to it, in a 5-month-old German shorthair pointer. (B) Saucer-shaped defect in a 6-month-old Great Dane. (C) Dystrophic calcification of the cartilage in a 7-month-old Great Dane. (D) Elevated calcified flap in a 17-month-old German shorthair pointer. (E) Calcified joint mice, roughened articular surface, and fracture of an osteophyte from the caudal glenoid of the scapula in a 2½-year-old Great Dane.

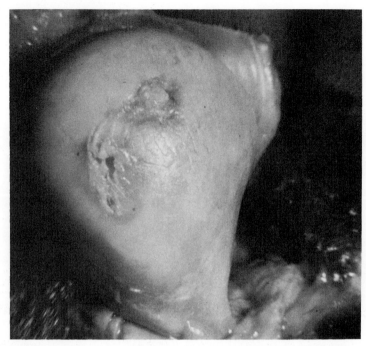

FIGURE 18–3

Humeral head of aged, stray Coonhound dog with bilateral involvement of its shoulder joints. Note the degenerative-looking fibrocartilage, which may represent the "healing" of a flap that never detached (see Figure 18–1B), or healing of the bed once the flap had detached.

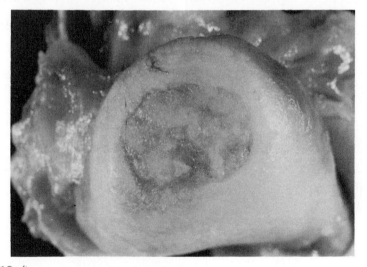

FIGURE 18–4

Humeral head of a 7-year-old Irish setter presented for forelimb amputation of an osteosarcoma of the radius. The dog had been lame all of its life. A rounded joint mouse 1″ in diameter was also found.

a better surface for long-term results.) This is especially true if the defect has dense sclerotic bone lining it. However, often a grayish material is already lining the defect (calcified cartilage layer) and may contribute to natural healing. Another alternative is to use a Kirschner drill wire to drill a few holes in the defect to allow neovascularization without disturbing some of the cartilage elements already there.

Controlled experimentation using cases of natural disease is needed to provide guidance as to the proper therapy of the bed. Currently, we do not agree on recommending curettage of the bed.

The appearance of the humeral defect several years after natural flap detachment is shown in Figure 18–3. An example of an incompletely "healed" lesion (unoperated) is shown in Figure 18–4.

REFERENCES

1. Olsson SE: Osteochondrosis—A growing problem to dog breeders. Gaines Dog Research Progress. White Plains, NY, Gaines Dog Research Center, Summer 1976, pp 1–11.
2. Cordy DR, Wind AP: Transverse fracture of the proximal humeral articular cartilage in dogs (so-called osteochondritis dissecans). Pathol Vet (Basel) 6:424–436, 1969.
3. Johnson KA, Howlett CR, Pettit GD: Osteochondrosis in the hock joints in dogs. J Am Anim Hosp Assoc 16:103–113, 1980.
4. Craig DH, Riser WH: Osteochondritis dissecans in the proximal humerus of the dog. J Am Vet Radiol Soc 6:40–49, 1965.
5. Leighton RL: Osteochondritis dissecans of the shoulder joint of the dog. Vet Clin North Am 1:391–401, 1971.
6. Olsson SE: Lameness in the dog: A review of lesions causing osteoarthrosis of the shoulder, elbow, hip, stifle and hock joints. Proceedings of the American Animal Hospital Association 42:363–370, 1975.
7. Van Sickle DC: Selected orthopedic problems in the growing dog. Atlas of the American Animal Hospital Association, 1975.
8. Rosenblum GP, Robins GM, Carlisle CH: Osteochondritis dissecans of the tibio-tarsal joint in the dog. J Small Anim Pract 19:759–767, 1978.
9. Mostosky UV: Osteochondritis dissecans of the canine shoulder. Gaines Veterinary Symposium 13:16–19, 1964.
10. Vaughan LC, Jones DGC: Osteochondritis dissecans of the head of the humerus in dogs. J Small Anim Pract 9:283, 1968.
11. Pedersen NC, Pool R: Canine joint disease. Vet Clin North Am 8:465–493, 1978.
12. Hedhammar A, Wu FM, Krook L, et al: Overnutrition and skeletal disease: An experimental study in growing Great Dane dogs. Cornell Vet 64 (Suppl 5):83–95, 1974.
13. Goedegebuure SA, Hazewinkle HA: Morphological findings in young dogs chronically fed a diet containing excess calcium. Vet Pathol 23:594–605, 1986.

19

Principles of Joint Surgery

The structure and function of joints, discussed in Chapter 16, should be well understood as a basis for surgery. An ever-increasing percentage of small-animal orthopedics cases have involved disorders of the joints, as stringent leash laws have limited the number of fractures seen in many urban practices. This chapter presents a few basic concepts necessary for success in arthroplastic procedures, defines some terms that will be used in Chapters 20 and 21, and illustrates some casts and splints used to immobilize joints of the limbs.

In small animals, diseases of the joints should be repaired as soon as possible to avoid permanent changes. Strict asepsis must be adhered to in order to avoid devastating infection. Hemostasis is of utmost importance.

The objective of the orthopedic surgeon is to minimize the amount of uneven wear and abnormal stress across joint surfaces. This is accomplished by realigning joint fractures perfectly, removing loose bone (e.g., ununited anconeal process, fragmented coronoid process), correcting angular deformities, stabilizing instability (e.g., cruciates, patellar luxations), reducing dislocations, removing repetitive microtraumata (e.g., meniscal tears), reconstructing joints with diseases of cartilage (e.g., osteochondritis dissecans, Legg-Calvé-Perthes disease), and arthrodesing nonreconstructible joints such as those with rheumatoid arthritis, severe osteoarthrosis, or chronic instability.

Correct diagnosis and understanding of the disease process are paramount in good patient care. All too often, the "grand old panacea" (cortisone or any pain medication) is given without diagnosing the problem correctly, sometimes at the expense of permanently crippling the animal. In other cases, when a correct diagnosis is made, eliminating the animal's signs may bring immediate relief to the owner and veterinarian; however, this may shorten the life span as the animal approaches old age and develops crippling arthritis as a result of misuse of the limb.

There are many treatments for any given disease, some directly contradictory. One has to bear in mind the client, the economic situation, the home care, the use and function of the animal, and the veterinarian's facilities and surgical abilities. The veterinarian has to adapt to those variables and may treat the same disease differently in different animals, depending on the circumstances.

Proper postoperative management is vital in achieving success. If the client is not advised on how to restrict the animal's activity for a certain length of time, how to take care of a splint (e.g., if a plaster of Paris cast gets wet), and how to look for complications, hours of the veterinarian's work may be wasted. If the patient or owner is uncooperative, longer hospitalization may be necessary. In all conditions in which osteoarthrosis is present or in which there is a potential for osteoarthrosis, the animal should be helped to reduce any excessive weight. To check for optimal weight, the owner should be advised to palpate and individualize each rib. When these ribs are palpable, and the abdominal area shows a discernible "waist," the animal has lost sufficient weight.

PRINCIPLES OF ARTHROTOMY

Surgical approaches to joints must be carefully planned to avoid damage to muscles, tendons, and major ligaments. Ideally, none of these structures would be incised, but in practice this is not always possible. It is very important, then, that these structures be properly sutured to maintain joint stability. Degenerative joint disease secondary to surgically induced instability of the joint is an unfortunate sequel to many otherwise successful procedures. Large ligaments and tendons should be detached, when necessary, by osteotomy of their bony origin or insertion rather than by incising and suturing. It is important to achieve adequate exposure for the proposed procedure; excessive retraction causes soft tissue trauma, and poor visualization of the joint usually results in an inadequate repair.

Incision into a joint often involves severing one or more fascial or fibrous tissue planes that function to stabilize the joint. These tissues are collectively known as the retinacula. The lateral retinaculum of the stifle, for instance, is composed of the fascia lata, the aponeurosis of the vastus lateralis and biceps femoris muscles, and the lateral patellar ligament. The fibrous joint capsule could also be considered part of the retinaculum. In some cases, these structures can be sutured collectively, and in some instances they need to be closed in layers to ensure normal function. The reader is referred to *An Atlas of Surgical Approaches to the Bones of the Dog and Cat*[1] for a discussion and illustration of specific approaches.

The actual incision into the joint capsule must be planned and executed to avoid damage to articular cartilage and to provide adequate tissue margins to allow suturing. Intraoperatively, damage to articular cartilage with retractors, knives, electrocautery, and other devices should be avoided. Frequent irrigation with saline or balanced electrolyte solution is valuable in maintaining superficial layers of articular cartilage in good condition. It is important to postoperative healing to maintain hemostasis to the extent possible and to remove large clots before closing the joint. Although the capsule is usually sutured, complete closure of the synovial layer is not necessary to prevent synovial fluid leakage. Like the peritoneum, the synovial membrane quickly seals itself by fibrin deposition and fibroplasia. Before a joint is closed, the joint space should be thoroughly irrigated to remove tissue debris and clotted blood.

Selection of suture material for joint capsule closure is the subject of a wide variety of opinions. Our general rules are as follows:

1. When the closure can be made without tension and the capsule is not important in stabilizing the joint, use continuous sutures of small gauge (sizes 2-0 to 4-0) absorbable material or an interrupted pattern with nonabsorbable materials. The synthetic absorbable materials such as polyglycolic acid (Dexon, Davis and Geck, Wayne, New Jersey) or polyglactin (Vicryl, Ethicon, Inc., Somerville, New Jersey) are more satisfactory than surgical gut, being initially stronger and more uniformly absorbed. The more slowly absorbed monofilament synthetic materials such as polydioxanone (PDS, Ethicon, Inc., Somerville, New Jersey) and polyglyconate (Maxon, Davis and Geck, Wayne, New Jersey) are also excellent materials for use in these applications.

2. If the capsule must be closed under tension or if it is being imbricated to add stability, use interrupted sutures of nonabsorbable material in sizes 3-0 to 1. The choice of material is not critical; however, monofilament materials such as nylon or polypropylene are not as prone to becoming infected as are the braided materials. Polydioxanone and polyglyconate sutures provide the long-lasting strength needed for healing of the capsule under tension as well as the advantage of ultimately being absorbed. This reduces the potential for long-lasting, suture-based infections to a very low level. For these reasons we are using these materials increasingly in joint surgery. It is important with any nonabsorbable material that the suture not penetrate the synovial membrane in an area that would allow the suture to rub on articular cartilage. Such contact will cause erosion of the cartilage. Lembert and mattress patterns allow slight imbrication due to eversion, whereas the simple interrupted pattern allows edge-to-edge apposition. The cruciate interrupted pattern is excellent for holding the tension on the first throw of a knot and so is very useful with suture material that is "slippery" to tie under tension.

The question is often raised regarding the usefulness of debridement of osteophytes in the arthritic joint. Experimental work has indicated that this procedure probably has little value.[2] In experimental dogs, osteophytes returned to 60 percent of predebridement level within 24 to 28 weeks, and there was no measurable clinical difference between treated and untreated dogs. Therefore, we remove osteophytes only when they mechanically interfere with joint motion, as commonly seen at the proximal trochlear sulcus of the stifle joint; however, partial synovectomy of hyperplastic synovial membrane is indicated to reduce inflammation within the joint.

LIGAMENTOUS INJURIES

A great deal of joint surgery in the dog and cat consists of treating various forms of ligamentous injury. We tend to think in terms of luxations or ruptured ligaments rather than in terms of sprain injury to ligaments. A brief review of the pathophysiology of sprain injury should help the clinician deal more confidently with these injuries.

Sprain

Although commonly used interchangeably, the terms sprain and strain have distinct definitions. A *strain* is an injury of the muscle-tendon unit, whereas a *sprain* is a ligamentous injury.

Ligaments are composed of longitudinally oriented bundles of collagen fibers that are so oriented as to have a much greater tensile strength in tension than in shear or torsion. Ligaments are very inelastic, however, and if tensile load exceeds the ligament's elasticity, the collagen fiber bundles will become permanently deranged at about 10 percent elongation. Damage to a ligament caused by external force is called a *sprain* (Fig. 19–1).

Sprains are conveniently categorized into three classes[3] (Table 19–1):

1. *First-degree* or *mild sprains* result from very short-lived application of moderate force. Relatively few collagen fibers are damaged, and minimal functional change results. Hematoma formation and edema occur in the parenchyma with rapid fibrin deposition. Invasion of the fibrin by fibroblasts results in rapid healing, with normal anatomy being restored and no functional deficit. Minimal or no treatment is needed.

2. *Second-degree* or *moderate sprains* (Fig. 19–2) are characterized by increased numbers of damaged collagen fibers, more extensive hematoma, and marked functional deficit. The ligament is grossly intact. Long-term restoration of normal function is unlikely without treatment.

3. *Third-degree* or *severe sprains* (Figs. 19–3, 19–4, and 19–5) are characterized by actual interstitial disruption (partial or complete) or avulsion of the ligament from bone. Avulsion fractures of the ligamentous origin or insertion may also be present. Function is completely lost and vigorous treatment is needed to restore function. Spontaneous healing by fibroplasia is virtually certain to result in an unstable joint.

TREATMENT

First-Degree (Mild) Sprains

Immediately following the injury, icing will reduce hemorrhage and minimize pain. Veterinarians rarely see the patient this early. Initial application of ice should be followed within a few hours by application of heat. External support is not necessary, although an elastic bandage may provide some comfort. Treatment is primarily directed at enforced rest for 7 to 10 days, followed by another 7 to 10 days of light exercise such as leash walking or the freedom of a small kennel-run. Nonsteroidal anti-inflammatories may be useful for a few days but may also encourage the animal to be overactive. By the end of the third week, most animals can be allowed unrestricted activity, although extremely vigorous exercise should be approached gradually.

Second-Degree (Moderate) Sprains

More aggressive and definitive therapy is required in these injuries to ensure full return to function. It is extremely important to realize that 6 to 10 weeks may be required for initial healing and that full stability may not be achieved until 3 to 6 months post injury. If no instability can be demonstrated, the limb is splinted for 2 to 3 weeks, followed by 2 weeks in a firm elastic bandage if possible. Light activity is started at the removal of the splint and slowly increased toward normal between 6 to 8 weeks post injury, although maximal effort activities should be delayed until at least 12 weeks.

If instability can be demonstrated either by palpation or radiography, the

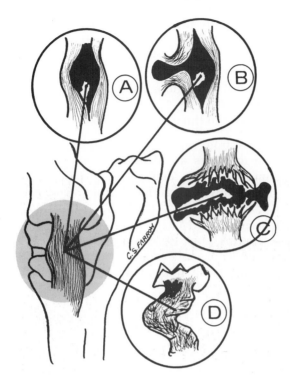

FIGURE 19–1

Sprain classification schemes generally focus on the qualitative aspects of the ligamentous injury. First-degree sprain injury involves minimal tearing of ligament and associated fibers, as well as a varying degree of internal hemorrhage (*A*). Second-degree sprain usually results in definite structural breakdown, as a result of partial tearing. Hemorrhage is both internal and periligamentous, with inflammatory edema being moderately extensive (*B*). Third-degree sprain is most severe and often involves complete rupture of the ligament body (*C*). Avulsion at the points of origin or insertion usually results in one or more small bone fragments, which may often be identified radiographically (*D*). (From Farrow CS: Sprain, strain, and contusion. Vet Clin North Am 8(2):169–182, 1978.)

TABLE 19–1

Characteristic Findings in *Sprain* Injury in the Dog

DISORDER	PHYSICAL FINDINGS	ROENTGENOLOGICAL FINDINGS
Chronic sprain	Regional soft-tissue alterations, lameness, and variable degrees of limb deformity unaccompanied by signs of inflammation. There is almost always a history of prior trauma.	Regional soft-tissue alterations often accompanied by signs of old bony trauma, osteoarthritis, and heterotopic bone formation.
Acute sprain Mild (first degree)	1. Minimal lameness 2. Mild to moderate regional soft-tissue swelling, which may be confined to the intracapsular location. 3. Tenderness on palpation. 4. Pain variable on manipulation.	1. Minimal regional soft-tissue swelling; may be entirely absent. 2. No bony lesions. 3. No apparent instability; stress radiographs fail to identify spatial derangement.
Moderate (second degree)	1. Obvious lameness. 2. Obvious swelling. 3. Frank pain on palpation. 4. Pain readily elicited on minimal manipulation.	1. Prominent regional soft-tissue swelling, usually both intra- and extracapsular in origin. 2. Bony lesions rarely present. 3. No apparent instability; stress radiographs may demonstrate spatial derangement (Fig. 19–2).
Severe (third degree)	1. Severe lameness often resulting in no weight-bearing by the affected limb. 2. Gross swelling, which may extend well into the proximal metacarpus and the digits of the affected paw (Fig. 19–3). 3. Extreme pain on palpation or manipulation, frequently accompanied by crepitus or abnormal mobility.	1. Gross regional soft-tissue swelling. 2. Bony lesions frequently present. Avulsion fractures are common and are often associated with subluxation. 3. Instability often apparent and readily demonstrable with stress radiographs (Figs. 19–4, 19–5).

From Farrow CS: Sprain, strain, and contusion. Vet Clin North Am 8(2):169–182, 1978.

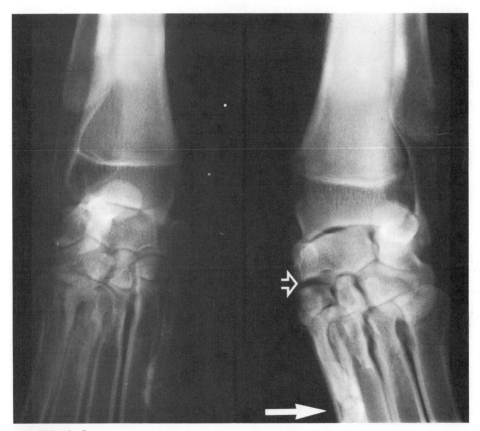

FIGURE 19-2

Second-degree sprain. This stressed radiograph (closed arrow) demonstrates slight instability on the medial side (open arrow) of the carpus, evidenced by excessive valgus deformity of the metacarpus. This view should be compared with a similar view of the contralateral limb to confirm the spatial derangement.

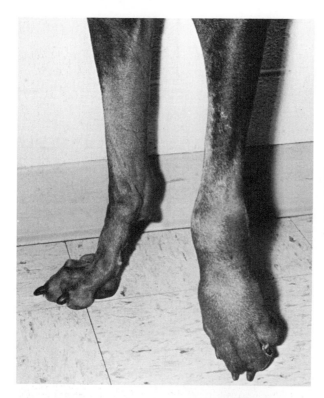

FIGURE 19-3

Third-degree sprain, showing marked swelling of the carpus and metacarpus and non–weight-bearing lameness.

FIGURE 19-4

Third-degree sprain. Stressing the metacarpus in the lateral direction indicates severe valgus deformity due to complete rupture of ligaments at the midcarpal and carpometacarpal joints (arrows).

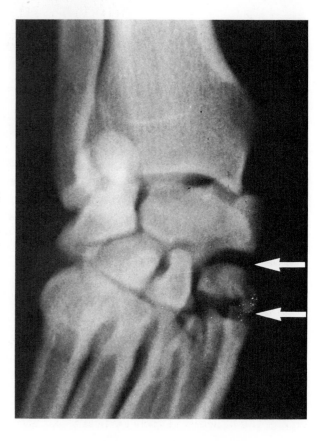

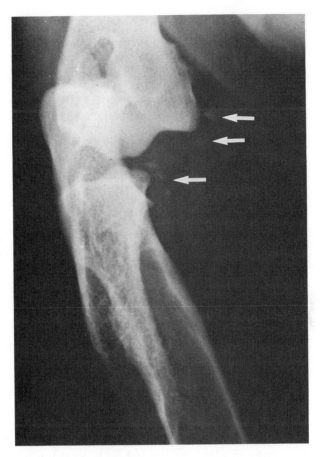

FIGURE 19-5

Third-degree sprain with avulsion of ligaments (arrows) on the medial aspect of the humeral condyle.

best chance of success lies with early surgical repair (see the following section on surgical repair). Since the ligament is basically intact, the technique of suture imbrication or plication is employed to make the ligament taut in its functional position and to support it during the healing phase. The joint capsule and retinaculum can also be imbricated for additional support. The limb must be immobilized postoperatively with the affected joint at a functional angle in some manner that will protect the ligament from severe stress initially. However, it is important not to stress shield the ligament completely for too long; four to six weeks in the splint/cast is adequate. (See the discussion of splints and casts below for more details.) Upon removal of the cast it is critical that the animal be closely confined until eight weeks postoperatively. Motion without undue stress will stimulate reorganization of collagen and produce more normal structure than will prolonged complete immobilization. An elastic padded bandage may be useful for the first two weeks after splint/cast removal.

Between 8 to 12 weeks post injury, a slowly progressive exercise program should be started. This may consist of short periods of leash walking or being turned loose in the yard for a few minutes. The activity level is gradually increased for another four to six weeks, at which point most patients will be able to return to near-normal activity.

Delayed surgery in the presence of instability is not as successful as early repair. The necessity of early surgical repair is directly related to the size and activity level of the patient. Small, sedentary animals may have a successful outcome when treated nonsurgically, whereas in the same type of situation a large, athletic dog would end up with a permanent instability and degenerative joint disease.

Third-Degree (Severe) Sprains

Suture repair (see Surgical Repair of Ligaments below) of the torn ligament is the primary method of treatment for this class of injuries. The locking-loop (Kessler)[4] and pulley suture patterns[5] have proven most reliable. Monofilament nylon or polypropylene in size 0-4/0 is most commonly used. Shredding of the ligament (a crabmeat-like appearance) may make it difficult to reappose the severed ends. In these cases, the ligament is augmented with strong suture material to support the joint while fibroplasia envelopes the suture and ligament. This fibrous tissue reorganizes in response to tension stress because of loosening or stretching of the suture and eventually can provide a functional substitute for the original ligament. Braided polyester sutures in size 0-2 are indicated. These sutures are usually anchored by means of bone screws or bony tunnels. It is important to make these anchor points of the ligament correspond to the normal origin or insertion point in order to allow a full and unrestricted range of motion. If a pedicle of nearby fascia or tendon can be harvested, it can be sutured to the remaining ligament to act as a source of fibroblasts and as a lattice for fibroplasia in the same manner that a bone graft functions.

If the ligament is avulsed close to a bony attachment, it can often be reattached with a screw and plastic spiked washer or a bone staple with a special insert. Likewise, it may be possible to anchor suture material in the ligament and then use the suture to pull the ligament into contact with the bone, following which the suture is tied around a screw or anchored through a bone tunnel.

Bony avulsions of ligaments can be reattached by small screws with or without spiked washers, multiple Kirschner wires driven through the fragment at divergent angles, tension band wire with or without a Kirschner wire, or stainless steel wire anchored through bone tunnels. Regardless of the method of fixation, reduction must be accurate in order to restore joint stability. If the joint is unstable following reduction, the ligament may need imbrication as described for second-degree injuries. Postoperative management is also as described for second-degree injuries.

Surgical Repair of Ligaments

Conservative treatment of many second- and most third-degree injuries with instability is discouraged because permanent joint laxity often results.[3] Ligamentous tissue shows little tendency to contract during healing, and very minor elongation, perhaps as little as 10 percent, causes loss of effective function and joint laxity. Additionally, scar tissue does not stand tension forces well and does not adequately substitute for ligamentous tissue.

Several basic methods are used in ligamentous reconstruction.

1. Stretched ligaments (second-degree injury) are imbricated by suturing (see Figs. 19–1 and 20–34G, H).

2. Torn ligaments are united by suturing as seen in Figures 19–6 and 19–7.

3. Avulsed ligaments are reattached as closely as possible to their original point of bony origin or insertion. If the ligament is pulled away from the bone cleanly, it can be reattached by a lag screw and plastic spiked washer (see Fig. 20–34C, D), or a suture placed in the ligament and then attached to either a bone screw (see Fig. 20–34F) or a tunnel through an adjacent bony prominence (see Fig. 20–43A).

4. When bony avulsion of a ligament occurs, a lag screw with or without a plastic spiked washer is ideal if the fragment is large enough (see Fig. 20–31A, B). Smaller fragments can be attached with stainless steel wire (Fig. 20–31C) or with three diverging Kirschner wires drilled through the fragment (see Fig. 20–31D).

5. Where the ligament is completely destroyed, as in shearing injuries of the carpus and tarsus, or in chronic injuries, the ligament must be prosthetically replaced. Such reconstruction is illustrated in Figures 20–44C, D and 21–38B, C. Large sizes of braided polyester suture and tape,* sizes 0 to 2, have been commonly used for this purpose, but polyester arterial grafts may be stronger. Carbon and stainless steel filaments show promise as extra-

---

*Polydek, Tevdek-Deknatel Inc., Queens Village, New York; Mersilene Ethicon, Inc., Somerville, New Jersey.

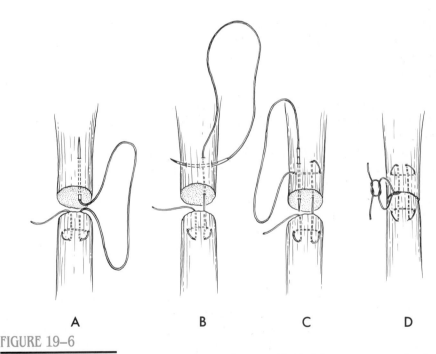

| A | B | C | D |

FIGURE 19–6

The locking loop tendon-ligament suture.[4] (A) The second half of the suture pattern is placed by entering the cut end with the suture needle and exiting the tendon at a distance from the cut end about equal to the width of the tendon. (B) A transverse bite is made superficial to the first bite. (C) The needle is passed deep to the transverse bite. The two corner loops surround and lock against a group of ligament-tendon fibers. (D) The suture is tied.

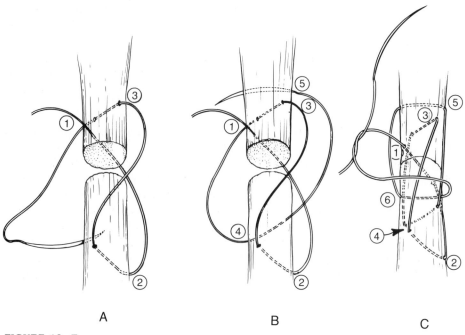

A   B   C

FIGURE 19–7

The pulley tendon-ligament suture.[5] A monofilament material such as nylon or polypropylene must be used to obtain proper tightening of this suture. In theory, bites 1, 3, and 5 are rotated 120 degrees from each other. In practice, as much rotation as possible is obtained. (A) The first bite is made in a near-far pattern. (B) The second bite is mid-length between the near-far pattern; the third bite is made in the far-near pattern. (C) The suture is tied.

TABLE 19–2

Characteristic Findings in *Strain* Injury in the Dog

DISORDER	PHYSICAL FINDINGS	ROENTGENOLOGICAL FINDINGS
Chronic strain	Comparatively nonspecific; lameness often accompanied by localized muscle spasm. Often there is little patient response to palpation of the affected muscle-tendon unit.	A generalized decrease in regional muscle mass, which depends on both severity and longevity of the injury. Disuse osteoporosis may be present in advanced cases.
Acute strain	Comparatively specific lameness usually associated with signs of localized inflammation. The area of involvement is often painful to touch and manipulation.	Regional soft-tissue swelling.
Mild (first degree)	Minimal lameness, which may be imperceptible to all but the owner.	Usually no radiographic abnormalities.
Moderate (second degree)	Easily perceived lameness, which appears to be the result of localized discomfort as opposed to frank, persistent pain.	Mild, often deceptively generalized regional soft-tissue swelling, frequently associated with abnormality of associated fascial planes.
Severe (third degree)	Obvious lameness, which is often rapidly progressive. Pain is easily elicited.	Mild to moderate regional soft-tissue swelling with distinct discrepancies of regional fascial planes.

From Farrow CS: Sprain, strain, and contusion. Vet Clin North Am 8(2):169–182, 1978.

articular ligamentous replacements because fibrous tissue infiltrates them well and can result in formation of a functional pseudoligament. However, carbon fibers have little initial strength.

6. Any type of repair may be augmented by transposition of adjacent fascia to add strength and more fibroblastic elements for repair (see Figs. 20–34I, J, K). Carbon fiber, sutured to the ligament, may also speed ingrowth of the fibrous structure.

Protection of the ligament during healing is necessary to prevent the sutures from tearing out and to prevent elongation of healing ligamentous fibers. None of the repair techniques available are able to withstand full weight-bearing stresses for several weeks. In some cases, internal support is supplied by prosthetic materials, as just described (see Fig. 20–34A). External skeletal fixators are often useful to support ligamentous repairs, particularly in the presence of open wounds (see Figs. 20–45 and 21–38D). Other cases are best supported by external casts and splints as detailed below. Casts and splints are generally maintained for four to six weeks, followed by six to eight weeks of very gradual resumption of activity. Swimming is an ideal form of physiotherapy.

MUSCLE-TENDON INJURIES

Injuries of the muscle-tendon unit are termed *strains* (Fig. 19–8). Strains can be chronic and multiple or acute and singular in nature, can occur anywhere in the muscle-tendon unit, and can vary in their severity from mild to complete rupture (Table 19–2). Milder forms produce minimal changes in gait and are

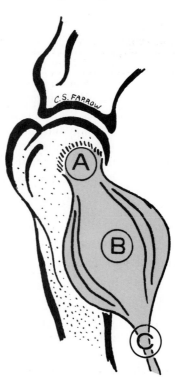

FIGURE 19–8

Strain injuries should always be considered in the context of *all* anatomical components associated with a muscle-tendon unit (MTU): origin or insertion (A), muscle belly (B), and muscle-tendon junction or tendon body (C). Injury to any part of the MTU is typically reflected by dysfunction of the unit as a whole. (From Farrow CS: Sprain, strain, and contusion. Vet Clin North Am 8(2):169–182, 1978.)

often overlooked except in animals such as the racing Greyhound, in which a slight falling off of speed may be noted. The affected muscles can be located by deep palpation of muscle bellies and tendons. Digital pressure in these areas evinces pain in the patient.

The majority of strains resolve with conservative management consisting of rest and confinement for several days. Complete rupture of a muscle-tendon unit can occur in the muscle belly, in the musculotendinous junction, or in the tendon. Such injuries are usually characterized by an inability to actively flex or extend the associated joints and to support weight. Since the affected muscles undergo spasm and contract, such injuries in the large muscles require surgical repair and external coaptation until primary healing can occur. Techniques for suturing tendons and for aftercare closely follow those described above for ligaments (see Figs. 19–6 and 19–7). Deficits in muscle tissue heal by unorganized scar tissue and, if large enough, can seriously interfere with function. In such cases it may be possible to resect the scar tissue and reappose the muscle tissue. In other cases the muscle is so extensively replaced by scar tissue and so severely restricts motion of the affected joint(s) that the only recourse is to section the tendon, thus freeing the bone. Contracture of the infraspinatus muscle (see Chapter 20) is one of the more common clinical conditions of this nature.

OPEN WOUNDS OF JOINTS

An open wound into a major joint is a surgical emergency and requires vigorous and early treatment to prevent the inevitable contamination from becoming an established infection. Septic arthritis is a devastating injury, often totally destroying articular cartilage.

The animal should be sedated or lightly anesthetized to allow surgical debridement under aseptic conditions. The wound is covered by sterile lubricating jelly while surrounding hair is clipped, after which the jelly and embedded hairs can be washed away. The wound is enlarged to allow removal of intrasynovial foreign material, and devitalized tissue is excised. A culture and sensitivity sample is obtained.

The joint is flushed copiously with sterile Ringer's or saline solution before closure. Tissues are closed in layers with fine monofilament interrupted sutures, and any ligament damage is repaired at this time. Stabilization of the joint is important in preventing infection because better blood supply is maintained in stable tissues. Drain tubes in the joint are not necessary in most cases and probably do more harm than good. Daily drainage and Ringer's or saline lavage by arthrocentesis are preferable. Pending culture results, antibiotic therapy is initiated with ampicillin and gentamicin. The joint should be immobilized for 7 to 10 days or longer if ligamentous damage is present.

IMMOBILIZATION OF JOINTS

Immobilization of major joints, especially of the elbow and stifle, is a double-edged sword. Although it can be very useful in protecting both hard and soft tissue during healing, it is also capable of producing undesirable side effects.

The most common side effect of joint immobilization is fibrosis and contracture of periarticular soft tissues, resulting in loss of range of motion. Articular cartilage is poorly nourished during periods of immobilization and will degenerate to a variable degree. Immobilization in rapidly growing animals, especially dogs of the large and giant breeds, often results in laxity of ligaments in the immobilized limb and in stretching (hence laxity) in the contralateral ligaments as a result of increased stress.

Despite these problems, the greater good is often done by immobilization of the joint following certain arthroplastic procedures. We specifically identify these situations and recommend appropriate immobilization devices in the procedures described in Chapters 20 and 21. There is probably a tendency on the part of most veterinarians to overuse, rather than underuse, external immobilization following joint surgery. The theoretical ideal would be to never immobilize a joint because all the periarticular structures, muscles, tendons, and joint cartilage thrive better in the presence of motion. Therefore, we should examine each situation to see if immobilization can be dispensed with or at least minimized, rather than slavishly adhering to any specific regimen. Remember, our patients are four-footed and get along quite well on three legs. It is often possible to delay immobilization until the animal shows signs of recovering from the initial pain and swelling and begins to touch the foot tentatively to the ground. Such delay can shorten the period of immobilization by 2 to 10 days in most instances. On the other hand, certain animals will overuse the limb and abuse the surgical repair, especially if the owners are not able to confine an active animal adequately. Good judgment is necessary in evaluating these situations.

Types of External Fixation (Coaptation)

External casts, splints, and bandages are often called coaptation fixation devices, the word "coapt" meaning to approximate. This is accomplished by simply immobilizing muscles, as with a bandage, or by transmitting compression forces to the bony structures by means of the interposed soft tissues as with casts and splints. Such pressure must be uniformly distributed throughout the cast or splint to avoid circulatory stasis.

Casts are generally considered to be molded tubular structures that, if removed, would form a mold from which a casting of the limb could be made. A splint is something less than a full cast and typically is molded only to one aspect of the limb. A wire frame structure such as the Schroeder-Thomas splint is a special case, using soft bandage materials to suspend the limb within the wire frame.

As a general rule, molded casts and splints are more satisfactory than premade ones or the Schroeder-Thomas splint, although good use can be made of both of the latter methods. The advantage of molded devices is that they fit the animal perfectly and therefore cause fewer soft-tissue problems and are better tolerated by the patient. For many years, plaster of Paris was the only moldable material available, but many such materials have become available. Of these, two have proved especially useful, Vet-Lite* and fiberglass/resin materials. Vet-Lite is a thermomoldable plastic material, impregnated onto an open-mesh fabric. When heated to 160° to 170° F, it becomes very soft and

---

*Runtech Medica, Micheroux, Belgium, and Jorgensen Laboratories Inc., Loveland, Colorado.

self-adherent and then hardens within a few minutes as it cools to room temperature. Vet-Lite is most useful in small animal patients for making splints.

Fiberglass materials have a resin-binding material impregnated into the roll of knitted fiberglass tape. The resin is activated by a 10- to 15-second immersion in water of room temperature, following which the material cures and hardens within a few minutes at room temperature. Fiberglass has proved very useful for full cylinder casts, although it can also be used for splints. Both of these products are lightweight, strong, porous, and waterproof. To obtain maximal usefulness, use them with polypropylene or other synthetic stockinet and cast padding, both of which shed water. Because these materials all "breathe" and do not retain water, there are few soft-tissue problems such as maceration of skin. Pressure sores are still possible when casts are incorrectly applied, but even this problem occurs less frequently than when cotton padding materials are used. Orthopedic felt used over bony prominences will do much to reduce pressure sores. In general, the middle toes should be left exposed to monitor swelling. The animal should be kept indoors to minimize damage to the external fixation device. If taken outside for eliminations in wet or damp conditions, a plastic bag or similar impervious material should be temporarily placed over the foot to keep the cast/splint or bandage material clean and dry. The owner should be instructed to have the device checked regularly at 7- to 10-day intervals or at any sign of foul odor, drainage, loosening, chafing, instability, or obsessive licking or chewing on the appliance.

LONG-LEG CYLINDER CAST ■ A long-leg cast is one that extends from the toes to the axilla or groin (Fig. 19–9).
Indications ■ Immobilization of the elbow and stifle, the radius and ulna, and the tibia and fibula.

These casts have to be removed with a cast-cutting oscillating saw whether they are made of plaster of Paris or fiberglass.

SHORT-LEG CYLINDER CAST ■ A short-leg cast extends only to the proximal tibia or radius (Fig. 19–10). The elbow and stifle joints are free to move normally.
Indications ■ Immobilization of the carpus and metacarpus and the tarsus and metatarsus.

As a general rule, short-leg casts are used primarily in large, active animals to provide more stabilization than short-leg splints.

SPICA SPLINT—FORELEG ■ Although this splint can be constructed with wood, rigid plastics, or aluminum, the molded splint is better tolerated and gives better immobilization (Fig. 19–11). This splint is named for the method of attaching it to the body by a spica (figure-8) bandage. In the dog the bandage is modified to be only half of a figure 8. It can be applied to the hip, but bandaging in this region is very difficult, especially in the male dog.
Indications ■ Immobilization of the shoulder, humerus, and elbow.

LONG LATERAL SPLINT ■ This splint is shorter than a spica, but otherwise it is constructed and attached similarly from the axilla or groin distally (Fig. 19–12).
Indications ■ Immobilization of the elbow and stifle joints.

Text continued on page 333

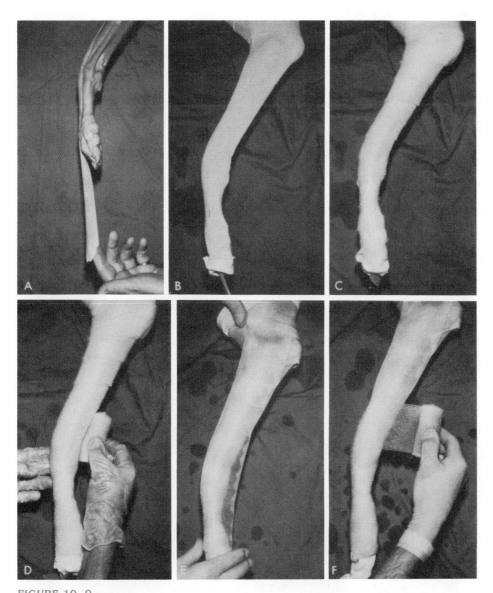

FIGURE 19-9

A long-leg cylinder cast extends from the toes to the axilla or groin. Application here is to the forelimb with fiberglass material. (A) Adhesive tape is applied to the lower limb and extends several inches beyond the toes. (B) Polypropylene stockinet is applied to the limb. The material should be long enough to extend distally beyond the toes and well into the axilla proximally. (C) Two to three layers of polypropylene cast padding are applied to the limb starting at the toes and proceeding proximally. (D) After the fiberglass tape is immersed in water at room temperature for 12 to 15 seconds, the roll of fiberglass is spiraled onto the limb; rubber or vinyl gloves are used to protect the hands. This material should be rolled on smoothly using even pressure, which is facilitated by rolling continuously around the limb in a spiral fashion and not raising the roll away from the skin. Two layers of cast material are produced by overlapping the spirals by half the width of the roll. The distal end of the cast should be at the level of the base of the distal phalanx of the middle toes. (E) A longitudinal splint is applied to both the medial and lateral sides. This material is cut from the roll and applied over the spiraled material. (F) A second spiraled layer is applied over the splints, resulting in four spiraled layers plus the medial and lateral splints.

Illustration continued on following page

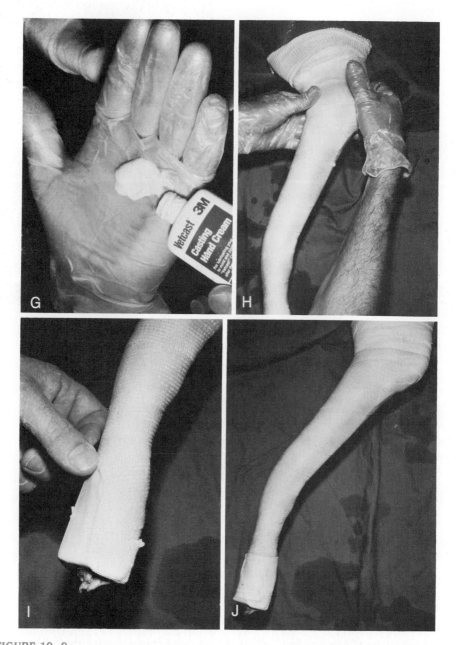

FIGURE 19–9

Continued (*G*) Hand lotion or lubricating jelly is used to treat the gloves to prevent them from sticking to the fiberglass resin. (*H*) After use of the lotion or jelly on the gloves, it is possible to smooth the fiberglass and conform it to the limb. The material begins to harden in 4 to 5 minutes under average temperature conditions. (*I*) After hardening of the fiberglass, the ends of the cast are dressed by folding the stockinet over the end of the fiberglass. At the distal end, the tape initially applied to the skin is folded over the end of the cast. This tape and the stockinet are secured with circular wraps of tape. The proximal end of the cast is similarly taped. (*J*) The completed cast. Note that both the elbow and the carpus have been maintained in moderate flexion.

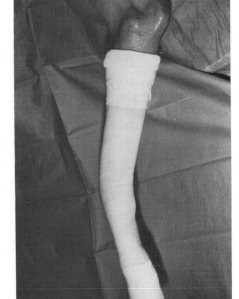

FIGURE 19–10

A short-leg cylinder cast is made in the same manner as the long-leg cast but does not cover the elbow or the stifle. In this case, the cast has been applied to the forelimb and ends just distal to the elbow joint.

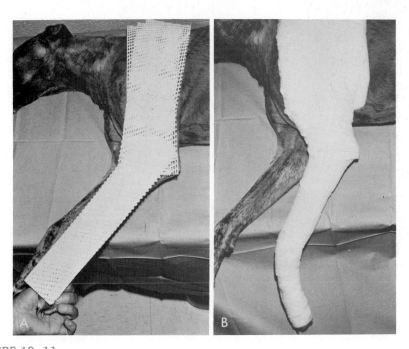

FIGURE 19–11

Spica splint for the foreleg. (A) Precut Vet-Lite splints are laid over the limb, and the area of overlap is noted. Three to six thicknesses are used, depending on the size of the animal and the degree of rigidity required. (B) The limb has been padded with two to three layers of polypropylene cast padding to the axilla, and sheet cotton is placed over the proximal humerus, shoulder joint, and scapula. This padding should extend dorsally to the midline.

Illustration continued on following page

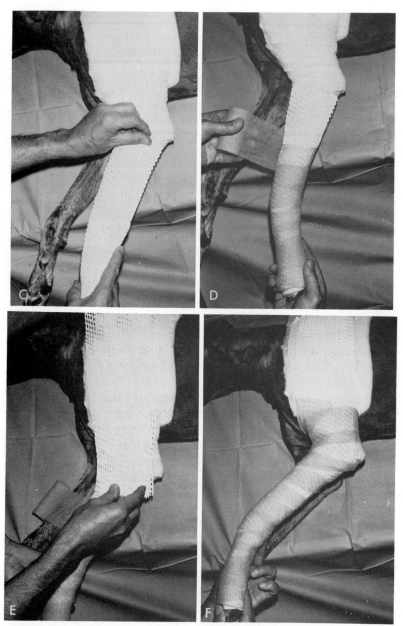

FIGURE 19–11

Continued (C) The distal splints have been heated by immersion in water at 170°F and are being placed over the lower limb, then molded by hand. (D) Conforming gauze is used to hold the softened splint material against the limb while it hardens. The proximal end of the splint is left exposed for attachment to the upper splints. (E) The upper splints have been heated and are placed over the shoulder and onto the more distal splints. The material will adhere to itself and form a continuous splint. These splints are then molded by hand to conform to the limb. (F) Conforming gauze has been rolled proximally to the axilla to complete molding of the proximal splints. The upper end of these proximal splints can be molded over the shoulder by hand pressure until sufficiently cooled to harden.

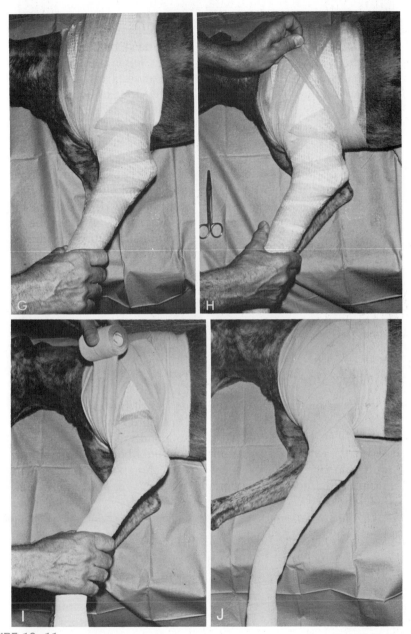

FIGURE 19–11

Continued (G) Conforming gauze is used to attach the splint to the chest wall. This gauze creates a half–figure 8 around the splinted limb but is carried behind the opposite axilla. (H) Bandaging has been completed. (I) The bandage is covered with wide elastic tape, applied in a pattern similar to that of the gauze. (J) Bandaging has been completed.

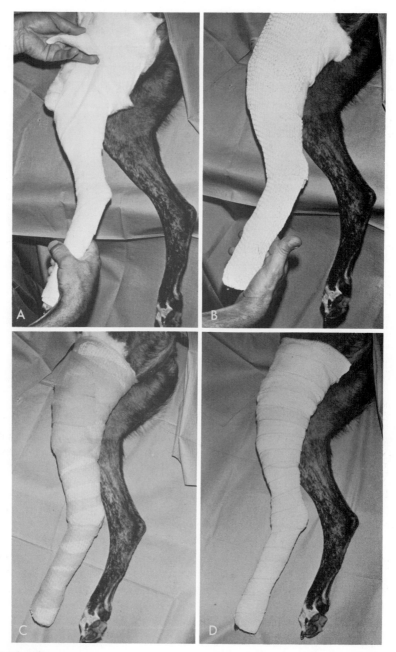

FIGURE 19–12

A long lateral splint applied to the hind limb. (*A*) The lower limb is padded with two to three layers of polypropylene cast padding to the level of the stifle, and sheet cotton is applied from the stifle to the level of the hip joint. The cast padding overlaps the lower end of the sheet cotton to help fix it in place. (*B*) Overlapping Vet-Lite splints are applied proximally and distally, with three to six thicknesses, depending on the size of the animal and rigidity required. The splints will stick together where they overlap, and the splints are initially molded by hand to conform to the limb. (*C*) The softened splints are covered with conforming gauze bandage to hold the splints conformed to the limb while they harden. (*D*) Following hardening, the splint material is covered with wide elastic tape to complete the splint.

SCHROEDER-THOMAS SPLINT ■ This versatile splint has been widely used for immobilization of fractures (see Fig. 1–13). Considerable artistry is required to construct a functional, well-tolerated, and effective splint.
Indications ■ Immobilization of the elbow and stifle, the radius and ulna, and the tibia and fibula.

SHORT LATERAL SPLINT—HIND LEG ■ Although this type of molded splint can be applied to any surface of the lower hind limb, the lateral surface has resulted in fewer soft tissue injuries (Fig. 19–13).
Indications ■ Immobilization of the tarsus and metatarsus.

SHORT CAUDAL SPLINT—FORELEG ■ This splint replaces the preformed rigid plastic and metal "spoon" splints in wide use. Such splints are not suitable to long-term use because of the incidence of soft-tissue problems and poor immobilization. The only way a curved limb can be put in a straight splint is with copious padding, and this destroys rigid immobilization. A properly made molded splint can often be left on for six weeks with no soft-tissue problems (Fig. 19–14).
Indications ■ Immobilization of the carpus and metacarpus.

PHALANGEAL SPLINT ■ This bivalved splint is designed to protect the toes while leaving the antebrachiocarpal or tarsocrural joints free to move normally (Fig. 19–15).

VELPEAU SLING BANDAGE ■ This bandage is generally well tolerated by most animals (Fig. 19–16). In addition to its main use for shoulder and scapular injuries, it can serve as a substitute for hard casts or splints when the objective is simply to prevent weight-bearing.

EHMER SLING ■ Primarily used to partially immobilize the hip joint, this bandage can also be used to prevent weight-bearing of any joint of the hind limb (see Fig. 5–24).

ROBERT JONES BANDAGE ■ This highly padded bandage is very versatile, being useful not only in immobilization, but also in decreasing or preventing edema. It is well tolerated, but because of the large volume of cotton, it can absorb considerable quantities of water and macerate skin or contaminate surgical incisions. It is generally used only for short-term immobilization. Additional rigidity can be obtained by adding a wire frame to the bandage (Fig. 19–17).
Indications ■ Immobilization of the elbow or stifle joints and structures distal to these joints.

Transarticular Skeletal Fixation

The Kirschner-Ehmer splint can be used to immobilize joints. It is particularly useful for open wounds, which make the use of casts and splints very difficult. In the case of multiple limb injuries, the pin splint provides rigid enough fixation to protect the joint, yet allows the animal to bear weight directly on the foot.

No standard patterns have evolved for the use of the Kirschner-Ehmer splint in this matter. Two such applications are illustrated in Figures 20–45 and 21–38D.

Text continued on page 339

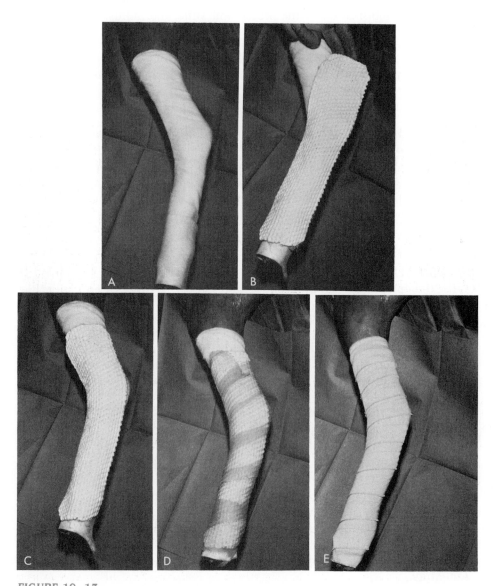

FIGURE 19–13

Short lateral splint for the hind leg. (A) The limb is padded with two to three layers of polypropylene cast padding to the level of the tibial tubercle. A small piece of orthopedic felt is placed on the tuber calcis and is secured by the cast padding. (B) Four to six thicknesses of Vet-Lite splints are placed on the lateral side of the limb. The distal end of the splint extends to the level of the base of the distal phalanx of the middle toes. (C) The splint is molded to the standing angle of the hock while the material is placed laterally to slightly dorsolaterally on the hock region. If the splint material extends more than 180 degrees around the limb, it should be trimmed. (D) The splint is held in position by a conforming gauze bandage while the material hardens. (E) The splint is completed by covering with elastic tape.

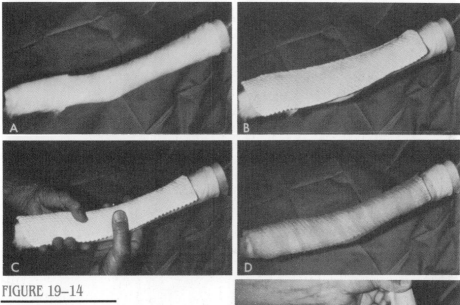

FIGURE 19-14

Short caudal splint for the foreleg. (A) The dog is positioned in dorsal recumbency to expose the caudal surface of the lower limb, which is padded with two to three layers of polypropylene cast padding. (B) Three to six Vet-Lite splints are heated and applied to the caudal surface of the limb. If the splint material extends more than 180 degrees around the limb, it should be trimmed. (C) The splints are conformed to the limb with the desired degree of carpal flexion. The distal end of the splint should extend to the level of the base of the distal phalanx of the middle toes. (D) The softened splints are held in position by a conforming gauze bandage. This bandage material must not be rolled too tightly, for it will create soft-tissue pressure sores along the edge of the splint. (E) After the splint hardens, it is completed by covering with conforming tape.

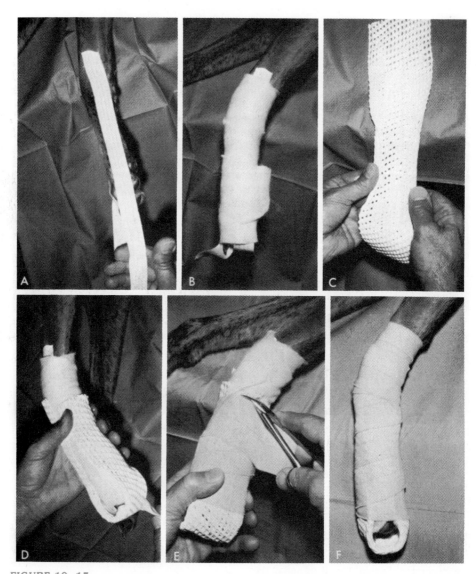

FIGURE 19–15

A phalangeal splint applied to the front foot. On the hind foot, the splint extends proximally to the level of the distal tarsal bones. (A) Adhesive tape is attached to the medial and lateral surfaces of the paw. (B) The paw and lower limb are covered with three to four layers of polypropylene cast padding to a point just proximal to the carpus. (C) Two to three thicknesses of Vet-Lite splints are heated to soften. The middle portion is then crimped on each edge to make the splints slightly narrower at this point and to create extra thickness at the end of the splint. (D) The soft splint material is applied on the dorsal and palmar sides of the foot with the splint material folded over the toes. There should be room to insert a finger between the claws and the end of the splint. The splint is conformed by hand pressure while the material cools and hardens. (E) The splint is covered with elastic tape. A portion of the proximal end of the palmar portion of the splint is trimmed when necessary to avoid pressure caused by flexion of the carpus. Wire-cutting scissors can be used for this trimming. (F) Elastic tape is applied over the splint and proximally to the end of the padding.

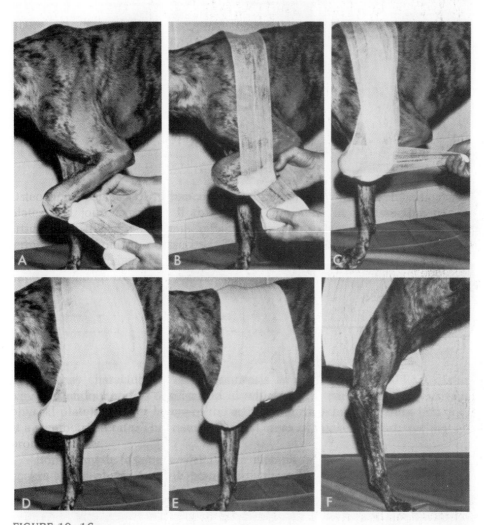

FIGURE 19–16

A Velpeau sling bandage used to immobilize the shoulder region. (*A*) Conforming gauze bandage material is wrapped loosely around the paw in a lateral to medial direction. (*B*) With the carpus, elbow, and shoulder all flexed, the gauze is brought from the paw over the lateral aspect of the limb and shoulder, over the chest, and behind the opposite axilla. It then continues under the chest, back to the starting point. (*C*) Several more layers of gauze are applied in a similar manner, and a few layers are brought around the flexed carpus to prevent extension of the elbow. Such extension could force the lower limb out of the bandage. (*D*) Gauze bandaging is completed. (*E*) Wide elastic tape is used to cover the gauze in a pattern similar to the gauze application. (*F*) On the opposite side of the animal, both gauze and adhesive tape are brought behind the opposite axilla.

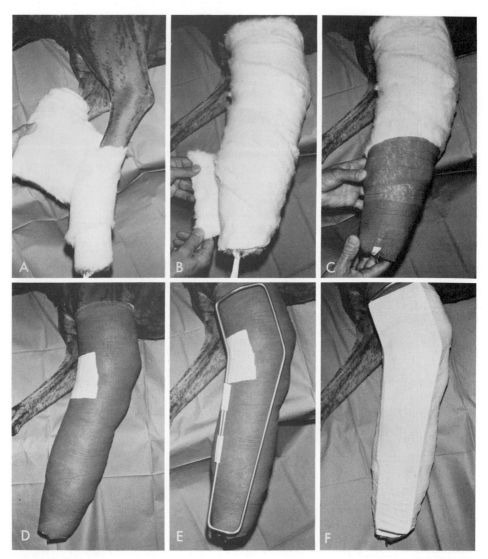

FIGURE 19–17

Robert Jones bandage. Application of the cotton for this heavily padded bandage is simplified by splitting a one-pound roll of cotton into two narrower one-half-pound rolls. (A) Adhesive tape has been applied to the lower limb and is used for traction while cotton is spiraled proximally. The tape is carried as high as possible into the axilla or groin. (B) One-half to two pounds of cotton are necessary to complete the padding, depending on the size of the animal. (C) Vetrap (Animal Care Products, 3-M, St. Paul, Minn.) is used to compress the cotton. The tape applied to the limb is folded back and incorporated into the four-inch-wide Vetrap. The first layer of Vetrap is used to conform and compress the cotton, and a second layer is used to further compress and firm the cotton padding. (D) Adhesive tape is used to secure the end of the Vetwrap. (E) Additional stability can be obtained by bending an aluminum splint rod to conform to the Robert Jones bandage. (F) The splint rod is attached to the Robert Jones bandage with nonelastic tape.

Arthrodesis

Surgical fusion of a joint to form a bony ankylosis is termed an *arthrodesis*. Spontaneous ankylosis rarely results in bony fusion of a joint in small animals; more often, it simply causes severe periarticular fibrosis and contracture. Arthrodesis relieves pain originating in articular and periarticular tissues, whereas ankylosis often does not.

Arthrodesis is a salvage procedure and an alternative to amputation in many situations:

1. Irreparable fracture of the joint.
2. Chronically unstable joint.
3. Chronic severe degenerative joint disease from any cause.
4. Neurological injury causing partial paralysis of the limb, especially of the carpal and tarsal joints. For arthrodesis to succeed, there must be cutaneous sensation in the palmar-plantar foot region or self-mutilation may result.

Functioning of the limb after arthrodesis is never normal, but in most instances, it is adequate to allow a reasonably active life for a pet. The more proximal the fusion, the more pronounced the disability. Stifle and elbow fusion produce severe disability, and the animal would, in most cases, probably function better with an amputation. The shoulder is an exception to the basic rule because the scapula becomes more mobile on the trunk and so allows considerable movement to replace normal shoulder motion. Arthrodesis of the more distal tarsal and carpal joints, on the other hand, produces almost no visible change in gait. The hip joint is never fused, since excision of the femoral head and neck is a more useful procedure. Assuring that the joint is fused in the proper angle is fundamental to success because the angle chosen is the primary means of producing correct leg length. Although a quadriped can make considerable compensation for lengthening or shortening of a single limb, function nevertheless suffers.

SURGICAL PRINCIPLES OF ARTHRODESIS

In order to achieve rigid and functional arthrodeses, the following principles should be observed:

1. The surgery should be performed only on a noninfected joint. Infection would lead to implant failure, loss of bone stock, and eventual loss of limb function.

2. Articular cartilage must be removed and subchondral bone exposed on what will be the contact surfaces at the fusion site (see Fig. 21–42A). Cartilage in noncontact areas can be left intact. Curettage, power-driven burs, and power saws are all useful.

3. Contact surfaces may be cut flat to produce the proper joint angle and to increase the contact area, or they may be prepared by following the normal contours of the joint (see Fig. 20–51A, B). The former provides more stability against shear stress but creates more shortening and is difficult to accomplish without power bone saws. Following the normal contour is the much easier method if working with hand instruments such as curettes and rongeurs.

4. Proper angle at the joint is assured by preoperative measurement of the opposite limb. Published ranges for each joint are only averages and may

not fit any specific animal. Intraoperative use of a goniometer will allow the chosen angle to be duplicated. In the absence of a goniometer, a short piece of splint rod can be bent to the contour of the normal limb, sterilized, and used intraoperatively as a template. In some fusions such as that of the stifle (see Fig. 20–40), debridement of cartilage causes noticeable loss of limb length and the angle may need to be increased 2 to 5 degrees to compensate. However, great care should be exercised to prevent an increase in leg length.

5. Fixation of the bones must be rigid and long lasting, with compression of the contact surfaces preferred. Bone plates, lag screws, and tension band wire fixation techniques are most useful. When the fixation device is being attached to the bones, care must be taken to maintain the chosen angle and rotational alignment of the limb. Temporary Kirschner wires may be driven on each side of the joint to help maintain normal relationships of the two bones (see Fig. 20–40A, B, C).

6. Bone grafting is useful to speed callus formation. Most commonly, autogenous cancellous bone is used to pack into and around the contact surfaces. See Chapter 3 for further discussion of bone grafting.

7. External cast-splint support is needed for six to eight weeks in certain cases, when the internal fixation device is not able to withstand weight-bearing loads before partial fusion has occurred.

REFERENCES

1. Piermattei DL: An Atlas of Surgical Approaches to the Bones of the Dog and Cat, 3rd ed. Philadelphia, W. B. Saunders Company, in preparation.
2. Nesbitt T: The effects of osteophyte debridement in osteoarthrosis. Presented at 17th Annual Meeting, American College of Veterinary Surgeons, San Diego, Calif., February 18, 1982.
3. Farrow CS: Sprain, strain, and contusion. Vet Clin North Am 8:169, 1978.
4. Pennington DG: The locking loop tendon suture. Plast Reconstr Surg 63:648, 1979.
5. Berg RJ, Egger EL: In vitro comparison of the three loop pulley and locking loop suture patterns for repair of canine weightbearing tendons and collateral ligaments. Vet Surg 15:107, 1986.

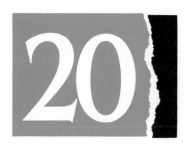

Diagnosis and Treatment of Orthopedic Conditions of the Hindlimb

Hindlimb Lameness

Following a history and lameness examination as described in Chapter 15, it is usually possible to localize the cause of lameness with some degree of accuracy. Following this comes the exercise of constructing a list of possible diagnoses and working through them until the correct one is found. The following listing is not exhaustive but includes the problems that are seen regularly.

HINDLIMB LAMENESS IN LARGE BREED, SKELETALLY IMMATURE DOGS

General/Multiple
- Trauma—fracture, luxation
- Panosteitis
- Hypertrophic osteodystrophy

Hip Region
- Hip dysplasia
- Luxation

Stifle Region
- Osteochondritis dissecans of femoral condyle
- Patellar luxation
- Avulsion of origin of long digital extensor muscle
- Avulsion of cruciate ligament
- Valgus or varus deformity due to premature physeal closure

Tarsal Region
- Valgus or varus deformity due to premature physeal closure
- Osteochondritis dissecans of talus

HINDLIMB LAMENESS IN LARGE BREED, SKELETALLY MATURE DOGS

General/Multiple
- Trauma—fracture, luxation, muscle and nerve injuries
- Spinal cord lesion
- Cauda equina lesion

- Bone or cartilage tumor
- Hypertrophic osteoarthropathy

Hip Region
- Degenerative joint disease, secondary to hip dysplasia
- Luxation

Stifle Region
- Degenerative joint disease, primary or secondary
- Rupture of cruciate ligaments
- Patellar luxation

Tarsal Region
- Ligamentous instabilities/hyperextension
- Avulsion of the gastrocnemius tendon
- Luxation of the tendon of the superficial digital flexor muscle
- Degenerative joint disease, primary or secondary

HINDLIMB LAMENESS IN SMALL BREED, SKELETALLY IMMATURE DOGS

General/Multiple
- Trauma—fracture, luxation

Hip Region
- Avascular necrosis/Legg-Calvé-Perthes disease

Stifle Region
- Patellar luxation

Tarsal Region
- Varus deformity due to premature physeal closure of distal tibia

HINDLIMB LAMENESS IN SMALL BREED, SKELETALLY MATURE
DOGS

General/Multiple
- Trauma—fracture, luxation, muscle and nerve injuries
- Spinal cord lesion—disk, tumor

Hip Region
- Degenerative joint disease, primary or secondary
- Luxation

Stifle Region
- Degenerative joint disease, primary or secondary
- Rupture of cruciate ligaments
- Patellar luxation

Tarsal Region
- Luxation of the tendon of the superficial digital flexor muscle
- Degenerative joint disease, primary or secondary
- Inflammatory joint disease

THE HIP

Luxations of the Hip

Coxofemoral luxations in dogs and cats are generally the result of external trauma, with 59 to 83 percent due to vehicular trauma.[1, 2] Most are unilateral injuries, and owing to the massive forces required to produce the luxation, about 50 percent have associated major injuries, often chest trauma.

Soft-tissue damage varies considerably; however, in all luxations, a portion of the joint capsule and the round ligament is torn. In some of the more severe cases, one or more of the gluteal muscles may be partially or completely torn. Rarely, portions of the dorsal rim of the acetabulum are fractured, or a portion of the femoral head may be fractured. This is usually an avulsion fracture at the insertion of the round ligament.

The aims of treatment for this condition are to reduce the dislocation with as little damage to the articular surfaces as possible and to stabilize the joint sufficiently to allow soft-tissue healing, with the expectation of normal clinical function. Most patients can be treated by closed reduction. More chronic cases and multiple injury may require open reduction, and some of these may need supplementary fixation to maintain reduction. In certain cases hip luxation is irreparable because of pre-existing dysplasia, severe abrasion to the articular cartilage of the femoral head, and irreparable concomitant fractures of the acetabulum or femoral head. Such patients are generally treated with excision arthroplasty or total hip replacement, which will be covered later in this chapter.

CLINICAL STUDIES

Because of the usual history of trauma, clinical signs are associated with sudden onset, pain, deformity, crepitus, and limited or abnormal movement of the limb. The specific signs vary somewhat, depending on the location of the femoral head in relation to the acetabulum. (See Chapter 15 for a discussion of physical examination of the hip.)

Craniodorsal Luxation

This is the most common injury, being seen in 78 percent of dogs and 73 percent of cats.[1] The head of the femur rests dorsal and cranial to the acetabulum (Fig. 20–1A,B). The limb is shorter than the opposite limb when positioned ventrally and extended caudally. The thigh is adducted and the stifle is rotated outward and the hock inward (Fig. 20–1C). On palpation, the trochanter major is elevated when compared with the normal side and the space between it and the tuber ischii is increased.

Caudodorsal Luxation

This is a rare condition and may simply be a craniodorsal luxation with a great deal of instability, allowing the femoral head to move caudally. In this case, the head of the femur rests caudal and dorsal to the acetabulum, and there is some risk of sciatic nerve injury (Fig. 20–1D,E). There is a slight increase in leg length when the limb is extended caudally but a decrease when the leg is positioned ventrally. The thigh is abducted, with inward

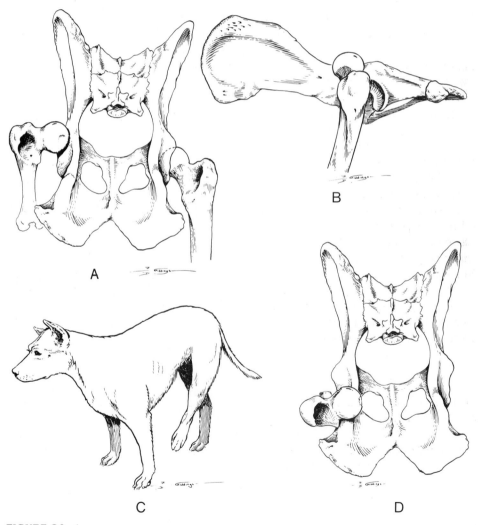

A

B

C

D

FIGURE 20–1

Luxation of the hip. *(A)* Craniodorsal luxation, dorsal view. *(B)* Craniodorsal luxation, lateral view. *(C)* Typical stance of a dog with a craniodorsal luxation. The leg is externally rotated and adducted. *(D)* Caudodorsal luxation, dorsal view.

Illustration continued on following page

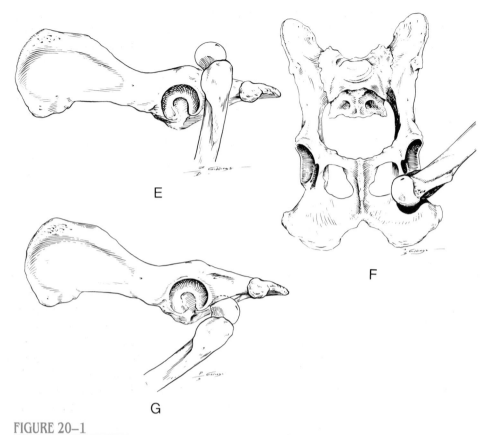

E

F

G

FIGURE 20–1

Continued *(E)* Caudodorsal luxation, lateral view. *(F)* Ventral luxation, ventral view. *(G)* Ventral luxation, lateral view.

rotation of the stifle and outward rotation of the hock. On palpation, there is a narrowing of the space between the trochanter major and the tuber ischii.

Ventral Luxation

This relatively rare luxation (1.5 to 3.2% in reported case studies[3, 4]) may occur as a separate entity or may be associated with an impaction fracture of the acetabulum. In nonfracture cases, the head of the femur rests ventral to the acetabulum, usually in the obturator foramen or cranial to it, hooked under the iliopectineal eminence. Cranioventral luxations are probably craniodorsal luxations that have been manipulated to the ventral position prior to diagnosis. Caudoventral luxations, however, occur spontaneously from trauma and not uncommonly are accompanied by fracture of the greater trochanter. The trochanter major is very difficult to palpate (Fig. 20–1F,G). There is a definite lengthening of the limb.

DIAGNOSIS

Although the presence of a luxation can usually be determined on the basis of clinical signs, it is imperative that radiographs be made for each case in order to rule out several other injuries that present similar clinical signs and that will not respond to treatment for luxation. These injuries include fractures of the acetabulum, luxation of the hip and fracture of the acetabulum, and fracture of the capital femoral physis or fracture of the head or neck. Additionally, the presence of dysplasia or Legg-Calvé-Perthes disease will generally prevent stabilization of a dislocated hip after reduction. Avulsion fracture of the insertion of the round ligament (see Fig. 6–2) generally prevents successful closed reduction; furthermore on the rare occasion when closed reduction is successful, the presence of the bone chip generally creates severe degenerative joint disease. All of the conditions mentioned require an open approach and specific treatment of the pathology present, as outlined in Chapters 5 and 6.

TREATMENT

Closed Reduction

When there are no complicating factors, most simple luxations can be reduced closed if they are treated within the first four to five days following the injury. As time passes, many factors will interfere with closed reduction. Reattachment of the round ligament to the gluteal muscles or to the shaft of the ilium will securely anchor the femoral head in some chronic cases. After several days, simple muscle contracture greatly limits the veterinarian's ability to reduce the luxation, particularly in large breeds. Soft tissue (such as joint capsule, hematoma, and hypertrophy of the round ligament and fat pad) within the acetabulum will block the acetabulum and prevent adequate reduction of the femoral head. For all these reasons, it is best to attempt closed reduction as soon as general anesthesia can be administered safely. Good relaxation of the animal is essential for the reduction process.

The manipulative technique for the *craniodorsal* luxation begins by anesthetizing the animal and placing it in lateral recumbency with the affected hip uppermost. A soft cotton rope is placed in the groin area, where it can be grasped by an assistant or anchored to the rail of the surgical table and serve as countertraction. This gives the operator a fulcrum with which to exert traction on the affected leg. With one hand on the trochanter major and the other hand grasping the leg in the hock region, the stifle is rotated inward (Fig. 20–2A). An alternate method favored by many involves first externally rotating the femur, followed by traction and internal rotation (Fig. 20–2B). This is followed in both methods by abduction of the limb and firm pressure on the trochanter to guide the femoral head toward the acetabulum. With this firm downward pressure on the trochanter and sufficient abduction and internal rotation combined with traction on the limb, the femoral head can usually be felt to "pop" into the acetabulum. The movement can be felt by the hand on the trochanter. The trochanter is pressed firmly toward the acetabulum with one hand while the hip is rotated, flexed, and extended with the other hand in order to force clots, joint capsule, or granulation tissue out of the acetabulum, all of which interfere with firm seating of the femoral head (Fig. 20–2B). Once this is accomplished, the hip joint is moved through a full range of motion with only light pressure on the trochanter major. In this way, the stability of the reduced joint can be determined. A similar technique is used for *caudodorsal* luxations. If the femoral head stays in position through a full range of motion without pressure being exerted on the trochanter, the

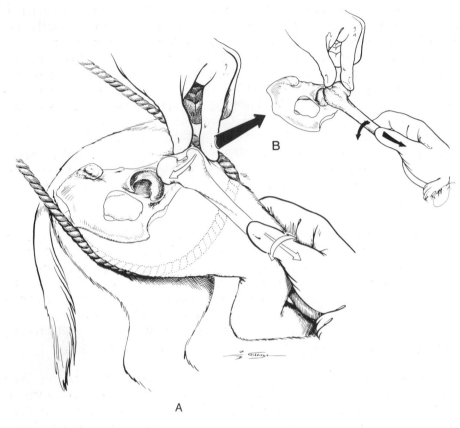

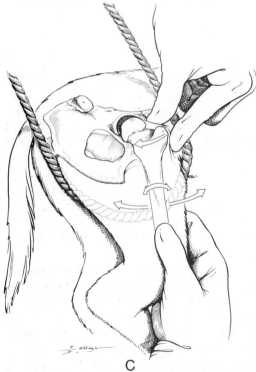

FIGURE 20–2

Closed reduction of a craniodorsal hip luxation. *(A)* The animal is secured to the table with a rope around the groin. The right hand pulls and internally rotates the femur to turn the femoral head toward the acetabulum while the fingers of the left hand are placed on the trochanter to help guide the femoral head. The right hand continues to pull and internally rotate the femur while abducting the limb. The left hand pushes by way of the trochanter to force the head over the acetabular rim. *(B)* Alternatively, the femoral head is first externally rotated as traction begins, followed by internal rotation. *(C)* Pressure is applied to the trochanter with the left hand while the femur is rotated, flexed, and extended to force soft tissue out of the acetabulum and to test stability of the luxation.

reduction is probably stable. If it luxates out of the acetabulum rather easily or seems to bind on flexion, indicating incomplete reduction, additional measures need to be taken. These will be explained later in this chapter.

Closed reduction of *ventral* luxations varies with the type. Cranioventral luxations can be either manipulated directly back into the acetabulum, or else they can be converted to craniodorsal luxations and reduced as above. No attempt should be made to similarly manipulate caudoventral luxations, however, as damage may be done to bone and soft tissues. The limb is placed in traction with one hand (left hand for left limb, right hand for right limb), while the other hand applies countertraction against the ischium. The traction hand then applies a levering or lifting action on the proximal femur which is aided by the thumb of the opposite hand. The effect is to lift the femoral head laterally into the acetabulum.[4]

AFTERCARE ■ If the dorsally luxated femoral head snaps in firmly, it may be unnecessary to use any external support for the limb; however, cage confinement for two to three days is advisable. In most cases, it is appropriate to apply an Ehmer sling (see Fig. 5–24) for five to seven days. If the femoral head snaps in somewhat loosely but seems to be reasonably stable, an Ehmer sling is always indicated and is generally left in place for 7 to 10 days.

To stabilize a ventral luxation, the leg is maintained in adduction by hobbling the rear legs together for five to seven days (see Fig. 15–24A).

PROGNOSIS ■ Failure rates of 47 to 65 percent have been reported for single attempts at closed reduction.[1, 2] The presence of degenerative joint disease or hip dysplasia significantly lowers the chance of success in closed reduction, but attempts at closed reduction probably do not reduce the success of later open reduction procedures.

Open Reduction—Dorsal Luxations

Situations in which the hip remains very unstable following reduction or in which the femoral head cannot be reduced require an open approach. Open reduction is also necessary to deal with avulsion fractures of the femoral head and in situations in which immediate mobility of the patient is needed in order to better deal with concurrent injuries. The method of choice for dorsal luxations is generally a dorsal or caudodorsal approach to the hip, either of which may be combined with osteotomy of the trochanter major.[5] Because the femoral head is most often luxated dorsally and cranially, the cranial approaches do not allow visualization of the acetabulum with the femoral head in the luxated position. Ventral luxations are exposed by means of a ventral approach to the hip.[5] If the hip can be reduced preoperatively, the soft tissues return to normal positions and surgical dissection is easier.

After the joint has been exposed, the objectives are to remove or reduce any soft tissue that may be blocking the acetabulum, to reduce the femoral head into the acetabulum, and to stabilize the femoral head in the acetabulum. Soft tissue in the acetabulum should be carefully identified. Hematomas, hypertrophic round ligaments or fat pads, and muscle fragments are excised, but all joint capsule tissue is preserved. Avulsed bone fragments are removed, except in rare cases where they are large enough to be fixed in place (see

Chapter 6). Following removal, a judgment must be made regarding the potential stability of the remaining femoral head. If it seems that the remaining head will not provide an adequate articular surface, a femoral head and neck excision arthroplasty or total hip replacement can be done. Fortunately it is rare that the fracture fragment is too large to simply excise.

Following reduction, several choices are available to maintain reduction. It is often sufficient to simply close the joint capsule and surrounding tissues with relatively heavy-gauge synthetic absorbable or nonabsorbable sutures (size 0 to 2–0) (Fig. 20–3A). A bone screw (or screws) and washer in the

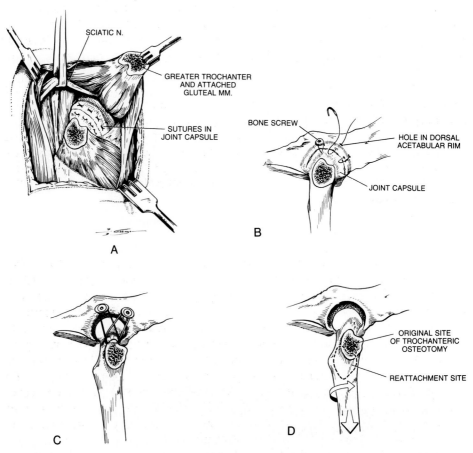

FIGURE 20–3

Open reduction of coxofemoral luxation. (A) The right hip has been exposed by osteotomy of the trochanter major.[5] The hip joint has been reduced and several mattress sutures are taken in the torn joint capsule. Size 3–0 to 0 synthetic absorbable or nonabsorbable suture material is used. (B) When the joint capsule cannot be reattached to the acetabular side, a bone screw on the dorsal acetabular rim or holes drilled in the labrum can be used to anchor sutures. Nonabsorbable material is used with the bone screw, and synthetic absorbable material is used in the bone tunnels. Usually two screws are necessary to get good attachment of the entire capsule. (C) When no joint capsule is available on either side of the joint, two bone screws are placed on the dorsal acetabular rim, at the 11:00 and 2:00 o'clock (or 10:00 and 1:00 o'clock for the left hip) positions. A hole is then drilled transversely through the bony bridge of the femoral neck. Size 1–5 nonabsorbable sutures are tied with the limb at a normal standing angle. Washers help prevent the sutures from slipping off the screw heads. (D) When the trochanter major is being reattached, additional stability may be gained by moving the trochanter slightly distal and caudal to its original site. Increased abduction and internal rotation of the femur results.

dorsal acetabular rim or holes drilled in the labrum can also be used to attach capsular tissue to the pelvis (Fig. 20–3B). When no joint capsule can be identified, suture material and bone screws can be used to prevent luxation until the capsule heals by fibroplasia (Fig. 20–3C). This method is described below in more detail (Synthetic Capsule Technique). In some cases, the joint capsule avulses at the femoral neck insertion and forms a virtual diaphragm covering the acetabulum. The opening must be found and retracted while the femoral head is reduced through it. The capsule is then sutured to the tendon of the internal obturator and gemellus muscles and to the origin of the vastus lateralis muscles.

If the capsule can be closed securely, fixation will often be sufficient, although additional stability may be provided by reattaching the trochanter major distal and caudal to its original position (Fig. 20–3D). This causes a temporary retroversion and a relatively more varus position of the femoral head as a result of femoral abduction and thus seats it more deeply in the acetabulum.[6]

When the capsule cannot be securely closed, additional measures must be taken to assure stability of the joint until the capsule is repaired by fibroplasia. The method chosen should artificially provide stability for three to four weeks, by which time the joint should have been restored to its original stability. The method chosen is not important to success, as all the methods suggested below have about the same rate of good to excellent results; the choice then is one that appeals to the surgeon and is compatible with the equipment at hand.

SYNTHETIC CAPSULE TECHNIQUE

This simple and effective technique is illustrated in Figure 20–3C.[7] After reduction as explained above, two bone screws of suitable diameter (2.7 to 4.0 mm) are inserted in the dorsal rim of the acetabulum, at the 10:00 and 1:00 o'clock positions for the left hip and the 11:00 and 2:00 o'clock positions for the right hip. Care must be taken to ensure that the screws do not penetrate the articular surface. Metal or plastic washers are placed on the screws to prevent the suture from slipping off the head of the screws. Two lengths of size 1–5 braided polyester or monofilament nylon or polypropylene suture are threaded through a hole drilled in the bony bridge between the trochanter and femoral head. The sutures are separated and then each is placed around a screw, under the washer. The femoral head is held firmly reduced with the hip at a normal angle of flexion and slightly abducted while the sutures are tied snugly tight. A few degrees of internal rotation of the limb is probably useful, as it creates femoral head retroversion, which adds stability, but external rotation must be avoided as the sutures are tied. A third screw and washer placed in the trochanteric fossa can be used to replace the drill hole.[8]

TOGGLE-PIN FIXATION

If the capsule has been severely damaged or if the luxation is chronic, it may not be possible to stabilize the joint sufficiently by suturing the remnants. In this case, other techniques must be used in addition to reconstruction of the joint capsule.

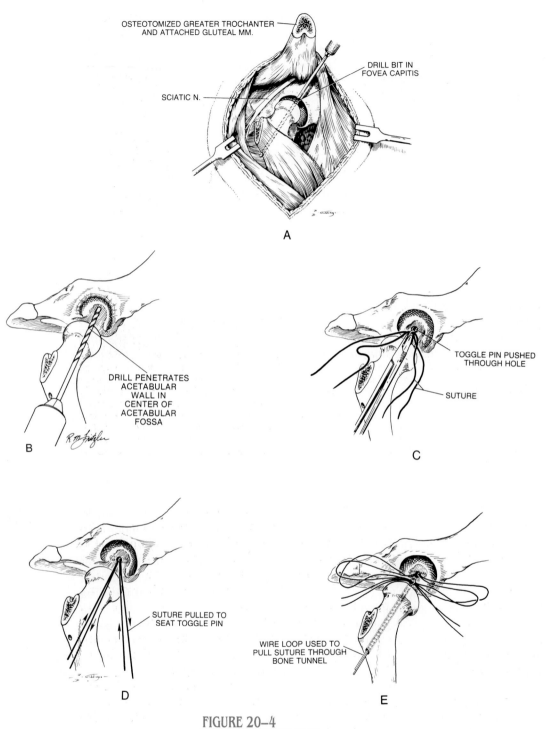

OSTEOTOMIZED GREATER TROCHANTER
AND ATTACHED GLUTEAL MM.

DRILL BIT IN
FOVEA CAPITIS

SCIATIC N.

A

DRILL PENETRATES
ACETABULAR
WALL IN
CENTER OF
ACETABULAR
FOSSA

B

TOGGLE PIN PUSHED
THROUGH HOLE

SUTURE

C

SUTURE PULLED TO
SEAT TOGGLE PIN

D

WIRE LOOP USED TO
PULL SUTURE THROUGH
BONE TUNNEL

E

FIGURE 20–4

See legend on opposite page

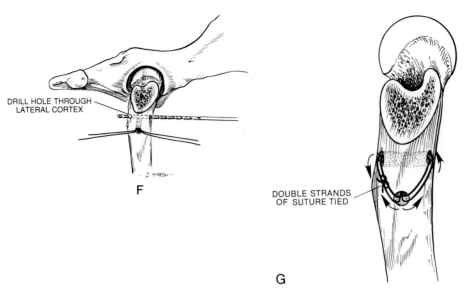

FIGURE 20–4

Toggle-pin fixation of a dislocated hip.[9] *(A)* The right hip has been exposed by means of a dorsal approach with osteotomy of the trochanter major.[5] A hole is drilled from the fovea capitis, through the neck to emerge along the crest of the third trochanter. (For proper drill size, see Fig. 20–5.) *(B)* With the hip luxated the drill is passed through the acetabular fossa wall. Care must be taken not to penetrate too deeply. *(C)* The hip has been reluxated. Two strands of braided polyester suture, size 0 to 5, are threaded through the toggle pin (see Fig. 20–5). With the pin held in forceps, it is then pushed through the acetabular hole. *(D)* The ends of the suture are alternately pulled back and forth to cause the toggle pin to turn 90 degrees and seat against the medial cortex of the acetabulum. *(E)* All four ends of the sutures are pulled through the bone tunnel with a piece of bent wire. The sutures are pulled taut, and the hip is reduced. *(F)* A small hole is drilled in the lateral cortex in the craniocaudal direction between the osteotomy and the bone tunnel. *(G)* One set of sutures is passed through the proximal bone tunnel and tied to the other suture set.

A modified Knowles toggle-pin technique has worked well in a variety of situations, even in chronic luxations.[9, 10] This technique is particularly useful when there is contralateral hindlimb injury and when early use of the luxated limb is desirable. The synthetic round ligament that is created is not expected to function indefinitely, but it will maintain stability until the soft-tissue damage in the region of the hip joint has undergone healing with maturation of the scar tissue and reformation of the joint capsule. No evidence has ever been seen in which the suture material used to create the synthetic round ligament has created a problem in the joint. In those cases that have reluxated and been reoperated, the broken suture material has been encapsulated in the regenerating round ligament and thus was no longer intrasynovial.

Following a dorsal open approach with osteotomy of the trochanter major,[5] a hole is drilled through the femoral head and neck starting at the fovea capitis and continuing laterally to exit the femoral shaft in the region of the third trochanter (Fig. 20–4A). The size of the hole is either 7/64 or 5/32 inch (2.8 or 4.0 mm), depending on the size of the toggle pin used (Fig. 20–5). This relatively small hole minimizes additional devascularization of the femoral head. The drill is then used to create a hole in the upper end of the acetabular fossa (Fig. 20–4B).

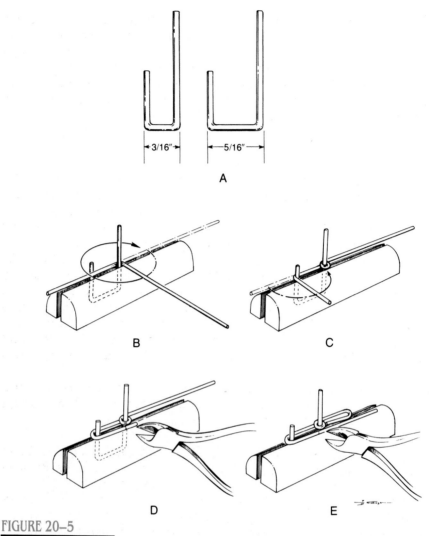

FIGURE 20–5

Fabrication of a toggle pin.[10] Small pins are used in animals weighing up to 9 kg., and large pins are used in animals weighing over 9 kg. *(A)* The pins are made from Kirschner wire bent around a jig that is clamped in a vise. The small jig is ³/₁₆ inch wide and is made of 0.035-inch Kirschner wire. The large jig is ⁵/₁₆ inch wide and is made of 0.045-inch Kirschner wire. *(B)* The pins are formed from the same-diameter wire as the jig. The long end of the wire is bent 360 degrees around the taller post of the jig. *(C)* The wire is repositioned on the jig. One end is bent 180 degrees around the short arm of the jig. *(D)* The wire is cut just short of the center hole. *(E)* The partially completed pin is rotated end-for-end and inverted to allow the second end to be formed, as in Figure 20–5D. The entire pin is then compressed with pliers to ensure that the small pin will pass through a ⅛-inch drill hole and that the large pin will pass through a ⁵/₃₂-inch drill hole.

The stainless steel toggle pin (Fig. 20–5) is attached to two lengths of size 0 to 5 braided polyester suture. The toggle pin is then placed in the acetabular hole and pushed through to the medial side (Fig. 20–4C). By means of alternate tugging on the suture ends, the toggle pin is made to turn 90 degrees to lock itself on the medial cortex of the acetabulum (Fig. 20–4D). These sutures are then pulled through the drill hole in the femoral neck (Fig. 20–4E) and held taut while the hip is returned to the reduced position (Fig. 20–4F). A hole is drilled from cranial to caudal through the lateral femoral cortex, slightly proximal to the exit hole of the sutures. One pair of sutures is pulled through the second drill hole and then tied to the opposite pair on the lateral side of the femoral cortex (Fig. 20–4G). The joint capsule is sutured to the extent possible (see Fig. 20–3A) and the trochanter major is reattached with two Kirschner wires or a tension band wire (see Fig. 6–9C,D).

TRANSARTICULAR PINNING[11]

This technique starts as described for the toggle pin, with a suitable size intramedullary pin or Kirschner wire (Table 20–1) being driven from the fovea capitis laterally through the neck and exiting the bone on the lateral cortex distal to the third trochanter (Fig. 20–6A). Following reduction the femoral head is held firmly reduced with the hip at a normal angle of flexion and slightly abducted while the pin is driven through the acetabular wall into the pelvic canal. A few degrees of internal rotation of the limb is probably useful, as it creates femoral head retroversion, which adds stability, but external rotation must be avoided as the pin is driven. The entire point of the pin (5 to 6 mm) should be within the pelvic canal, and this is checked by rectal palpation by an assistant. The protruding (lateral) end of the pin is cut short but long enough to allow later removal (Fig. 20–6B). The joint capsule is closed to the extent possible.

An Ehmer sling is applied postoperatively for 10 to 14 days, at which time the sling and the pin are removed. If the hip is very unstable at the time of reduction, the pin can be left in for three weeks.

AFTERCARE ■ Following all techniques, the limb is usually supported in an Ehmer sling (see Fig. 5–24) for 7 to 10 days unless otherwise noted. Exercise is limited to the house or leash for three weeks, then gradually increased to normal over a two- to three-week period. Sometimes when limb fractures are on the opposite side, no sling bandage is used, and early, limited weight-bearing is allowed. Bilateral luxations have also been repaired without the use of postoperative slings but require meticulous postoperative care.

PROGNOSIS ■ The prognosis for open reduction varies with the stability achieved following reduction and with the time interval between luxation and reduction. Cases that are reduced early with adequate stability carry a good prognosis, and essentially normal function may be anticipated in 70 to 75 percent of these cases. Those cases that have been luxated for a considerable

TABLE 20–1

Pin Selection According to Body Weight[12]

WEIGHT (KG)	DIAMETER (MM)	DIAMETER (INCHES)
4–7	1.6	1/16
8–11	2.0	5/64
12–19	2.3	3/32
20–29	2.7	7/64
≥ 30	3.1	1/8

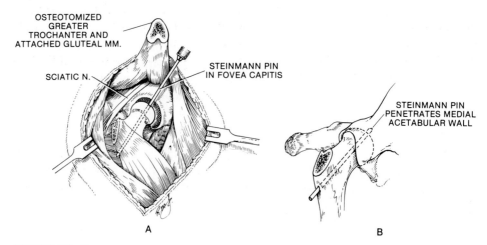

OSTEOTOMIZED
GREATER
TROCHANTER AND
ATTACHED GLUTEAL MM.

SCIATIC N.

STEINMANN PIN
IN FOVEA CAPITIS

STEINMANN PIN
PENETRATES MEDIAL
ACETABULAR WALL

A

B

FIGURE 20–6

(A) Transarticular pinning of the hip joint. Following an open approach (here a dorsal approach with osteotomy of the trochanter major), cleaning of the acetabulum, and a trial reduction of the femur, a small Steinmann pin (see Table 20–1) is driven from the fovea capitis laterally through the head and neck. It should exit the lateral cortex distal to the trochanter major. *(B)* With the hip reduced and the limb fixed at a normal standing angle, the pin is carefully driven through the acetabular wall. It should protrude not more than ¼ inch (6 mm) into the pelvic canal. The joint capsule is then sutured to the extent possible before closing.

length of time, most especially in skeletally immature animals, may result in avascular necrosis of the femoral head. Occasionally, a hip may reluxate after reduction, although this is rare if reduction is maintained for seven to eight days. Varying degrees of osteoarthritis may develop if there has been sufficient damage to the acetabulum or femoral head. Hips that are even slightly dysplastic usually will reluxate. Reluxation is an indication for femoral head and neck resection arthroplasty or for a prosthetic hip joint.

Open Reduction—Caudoventral Luxations

Although most caudoventral luxations can be handled by closed reduction,[4] nevertheless some cases require open reduction. Typically, a craniodorsal approach[5] is used if the greater trochanter is fractured, as it allows access to the acetabulum as well as to the trochanter. The joint is debrided as described above, the hip is reduced, and any available soft tissues are sutured. Once the greater trochanter is repaired (see Chapter 6), the joint is usually very stable.[3]

There are cases, however, that remain very unstable following reduction, and it has been suggested that a deficiency in the ventral transacetabular ligament is responsible.[13] A ventral approach will allow inspection of this area.[5] Two techniques have been reported for stabilizing these luxations. An autogenous corticocancellous bone graft from the iliac crest was implanted on the ventral acetabular region with success in four cases.[13] In another case, the pectineus muscle was used to stabilize the femoral head.[14] The muscle was detached distally and directed caudally ventral to the femoral neck, then dorsally and cranially over the femoral neck and deep to the gluteal muscles. The remaining free portion of the muscle was then sutured to any soft tissue available to hold the pectineus in position.

Remaining portions of the joint capsule are sutured and the hindlimbs are hobbled together (see Fig. 5–24A) for two to three weeks postoperatively. Slow return to normal activity is allowed over the next two to three weeks. Owing to the small number of cases available for evaluation, the prognosis in this situation is uncertain.

Hip Dysplasia

Hip dysplasia is an abnormal development or growth of the hip joint, usually bilaterally. It is manifested by varying degrees of laxity of surrounding soft tissues, instability, malformation of the femoral head and acetabulum, and osteoarthrosis.

INCIDENCE

One of the most prevalent disorders of the canine hip, hip dysplasia is the most important cause of osteoarthritis of the hip in the dog. Incidence ranges from 0.9 percent in the Borzoi to 47.4 percent in the St. Bernard in dogs radiographically evaluated by the Orthopedic Foundation for Animals.[15] This is not the true incidence for any breed or the general population, as most radiographs with recognizable dysplasia are not submitted, but it does indicate the relative incidence among the breeds, and most of the large working and sporting breeds are well represented.

The disease rarely occurs in dogs that have a mature body weight of less than 11 to 12 kg. Although hip dysplasia has been observed in toy breeds and cats, their unstable hips do not typically produce the bony changes common in heavier dogs.

PATHOGENESIS

Recent comprehensive reviews of hip dysplasia have brought together most of the known facts regarding this disease and are the basis for most of the discussion that follows.[16, 17] A book intended for the lay public is an excellent source for dog owners and breeders.[18]

Many observations have been made regarding the etiology of this complex disease. Among the more important are the following:

1. There is a polygeneic predisposition to congenital dislocation of the hip with multiple factors that influence and modify the disease.

2. Environmental factors are superimposed on the genetic susceptibility of the individual.

3. The genes do not affect the skeleton primarily but rather the cartilage, supporting connective tissue, and muscles of the hip region.

4. The biochemical explanation of the disease is that it represents a disparity between primary muscle mass and disproportionately rapid skeletal growth.

5. The hip joints are normal at birth. Failure of muscles to develop and reach functional maturity concurrently with the skeleton results in joint instability. Abnormal development is induced when the acetabulum and

femoral head pull apart and initiate a series of changes that end in the recognizable disease of hip dysplasia.

6. Bony changes of hip dysplasia are a result of failure of soft tissue to maintain congruity between the articular surfaces of the femoral head and acetabulum.

7. The disease is preventable if hip joint congruity is maintained until ossification makes the acetabulum less plastic and the surrounding soft tissues become sufficiently strong to prevent femoral head subluxation. Under usual circumstances, tissue strength and ossification progress sufficiently to prevent the disease by 6 months of age.

8. Dogs with greater pelvic muscle mass have more normal hip joints than those with a relatively smaller pelvic muscle mass.

9. The onset, severity, and incidence of hip dysplasia can be reduced by restricting the growth rate of puppies.

10. The occurrence of hip dysplasia can be reduced, but not eliminated, by breeding only dogs that have radiographically normal hips. Only 7 percent will be normal if both parents are dysplastic.[18]

HISTORY AND CLINICAL SIGNS

Clinical findings in hip dysplasia vary with the age of the animal.[16] There are two recognizable clinical groups of dogs:

1. Young dogs between 4 and 12 months of age.
2. Animals over 15 months of age with chronic disease.

Young dogs often show sudden onset of unilateral disease (occasionally bilateral), characterized by sudden reduction in activity associated with marked soreness of the hindlimbs. They will show sudden signs of difficulty in arising with decreased willingness to walk, run, and climb stairs, and the muscles of the pelvic and thigh areas are poorly developed. Most will have a positive Ortolani sign. This is the click produced by the movement of the femoral head as it slips in and out of the acetabulum with adduction and proximal pressure applied to the femur followed by abduction (see Figs. 20–8C and D and 15–7). Radiographically, the conformation of the femoral heads usually appears normal; however, some degree of subluxation can be seen, and if the process has been present for a few months, the angle of inclination of the femoral neck may increase beyond 146 degrees (valgus), and occasionally some lipping of the ventral aspect of the femoral head will be seen radiographically.

The sudden onset of signs in young dogs is caused by occurrence of microfractures of the acetabular rims. When femoral heads are subluxated, the area of contact of the femoral head with the dorsal acetabulum is limited to the area between 10 o'clock and 2 o'clock, with an extreme buildup of stress in that area. This eventually overloads the acetabular rim, producing tissue fatigue, loss of tissue elasticity and contour, and eventual microfracture. Pain results from tension and tearing of nerves of the periosteum. Sharpey's fibers rupture, bleed, and form osteophytes on the acetabulum and femoral neck. These usually do not become radiographically visible until 17 or 18 months of age, but may be seen as early as 12 months.[16] These fractures heal by the time of skeletal maturity, with the result that the hip joints become more stable and pain is markedly decreased. Most dysplastic dogs between 12 and 14 months of age walk and run freely and are free of significant pain, despite the radiographic appearance of the joint. Most exhibit a "bunny hopping" gait when running.

Older dogs present a different clinical picture because they suffer from chronic degenerative joint disease and its associated pain (see Chapter 17). Lameness may be unilateral but is usually bilateral. The signs may have become apparent over a long period of time, or they suddenly occur after brisk activity that results in a tear or other injury of soft tissues of the abnormal joint. Most clinical signs result from prolonged degenerative changes within the joint. There is lameness after prolonged or heavy exercise, a waddling gait, and often crepitus and restricted range of motion of the joint. The dog often prefers to sit rather than stand and arises slowly and with great difficulty. Thigh and pelvic muscles atrophy markedly with the result that the greater trochanters become quite prominent and even more so if the hip is subluxated. Concurrently, shoulder muscles hypertrophy because of the cranial weight shift and increased use of the forelimbs. The Ortolani sign is rarely present owing to the shallowness of the acetabulum and fibrosis of the joint capsule.

Hip dysplasia may be only the most prominent manifestation of a disease that affects several joints. In one study about 30 percent of young dogs predisposed to hip dysplasia had pathological changes in the shoulder and stifle joints. These changes were typical of degenerative joint disease and included mild synovitis, increased synovial fluid, and cartilage abrasions.[19]

DIAGNOSIS

Radiology

Radiographic confirmation is essential in establishing a positive diagnosis. The Orthopedic Foundation for Animals has formed a hip dysplasia registry (University of Missouri, Columbia, Missouri) and, as a result of examining many radiographs, has established seven grades of variation in congruity of the femoral head and acetabulum. The first three are considered within the range of normal:

1. Excellent—Nearly perfect conformation.
2. Good—Normal conformation for age and breed.
3. Fair—Less than ideal but within normal radiographic limits.
4. Near normal—A borderline category in which minor hip abnormalities often cannot be clearly assessed because of poor positioning during radiographic procedures.

Dysplastic animals fall into three categories:

1. Mild—Minimal deviation from normal with only slight flattening of the femoral head and minor subluxation.
2. Moderate—Obvious deviation from normal with evidence of a shallow acetabulum, flattened femoral head, poor joint congruency, and in some cases subluxation with marked changes of the femoral head and neck.
3. Severe—Complete dislocation of the hip and severe flattening of the acetabulum and femoral head.

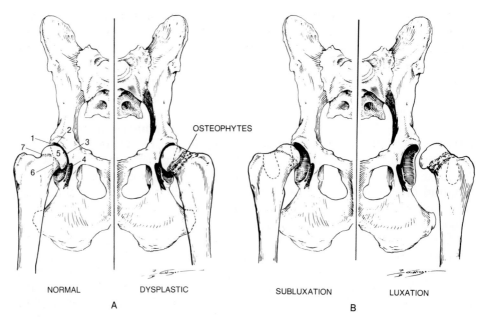

FIGURE 20–7

Hip dysplasia. (A) The right side is normal with several landmarks identified: (1) craniolateral rim; (2) cranial acetabular margin; (3) fovea capitis; (4) acetabular notch; (5) femoral head; (6) dorsal acetabular rim; and (7) physeal scar. (See text for details.) The left side is dysplastic: The femoral head is flattened and not congruent with the cranial acetabular margin; the intersection of the physeal scar and the dorsal acetabular rim shows only about 40 percent of the femoral head under the acetabular rim; osteophytes have formed at the intersection of the joint capsule and the femoral neck, giving it a very thickened appearance. (B) The right side shows obvious subluxation. Dramatic incongruency is noted between the femoral head and the cranial acetabular margin, and the intersection of the physeal scar and dorsal acetabular rim shows less than one third of the femoral head under the acetabular rim. The femoral head has become flattened and remodeled. The left side shows complete luxation with secondary changes of the femoral head and neck.

Dogs in moderate and severe grades are most likely to be clinically affected. Examples taken from radiographs are shown in Figure 20–7.

Radiographic evaluation of dysplasia requires adequate relaxation for proper positioning in dorsal recumbency with the femurs extended parallel to each other and to the cassette and the patellae centered on the femoral condyles.[20] Evaluation of properly exposed radiographs is done by reference to several landmarks that are illustrated in Figure 20–7A. The more important points are:

- The femoral head should be congruent with the cranial acetabular margin, which should in turn be perpendicular to the midline.
- The intersection of the physeal scar with the dorsal acetabular rim defines the amount of the femoral head that is under the acetabular rim. At least 50 percent of the head should be covered by the acetabulum.
- Variable amounts of femoral head flattening and remodeling may obscure the fovea capitis. The head becomes more oval in outline as osteophytes build on the femoral neck, at the insertion of the joint capsule. In later stages the acetabulum becomes filled with bone and the medial wall appears very thickened.

Reliability of radiographic evaluation for dysplasia is a function of age of the dog. In the German shepherd dog (Alsatian), it is 70 percent at 12 months, 83 percent at 18 months, and 95 percent at 24 months. In general, evaluation between 12 and 18 months has a reliability of 85 percent compared with evaluation at 24 months.[15]

Physical Examination

The ability to diagnose hip dysplasia early in life is economically useful to breeders and could eliminate considerable distress for owners who become very attached to a pet only to find later that the dog has hip dysplasia. Palpation of 6- to 8-week-old puppies for hip joint laxity by the method of Bardens[21] has been demonstrated to be statistically significant in predicting hip dysplasia in at-risk breeds.[22] Bardens reported an accuracy of 83 percent in predicting dysplasia in puppies. The technique is best done on 8- to 9-week-old puppies and requires deep sedation or light general anesthesia. With the pup on its side, the thumb of one hand is rested on the tuber ischii and the middle finger on the dorsal iliac spine. The index finger of the same hand is placed on the greater trochanter as the opposite hand lifts the femur laterally, raising the femoral head out of the acetabulum. The amount of lift can be estimated by observation of the index finger on the acetabulum. Although this is a very subjective measurement, a simple lever device has been described to allow an objective measurement.[22] There is a correlation between the degree of laxity and the presence of hip dysplasia at 12 months of age.

The usefulness of the Ortolani sign (Figs. 20–8C and D and 15–7) as a predictor of dysplasia has not been documented in puppies of this age range, but a similar correlation would be expected since both methods measure hip joint laxity. Palpation for joint laxity in mature animals is usually unrewarding owing to the fibrosis of the joint capsule and shallowness of the acetabulum. The general orthopedic and radiographic examination is more important in this situation.

TREATMENT

Conservative Therapy

Many dogs with hip dysplasia show no signs of pain; others have only mild, intermittent signs. Indeed, in 68 dogs in which hip dysplasia was diagnosed at an early age, 76 percent had minimal gait abnormalities at a mean of 4.5 years later.[23] A large number of these animals can be treated by conservative methods that include minimizing activity to restrict exercise below the threshold level that the hips can tolerate without clinical signs of pain and fatigue. This will often cause relief of signs with no other treatment. Weight reduction, for instance, is essential for obese animals.

The use of analgesics and other anti-inflammatory agents is indicated in many animals. Aspirin and sodium salicylate do much to improve the well-being of the dog and improve the quality of life. Buffered aspirin is generally the first choice in a twice-daily dose of 325 mg (5 grains) for a 25- to 30-pound animal (25 mg/kg). Phenylbutazone is useful and seems to be more effective than aspirin in some dogs. For chronic use, a therapeutic dosage is 1 mg/kg divided into two or three daily doses, but doses as high as 4 to 5 mg/kg can be used for short periods of time. Corticosteroids hasten degenerative changes in the joint and should be avoided for chronic use. Meclofenamic acid (Arquel, Parke-Davis) has worked well in dogs who tolerated it without gastric or intestinal irritation. It is available only as an equine powder but works well mixed in dog food. Dosage is 1 mg/kg daily for four to seven days, then ½ mg/kg. One teaspoon of the equine powder equals 160 mg.

Surgical methods of treating hip dysplasia include pectineal myectomy, pelvic osteotomy, intertrochanteric osteotomy, excision arthroplasty, and total hip prosthesis. These are discussed later in this chapter.

Hannan and associates[24] have demonstrated a chondroprotective effect by polysulfated glycosaminoglycan (Arteparon, Luitpold Werk, Munich, FRG; Adequan, Luitpold Pharmaceutical Inc., Shirley, N.Y.) following experimental meniscectomy. This is also supported by limited clinical experience in treating hip dysplasia. Dosage of 1 mg/kg intramuscularly every four days for six doses often produces clinical improvement. This dose is then repeated to effect, usually every four to six weeks. The drug is not yet approved for use in dogs in the United States, so the equine variety must be used.

Surgical Therapy

PECTINEAL MYECTOMY

A variety of operations on the pectineus muscle have been proposed to treat hip dysplasia and to prevent it. These surgeries include myectomy, myotomy, tenectomy, and tenotomy. All are designed to relieve tension produced by the muscle and transmitted to the hip joint. It has been speculated that this dorsal force on the femoral head pushes it against the dorsal acetabular rim and thus contributes to development of hip dysplasia.[25] Subsequent studies have indicated no effect in preventing dysplasia as a result of pectineal tenotomy[95] or myotomy.[96] Nevertheless, symptomatic improvement does result in many mature dogs for a variable length of time following pectineal resection.

Pectineal resection does not affect the radiographic changes associated with hip dysplasia; the degenerative changes progress at least as fast after surgery as would be expected without surgery. It is possible that increased abduction of the femur results, with a more varus position of the femoral head relative to the pelvis, which places the head more deeply in the acetabulum (see the discussion of the intertrochanteric varus osteotomy following). Relief of pain possibly results from increasing the load-bearing areas of the femoral head and neck, thus decreasing the load/unit area of articular cartilage. Stress on the joint capsule may also be lessened. Because the joint is still unstable, however, degenerative changes continue and pain usually returns after a variable period of time ranging from a few months to years.

There is no way of predicting how long the effects of surgery will be beneficial; therefore, pectineal surgery has only limited value in treating hip dysplasia. It is useful under conditions in which short-term effects are acceptable, such as completing a field trial campaign.

SURGICAL TECHNIQUE ■ The pectineal muscles are exposed by means of the ventral approach to the hip joint.[5] The pectineus tendon is transected distally at the point where a neurovascular bundle crosses the musculotendinous junction. The tendon of origin is cut close to its origin on the prepubic tendon, and the muscle is removed. Subcutaneous tissues and skin are closed only after attaining perfect hemostasis in the field.

AFTERCARE ▪ Moderate exercise should be started two to three days after surgery to minimize the possibility of fibrous bands forming in the excision site; this could restrict the femur. Such bands are minimized by total myectomy; however, they are not totally eliminated.

TRIPLE PELVIC OSTEOTOMY

Pelvic osteotomy with axial rotation of the acetabulum to stabilize the femoral head within the acetabulum in a functional position (Fig. 20–8A and B) is an effective method of treating dysplasia, especially in young animals. The operation should be done early, most commonly between 4 and 8 months of age, in order to take advantage of the remodeling capacity of immature bone. With instability and subluxation over a period of time, the acetabulum becomes filled with osteophytes and new bone that covers the original surface, thus preventing congruency between the femoral head and acetabulum. These changes become increasingly severe by the age of 10 to 12 months.

Age is, however, not the most important criterion determining success. The primary consideration is the condition of the joint surfaces, i.e., the amount of degeneration that has occurred. If the acetabulum is filled with bone, or the dorsal acetabular rim (labrum) is lost due to eburnation, or the cartilage of the femoral head is destroyed, pelvic osteotomy will fail.[26, 27]

In selecting patients for this procedure, standard ventrodorsal and lateral radiographs are taken and analyzed for the pathology described above. Equally as important as the radiographs is palpation of the hips with the dog anesthetized or deeply sedated. With practice one can recognize breakdown of the dorsal acetabular rim and the condition of the cartilage of the femoral head. This surgery is contraindicated when there are radiographic or palpable signs of advanced degenerative joint disease, breakdown of the dorsal acetabular rim, or shallow acetabulum. The sign of Ortolani is elicited (Fig. 20–8C, D, and E) with the dog on its back, with the femur held vertically, and the stifle flexed. The femurs are grasped distally, pressure is applied proximally (toward the table), and as the femur is abducted, a distinct "click" is heard when the femoral head reduces. The angle of the femur from vertical is measured, and this angle of reduction is the maximum angle the acetabulum needs to be rotated to achieve stability. Reversing the procedure by adducting the femur results in another click when the head subluxates from the acetabulum. The angle of the femur from vertical at this point is the angle of luxation and represents the minimal angle of rotation of the acetabulum that will produce stability of the hip. These two angles are used to select the appropriate implant for axial rotation of the acetabular segment of the pelvis.[27] In order to prevent overrotation of the pelvis and subsequent impingement of the dorsal acetabular rim on the femoral neck, the angle selected should usually be closer to the angle of luxation than to the angle of reduction.

SURGICAL TECHNIQUE ▪ Two surgical techniques have emerged in recent years, the triple pelvic osteotomies of Schrader[28] and Slocum.[26, 27] Slocum has devised a bone plate for this procedure (Canine Pelvic Osteotomy Plate, Slocum Enterprises, 621 River Ave., Eugene, Oregon 97404, USA), using 3.5-mm screws, which is made in three angles of rotation: a 20-degree plate with a fixed angle; a 30-degree plate that can be twisted to angles between 20 and 40 degrees; and a 45-degree plate that can be molded between 35 and 60 degrees. This device has proved most satisfactory and easy to use in our hands and is our method of choice (Fig. 20–8I and J). It is superior to a twisted conventional bone plate because it provides eight potential points of fixation (six screws, two cerclage wires) and thus minimizes fixation failure. It also lateralizes the acetabular portion of the pelvis and so widens the pelvic canal. A standard 5–7 hole, 2.7 or 3.5 mm straight plate can be used with good success, although more work is involved in twisting the plate. It is probably best to preoperatively twist several plates to the 20-, 30-, and 45-degree angles than to spend the time needed to do this intraoperatively.

The procedure is performed in three stages. The pubic ramus is exposed through a ventral approach[5] (Fig. 20–8F). The pectineus muscle is severed close to its origin on the iliopectineal eminence and the prepubic tendon and again as far distally as possible. The muscle belly is discarded. Elevation of the gracilis muscle caudally and the abdominal muscles and prepubic tendon cranially exposes the pubic ramus. Most of the ramus is removed after two cuts in the bone, one near the medial limit of the obturator foramen and the other at the junction of the pubis with the ilium, lateral to the iliopubic eminence. The obturator nerve must be protected during the lateral cut as it lies very near the caudal limit of this cut. The abdominal muscles and prepubic tendon are sutured to the cranial border of the gracilis muscle and the rest of the tissues are sutured in layers.

The second incision is made sagittally over the medial angle of the ischiatic tuberosity. After elevation of the internal obturator dorsally and the semimembranosus and quadratus muscles ventrally, the ischiatic table is osteotomized in a paramedian plane, beginning cranially at the lateral aspect of the obturator foramen (Fig. 20–8F and G). Drill holes are placed 5 mm from the cut edges, and a 1-mm (18 gauge) wire is threaded through the holes but not tightened. A lateral approach is next made to the shaft of the ilium,[5] and the gluteal muscles are elevated from the body and ventral wing of the ilium. Taking care to protect the cranial gluteal, obturator, and sciatic nerves, all tissues are elevated from the iliac shaft ventrally, medially, and dorsally. An iliac osteotomy is performed just caudal to the sacrum (Fig. 20–8H). The cut is made perpendicular in both planes to a line between the dorsal side of the ischiatic tuberosity and the ventral third of the iliac crest. This line is established by inserting a small Steinmann pin from the dorsal surface of the tuber ischium cranially toward the cranial ventral iliac spine, where it is positioned by palpation. The pin can then be used to establish the proper angle for the iliac osteotomy.

Following this osteotomy the acetabular segment is moved cranially and laterally with bone-holding forceps to allow fixation of the plate to the caudal segment with 3.5-mm screws. If the Pelvic Osteotomy Plate is used, at least one of these screws is placed in the load position to compress the angular step against the bone. The sharp spike of ilium dorsal to the plate is removed to prevent irritation of the gluteal muscles. The acetabular segment is rotated laterally and the plate temporarily clamped to the iliac crest portion. The hip should now be stable with no Ortolani sign; if not, the plate is removed and

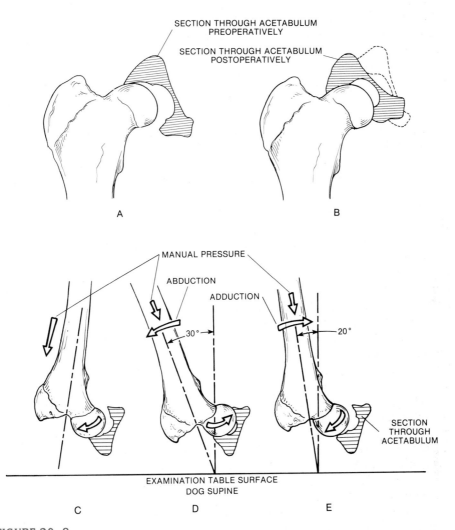

FIGURE 20–8

Triple pelvic osteotomy. *(A)* Preoperatively the femoral head is riding loosely in the acetabulum and contacting only a small area of the dorsal acetabular rim, setting the stage for the structural changes we identify as hip dysplasia. *(B)* Following osteotomy the acetabular portion of the pelvis has been rotated laterally over the femoral head, greatly increasing the contact area between head and acetabulum and thus decreasing local bone and cartilage loads. *(C, D, and E)* Finding the acetabular rotation angle.[26, 27] *(C)* With the dog supine, the Ortolani sign (subluxation of the femoral head) is elicited by *adduction* and pressure on the femur directed toward the table. This is most easily done bilaterally, which eliminates the problem of the dog rotating when pressure is applied. *(D)* While continuing to apply pressure to the femur, the femur is slowly *abducted*. At some point a distinct click or popping sensation will be felt and perhaps heard as the femur reduces into the acetabulum. In addition, a visible motion will be seen in the inguinal region as the femur returns medially. The angle of the femur relative to the sagittal plane (i.e., the plane 90 degrees to the table top) is identified as the reduction angle and represents the maximum angle the acetabulum would need to be rotated to stabilize the femur. In this example the angle measured 30 degrees. The optimal angle of rotation is about 5 to 10 degrees less than the angle of reduction. *(E)* With the femur in the reduced position, it is slowly *adducted* while maintaining pressure toward the table. Again a distinct point will be appreciated visually, audibly, and by palpation that represents the femur luxating from the acetabulum. This is measured as in *D* and is called the angle of luxation, 20 degrees here, and represents the minimum angle of rotation of the acetabulum.

Illustration continued on following page

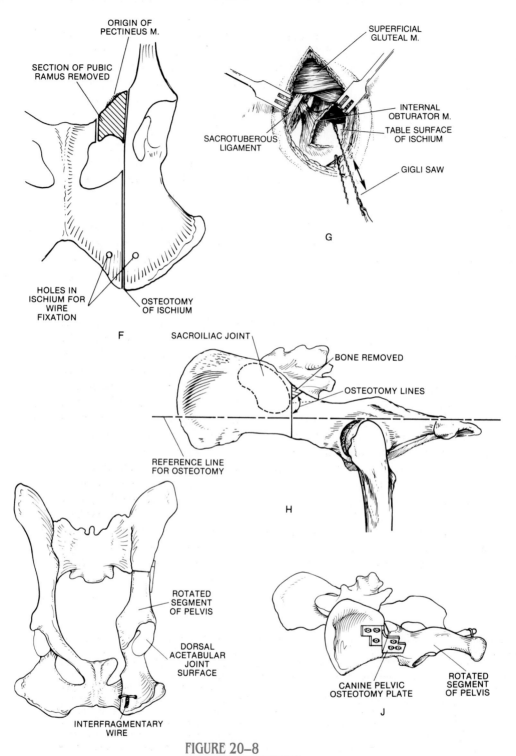

ORIGIN OF
PECTINEUS M.

SECTION OF PUBIC
RAMUS REMOVED

SUPERFICIAL
GLUTEAL M.

INTERNAL
OBTURATOR M.

TABLE SURFACE
OF ISCHIUM

SACROTUBEROUS
LIGAMENT

GIGLI SAW

G

HOLES IN
ISCHIUM FOR
WIRE
FIXATION

OSTEOTOMY
OF ISCHIUM

F

SACROILIAC JOINT

BONE REMOVED

OSTEOTOMY LINES

REFERENCE LINE
FOR OSTEOTOMY

H

ROTATED
SEGMENT
OF PELVIS

DORSAL
ACETABULAR
JOINT
SURFACE

INTERFRAGMENTARY
WIRE

CANINE PELVIC
OSTEOTOMY PLATE

ROTATED
SEGMENT
OF PELVIS

J

FIGURE 20–8

See legend on opposite page

twisted more or replaced with another plate of increased angle. If the Ortolani sign is eliminated but there is still lateral movement of the femoral head in the acetabulum (Bardens' sign[21]), transposition of the greater trochanter (see Fig. 20–3D) will usually provide the stability needed for the femoral head. After the proper angle is found for the acetabular segment, the ischial wire is tightened, and the plate is then fixed to the cranial iliac bone (Fig. 20–8I and J). In very young dogs, the screw fixation can be supplemented with a hemicerclage wire through holes in each end of the Pelvic Osteotomy Plate. The triangular bone fragment previously removed can be cut into small fragments and used as bone graft in the osteotomy site. Both surgery sites are closed routinely by layers.

AFTERCARE ■ Postoperatively the dog is confined to the house or leash exercise for six weeks, at which time the opposite side is operated if indicated. In severely dysplastic puppies in the 4- to 7-month range, the second osteotomy should be done in two to three weeks as the bony structures and joint cartilage are breaking down rapidly.

PROGNOSIS ■ Slocum has reported on follow-up evaluation of 138 dogs that underwent triple pelvic osteotomy. Of these dogs, 122 had hip dysplasia: 30 percent had grade 4 dysplasia; 33 percent grade 3; and 34 percent grade 2. In age at surgery, 13 percent were < 6 months of age; 47 percent were 6 to 12 months; 22.5 percent were 1 to 2 years; and 17 percent were > 2 years. At the time of postoperative evaluation, 86.2 percent were fully active with normal weight-bearing and activity.[27] Schrader found satisfactory functional ability in 93 percent of his cases, and a satisfactory functional, physical, and radiographic result in 73 percent of the cases.[28]

The veterinary orthopedist is truly in a quandary when trying to decide on a course of treatment for an individual dog when the clinical signs of dysplasia develop at an early age. Although the results of triple pelvic osteotomy are very encouraging, they must be balanced against the observation of Barr, Denny, and Gibbs that 76 percent of dogs diagnosed with hip dysplasia at a young age never had serious clinical signs of dysplasia at follow-up 4½ years later.[23] One might ask if these dogs would not develop problems later in

---

FIGURE 20–8

Continued (F and G) Pubic ostectomy and ischial osteotomy. *(F)* A section of the pubic ramus is removed via a ventral approach and detachment of the pectineus muscle at its origin (see text). *(G)* A caudal approach to the ischium allows elevation of the internal obturator muscle and osteotomy of the ischial table from the lateral border of the obturator foramen caudally on a line parallel to the midline. The results of this osteotomy are seen in *(F)* as are the 2-mm drill holes, through which 20- or 18-gauge (0.8 to 1 mm) wire is threaded but not tightened at this time. *(H)* Osteotomy of the iliac shaft. A horizontal reference line is created by passing a small blunted Steinmann pin from the dorsal surface of the tuber ischii cranially to a point one-third the distance from the ventral to the cranial dorsal iliac spines. The transverse osteotomy is 90 degrees to the horizontal line and at the caudal aspect of the sacroiliac joint. The sciatic nerve must be protected when the osteotomy is made (see text). A triangular piece of bone will be removed dorsally after the plate is attached. *(I and J)* The completed triple pelvic osteotomy procedure. The iliac osteotomy is stabilized with a Canine Pelvic Osteotomy Plate (Slocum Enterprises) and the ischial osteotomy with a twisted interfragmentary wire. A standard 2.7- or 3.5-mm plate can be twisted to provide a similar effect. Note how the rotated acetabular segment would provide greater dorsal coverage for the femoral head.

life. However, if these figures hold true, only between 10 and 17 percent of the affected puppies really will benefit from triple pelvic osteotomy or intertrochanteric femoral osteotomy (see below). Conversely, it is impossible to predict how any individual puppy will fare later in life, and so the decision to pursue surgical treatment needs to be carefully considered since the results are predictable. If the animal is destined to be primarily a house/yard pet, a conservative approach is probably rational. If the dog is wanted as a sporting or working "canine athlete," a more aggressive approach should be pursued at an early age, when the chances for a reconstructive approach are best.

INTERTROCHANTERIC VARUS OSTEOTOMY OF THE FEMUR

The true angle of inclination of the canine femoral neck in relation to the diaphysis is about 146 ±5 degrees.[29] In animals with hip dysplasia, this angle increases as much as 30 to 35 degrees, leading to the condition known as coxa valga (Fig. 20–9C). This is due to subluxation of the hip joint and subsequent lack of normal stress on the femoral neck, which is apparently necessary for development of the normal angle. This valgus angle of the head and neck contributes to further subluxation and instability, perpetuating a vicious circle. Additionally, the femoral neck inclines farther cranially (anteversion) from the normal angle of about 27 ±6.5 degrees[29] and again contributes to subluxation and instability.

The principle of varus derotational osteotomy for treatment of congenital hip luxation and instability is well established in humans and, recently, in the dog.[30] By making the femoral neck more perpendicular to the femoral shaft (varisation) and reducing anteversion, the femoral head can be placed more deeply within the acetabulum and forces acting on the bone and cartilage of the acetabulum and femoral head can be reduced by distributing weight-bearing loads through greater congruency over a greater percentage of the articular cartilage. When the osteotomy is done in an immature animal with a high potential for bony remodeling, there can be permanent improvement in joint congruity. In the mature animal with degenerative joint disease and instability, pain may be relieved by reduced forces on the acetabulum and femoral head and distributing weight-bearing forces more uniformly over the diseased cartilage.

The purpose of intertrochanteric osteotomy is to improve the biomechanics of the hip and to reduce hip pain.[30] It is more effective when done before

---

FIGURE 20–9

Intertrochanteric varus osteotomy. (A) Finding the angle of inclination of the femoral neck. These measurements are made from the ventrodorsal pelvic radiograph, with the hips extended (femurs parallel to table) and the patellae centered. See text for explanation. (B, C, and D) Intertrochanteric varus osteotomy using AO/ASIF 3.5-mm double hook plates (Synthes). (See text for details.) (B) The hooks on the proximal end of the plate are placed in holes in the trochanter major. (C) Instability of the hip joint is created by the valgus angle of inclination of the femoral neck. Removal of the wedge of bone will create a slightly varus 135-degree angle and restore stability. (D) The bone wedge has been removed and the intertrochanteric osteotomy fixed with the double hook plate. Note the improved congruity of the joint surfaces and compare with Figure 20–8B. (E) In dogs too small for the double hook plate, a multiple pin and tension band wire fixation technique can be used.

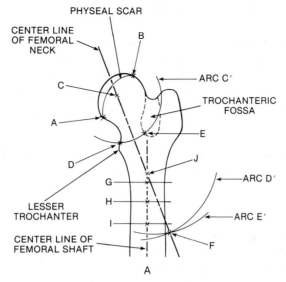

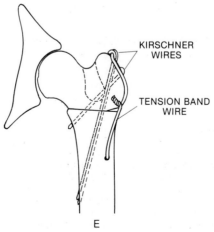

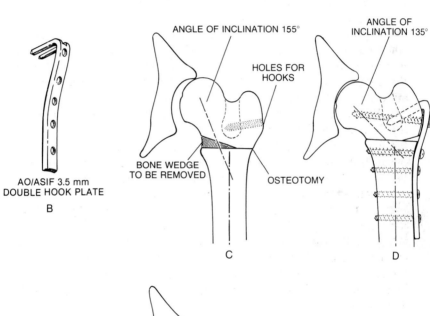

FIGURE 20-9

See legend on opposite page

degenerative joint disease is present, between the ages of 4 and 10 months in most patients. As with triple pelvic osteotomy, careful radiographic evaluation and palpation of the joints will aid in evaluating the condition of the joint surfaces. Contraindications include degenerative joint disease that is radiographically obvious, shallow acetabulum, and loss of the dorsal acetabular rim.

PREOPERATIVE PLANNING ■ Extensive planning[30] is necessary to establish the proper angles for osteotomizing the femoral neck in order to end with an inclination angle of 135 degrees. This is about 10 degrees less than normal, hence a varus position. In this position the femoral head is more deeply placed within the acetabulum and hence more stable (Fig. 20–9D).

It is first necessary to establish the angle of inclination of the femoral head and neck.[31] A well-positioned radiograph, as detailed above (see Fig. 20–7) is needed. It is particularly necessary that the patella be well centered on the femoral condyle. Tracing paper can then be used to produce a drawing similar to Figure 20–9A. Line A B is the physeal scar, and point C, the center of the femoral head, is midway between. Arc C' is struck from C to intersect the femoral neck at the base of the trochanteric fossa at points D and E. Arcs D' and E' are struck to intersect each other lateral to the femoral shaft and thereby form point F. Connecting point F with point C delineates the center line of the femoral neck. Three lines, G, H, and I, are next drawn across the proximal femur. These lines are spaced 1 to 1.5 cm apart and are used to find the centerline of the femur by marking the midpoint of each line and then connecting the points and extending the line to intersect the femoral neck midline at point J. The angle formed by the femoral neck and femoral midlines is the *angle of inclination* of the femoral head and neck.

The apparent angle of inclination is influenced by the degree of anteversion; increasing anteversion increases the projected angle of inclination seen in the radiograph. Measurement of anteversion can be performed,[31] but it is not essential to do so. If anteversion is normal, the lesser trochanter will protrude only slightly beyond the medial cortex if the patella is centered on the femoral condyle. If the lesser trochanter is very prominent, as in Figure 20–9A, it can be assumed that anteversion is increased and that the measured angle is larger than the true angle. Experience has shown that reducing the measured angle by 5 degrees is satisfactory for planning purposes. Surgical reduction of anteversion does not depend on measurements, as it is only possible to estimate the angle intraoperatively.

Planning continues by drawing a line transversely across the femur from point D, just proximal to the lesser trochanter (Fig. 20–9C). This represents the first osteotomy of the femur. The angle of the wedge of bone to be removed is determined by subtracting 135 from the final determined angle of inclination. Using a protractor, this angle is drawn so that the wide end of the wedge is medial, and the proximal line intersects the medial cortex just distal to the femoral neck. A new drawing can now be made by tracing the femoral head with the bone wedge removed and placing it on the femoral shaft in its final position (Fig. 20–9D). The bone plate, or a tracing of it, can be superimposed on the final drawing to determine the position of the holes for the hooks. This is transferred back to the original drawing to indicate the position of the holes in the proximal segment before the first osteotomy.

SURGICAL TECHNIQUE ■ Special AO/ASIF 3.5-mm hook plates (Fig. 20–9B), drill jigs, and cutting jigs are available from Synthes, and the technique of using them has been described.[30, 32, 33] Application of this hook plate for other osteotomies and certain fractures has also been reported.[34] In principle, an intertrochanteric osteotomy is performed, a wedge of bone is removed from the medial side of the base of the femoral neck, and the hook plate is used to create rigid internal fixation of the osteotomy (Fig. 20–9D). The femoral head is also rotated caudally (retroverted) until the anteversion angle is about 5 to 10 degrees in relation to the femoral shaft.

Although the double hook plate and its accompanying instrumentation represent an elegant and precise method of accomplishing this osteotomy, the plate is too large for use on most dogs under 20 kg. Multiple pin and tension band wire fixation is a satisfactory fixation method in these animals (Fig. 20–9E). Preoperative planning is similar to that explained above, and the AO/ASIF jigs can be used to assist in the osteotomies, although with some practice they can be done "free-hand" with good accuracy.

AFTERCARE ■ Postsurgical care is uncomplicated and consists primarily of restricted exercise for three to four weeks, followed by a slow return to normal exercise by six weeks. The opposite hip can be operated as early as three weeks postoperatively if indicated.

PROGNOSIS ■ Walker and Prieur reported on follow-up, between 1 and 7 years postoperatively, of 183 dogs with hip dysplasia that received intertrochanteric femoral osteotomies.[30] At the time of follow-up, 89.6 percent of these dogs had good to excellent function. Most animals had only one hip operated. Those animals operated on before degenerative joint disease was present did better than those in which the disease was established at the time of surgery. Thus the results are very similar to Slocum's triple pelvic osteotomy series[27] and present the surgeon with the same dilemma regarding treatment of a young dysplastic dog as was discussed above for triple pelvic osteotomy.

TOTAL HIP REPLACEMENT

Total hip replacement (THR) consists of implanting a high-density polyethylene acetabular cup and stainless steel femoral head component (Richards Canine II total hip prosthesis, Richards Manufacturing Inc, Memphis, TN), after removing the femoral head and neck and preparing the acetabulum by reaming. These prostheses are permanently bonded to bone by polymethylmethacrylate bone cement (Fig. 20–10). At present, two sizes of prostheses are available, allowing replacement in most dogs over 18 kg (40 lb). The procedure should not be done before the physes are closed. Thus, most large breeds cannot be operated before 12 to 14 months of age, but there are no specific upper age limits.

INDICATIONS ■ In addition to hip dysplasia, THR can be used to replace hip joints damaged by degenerative joint disease from causes other than hip dysplasia; nonunion or malunion of femoral head, neck, or acetabular fractures; traumatic hip luxation; or avascular necrosis of the femoral head.

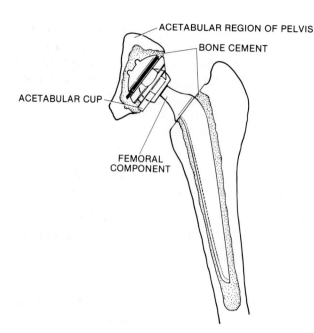

ACETABULAR REGION OF PELVIS

BONE CEMENT

ACETABULAR CUP

FEMORAL
COMPONENT

FIGURE 20–10

The Richards Canine II Total Hip Replacement (Richards Manufacturing Co., Memphis, TN). Polymethylmethacrylate bone cement anchors the high-density polyethylene acetabular cup to the pelvis and the cobalt-chrome alloy femoral component to the femur.

CONTRAINDICATIONS ■ Not every dog with hip dysplasia is a candidate for THR because not all dysplastic dogs show clinical signs. Such animals should be periodically re-evaluated for deterioration of their condition. It is often suggested that THR might be done in cases in which function is not satisfactory following femoral head and neck excision (discussed below). The bone remodeling that follows excision arthroplasty makes this procedure extremely difficult to do in this situation and is not recommended. Neurological causes of abnormal gait must be carefully eliminated as a cause of the dog's problems. Degenerative myelopathy is the most common problem in these patients, but ruptured intervertebral disk, spinal or nerve root tumor, and cauda equina disease are other possibilities. When there is a sudden worsening of hindlimb lameness in a known dysplastic dog, there is a strong tendency to blame it on the dysplasia, but rupture of the cranial cruciate ligament is a far more common cause. Any infectious process, such as dermatitis, otitis, anal sac disease, dental disease, cystitis, or prostatitis, must be cleared before THR, to prevent contamination of the surgical site.

SURGICAL TECHNIQUE ■ The technique most widely used in North America was perfected by Olmstead and Hohn.[35, 36] The operation is technically demanding and unforgiving of errors in technique. Adequate instrumentation and assistance must be available to the surgeon to allow the procedure to be completed within 1.5 to 2 hours, or the infection rate will be unacceptable. Special training should be obtained before attempting this operation.

PROGNOSIS ■ Most dogs return to full function by eight weeks postoperatively. Satisfactory function occurred in 95 percent of 362 cases followed three months or more.[36] This is defined as full weight-bearing, normal range of motion, normal gait, and normal level of activity with no signs of pain in the hip. Similar results have been experienced at Colorado State University. Late infection with loosening of the acetabular prosthesis accounts for most of the failures. There seems to be no tendency for the prosthesis to break down or loosen with time as in humans. Thus, at this point, the procedure does not appear to be time limited. This indicates that the technique has established itself as a reliable clinical procedure for the treatment of a variety of abnormal conditions of the hip.

FEMORAL HEAD AND NECK EXCISION

Femoral head and neck excision to allow formation of a fibrous false joint is also termed *excision arthroplasty* or *femoral head and neck ostectomy*. Pain is relieved by elimination of bony contact between the femur and the pelvis as scar tissue interposes. Because of slight limb shortening and some loss of range of motion, some gait abnormality persists. The procedure may be performed bilaterally, preferably with procedures separated by an interval of 8 to 10 weeks.

PATIENT SELECTION ■ Excision arthroplasty is a nonreversible procedure and must be considered a salvage operation. Nevertheless, it is a valuable method for improving the quality of life for many pets by elimination of pain. Indications will vary with the skill of the surgeon, internal fixation devices available, and financial considerations. There is some tendency to overuse the procedure for conditions that are reparable.

Degenerative joint disease resulting from dysplasia is the most common indication for excision arthroplasty. The procedure is often the first choice of treatment for a mature animal that is basically a house or yard pet only; it is also the treatment of choice for Legg-Calvé-Perthes disease. Other common indications include chronic osteoarthrosis from any cause, comminuted fractures of the acetabulum or femoral neck, fractures of the femoral head, and chronic luxation of the hip with erosion of the femoral head. In summary, the procedure is suitable for any condition in which the integrity of the hip joint has been compromised and primary repair is not feasible[37] or in which osteoarthrosis is well established.

SURGICAL TECHNIQUE ■ A craniolateral approach to the hip (Fig. 20–11A and B) is preferred because it does not involve transection of the gluteal muscles, as do the dorsal approaches.[5] Some surgeons favor a ventral approach (Fig. 20–11C and D) because it is more cosmetic. In the craniolateral approach, it is important to incise and reflect the joint capsule and origin of the vastus lateralis muscle to expose the cranial aspect of the femoral neck adequately. The gluteal muscles are retracted dorsally by inserting a Hohman retractor inside the joint capsule. Bone-holding forceps attached to the region of the trochanter may be used to subluxate the femur. This facilitates cutting of the round ligament with curved scissors and elevation of the rest of the joint capsule from the femoral head.

The neck is best cut with an osteotome, with the leg externally rotated 90 degrees. In a large dog, this osteotome should be at least 1 inch wide (2.5 cm). The cut should extend from the base of the trochanter major across the neck in a line that will intersect the medial cortex of the femur without leaving a sharp angle (Fig. 20–12A). The cut may include the trochanter minor in some cases.

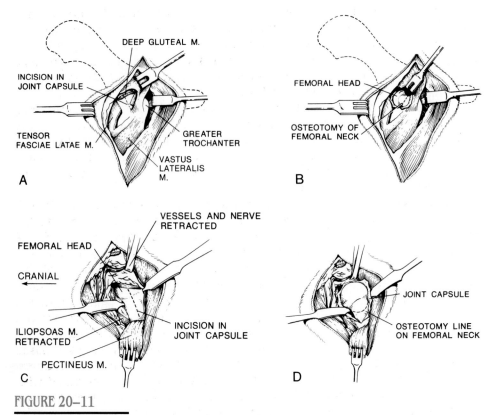

FIGURE 20–11

Approaches for femoral head and neck excision. (A) Incision of the joint capsule in the craniolateral approach[5] in the left hip. The incision starts on the acetabulum and extends over the center of the femoral head and neck into the origin of the vastus lateralis muscle. (B) The joint capsule has been retracted and the femoral head luxated by cutting the round ligament. The position of the femoral neck osteotomy can now be visualized. (C) Incision of the joint capsule in the ventral approach[5] in the right hip. (D) The joint capsule has been retracted and the femoral head luxated by cutting the round ligament. The position of the femoral neck osteotomy can now be visualized.

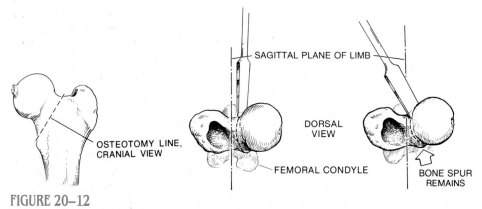

FIGURE 20–12

Femoral head and neck excision. (A) The osteotomy line as seen from the cranial aspect (frontal or transverse plane) of the femur. (B) Once the proper angle of cut in the transverse plane is established the osteotome is moved toward the animal's trunk until it is parallel to the sagittal plane of the femur. (C) If the osteotome is directed perpendicular to the femoral neck, a spur of the caudal neck (arrow) will be left on the femur.

Once this line of cut has been established, the handle of the osteotome is moved toward the animal's body until it is parallel to the sagittal plane of the thigh (Fig. 20–12A). This plane is best visualized by observing the position of the patella and tibial tubercle. The tendency is to align the osteotome perpendicular to the femoral neck as shown in Figure 20–12B. Because of the anteversion of the neck, such a cut will result in a spur of the caudal neck being left on the femur, which then rubs on the acetabular rim and prevents fibrous tissue interposition between the bones. The cut is made from a slightly distal to proximal direction to avoid splitting the medial cortex of the femur. Once the femoral head and neck are free, they can be grasped with bone-holding forceps or a towel clamp to allow cutting the remaining soft tissue attachments with curved scissors.

The femoral neck is palpated for irregularities, splinters, or a shelf of neck on the caudal surface. If any of these are found, they are removed with the osteotome or rongeurs. Leaving too long a neck that rubs on the dorsal acetabular rim is the most common reason for failure to achieve good function. Some recommend use of a rasp, but it is awkward to use. Exposure of this area of the femoral neck is facilitated by externally rotating the femur until the lateral aspect of the hock can be placed against the thoracic or abdominal wall. In some animals, osteophyte production on the dorsal acetabular rim results in excessive bone deposition, which should also be debrided.

Some reports indicate better results are obtained by interposing soft tissue between the femoral neck and the acetabulum.[37, 38] Experimental observations have not shown any objective difference when this method is compared with the conventional noninterpositional method,[39] but the study was done on normal dogs, so its application to clinical situations is open to question. The authors have observed a more rapid return to active use of the limb but generally no difference in long-term results when the deep gluteal muscle pedicle is used. The exception is when excision arthroplasty is done in the presence of irreparable acetabular fractures. Here, deep gluteal interposition has been helpful. The joint capsule may be closed over the acetabulum if possible. Two methods have been proposed for further soft-tissue interposition. Berzon and colleagues[37] recommend detaching the cranial third of the deep gluteal muscle from the trochanter major and suturing its tendon to the insertion of the iliopsoas muscle on the trochanter minor (Fig. 20–13). Lippincott[38] detached a pedicle of biceps femoris muscle, wrapping it around the femoral neck and suturing it to the gluteal and vastus lateralis muscles. This technique is shown in Figure 20–14.

AFTERCARE ■ Early, active use of the limb is necessary. Passive range-of-motion exercises, prescribed 20 to 30 times four times per day, are started immediately. Leash walking and freedom for the animal to move about a confined area are encouraged until suture removal. After two weeks postoperatively, active exercise such as running and swimming, is encouraged. Animals will ordinarily be toe-touching in 10 to 14 days, partially weight-bearing in three weeks, and actively using the leg by four weeks. When bilateral operations are indicated, they should be done 8 to 10 weeks apart. In some cases, it will be necessary to delay the second surgery even further until active use of the first limb has been achieved. In cases of severe pain from bilateral hip problems, bilateral excisions can be done simultaneously.

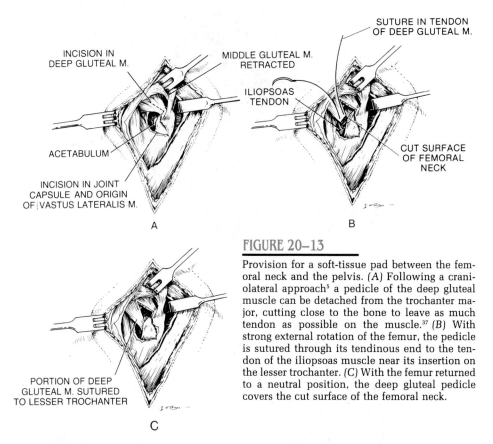

**INCISION IN
DEEP GLUTEAL M.**

**MIDDLE GLUTEAL M.
RETRACTED**

ACETABULUM

**INCISION IN JOINT
CAPSULE AND ORIGIN
OF VASTUS LATERALIS M.**

A

**SUTURE IN TENDON
OF DEEP GLUTEAL M.**

**ILIOPSOAS
TENDON**

**CUT SURFACE
OF FEMORAL
NECK**

B

**PORTION OF DEEP
GLUTEAL M. SUTURED
TO LESSER TROCHANTER**

C

FIGURE 20-13

Provision for a soft-tissue pad between the femoral neck and the pelvis. *(A)* Following a craniolateral approach[5] a pedicle of the deep gluteal muscle can be detached from the trochanter major, cutting close to the bone to leave as much tendon as possible on the muscle.[37] *(B)* With strong external rotation of the femur, the pedicle is sutured through its tendinous end to the tendon of the iliopsoas muscle near its insertion on the lesser trochanter. *(C)* With the femur returned to a neutral position, the deep gluteal pedicle covers the cut surface of the femoral neck.

PROGNOSIS ■ Return to active and pain-free use of the limb depends on surgical skill, length of time the hip pathology has been present, and severity of the pathology. Animals receiving operations for acute trauma, such as head and neck fractures, may be functional within 30 days. Those having chronic dysplasia with long-standing pain and muscle atrophy may require six months or more. These animals benefit particularly from swimming as an exercise. Patients with markedly displaced acetabular fractures and some with chronic dysplasia may never regain good function.

Reported results vary considerably. Gendreau and Cawley's[40] analysis of 32 cases indicated only 37 percent excellent results and 26 percent good results, with only three of seven dogs weighing over 25 kg experiencing excellent results. Yet the Berzon series showed 90 to 100 percent use of the limb in 83 percent of all cases with no significant difference in results between large and small breeds.[37] There is no doubt that smaller breeds experience less change in gait but the operation is usually successful in large breeds for relieving pain and restoring the animal's quality of life.

FIGURE 20-14

(A) Another method of soft-tissue interposition involves freeing a pedicle of biceps muscle *(dashed line).*[38] *(B)* A suture is attached to the muscle pedicle and is pulled under the gluteal muscles from a caudal to cranial direction. *(C)* The muscle pedicle is sutured to the elevated vastus lateralis in a position that holds it across the femoral neck ostectomy.

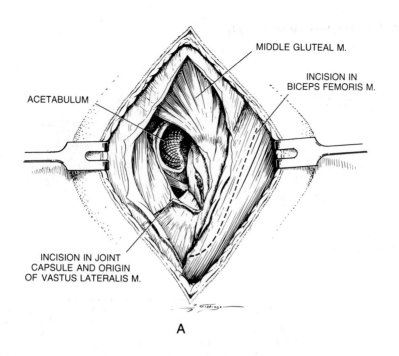

ACETABULUM

MIDDLE GLUTEAL M.

INCISION IN
BICEPS FEMORIS M.

INCISION IN JOINT
CAPSULE AND ORIGIN
OF VASTUS LATERALIS M.

A

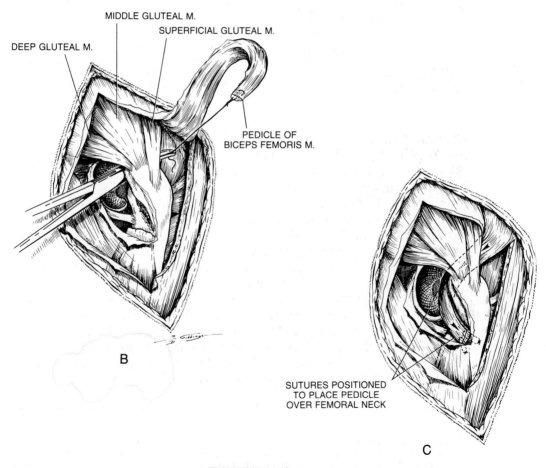

DEEP GLUTEAL M.

MIDDLE GLUTEAL M.

SUPERFICIAL GLUTEAL M.

PEDICLE OF
BICEPS FEMORIS M.

B

SUTURES POSITIONED
TO PLACE PEDICLE
OVER FEMORAL NECK

C

FIGURE 20–14

See legend on opposite page

Legg-Calvé-Perthes Disease

Known by several other names such as Legg-Perthes or Calvé-Perthes disease, osteochondritis juvenilis, avascular necrosis, and coxa plana, Legg-Calvé-Perthes disease is a noninflammatory aseptic necrosis of the femoral head and neck in small-breed dogs (Fig. 20–15). The cause of such necrosis is not known with certainty, but ischemia resulting from vascular compression[41] and precocious sex hormone activity[42] have been proposed. A genetic cause, homozygosity for an autosomal recessive gene, has been reported.[43]

In all cases, the bone of the femoral head and neck undergoes necrosis and deformation, during which time pain is manifested by the animal. The

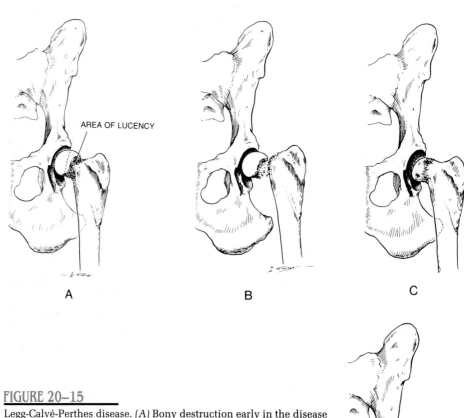

AREA OF LUCENCY

A   B   C

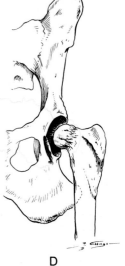

D

FIGURE 20–15

Legg-Calvé-Perthes disease. (A) Bony destruction early in the disease causes both radiographic lucency and actual loss of substance in the femoral neck. The epiphysis seems unaffected in this early stage. (B) Fracture and collapse of the femoral neck. The epiphysis remains in the acetabulum, but the deformed neck is displaced. (C) Early remodeling stage. Bone is again being deposited, but the head and neck remain deformed. (D) Late, remodeled stage. The femoral head is flattened and wrinkled, leading to instability and degenerative joint disease.

articular cartilage cracks as a result of the collapse of subchondral bone. Bone eventually returns to the necrotic area, but the femoral head and neck are deformed, with resulting joint incongruity and instability. This condition leads to severe degenerative changes within the entire hip joint and to development of marked osteoarthrosis.

Male and female animals are equally affected. Bilateral involvement has been reported as 16.5 percent[44] and 12 percent.[45] The toy breeds and terriers are most susceptible. The peak incidence of onset is 5 to 8 months of age, with a range of 3 to 13 months.[44]

CLINICAL SIGNS

Often the first abnormality noted is irritability. The animal may chew at the flank and hip area. Pain can be elicited in the hip, especially on abduction. Later, crepitus may be present, with restricted range of motion and shortening of the limb. Atrophy of the gluteal and quadriceps muscles becomes apparent. Onset of lameness is usually gradual, and 6 to 8 weeks are required to progress to complete carriage of the limb,[44] although pain can be acute when there is fracture of the femoral head at lytic areas.

Radiographic signs (Fig. 20–15) include increased joint space and foci of decreased bone density in the head and neck. The femoral head flattens where it contacts the dorsal acetabular rim, then distorts further to a variable degree. Osteophytes, as well as subluxation and fracture of the femoral head and neck, may be seen occasionally.

TREATMENT

Excision of the femoral head and neck produces more favorable results than does conservative treatment consisting of rest and analgesics.[44, 45] Results are better, and recovery time is much shorter. With the proper surgical technique, virtually 100 per cent of these animals will become ambulatory and free of pain. A slight limp may remain because the leg is shortened by removal of the femoral head and neck, and the thigh and hip muscles remain somewhat atrophied.

THE STIFLE

Patellar Luxation

Patellar luxations occur frequently in dogs and occasionally in cats and are commonly seen in most small animal practices. These luxations fall into several classes:

1. Medial luxation—toy, miniature, and large breeds.
2. Lateral luxation—toy and miniature breeds.
3. Medial luxation resulting from trauma—various breeds.
4. Lateral luxation—large and giant breeds.

MEDIAL LUXATION IN TOY, MINIATURE, AND LARGE BREEDS

These luxations are often termed "congenital" because they occur early in life and are not associated with trauma. Although the luxation may not be present at birth, the anatomical deformities that cause these luxations are present at that time and are responsible for subsequent recurrent patellar luxation. The only well-researched investigation into the cause of these luxations concluded that the occurrence of medial patellar luxation is characterized by coxa vara (a decreased angle of inclination of the femoral neck) and a decrease in femoral neck anteversion (relative retroversion).[46] These basic skeletal changes were considered to be the cause of the complex series of derangements of the pelvic limb that characterize medial patellar luxations in the small breeds. The changes are depicted in Figure 20–16A and B. Patellar luxation in these breeds should be considered an inherited disease. Breeding of affected animals is not advisable.[47]

Medial luxation is far more common than lateral luxation in all breeds, representing 75 to 80 percent of cases, with bilateral involvement seen 20 to 25 percent of the time. We have noted a dramatic increase in medial luxation in large and giant breeds in recent years. Concurrent rupture of the cranial cruciate ligament is present in 15 to 20 percent of the stifles of middle-aged and older dogs with chronic patellar luxation. In this situation, the cruciate ligament is placed under increased stress because the quadriceps mechanism is ineffective in stabilizing the joint. In the cat, medial luxation is also more common than lateral luxation. One series of 21 cases included 52.4 percent bilateral medial, 33.3 percent unilateral medial, and 14.3 percent unilateral lateral luxations.[48]

A method of classifying the degree of luxation and bony deformity is useful for diagnosis and for deciding on the method of surgical repair. Such a classification was devised by Putnam[46] and adapted by Singleton.[49] The following is adapted from Singleton (see Fig. 20–16C).

Grade 1

Intermittent patellar luxation causing the limb to be carried occasionally. The patella easily luxates manually at full extension of the stifle joint, but returns to the trochlea when released. No crepitation is apparent.

The medial, or very occasionally, lateral deviation of the tibial crest (with lateral luxation of the patella) is only minimal, with very slight rotation of the tibia. Flexion and extension of the stifle is in a straight line with no abduction of the hock.

Grade 2

There is *frequent patellar luxation* which, in some cases, becomes more or less permanent. The limb is sometimes carried, although weight bearing routinely occurs with the stifle remaining slightly flexed.

Especially under anesthesia it is often possible to reduce the luxation by manually turning the tibia laterally, but the patella reluxates with ease when manual tension of the joint is released.

As much as 30 degrees of medial tibial torsion and a slight medial deviation of the tibial crest may exist.

When the patella is resting medially the hock is slightly abducted. If the condition is bilateral, more weight is thrown onto the forelimbs.

Many cases in this grade "live" with the condition reasonably well for many years, but the constant luxation of the patella over the medial lip of the trochlea causes erosion of the articulating surface of the patella and also the proximal area of the medial lip. This results in crepitation becoming apparent when the patella is luxated manually.

Grade 3

The *patella is permanently luxated* with torsion of the tibia and deviation of the tibial crest of between 30 degrees and 60 degrees from the cranial/caudal plane. Although the luxation is not intermittent, many animals use the limb with the stifle held in a semi-flexed position.

Flexion and extension of the joint causes abduction and adduction of the hock.

The trochlea is very shallow or even flattened.

Grade 4

The tibia is medially twisted and the tibial crest may show further deviation medially with the result that it lies 60 degrees to 90 degrees from the cranial/caudal plane.

The *patella is permanently luxated.*

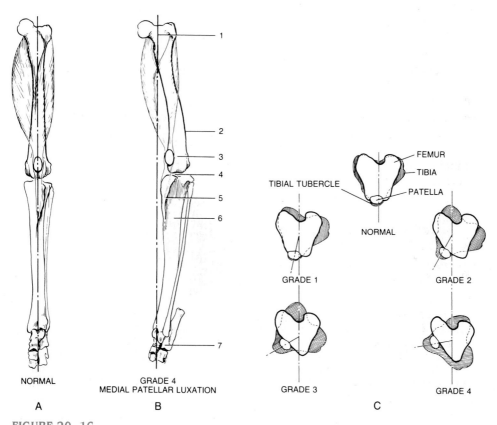

FIGURE 20–16

Skeletal abnormalities associated with severe congenital medial patellar luxation. *(A)* Normal left hindlimb, cranial view. Note that the quadriceps mechanism is centered over the femur and that the dashed line through the proximal femur and distal tibia also runs through the patella. *(B)* Deformities typical of medial patellar luxation. Note the position of the quadriceps mechanism and patella; the dashed line from proximal femur to distal tibia lies well medial to the stifle joint. *(1)* Coxa vara. *(2)* Distal third of femur bowed medially (genu varum). *(3)* Shallow trochlear sulcus with poorly developed or absent medial ridge. *(4)* Medial condyle hypoplastic; joint tilted. *(5)* Medial torsion of the tibial tubercle, associated with medial rotation of the entire tibia. *(6)* Medial (valgus) bowing of the proximal tibia. *(7)* Internal rotation of foot despite lateral torsion of distal tibia. *(C)* Position of the tibia relative to the femur and shape of femoral trochlea in grades 1 through 4 of medial patellar luxation. The femoral cross section in the region of trochlear sulcus is shown in dark outline, and the proximal tibial cross section is shaded. Progressive medial rotation of the tibia and deformity of the medial trochlear ridge are noted. (See the text for a complete explanation of grades 1 through 4, according to Singleton.[49])

The patella lies just above the medial condyle and a "space" can be palpated between the patellar ligament and the distal end of the femur.

The limb is carried, or the animal moves in a crouched position, with the limb partly flexed.

The trochlea is absent or even convex.

Clinical Signs

Three classes of patients are identifiable:

1. Neonates and older puppies often show clinical signs of abnormal hind-leg carriage and function from the time they start walking; these represent grades 3 and 4 generally.

2. Young to mature animals with grade 2 to 3 luxations usually have exhibited abnormal or intermittently abnormal gaits all their lives but are presented when the problem symptomatically worsens.

3. Older animals with grade 1 and 2 luxations may exhibit sudden signs of lameness because of further breakdown of soft tissues as a result of minor trauma or because of worsening of degenerative joint disease pain.

Signs vary dramatically with the degree of luxation. In grades 1 and 2, lameness is evident only when the patella is in the luxated position. The leg is carried with the stifle joint flexed but may be touched to the ground every third or fourth step at fast gaits. Grade 3 and 4 animals exhibit a crouching, bowlegged stance (genu varum) with the feet turned inward and with most of the weight transferred to the front legs. Permanent luxation renders the quadriceps ineffective in extending the stifle. The position of the patella can most easily be palpated by starting at the tibial tubercle and working proximally along the patellar ligament to the patella. (See Chapter 15 for further comments on examining the stifle joint.) Extension of the stifle will allow reduction of the luxation in grades 1 and 2. Pain is present in some cases, especially when chondromalacia of the patella and femoral condyle is present. Most animals, however, seem to show little irritation upon palpation.

Drawer motion should always be checked with the patella reduced to determine the status of the cruciate ligaments. With patellar luxation joint effusion is rarely present; these joints show amazingly few signs of degenerative disease such as periarticular fibrosis and osteophyte formation, which are very common in other instabilities of the stifle. Radiological examination is rarely necessary to confirm a diagnosis, but it is useful in grade 4 cases in which corrective osteotomies of the femur and tibia may be indicated.

SURGICAL REPAIR OF PATELLAR LUXATION

Arthroplastic techniques applicable to stabilization of patellar luxations can be divided into two classes; soft-tissue reconstruction and bone reconstruction. Considerable judgment and experience are necessary to decide the best procedure or combination of procedures for a given case. Although we have listed specific procedures for each condition, clinical cases do not always fall into definitive categories. Indeed, it may be difficult to assign a specific case to one of the grades we have listed. In such cases, surgical repair must proceed through the list of procedures until stability is achieved. The following section,

Treatment Plan, gives an overview of how these surgical procedures are combined in a given case.

A cardinal principle is that skeletal deformity, such as deviation of the tibial tuberosity and shallow trochlear sulcus, must be corrected by bone reconstruction techniques. Attempting to overcome such skeletal malformation by soft-tissue reconstruction alone is the most frequent cause of failure. Soft-tissue procedures, by themselves, *must be limited* to obvious grade 1 cases. Failure to transpose the tibial tubercle is perhaps the most common cause of failure. The surgeon must be aggressive in moving the tubercle without moving it too great a distance. Sometimes 2 to 3 mm is a sufficient amount to realign the quadriceps mechanism with the femoral trochlea and thus stabilize the patella. Both stifles are routinely operated on at the same time in small dogs and cats, regardless of the types of procedures done. With practice, the surgeon will not find these to be lengthy procedures, and the extra costs and dangers of a second operation outweigh the slightly more difficult postoperative course with bilateral surgery.

Soft-Tissue Reconstructive Procedures

OVERLAP OF THE LATERAL OR MEDIAL RETINACULUM ■ This method can be used on either the lateral side for a medial luxation or on the medial side for a lateral luxation. The retinacular fascia and joint capsule are incised 3 to 5 mm from and parallel to the patella. This incision extends from the tibia proximally to a point 1 to 2 cm above the patella. An incision of the fascia lata continues to the midfemur level (Fig. 20–17A). With size 2–0 or 3–0 nonabsorbable suture, the cut edge of the fascia attached to the patella is sutured beneath the more lateral fascia with several mattress sutures placed through the fornix of the capsule (Fig. 20–17A,B). The superficial layers of fascia and capsule are next sutured to the fascia that remains attached to the patella. In some cases, this fascia will extend beyond the cranial midline of the joint and will be sutured to fascia on the opposite side of the patella (Fig. 20–17B). Suturing continues the length of the fascial incision (Fig. 20–17C).

This technique can be combined with patellar and tibial antirotational suture ligaments (see Fig. 20–19). For lateral luxation, a similar procedure is performed on the medial side. The fascial incision is made through fascia between the caudal belly of the sartorius and the vastus medialis and cranial belly of the sartorius.

FASCIA LATA OVERLAP ■ This technique, described by Flo and Brinker,[50] is applicable only to medial luxations; when the procedure is used alone, it is indicated only in the limb that has normal conformation (grade 1 luxation). This overlap is opposite that of the retinacular overlap. It can be combined with patellar and tibial antirotational sutures (see Fig. 20–20).

Subcutaneous tissues are reflected to expose the lateral retinaculum and fascia lata to the midpoint of the femur. The fascia lata is incised at its junction with the biceps femoris muscle from the level of the patella proximally as far as possible. Distal to the patella, the incision runs parallel to the patellar ligament over the tendon of the long digital extensor (Fig. 20–18A). The fascia lata proximal to the patella is reflected cranially and bluntly elevated off the underlying vastus lateralis until the white aponeurosis between

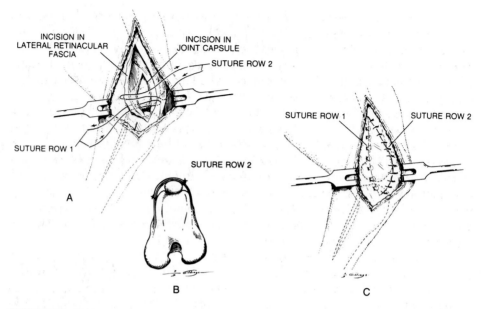

FIGURE 20-17

Lateral retinacular overlap. *(A)* A lateral parapatellar incision has been made through lateral fascia and joint capsule. The superficial fascia (fascia lata) has been incised from the tibia to the midfemoral level. Suture row 1 is started well back from the edge of the fascia caudally; it passes through the fornix of the joint capsule, through the cranial fascia close to the incision, and back through the caudal fascia like a mattress suture. All these sutures are placed before row 2 is placed. Size 2–0 or 3–0 nonabsorbable suture is preferred. *(B)* A cross-sectional view shows the two suture rows. Note that row 2 may actually be medial to the midline, depending on the looseness of the caudal fascia. *(C)* Row 1 and 2 sutures are complete. The biceps creates increased tension on the patellar ligament, the patella, and the distal half of the quadriceps.

the vastus lateralis muscle and the rectus femoris muscle is visualized. Nonabsorbable size 2–0 and 3–0 sutures are placed between the cranial edge of the biceps muscle and the exposed aponeurosis. The first suture is in the patellar tendon at the proximal end of the patella, with three to four more sutures placed proximally (Fig. 20–18A,B). If the patella can still be luxated, one or two more sutures are placed just proximal to the patella to further tighten the biceps muscle. Distal sutures are placed in the patellar ligament. The cranial fascia lata is pulled caudally over the surface of the biceps muscle and sutured in place with a combined simple pattern and a Lembert pattern (Fig. 20–18B, C).

PATELLAR AND TIBIAL ANTIROTATIONAL SUTURE LIGAMENTS ■ An adaptation of Rudy's technique creates a synthetic lateral patellar ligament by anchoring the lateral fabella to the patella with nonabsorbable suture (Fig. 20–19A,B). Medial tibial rotation can be prevented by another suture passing from the lateral fabella to the tibial tubercle or distal patellar ligament (Fig. 20–19B). The two sutures can also be combined, as in Figure 20–19C. Similar placement of sutures around the medial fabella is used for lateral patellar luxations. Such sutures are most commonly used in conjunction with trochleoplasty in grade 2 older dogs and also work well as primary treatment in neonates as young as five days.[51]

The fabella is the center of the arc of rotation of the patella; hence, the suture remains relatively taut during both flexion and extension of the stifle. By adjusting the point of insertion on the distal patellar ligament or tibial tubercle (Fig. 20–19B), the surgeon can make the suture taut at whatever degree of flexion produces the most medial tibial rotation. In many cases, particularly in dogs that are several years old before patellar luxation occurs, the tibial tubercle is not truly displaced or rotated relative to the rest of the tibia and foot (grades 1 and 2). In this situation it will be noted that when the stifle is flexed, the patella tends to luxate medially and the whole tibia rotates medially. This phenomenon is particularly noticeable in lateral luxation, a condition in which the tibia rotates laterally. Prevention of tibial rotation will markedly reduce the tendency of the patella to luxate. These sutures will probably break or loosen eventually in most cases; however, the fibrous tissue formed around the suture, plus realignment of soft tissues, will maintain the new position of the tibia or patella.

The fascia lata is incised along the cranial edge of the biceps muscle to allow retraction of the biceps caudally (Fig. 20–19A). Braided polyester (suture size 2–0 to 0 for small breeds, 0 to 2 for large breeds) is carried around the fabella on a half circle Mayo catgut or Martin's uterine suture needle. The needle passes around the fabella in a distal-to-proximal or cranial-to-caudal direction most easily. The joint capsule can be opened on the lateral side to

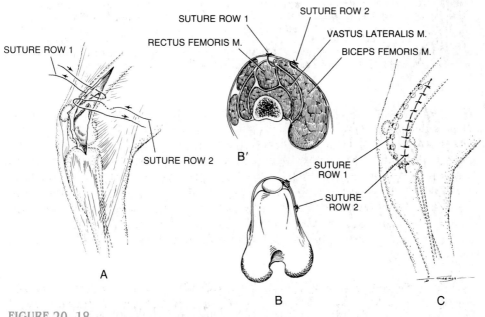

FIGURE 20–18

Fascia lata overlap[50] (A) A lateral parapatellar incision has been made through the fascia lata and joint capsule. This incision follows the cranial edge of the biceps muscle proximally, and distally it ends over the long digital extensor tendon. The cranial fascia is reflected and elevated in order to identify the white aponeurosis between the rectus femoris and vastus lateralis muscles. Row 1 sutures are placed to pull the biceps to this aponeurosis proximal to the patella and to the lateral border of the patella and patellar ligament distally. Row 2 sutures complete the overlap. (B, B') Two cross-sectional views show the relationship of the biceps muscle and fascia lata to the rectus femoris muscle and patella. The biceps has been pulled cranially to exert lateral tension on the quadriceps and patella. (C) Suture rows 1 and 2 are completed.

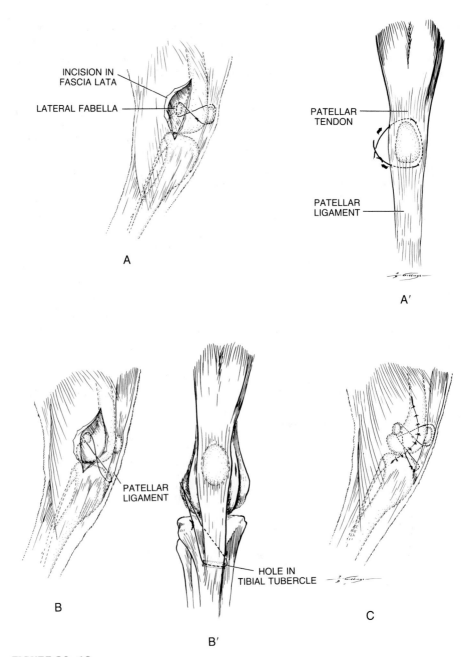

FIGURE 20–19

Patellar and tibial antirotational suture ligaments[51] (A) The fascia lata is opened along the cranial border of the biceps muscle to expose the lateral fabella by caudal retraction and elevation of the biceps. Braided polyester suture material (size 2–0 in toy breeds to size 2 in large breeds) is passed behind the lateral fabella and around the patella, as shown in A'. The suture is tied just tight enough to stabilize the patella. (B) To prevent medial tibial rotation, a suture can be passed around the fabella as in A, then placed either in the distal patellar ligament or in the tibial tubercle (B'). Various locations are tried in order to find one that results in the suture's being tightest when the stifle is flexed to the degree that causes greatest internal tibial rotation. The suture is tied tight enough to prevent rotation. (C) The two sutures can be combined. The caudal fascia lata has been overlapped in closing.

allow inspection of the joint and to perform trochlear arthroplasty if indicated. The suture is attached around the patella in semipurse-string fashion by a bite taken into the patellar tendon from lateral to medial at the proximal end of the patella. The suture is then passed distally along the medial border of the patella and laterally along the distal end of the patella (Fig. 20–19A).

All bites are placed deeply and as close to the patella as possible. With the suture passing medial to the patella, it cannot pull out. The lateral joint capsule is closed and sometimes imbricated if there is redundant tissue. The patellar suture must not lie on exposed articular cartilage. With the patella in place, the suture is tied with enough tension to prevent patellar dislocation.

The same method can be used on the medial side for lateral luxation. An incision is made along the cranial border to the caudal belly of the sartorius muscle, which is retracted caudally to expose the medial fabella. Suture placement is similar to that described for medial luxation.

The tibial antirotational suture is placed around either the medial or the lateral fabella. The suture can be attached either to the distal patellar ligament or through a hole in the tibial tubercle (Fig. 20–19B). The leg is positioned in various degrees of flexion to find the angle of maximal tibial rotation. The suture material is then tied tightly enough to prevent tibial rotation. Lateral or medial retinacular overlap can be performed to imbricate the joint (Figs. 20–17, 20–19C), or the fascia lata overlap method can be used (Fig. 20–20).

DESMOTOMY ■ A desmotomy is simply a release of the medial or lateral retinaculum on the side toward which the patella was luxated (see Fig. 20–

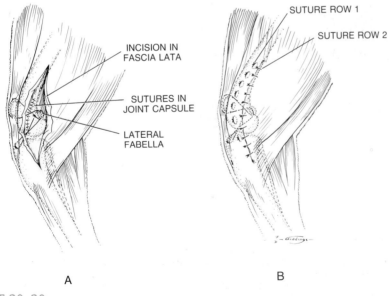

A   B

FIGURE 20–20

Combining patellar and tibial suture ligaments with fascia lata overlap. *(A)* The lateral fascia has been excised (see Fig. 20–18). The joint capsule has been sutured before the suture ligaments are placed (see Fig. 20–32) in order to prevent suture material from rubbing on articular cartilage. *(B)* After the fascia lata overlap, the suture ligaments are almost completely covered by fascia, emerging only for a short distance before being inserted around the patella or in the patellar ligament.

22F). When the patella luxates medially, retinacular tissues on that side contract and either prevent reduction of the luxation or provide enough tension to easily reluxate the patella. The incision commences at the tibial plateau and continues proximally through both layers of the joint capsule and retinacular tissues as far proximally as needed to relieve all tension on the patella. The incision is usually left open to prevent tension from redeveloping. Synovium will quickly seal the joint to prevent synovial fluid leakage.

QUADRICEPS RELEASE ■ In some grade 3 and most grade 4 luxations, the quadriceps is so misaligned that it causes displacing tension on the patella after reduction of the luxation. In this situation, the entire quadriceps mechanism must be dissected free to the midfemoral level.

Bilateral parapatellar incisions are made through the joint capsule and retinaculum, as in the bilateral approach to the stifle joint.[5] These indications are continued proximally along the borders of the quadriceps muscle groups. Laterally, the separation is made between the vastus lateralis and biceps muscles; medially, it is made between the vastus medialis and caudal belly of the sartorius. The entire quadriceps is then elevated from the femur, freeing the insertion of the joint capsule proximal to the trochlea. The superficial fascial incisions are sutured after the rest of the reconstructive procedures are completed.

Bone Reconstructive Procedures

TROCHLEOPLASTY ■ Arthroplastic procedures to deepen the trochlear sulcus take three forms:

1. *Trochlear sulcoplasty.*[52] Articular cartilage is removed to the level of subchondral bone to create a sulcus deep enough to prevent patellar luxation (Fig. 20–21A, B). By cutting completely through articular cartilage to subchondral bone, fibroplasia will result in a sulcus lined with fibrocartilage, which is an acceptable substitute for hyaline cartilage in nonweight-bearing areas. This method has been replaced in our hands by the following technique.

2. *Recession sulcoplasty.*[53] A V-shaped wedge, including the sulcus, is removed from the trochlea with a saw. The resulting defect in the trochlea is widened by another saw cut on one edge to remove a second piece of bone. When the original bone wedge is replaced, it is recessed into the defect, creating a new sulcus composed of hyaline cartilage[54] (Fig. 20–21C–E). The sides of the defect become lined with fibrocartilage. This method is preferred in mature animals.

3. *Trochlear chondroplasty.*[55, 56] This technique is useful only in puppies to the age of 4 to 6 months. A cartilage flap is elevated from the sulcus (Fig. 20–21F, G) and subchondral bone removed from beneath it. The flap is then placed back in position to line the new sulcus (Fig. 20–21H). As with recession sulcoplasty, hyaline cartilage remains in the bottom of the sulcus with fibrocartilage only along the sides. The cartilage flap has been shown to survive this transposition, and experimental dogs have shown no ill effects from the procedure.

Owing to the relatively wide patella in the cat, it does not fit into the trochlea well. The patella can be narrowed by removing bone from the medial and lateral sides.

TRANSPOSITION OF THE TIBIAL TUBERCLE ■ When the tibial tubercle is rotated, the quadriceps is realigned so that the patella is not pulled toward either side of the joint but so that it lies on a straight line from the proximal femur to the distal tibia. Visualization of this relationship is enhanced if the animal is placed in dorsal recumbency with the surgeon standing at the end of the table near the animal's feet. The procedure shown here is based on techniques of Brinker[57] and Singleton[58] (Fig. 20–22).

A medial or lateral skin incision can be used, and a lateral parapatellar joint incision is made.[5] The cranial tibial muscle is elevated from the proximolateral tibia starting at the distal end of the tubercle and continuing to the sulcus of the long distal extensor tendon (Fig. 20–22A). An incision is made through periosteum on the medial side of the tubercle along the line of the proposed osteotomy and continued proximally into the medial joint capsule. The patellar ligament must be freed from the infrapatellar fat pad.

A lateral view of the osteotomy is shown in Figure 20–22A. The tubercle is partially osteotomized with an osteotome, bone cutter, or a scalpel in the case of puppies. The osteotomy is usually not complete distally in order to leave periosteum and fibrous tissue intact (Fig. 20–22B). The osteotome or a periosteal elevator is used to pry the tubercle medially and expose the osteotomy site, where a rongeur is used to cut off the sharp corner on the lateral edge of the tibial osteotomy site (Fig. 20–22C). When prepared in this way, the osteotomy surface angles laterally and smoothly blends with the intact lateral tibial cortex, as in Fig. 20–22D.

The proximal end of the tubercle is now pried laterally until the patella and quadriceps are aligned with the femur and tibia. This relationship is shown in Figure 20–16A. When the proper position is found, a Kirschner wire is driven through the thickest part of the tubercle at an angle perpendicular to the osteotomy surface of the tubercle (Fig. 20–22E). The pin will cross the tibia at an angle and will be drilled through the caudomedial cortex. The pin is then backed out 1 cm and cut; the end is bent to form a hook and is then tapped back flush with the tubercle (Fig. 20–22F). Bending the end may lead to cracking very small tubercles and can be skipped. The Kirschner wire is usually 0.045 inch in diameter in toy and miniature breeds, but 0.035-inch wire is better for puppies. Two 0.062-inch wires are used in large breeds. If the tubercle should accidentally be completely broken free, a small tension band wire is added to the fixation.

Leaving the tubercle attached distally limits lateral transposition and thus may be insufficient in some cases. In this situation, it is best not to elevate the cranial tibial muscle from the tubercle in order to better preserve the tubercle's blood supply. The tubercle is completely osteotomized from the medial side and then pried laterally while the cranial tibial muscle is elevated from the tibia laterally to the long digital extensor sulcus. A triangular-shaped notch is cut in the tibial cortex to accommodate the triangular cross section of the tubercle. This notch is positioned in such a way that when the proximal end of the tubercle is inserted into it, the quadriceps will be properly positioned. The tubercle is pinned to the tibia as already described, but the pin is angled slightly proximally toward the caudomedial tibial cortex.

Closure commences by suturing of the external fascia of the cranial tibial muscle to the periosteum medial to the tubercle. The lateral retinaculum is overlapped and sutured to the patellar ligament and quadriceps fascia (Fig. 20–22F).

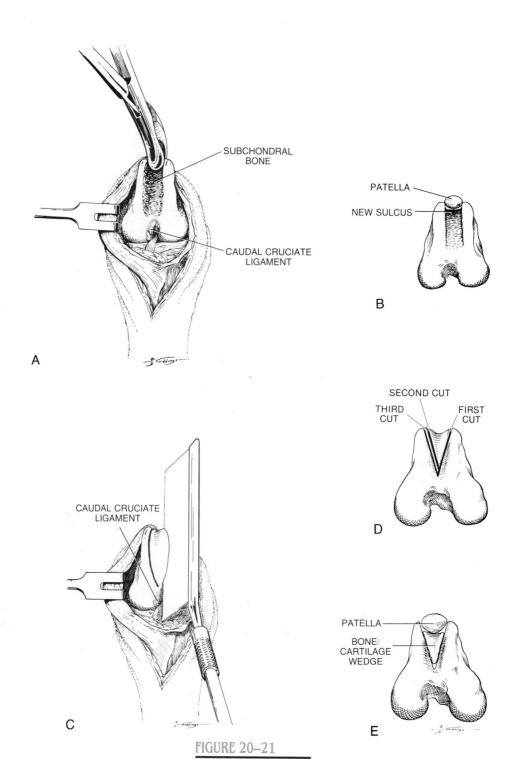

SUBCHONDRAL
BONE

CAUDAL CRUCIATE
LIGAMENT

A

PATELLA

NEW SULCUS

B

CAUDAL CRUCIATE
LIGAMENT

C

SECOND CUT

THIRD
CUT

FIRST
CUT

D

PATELLA

BONE/
CARTILAGE
WEDGE

E

FIGURE 20–21

See legend on opposite page

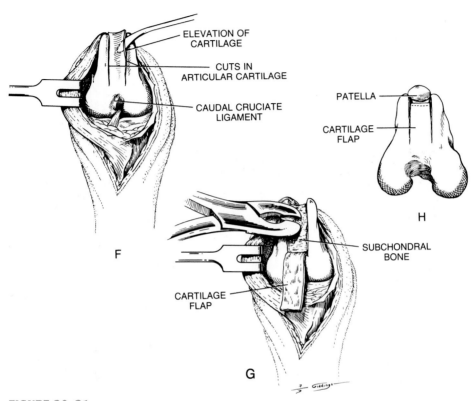

ELEVATION OF
CARTILAGE

CUTS IN
ARTICULAR CARTILAGE

CAUDAL CRUCIATE
LIGAMENT

PATELLA

CARTILAGE
FLAP

H

F

SUBCHONDRAL
BONE

CARTILAGE
FLAP

G

FIGURE 20–21

Trochleoplasty techniques. (A, B) Trochlear sulcoplasty. An outline of the proposed sulcus is made in the cartilage with a scalpel along the condylar ridges. Then articular cartilage is removed (A) within the outlined area to create a straight-sided, flat-bottomed trough as shown in (B). The distal end of the trough is near the origin of the caudal cruciate ligament, and it extends to the proximal trochlear ridges. The trough should be deep enough so that the patella does not touch bone in the bottom of the trough and wide enough so that the patella rides deeply in the new sulcus. Done in this manner, articular cartilage of the patella is not damaged by abrasion on subchondral bone, and fibrocartilage can fill in the gap and conform to the excursions of the patella. (C) Modified recession sulcoplasty.[53] A thin-blade hobby saw (X-Acto, Long Island City, NY), ethylene oxide or chemically sterilized, is used to cut a V-shaped wedge from the trochlea, extending from the caudal cruciate origin to the proximal trochlear ridges. (D) Cuts made in the indicated order create a V-shaped defect and slightly smaller wedge. (E) When the original bone and cartilage wedge is replaced in the defect, it is recessed and hence creates a deeper sulcus. No fixation of the wedge is required. (F) Trochlear chondroplasty. For this technique, the animal must be less than 6 months old. The new sulcus is outlined by cuts through the thick adolescent cartilage. The transverse cut proximally is at the level of the proximal trochlear ridges. A sharp periosteal elevator is used to raise cartilage from subchondral bone. (G) The cartilage flap is hinged distally to allow removal of subchondral bone with rongeurs. (H) When the cartilage flap is replaced, the sulcus is deep enough to retain the patella. Fixation of the cartilage is not required.

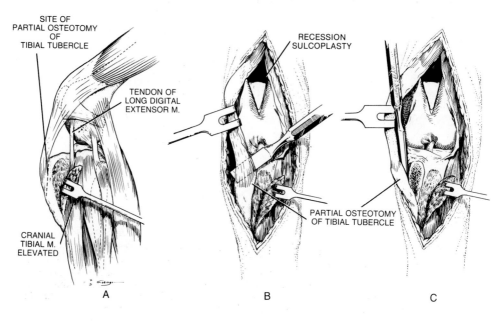

SITE OF
PARTIAL OSTEOTOMY
OF
TIBIAL TUBERCLE

TENDON OF
LONG DIGITAL
EXTENSOR M.

CRANIAL
TIBIAL M.
ELEVATED

A

RECESSION
SULCOPLASTY

PARTIAL OSTEOTOMY
OF TIBIAL TUBERCLE

B

C

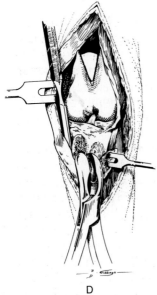

D

FIGURE 20–22

Transposition of the tibial tubercle.[57, 58] (A) A lateral approach is made to the stifle joint.[5] The left stifle is illustrated here. Elevation of the cranial tibial muscle exposes the area into which the tubercle will be moved. The osteotomy is planned to include all of the insertion of the patellar ligament. (B) Recession sulcoplasty and medial desmotomy have been performed. An osteotome is being used to osteotomize the tubercle partially, leaving distal periosteum and fibrous tissue intact. (C and D) The tubercle is pried medially, bending the distal intact tissues, to allow shaping the tibial osteotomy site with rongeurs by removing the square lateral edge. A smooth surface that blends with the tibial cortex is created as a bed for the tubercle.

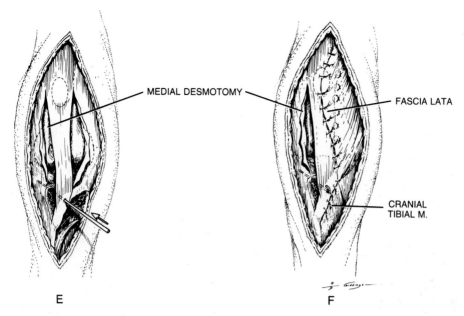

MEDIAL DESMOTOMY

FASCIA LATA

CRANIAL TIBIAL M.

E

F

FIGURE 20–22

Continued (E) After the tubercle is pried laterally to a point that aligns the quadriceps mechanism with the femur and tibia (see Fig. 20–16A), a Kirschner wire is used to pin the tubercle to the proximal tibia. The pin crosses the tibia at an angle and is embedded in the caudomedial cortex. (F) A hook has been placed in the Kirschner wire, which is then tapped flat against the bone. The external fascia of the cranial tibial muscle has been sutured to the periosteum of the tubercle and the lateral fascia has been overlapped. The medial desmotomy is not sutured.

OSTEOTOMY, ARTHRODESIS ■ Some grade 4 cases have such severe deformities that the procedures we have described are not sufficient to create a functional joint. Osteotomy of the distal femur and sometimes of the proximal tibia has been proposed to straighten the limb enough to allow the other reconstruction to be effective.[49] Because of the complexity of these procedures and the possibility that the joint still will not function well, arthrodesis is probably a more feasible procedure. (Arthrodesis will be described later in this chapter.)

FEMORAL OSTEOTOMY FOR LATERAL LUXATION ■ In the large and giant breeds, lateral luxation (see further discussion below) may be associated with valgus deformity and rotation of the femur, and if these deformities are severe enough the bone corrective procedures described above may not be sufficient to stabilize the patella. In such a situation a midshaft opening wedge osteotomy is done, the femur is derotated and placed in sufficient varus position to allow the patella to center in the trochlear sulcus, and a bone plate is used for fixation (Fig. 20–23). The defect created in the lateral cortex is filled with autogenous cancellous bone graft (see Chapter 3). Lateral desmotomy, various soft-tissue reconstructions, and recession trochleoplasty as detailed above, may be necessary in addition to the osteotomy.

Aftercare for All Surgical Techniques

External splinting is usually not needed in any of the procedures mentioned. Early, active use of the limb is beneficial if trochlear sulcoplasty has been

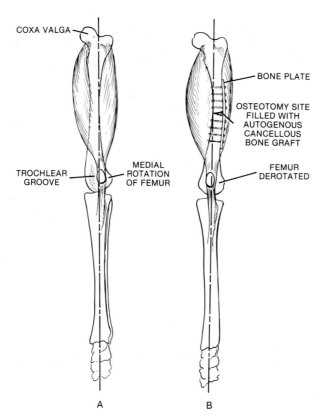

COXA VALGA

TROCHLEAR
GROOVE

MEDIAL
ROTATION
OF FEMUR

BONE PLATE

OSTEOTOMY SITE
FILLED WITH
AUTOGENOUS
CANCELLOUS
BONE GRAFT

FEMUR
DEROTATED

A   B

FIGURE 20–23

Correction of lateral patellar luxation in large and giant breeds. (A) The deformities associated in variable degrees with this condition are coxa valga (increased angle of inclination), genu valgum (knock knee), and internal rotation of the distal femur. The quadriceps mechanism and patella are shifted laterally. (B) Surgical correction involves a midshaft transverse osteotomy, external rotation of the distal femur, creating a varus bowing of the femur sufficient to realign the quadriceps mechanism, and stabilization with a bone plate. The osteotomy gap is filled with autogenous cancellous bone graft.

performed, but exercise should be limited for three to four weeks, and jumping should in particular be prevented. Since many of these breeds are "jumpers," padded bandage support for 10 to 14 days may be useful in the active patient. If bilateral surgery has been performed, postoperative pain may seriously inhibit attempts to use the limbs. Appropriate aspirin or phenylbutazone dosage for five to seven days is useful.

Because toy and miniature breeds are not especially tolerant of pain, some difficulties are occasionally encountered. If the dog is not starting to bear weight by four weeks, active physiotherapy must be started. Swimming is best but often is not possible. Passive flexion-extension, 20 to 30 times, four times a day may be helpful. Leash walking, ball throwing, and other activities to tempt the animal into a running gait are also useful. Taping a small plastic syringe cap or glass marble between the toes and metatarsal pad of the opposite limb for a few hours at a time also works very well on some dogs. Placing the opposite leg in an Ehmer sling for several days may be done as a last resort.

Prognosis

Willauer and Vasseur have reported on the follow-up evaluation of medial patellar luxation repair in 52 stifles.[59] No lameness was observed in 92 percent of the stifles, although 48 percent had recurrent patellar luxation. The recurrent luxations were always of a lesser grade than the preoperative grade, 17 of the

25 being grade 1. Regardless of the degree of lameness or stability of the patella, most dogs had radiographic signs of degenerative joint disease. It must be inferred from these findings that stability of the femoropatellar joint is not essential to good function in the small breeds, and this conforms to the common clinical observation of small breed dogs with medial patellar luxations who never show clinical signs. Early correction of severe deformities will undoubtedly go a long way toward ensuring good function.

TREATMENT PLAN

Although not all cases can be fitted into rigid categories, we have attempted to outline procedures that may be useful for each grade of luxation. Treatment is aimed at reducing the anatomical defects. The procedures are done in the following order until patellar stability is achieved.

Grade 1
1. If the extensor mechanism is straight:
   a. Lateral fascia lata overlap (see Fig. 20–18).
   b. Tibial antirotational suture (see Figs. 20–19B, 20–20).
2. If the tubercle is deviated:
   Tibial tubercle transposition (see Fig. 20–22), with or without retinacular or fascia lata overlap (see Figs. 20–17, 20–18).

Grade 2
1. Medial desmotomy if the medial retinaculum prevents easy patellar reduction (see Fig. 20–22F).
2. Tibial tubercle transposition (see Fig. 20–22) and lateral retinacular or fascia lata overlap (see Figs. 20–17, 20–18).
3. If the patella is still unstable, add:
   Trochleoplasty (see Fig. 20–21).

Grade 3
1. Medial desmotomy (see Fig. 20–22F).
2. Tibial tubercle transposition (see Fig. 20–22).
3. Trochleoplasty (see Fig. 20–21).
4. Lateral retinacular or fascia overlap (see Figs. 20–17, 20–18).
5. Lateral patellar and tibial antirotational sutures (see Figs. 20–19, 20–20) if the patella is still unstable.

Grade 4
1. Procedures for grade 3.
2. Release of quadriceps.
3. If still unstable, consider:
   a. Femoral and tibial osteotomy, or
   b. Arthrodesis (see Figs. 20–41, 20–42).

The limiting factor in grade 4 luxation repair is flexure contraction at the stifle. If the joint cannot be extended to a normal angle, arthrodesis may be the only viable option.

LATERAL LUXATION IN TOY AND MINIATURE BREEDS

Lateral luxation in small breeds is most often seen late in the animal's life, from 5 to 8 years of age. Skeletal abnormalities are relatively minor in this syndrome, which seems to represent a breakdown in soft tissue in response to, as yet, obscure skeletal derangement. Thus, most lateral luxations are grades 1 and 2, and the bony changes are similar, but opposite, to those described for medial luxation. The dog has more functional disability with lateral luxation than with medial luxation.

Clinical Signs

In mature animals, signs may develop rapidly and may be associated with minor trauma or strenuous activity. A knock-knee or genu valgum stance, sometimes described as seal-like, is characteristic. Sudden bilateral luxation may render the animal unable to stand and so simulate neurological disease. Physical examination is as described for medial luxation.

Treatment

Surgical treatment is as follows:

Grade 1
1. Medial retinacular overlap (see Fig. 20–17) in all cases.
2. Medial tibial antirotational suture (see Fig. 20–19B) if the patella is still unstable after 1.

Grades 2 and 3
1. Lateral desmotomy if the lateral retinaculum prevents easy patellar reduction (see Fig. 20–22F).
2. Medial tibial tubercle transposition (see Fig. 20–22).
3. Medial retinacular overlap (see Fig. 20–17).
4. If the patella is still unstable, add:
    a. Trochleoplasty (see Fig. 20–21).
    b. Medial patellar and tibial antirotational sutures (see Figs. 20–19B, 20–20).

COMBINED MEDIAL AND LATERAL LUXATION

Occasionally, this patellar instability is seen in dogs without obvious bony deformity. Clinical signs are similar to grade 1 signs for both medial and lateral luxation.

Treatment

Surgical procedures are as follows:

1. Trochleoplasty (see Fig. 20–21).
2. Combined medial and lateral retinacular overlap (see Fig. 20–17).

MEDIAL LUXATION RESULTING FROM TRAUMA

All breeds are subject to this relatively rare injury, although minor skeletal changes and mild patellar instability predispose to the problem. Luxation of the hip can be accompanied by medial patellar luxation. In our experience, we have not seen traumatic lateral luxation.

Clinical Signs

Mechanically, the situation is similar to that of a grade 1 luxation, with signs of acute inflammation superimposed. Pain is severe, and anesthesia or deep sedation is usually required for palpation. The limb is carried in flexion and internal rotation. Joint effusion and swelling of soft tissue are evident.

Radiographic examination to rule out patellar fracture and avulsion or tearing of the patellar ligament is indicated. (See Chapter 6 for a discussion of these injuries.)

Treatment

Closed reduction and immobilization in a sling or Schroeder-Thomas splint may be indicated if the patella is reasonably stable following reduction. If the patella is markedly unstable or if luxation recurs after immobilization, surgical treatment should be undertaken.

1. Fascia lata overlap.
2. Lateral patellar suture (see Figs. 20–19, 20–20) if stability is not achieved by 1.

LATERAL LUXATION IN LARGE AND GIANT BREEDS

Also called genu valgum, this condition is seen in the same breeds that are affected by hip dysplasia. We have noted an unusual incidence in certain strains of flat-coated retrievers. Rudy[51] postulated a genetic pattern of occurrence and noted Great Danes, St. Bernards, and Irish wolfhounds as being the most commonly affected.

Components of hip dysplasia, such as coxa valga (increased angle of inclination of the femoral neck) and increased anteversion of the femoral neck,[97] are related to lateral patellar luxation. These deformities cause internal rotation of the femur with lateral torsion and valgus deformity of the distal femur, which displaces the quadriceps mechanism and patella laterally (see Fig. 20–23A).

Clinical Signs

Bilateral involvement is most common. Animals appear to be affected by the time they are 5 to 6 months of age. The most notable finding is a knock-knee (genu valgum) stance. The patella is usually reducible, and laxity of the medial collateral ligament may be evident. The medial retinacular tissues of the stifle joint are often thickened, and the foot can often be seen to twist laterally as weight is placed on the limb.

Treatment

The following procedures are used:

1. Mildly affected—lateral luxation without marked rotational deformity of the femur.
   a. Trochleoplasty (see Fig. 20–21).
   b. Tibial tubercle transposition (see Fig. 20–22).
   c. Retinacular overlap (see Fig. 20–17).
2. Markedly affected—lateral luxation with marked valgus deformity of femur.
   a. Corrective osteotomy of the femur (see Fig. 20–23).

PATELLAR LUXATION WITH SEVERE EROSION OF THE PATELLA

In long-standing cases of patellar luxation, the articular surface of the patella can become severely eroded and eburnated. This condition is infrequent, but when it is present, stabilization of the patella is of little value. Treatment is by patellectomy (see Fig. 20–24).

Patellectomy

A parapatellar approach from either side is used to expose the patella. Stay sutures are placed in the patellar tendon and ligament to aid in rotating the patella 90 degrees to expose its articular surface (Fig. 20–24A). Sharp dissec-

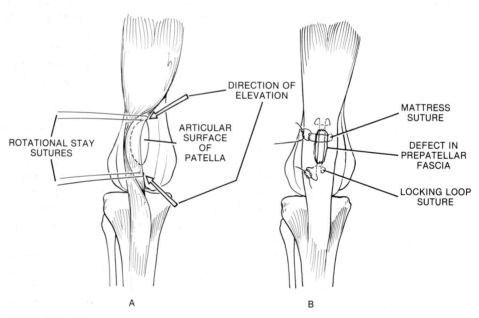

FIGURE 20–24

Patellectomy. *(A)* A medial or lateral parapatellar approach is used to gain access to the joint. The patella is rotated 90 degrees to expose the articular surface; stay sutures are helpful to hold it in this position. Sharp dissection of the patella from the tendon/ligament proceeds from each pole toward the center in an attempt to save as much prepatellar fascia and periosteum as possible and minimize the defect created. *(B)* Nonabsorbable suture size 2/0–0 is used to first place one or more locking-loop sutures (see Fig. 19–1), followed by several mattress or cruciate pattern sutures placed transversely.

tion to elevate the tendon, ligament, and prepatellar fascia proceeds from each pole of the patella toward the center. Extreme care must be taken to keep the dissection plane on the periosteal surface of the bone in order to minimize the defect produced in the soft tissues.

Closure of the defect starts with one or more locking loop sutures placed longitudinally, trying to pull the tendon into apposition with the ligament. This is followed with mattress sutures placed transversely. All sutures are nonabsorbable size 2–0 to 0. If a considerable defect remains after attempts at suturing, a pedicle of fascia lata is freed, with its base proximolateral to the patella. The pedicle is reflected distally and sutured into the defect. The parapatellar defect is sutured routinely.

Postoperative support in a long leg lateral splint (see Fig. 19–12) or Schroeder-Thomas splint (see Fig. 1–13) is maintained for three weeks, and normal activity is resumed after six to eight weeks.

Rupture of the Cranial Cruciate Ligament

Cranial cruciate ligament ruptures are one of the most common injuries in the dog and the major cause of degenerative joint disease in the stifle joint. The ligamentous injury may be a complete rupture with gross instability or a partial rupture with minor instability. In either case, untreated animals show degenerative joint changes within a few weeks and severe changes within a few months. The severity of degeneration seems to be directly proportional to the body size, with those animals over 15 kg showing the most changes. Indeed, Vasseur has consistently demonstrated degenerative changes and decline in material properties (strength) of the ligament in dogs over 5 years of age.[60] The intensity of the changes became worse with age, but animals of less than 15 kg body weight had significantly less change in material properties than did larger dogs. This confirms the earlier observations of Paatsama[61] and Rudy.[51]

The function of the cranial cruciate ligament is to constrain the stifle joint so as to limit internal rotation and cranial displacement of the tibia relative to the femur and to prevent hyperextension.[62] The ligament is composed of two functional parts: the small craniomedial band (CMB) and the larger caudolateral band (CLB). Mechanisms of injury can be related to these normal functions: most commonly the ligament is injured when the stifle is rotated rapidly with the joint in 20 to 50 degrees of flexion or when the joint is forcefully hyperextended.[63] The former happens when the animal suddenly turns toward the limb with the foot firmly planted. This causes extreme internal rotation of the tibia with stress on the cranial cruciate ligament. Hyperextension probably occurs most commonly by stepping into a hole or depression at a fast gait.

The medial meniscus may be torn acutely at the time of injury but is more often damaged as a result of chronic instability of the joint, producing folding and eventual shredding of the caudal horn of the medial meniscus. Some type of meniscal injury is present in about 50 percent of the animals we have seen. These injuries are discussed later in this chapter. Concurrent patellar luxation is fairly often seen in toy breeds of dogs. It seems most likely in these cases that the patellar luxation is probably the initial condition and that the cruciate ligament ruptures are due to the tibial instability produced by the luxated patella and subsequent stretching of the cruciate ligament.

CLINICAL SIGNS AND DIAGNOSIS

Although pain is noted early with nonweight-bearing, most animals will start to use the limb within two to three weeks and apparently improve for several months until a gradual or sudden decline in the use of the limb is noted, often as a result of secondary meniscal damage. At this time, the degenerative changes of osteoarthrosis are present and functional decline is continuous. Diagnosis is based upon demonstration of cranial drawer motion (see Chapter 15). Drawer motion should be tested in both flexion, normal standing angle, and extension. With acute injuries and gross instability, drawer motion may be evident. Joint effusion may be noted for several days after injury. With chronic injuries and with partial tears, drawer motion is much less evident and requires very careful examination. With chronic cruciate ligament instability, periarticular tissues become thickened and fibrotic with only limited stretching possible. Drawer motion in these cases may be almost imperceptible, but any motion that ends gradually as a result of tissue stretching is abnormal. In skeletally immature dogs especially, slight drawer motion may be possible, but such motion stops abruptly as the ligament is stretched taut. This abrupt stoppage of cranial drawer motion is also noted in cases of isolated caudal cruciate rupture.

With partial cruciate ruptures, a small amount of drawer motion will be appreciated only in flexion. This injury and its diagnosis are discussed in more detail later in this chapter. Testing the joint for increased internal rotation of the tibia is also helpful in chronic cases and in partial rupture cases. The amount of torsion of the tibia can be compared with the opposite limb.

Fibrosis of the joint capsule and associated structures partially stabilizes the joint but not sufficiently to prevent its continual deterioration. Radiographs are of little value other than to document the degree of osteoarthrosis present; thus, they may be useful in the prognosis. An experienced clinician will be able to palpate large osteophytes. Opacity of the infrapatellar fat pad is often seen, and any skeletally immature animal with gross drawer motion should be radiographed to look for avulsion of the cruciate ligament. In animals of all ages there is often a nonradiopaque, firm swelling of tissues on the medial surface of the joint between the medial collateral ligament and the tibial tubercle. The significance of this swelling is uncertain, but we believe it to be associated with chronic meniscal injury.

MODES OF THERAPY

Controversy exists regarding the best treatment for ruptured cranial cruciate ligament. More than a hundred techniques have been reported, but certain facts have been established. It is well agreed that once instability resulting from cranial cruciate insufficiency occurs, progressive degenerative changes such as periarticular osteophytes, articular erosions, and meniscal damage begin within a few weeks. Extra-articular methods embrace a wide variety of stabilization techniques for the cruciate-deficient stifle joint. Most of these methods involve use of heavy gauge suture to imbricate the joint and restore stability, although some rely instead on transposition of soft or bony tissues. The indication for these approaches as opposed to the reconstructive intra-articular methods has been the subject of endless debates in the last 30 years. Regardless of the type of repair done, most published reports indicate between 85 and 90 percent good to excellent function at follow-up. An in vitro examination of various methods of repair indicated that intra-articular methods of repair result in more normal joint motion than extra-articular methods.[64] This seems to be particularly important in dogs weighing over 17 to 20 kg and most especially in the athletic animal. Extra-articular methods work well in smaller breeds but have not generally been considered as satisfactory in the larger, athletic animal with an acute cruciate rupture. Stability with extra-articular suture is attributed to thickening of the joint capsule and retinaculum owing to inflammation from the surgical procedure and implanted sutures. Recent experience of one of us (DLP), however, suggests that the fibular transposition method discussed later in this chapter is highly satisfactory for large dogs. Recent experience also indicates that extra-articular techniques are the method of choice when the cruciate injury is chronic. In this situation the inflammatory response and chronic changes within the joint create an adverse environment for transposed autologous tissue. Synthetic replacements for the cranial cruciate ligament have had some success in humans, but none of the available prostheses are economically feasible for widespread veterinary use.

Conservative treatment by splintage has been advocated. Close confinement for four to eight weeks was reported to yield satisfactory function in the majority of small dogs (body weight less than 20 kg).[64a] Vasseur reported similar results.[65] He found that dogs of 15 kg or less had satisfactory function several months after injury, while larger breeds uniformly functioned poorly. All animals had evidence of degenerative joint disease, and one has to speculate how well they would function several years later. Despite this evidence to the contrary, if the owner wants the best treatment for his or her pet, our clinical experience leads us to recommend surgical treatment of all dogs and cats with this injury.

A question arises as to the advisability of operating on an animal with very chronic instability and severe degenerative joint disease. Simply providing stability will not cause the degenerative joint disease to disappear, but the animal will improve dramatically in function. Because most chronic cases suffer from torn menisci, they will be greatly improved, and inflammatory reaction in the joint will decrease in intensity if the torn meniscus is removed (see discussion later in this chapter). Attention must be given to medical management of the joint disease as discussed in Chapter 17.

Extra-articular Stabilization

THREE-IN-ONE TECHNIQUE

The technique shown here is a slight modification of Flo's original procedure.[66] The objective of surgery is to pass one suture from the lateral fabella and one suture from the medial fabella to a hole created in the tibial tubercle or through the distal patellar ligament. These sutures approximate the plane of the cranial cruciate origin and insertion and eliminate drawer movement when tightened.

A medial arthrotomy is performed (Fig. 20–25A). Fragments of the cruciate ligament are removed and menisci are inspected and removed only if severely torn or fragmented (see discussion of meniscus below). The medial joint capsule is closed with synthetic absorbable or nonabsorbable suture material (Fig. 20–25B). To expose the medial fabella, an incision is made through the fascia on the cranial edge of the caudal belly of the sartorious muscle and extended distally into the proximal portion of this muscle's insertion on the tibial crest (Fig. 20–25A,B). A large braided polyester suture (size 0 to 1 for small breeds and 2 to 4 for larger breeds) is passed around the medial fabella with a half circle Mayo catgut or Martin's uterine suture needle. Another source of heavy gauge suture material is monofilament nylon fishing leader material in the 30 to 60 pound test, or .030- to .040-inch sizes. This material is carefully cleaned, rinsed, and sterilized with ethylene oxide. No adverse reactions to the material have been noted in our hands.

The skin is then undermined and reflected laterally to expose the lateral side of the joint (Fig. 20–25C). The fascia lata is incised on a line from the cranial edge of the biceps femoris muscle toward the patella, where the incision is angled toward the proximal tibia, paralleling the patellar ligament. The fascia lata is reflected caudally to expose the lateral fabella and collateral ligaments without incising the synovial capsule (Fig. 20–25D). Two sutures are placed around the lateral fabella. A small hole is drilled transversely through the tibial tuberosity near the insertion of the patellar ligament (Fig. 20–25E). One end of the medial suture is brought through the bone tunnel from a medial to lateral direction, then taken back toward the medial fabella under the patellar ligament (Fig. 20–25F). A similar but opposite maneuver is performed with one of the two lateral sutures. The suture can also be placed through the patellar ligament near the tibial tuberosity if braided suture is used. Placement in this manner is illustrated in Figure 20–25G. Monofilament nylon in the larger sizes is too stiff to use in this manner and is best placed through the tuberosity. With the stifle held at a standing angle and all drawer motion removed (i.e., the tibia externally rotated and forced caudally), these sutures are then tied snugly, thus eliminating drawer movement. The lateral suture is tied first. The second lateral suture is used to further imbricate the joint by placing it in the lateral third of the distal end of the patellar ligament.

The fascia lata is closed by overlapping it onto the patellar ligament and quadriceps fascia (see Fig. 20–27G). The previously detached portion of the caudal belly of the sartorius and medial fascia are sutured to the patellar ligament medially. The proximal portion of the medial fascial incision is closed conventionally.

This technique of closing the medial and lateral incisions places a caudal pull on the tibia and in this way helps stabilize the joint. Soaking the imbrication sutures in chlorhexidine solution a few minutes before implantation reduces the number of infections and drainage tracts associated with burying large-gauge, braided nonabsorbable sutures, which has been reported to be as high as 21 percent.[67]

POSTOPERATIVE CARE ■ The limb is not splinted postoperatively. Very restricted exercise is allowed for the first four weeks with a slight increase in activity between four and six weeks and then unrestricted activity after eight weeks.

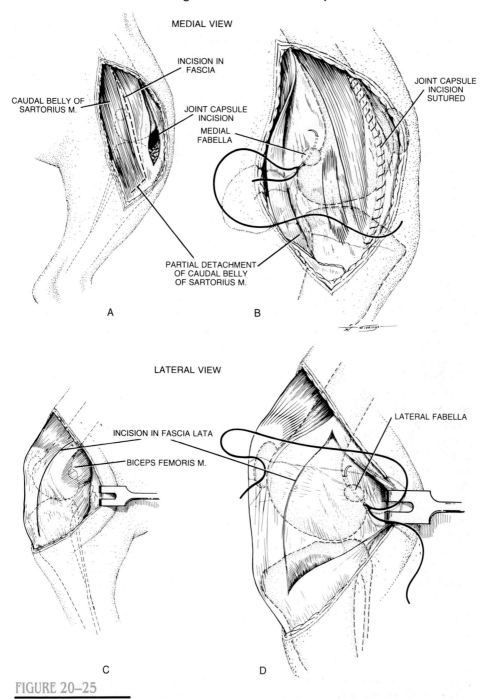

MEDIAL VIEW

INCISION IN FASCIA

CAUDAL BELLY OF SARTORIUS M.

JOINT CAPSULE INCISION

MEDIAL FABELLA

JOINT CAPSULE INCISION SUTURED

PARTIAL DETACHMENT OF CAUDAL BELLY OF SARTORIUS M.

A   B

LATERAL VIEW

INCISION IN FASCIA LATA

BICEPS FEMORIS M.

LATERAL FABELLA

C   D

FIGURE 20–25

Extra-articular cranial cruciate stabilization. *(A)* A medial approach has been made to the left stifle joint.[5] After removal of any remnants of the cruciate and exploration of the joint, the fascia is incised along the cranial border of the caudal belly of the sartorius. *(B)* The fascial incision continues distally and a part of the tibial insertion of the caudal sartorius is detached. The joint capsule has been closed. Heavy-gauge braided polyester suture (size 0–1 for small breeds, 1–4 for larger breeds) is passed behind the medial fabella. *(C)* An incision is made only through the fascia lata on the lateral side of the joint. The incision parallels the cranial edge of the biceps proximally. *(D)* Elevation and retraction of the biceps expose the lateral fabella. A double length of heavy suture (as in *B*) is passed around the medial fabella. After passage, the suture is cut near the needle to form two pieces.

Illustration continued on following page

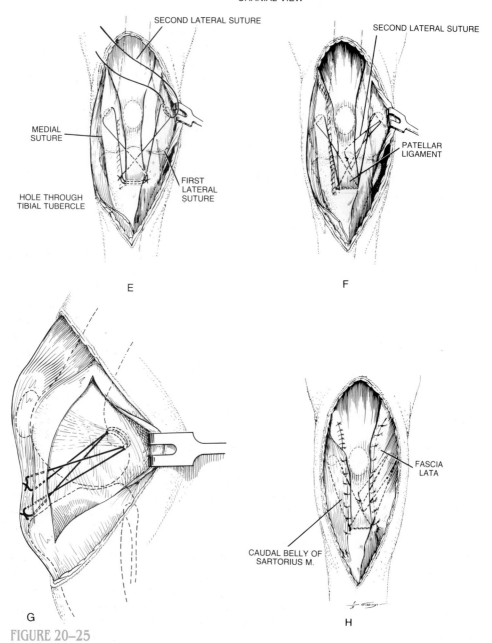

CRANIAL VIEW

FIGURE 20–25

Continued (E) A small hole has been drilled transversely in the tibial tubercle close to the insertion of the patellar ligament. The medial suture and one lateral suture are passed through this hole. *(F)* The fabellar sutures are tied tightly with drawer motion reduced and the stifle at a standing angle. The lateral suture is tied before the medial suture is tightened. The second lateral suture is placed through the midportion of the patellar ligament to further imbricate the joint. Tying the knots in the indicated positions will help prevent the first throw from slipping during tying. *(G)* Lateral view. Sutures may alternatively be placed in the patellar ligament close to the tibial tuberosity. Note the slight caudal displacement of the patellar ligament. *(H)* The detached portion of the caudal sartorius is sutured, with other medial fascia, to the patellar ligament proximally to the level of the patella. From that point proximally, the sartorius is not included in the medial fascial closure. The fascia lata is overlapped laterally to place the biceps muscle under increased tension (see also Fig. 20–17).

An alternative extra-articular technique, and one that appears to be more suitable in large breeds than the suture method, is the fibular head transposition of Smith and Torg.[68] By freeing the fibular head and attached lateral collateral ligament, the fibula can be moved cranially and attached to the tibia. The collateral ligament is placed under tension and functions similarly to the sutures in the three-in-one method. Drawer motion and internal tibial rotation are resisted by the transposed ligament. Smith and Torg found the method produced better results than an intra-articular fascial strip repair, when the two procedures were compared using an identical grading system. Good to excellent clinical grades were achieved in 90 percent of the cases. Our experience with the technique over a two-year period is similar.

SURGICAL TECHNIQUE ■ The technique described is modified from the original description. A lateral skin incision and medial parapatellar approach to the joint is made. Following inspection of the joint, with removal of the remnants of the cranial cruciate ligament and inspection of the meniscus (see discussion below), the medial capsule and retinaculum are closed, including the caudal belly of the sartorius muscle in the closure, as in Figure 20–27F. The fascia lata is next incised as in Figure 20–25D, except that the incision continues distally along the lateral edge of the tibial tuberosity for 2 to 3 cm. Caudal retraction of the fascia lata and biceps femoris muscle exposes the fibular head, collateral ligament, and the underlying muscles (Fig. 20–26A). The fibular nerve should be identified and protected.

Incisions are made in the intermuscular fascia between the peroneus longus and tibialis cranialis muscles, and then cranially through the origin of the tibialis cranialis until the tendon of the long digital extensor muscle is exposed. Incisions are then made through fascia and superficial layers of the joint capsule cranial and caudal to the lateral collateral ligament. These incisions are only deep enough to allow undermining and freeing of the ligament from the underlying tissues. The caudal incision is continued distally over the caudal aspect of the fibular head. The ligaments of the fibular head (Fig. 20–26B) are incised to free it from the tibia by working from the cranial aspect of the fibular head while retracting the peroneus longus muscle. Some of the fibular origin of the peroneus longus may have to be elevated to expose the fibular head. Incision of the ligaments can be done with a variety of instruments such as a sharp periosteal elevator or osteotome, but the most useful instrument has been a canine meniscus knife (Veterinary Instrumentation, Sheffield, England; Jorgensen Laboratories Inc, Loveland, Colorado: see Fig. 20–33E). This instrument follows the plane between the bones without cutting bone and greatly reduces the chance of accidental fracture of the fibular head. The dissection plane between the tibia and fibular head is approximately 45 degrees caudal from the sagittal plane of the tibia.

After the fibula is freely movable, a 0.62-inch (1.5-mm) Kirschner wire is driven into the caudal half of the head of the fibula and is then used to move the fibula laterally and then cranially under the caudal edge of the tibialis cranialis muscle. The tibia is externally rotated, and the stifle is held at a standing angle with drawer movement removed during the transposition maneuver. A Schroeder vulsellum forceps or an AO/ASIF pointed reduction

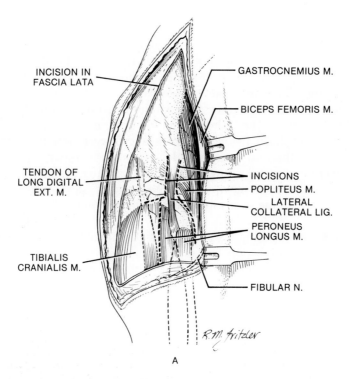

INCISION IN
FASCIA LATA

GASTROCNEMIUS M.

BICEPS FEMORIS M.

TENDON OF
LONG DIGITAL
EXT. M.

INCISIONS
POPLITEUS M.
LATERAL
COLLATERAL LIG.

PERONEUS
LONGUS M.

TIBIALIS
CRANIALIS M.

FIBULAR N.

R.M. Fritzler

A

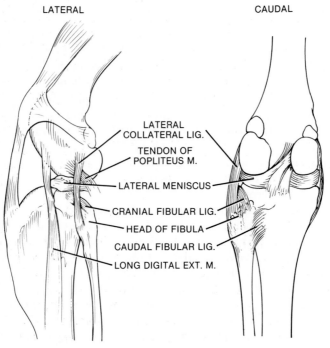

LATERAL

CAUDAL

LATERAL
COLLATERAL LIG.

TENDON OF
POPLITEUS M.

LATERAL MENISCUS

CRANIAL FIBULAR LIG.

HEAD OF FIBULA

CAUDAL FIBULAR LIG.

LONG DIGITAL EXT. M.

B

FIGURE 20–26

See legend on opposite page

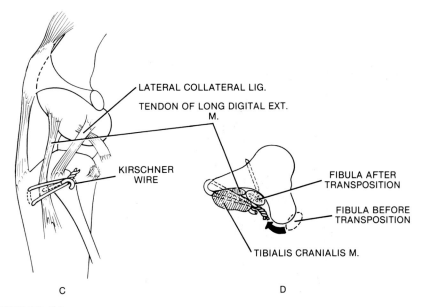

LATERAL COLLATERAL LIG.

TENDON OF LONG DIGITAL EXT. M.

KIRSCHNER WIRE

FIBULA AFTER TRANSPOSITION

FIBULA BEFORE TRANSPOSITION

TIBIALIS CRANIALIS M.

C

D

FIGURE 20–26

Fibular transposition technique, modified from method of Smith and Torg.[68] (A) A lateral skin incision and medial parapatellar approach to the joint has been made. The medial capsule and retinaculum has been closed as in the three-in-one technique, but without a suture around the medial fabella (see Fig. 20–25). The fascia lata is incised as in Figure 20–25D except that the incision continues distally along the lateral edge of the tibial tuberosity for 2 to 3 cm. Caudal retraction of the fascia lata exposes the fibular head, collateral ligament, and the underlying muscles. The fibular nerve should be identified and protected. An incision is made in the intermuscular fascia between the peroneus longus and tibialis cranialis muscles. (B) The lateral collateral ligament and tibial ligaments of the fibular head. The collateral ligament is dissected free from the joint capsule and the ligaments of the fibula incised to free it from the tibia. (C, D) A 0.62-inch (1.5-mm) Kirschner wire is driven into the caudal half of the head of the fibula and is then used to move the fibula cranially under the caudal edge of the tibialis cranialis muscle. The tibia is externally rotated, and the stifle is flexed to a standing angle during the transposition maneuver. When the collateral ligament is taut, the Kirschner wire is driven into the tibia to penetrate the transcortex. A hole is drilled in the tibial tuberosity for an 18- or 20-gauge (1.0 to 0.8 mm) wire, which is passed through the tibialis cranialis muscle, around the pin, and back through the muscle. The ends of the wire are twisted, and as the wire is tightened, the pin will bend and produce more tension on the collateral ligament. When cranial drawer motion is abolished, the wire is cut and the twisted end is bent toward the bone.

forceps (Synthes) is useful to maneuver and hold the fibula in the desired position. One jaw of the forceps is placed caudal to the fibular head, and the other jaw is engaged on the tibial tuberosity. This fixes the fibular head and collateral ligament and allows testing of drawer motion before drilling the Kirschner wire into the tibia. Most of the motion should be neutralized at this time. When the collateral ligament is taut, the Kirschner wire is driven into the tibia to penetrate the transcortex (Fig. 20–26C). A 5/64-inch (2-mm) hole is drilled in the tibial tuberosity, and a 16-gauge hypodermic needle is passed through the hole and through the tibialis cranialis muscle toward the surface of the fibula where the Kirschner wire penetrates it.

An 18 to 20 gauge (1.0 to 0.8 mm) wire is inserted into the needle, which is then withdrawn, leaving the wire in place. The other end of the wire is looped around the pin and then passed through the tibialis cranialis muscle

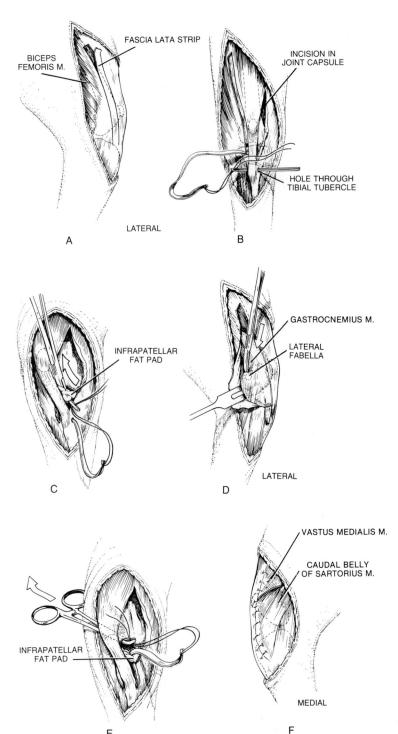

A

FASCIA LATA STRIP

BICEPS
FEMORIS M.

LATERAL

B

INCISION IN
JOINT CAPSULE

HOLE THROUGH
TIBIAL TUBERCLE

C

INFRAPATELLAR
FAT PAD

D

GASTROCNEMIUS M.

LATERAL
FABELLA

LATERAL

E

INFRAPATELLAR
FAT PAD

F

VASTUS MEDIALIS M.

CAUDAL BELLY
OF SARTORIUS M.

MEDIAL

FIGURE 20–27

Intra-articular cranial cruciate stabilization: four-in-one over-the-top.[69] (A) Lateral view of right stifle. A medial arthrotomy has already been performed, the ligament remnants removed, and the joint explored. A fascia lata strip is developed, based on the tibial-patellar ligament junction. The strip is 1 to 1.5 cm wide at the base and slightly wider proximally. Its total length is 2.5 to 3 times the distance from the tibial tubercle to midpatella. (B) A $\frac{5}{32}$- to $\frac{3}{16}$-inch hole has been drilled transversely through the tibial tubercle, close to the tibial plateau. A heavy monofilament suture has been attached to the fascial strip, which is then reflected distally and pulled through the hole from lateral to medial. (C) The fascial strip is pulled into the joint by tunneling it through the fat pad. (D) The lateral edge of the fascia lata incision is dissected and retracted to expose the lateral fabella. The portion of the gastrocnemius muscle originating proximal to the fabella is elevated, and a curved forceps is passed medial to the fabella, through the caudal joint capsule, and into the intercondylar notch of the femur. (E) The curved forceps must emerge in the intercondylar space lateral to the caudal cruciate ligament. One end of the monofilament suture attached to the fascial strip is grasped so that the strip can be pulled proximally through the joint. (F) The medial arthrotomy is closed in one layer. The caudal sartorius muscle is partially detached from the tibia, then sutured with the joint capsule and medial fascia to the patellar ligament, creating increased tension in the muscle (see also Fig. 20–25B).

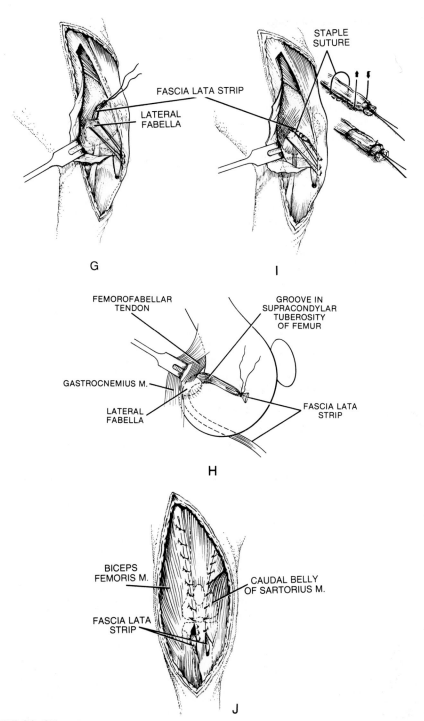

FIGURE 20–27

Continued (G) Two sutures of No. 2–4 nonabsorbable material are placed from the lateral fabella to the distal patellar ligament and tied under tension with drawer motion reduced (see Fig. 20–25). (H) The femorofabellar ligament is elevated from the supracondylar tuberosity of the femur to allow a groove to be produced in the cortical bone of the tuberosity by rongeur, rasp, or osteotome. A wire loop can then be used to fish the suture attached to the fascia strip through this opening. (I) The fascial strip is pulled tight and attached to joint capsule or patellar ligament with the suture attached to its end. The strip is then sutured to the femorofabellar tendon, fascia, and joint capsule with 3–4 cruciate "staple" sutures (see inset). (J) This cranial view shows the bilateral closure that places caudal traction on the tibia as a result of increased tension from the biceps femoris and caudal sartorius muscles. Because of the removal of the fascial strip, the lateral closure places the biceps femoris muscle under tension.

to pass over the tibial tuberosity. The ends of the wire are twisted at either the Kirschner wire or the tuberosity end, and as the wire is tightened, the pin will bend cranially and produce more tension on the collateral ligament. When cranial drawer motion is abolished, the twist is cut and bent flush with the bone. A hook is bent in the Kirschner wire, which is then driven flush with the fibula. The fascia lata is sutured by advancing it as far craniomedially as possible, thereby placing the biceps femoris muscle under tension (see Fig. 20–27J).

AFTERCARE ■ The limb is not splinted postoperatively. Very restricted exercise is allowed for four weeks, then gradual increase of activity and full resumption of activity at eight weeks.

Intra-articular Stabilization

FOUR-IN-ONE OVER-THE-TOP TECHNIQUE

This technique[69] is indicated for animals weighing over 15 kg and can be used for smaller breeds if they are athletic, such as hunting beagles. The procedure is a modification of the over-the-top technique of Arnoczky and associates.[70] Although the original technique (see Fig. 20–28) results in excellent stabilization, some surgeons have experienced technical difficulties in collecting the patellar ligament–fascia strip used for cruciate ligament replacement. An attempt has been made to simplify the procedure by using a fascia strip collected entirely from the fascia lata. Additionally, lateral stabilizing sutures (as in the three-in-one technique above) provide immediate stability and protection for the fascial strip. The procedure is described as done in dogs weighing more than 20 kg. The next smaller suture sizes can be used in dogs between 15 and 20 kg.

A medial arthrotomy following a lateral skin incision is made to allow inspection of the joint, removal of ligament fragments, and meniscectomy (see Fig. 20–33) when needed. A strip of fascia 1.5 to 2 cm wide at the base is isolated from the lateral aspect of the joint and remains attached at the junction of the patellar ligament with the tibial tubercle distally (Fig. 20–27A). The strip is fashioned by cutting its cranial edge from the lateral border of the patellar ligament and is continued proximally a few millimeters lateral to the patella. This incision, which is made with a scalpel, is ended just proximal to the patella, and the caudal edge of the strip is formed by incising 1.5 to 2 cm caudal and parallel to the first incision. Care is taken to avoid incising the underlying synovial membrane. Proximal to the patella, the fascia lata is easily elevated from the quadriceps and dissection is continued with scissors. The caudal cut is continued proximally first and follows the cranial border of the biceps femoris muscle. The cranial border from the proximal patella is cut next, taking care to maintain or slightly increase the strip's width at the proximal end. The length of this strip is equal to 2½ to 3 times the distance from the tibial tubercle to the midpatella.

A ⁵⁄₃₂-inch to ³⁄₁₆-inch (4 to 4.8 mm) hole is drilled transversely through the tibial tubercle close to the tibial plateau, and the proximal end of the fascial strip is drawn through the hole, thus transferring the strip to the medial side of the tibia (Fig. 20–27B). Size 0 to 1 monofilament suture is attached to the fascia strip to aid in pulling it through the bone. The ligament is pulled into the medial arthrotomy through the fat pad into the joint, medial to the patellar ligament (Fig. 20–27C).

On the lateral side of the joint, the lateral edge of the fascia lata incision is dissected and retracted to expose the lateral fabella. The portion of the gastrocnemius muscle originating proximal to the fabella is elevated from the femur and a 7-inch curved Crile or Kelly hemostatic forceps is passed through this opening medial to the fabella with the curve facing cranially, through the caudal joint capsule, and into the intercondylar notch of the femur (Fig. 20–27D). The tips of the forceps are positioned lateral to the caudal cruciate ligament, where one end of the suture attached to the fascial strip is grasped within the jaws of the forceps (Fig. 20–27E). The forceps are pulled proximally, and the suture is used to pull the ligament "over-the-top" of the lateral fabella.

The medial arthrotomy is now closed in one layer. The insertion of the caudal belly of the sartorius is partially detached from the tibia and sutured to the patellar ligament along with the joint capsule and medial fascia as far proximally as the patella. From that point proximad, the sartorius is not included in the remainder of the medial closure (Fig. 20–27F).

Two sutures of size 2 to 4 braided polyester or monofilament suture material are placed from the lateral fabella to the distal portion of the patellar ligament and tied tightly to eliminate drawer movement and to act as internal splints (Fig. 20–27G). The femorofabellar ligament is elevated from the supracondylar tuberosity of the femur to allow a groove to be produced in the cortical bone of the tuberosity by rongeur, rasp, or osteotome (Fig. 20–27H). A wire loop can then be used to fish the suture attached to the fascia strip through this opening. The fascial strip is pulled taut and then sutured to the femorofabellar fascia and joint capsule with a "staple" suture (Fig. 20–27I). The lateral fascial incision is closed. Because of the strip of fascia removed, this closure results in tightening of the lateral retinaculum (Fig. 20–27J).

Four separate procedures have served to stabilize the joint: Advancement of the caudal sartorius and biceps muscles create caudal traction on the tibia; fabellar-patellar ligament sutures prevent drawer motion immediately and serve as an internal splint for the fascial strip; and the fascial strip replaces the cruciate ligament.

OVER-THE-TOP TECHNIQUE

This procedure, developed by Arnoczky and co-workers,[70] is similar to the four-in-one procedure except for preparation of the ligament replacement.

Following a medial arthrotomy the medial third of the patellar ligament is split away from the rest of the ligament but is left attached to the tibia and patella. Incisions in the patellar tendon and fascia lata continue proximally (Fig. 20–28A). A portion of the medial edge of the patella is split away from the patella with a small osteotome. Care should be taken not to penetrate the articular cartilage of the patella. The attachments of the patellar tendon proximally and patellar ligament distally must be preserved (Fig. 20–28B). When the bone fragment is free, dissection is continued proximally into the fascia lata, where the strip is prepared as described above (Fig. 20–28C). The fascia-bone-ligament strip needs to be only two times as long as the tibial tubercle–patella distance. The medial capsule incision is continued as far

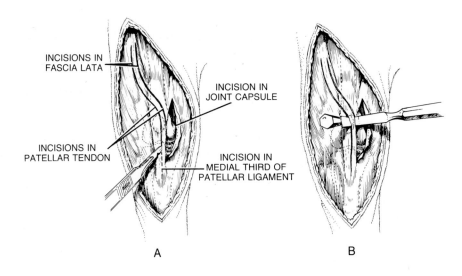

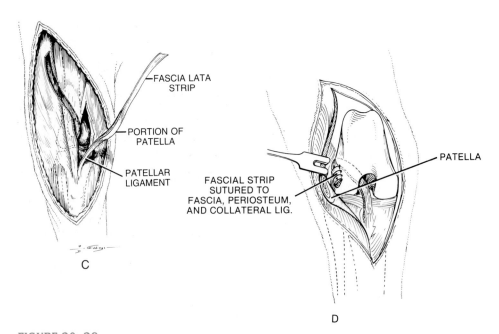

FIGURE 20–28

Intra-articular cranial cruciate stabilization: over-the-top technique.[70] (A) A medial approach[5] with a lateral skin incision has been made to the right stifle. The medial arthrotomy is made on the medial edge of the patellar ligament and patella and continues proximally into the cranial sartorius and vastus medialis. The medial third of the patellar ligaments is split away from the remainder of the ligament. Incisions in the patellar tendon and fascia lata define the fascial strip proximal to the patella. (B) A portion of the patella is removed with an osteotome, and care is taken not to cut into the articular surface. The patellar ligament attachment distally and the patellar tendon proximally must be preserved. (C) The patellar ligament–patella–fascia lata strip is freed. (D) The medial incision is continued as far proximally as necessary to allow lateral luxation and retraction of the patella and exposure of the lateral condyle. The fascial strip is pulled through the joint as in Figure 20–27D,E, except that the forceps are passed from inside the joint capsule. Following fixation of the fascial strip to the periosteum, fascia, and the lateral collateral ligament (see Fig. 20–27H,I), the joint is closed as in Figure 20–27F.

proximally as necessary to allow lateral luxation and retraction of the patella and exposure of the lateral condyle. The fascial strip is pulled through the joint similarly to Figure 20–27D,E except that the forceps is passed from inside the joint capsule. Following fixation of the fascial strip to periosteum, fascia, and the lateral collateral ligament (see Fig. 20–27H,I), the joint is closed as in Figure 20–27F.

AFTERCARE ■ No postoperative splinting is used with either technique, but very restricted exercise (confining the animal to the house and walking the animal with a leash) is ordered for 12 weeks, followed by gradual return to activity and freedom for moderate exercise after 18 weeks. Intensive training of working dogs should not start until six months postoperatively.

Evaluation of Over-the-Top Procedures ■ Both techniques generally provide a more anatomically placed pseudoligament than does Paatsama's original method involving the fascia lata.[61] Although in theory Paatsama's technique should result in anatomical placement of the fascial strip, in fact it has proved difficult for most surgeons to accurately drill from the lateral surface of the condyle to the point of the ligament's femoral origin. Additionally, the fascia usually made a sharp bend as it emerged from the bone tunnel and then turned distally, thus subjecting it to shearing forces. Arnoczky and colleagues demonstrated that the fascial strip placed "over-the-top" almost perfectly mimics the normal ligament, remaining taut during the complete range of motion of the stifle.[70] Because the pseudoligament is subjected only to tension and not shearing stress, it is not as apt to break. The fascial strip becomes vascularized, then undergoes fibroplasia and reorganization of collagen to resemble a normal ligament. This process appears to take five to six months; however, the animal is at risk until the tissue transfer regains strength and is the reason for using the lateral support sutures in the four-in-one procedure. Occasionally, an animal will stretch the ligament between three and six months postoperatively and will redevelop drawer motion. Such cases have undergone reoperation using extra-articular stabilization because the remaining fascia was unfit for use again. Previously these cases were reoperated by replacing the lateral sutures and adding a medial suture, as in the three-in-one technique described above. More recently, reoperation has been done with the fibular transposition method.

Partial Rupture of the Cranial Cruciate Ligament

A surprising number of stifle lamenesses are due to partial rupture of the cranial cruciate ligament. The veterinarian has only to explore joints in the face of minimal physical findings to verify this. Clinical signs and history mimic those of complete rupture but are not as dramatic, and secondary arthrosis is much slower in developing, probably because the meniscus is not damaged as often as in complete ligament rupture. Degenerative changes can be extensive given enough time.

The cranial cruciate functionally is composed of two parts: the small craniomedial band (CrMB) and the larger caudolateral band (CLB). The CrMB is taut in both flexion and extension, while the CLB is taut only in extension. The ability to diagnose these injuries by examination for drawer motion depends on which part of the ligament is damaged. If the injury is due to hyperextension, it is most likely to damage the CLB, and no drawer motion will be present since the CrMB is intact. An injury caused by rotation or twisting with flexion is more likely to injure the CrMB. Under these circumstances there is a small amount of drawer motion in flexion (the CLB is relaxed) but no motion in extension (the CLB is taut). Partial rupture of the CrMB in a single case was first reported by Tarvin and Arnoczky,[71] and more recently a series of cases has been described by Scavelli and associates.[72] In this series partial ruptures accounted for 8 percent of 320 cases of isolated cranial cruciate rupture. Drawer motion was detected in 52 percent of the cases and, when present, was found in flexion only 69 percent of the time. At surgery 80 percent of the injuries were to the CrMB, 4 percent were CLB, and 16 percent were interstitial tears (grade 2 sprain), where the ligament was grossly intact but had suffered damage sufficient to render it functionally incompetent. Medial meniscus damage requiring surgical treatment was present in 20 percent of these cases.

As can be seen from these figures, the incidence of partial tears of the cranial cruciate ligament is not insignificant and should be carefully considered as a cause of lameness in midsize to large breeds with pain in the stifle region and minimal or no drawer motion. When operating these injuries they should be handled as if they were complete ruptures, since the ligament is no longer functional.[63]

Avulsion of the Cranial Cruciate Ligament

As with most avulsions, this is a disease of skeletally immature dogs. Ligamentous attachments to bone by means of Sharpey's fibers are in some cases stronger than the bone; hence, an avulsion rather than a tear of the

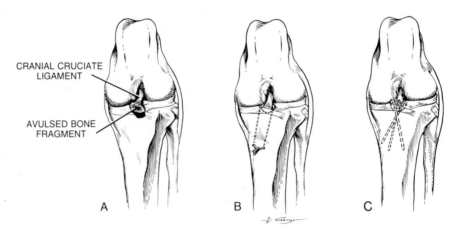

CRANIAL CRUCIATE
LIGAMENT

AVULSED BONE
FRAGMENT

A   B   C

FIGURE 20–29

Avulsion of the tibial insertion of the cranial cruciate ligament. (A) A bone fragment with the cranial cruciate attached has been elevated from the tibial plateau of the left tibia. A medial approach to the stifle is used for exposure.[5] Lag screw fixation is ideal if the bone fragment is large enough (see Fig. 20–31B. For smaller fragments: (B) Stainless steel wire, 20 to 22 gauge, is placed through the ligament insertion and through two drill holes that exit through the medial tibial cortex where the wire is twisted. (C) Three Kirschner wires, inserted at diverging angles, provide good fixation.

ligament results (Fig. 20–29). Usually seen as an avulsion of the insertion, this lesion is very rare in the dog.

Physical examination findings are similar to those described for rupture of the ligament, except that drawer motion is very obvious and joint effusion is marked. Radiographs demonstrate the avulsed bone fragment in the intercondylar space.

SURGICAL TECHNIQUE

The joint is exposed by a medial approach.[5] Hematoma and granulation tissue are removed from the bone fragment so that it can be identified (Fig. 20–29A). Two small holes are drilled from the medial and lateral sides of the tibial defect toward the medial tibial cortex (Fig. 20–29B). Stainless steel wire (size 20 to 22 gauge, 0.8 to 0.6 mm) is placed through the ligament close to the bone. Each end is then passed through the bone tunnels and twisted tightly on the medial tibial cortex. Alternatively, three diverging Kirschner wires can be used (Fig. 20–29C). In rare instances, the bone fragment is large enough to allow lag screw fixation (see Fig. 20–31B).

AFTERCARE ■ The limb must be immobilized for four weeks to allow healing of the fracture. A Thomas splint (see Fig. 1–11) or a long lateral splint is suitable (see Fig. 19–12). The stifle must be fixed at the standing angle to minimize complications of immobilization such as periarticular fibrosis and quadriceps contracture. Full exercise should not be allowed until four weeks after splint removal.

Rupture of the Caudal Cruciate Ligament

The caudal cruciate ligament is slightly larger than the cranial ligament and is an important stabilizer of the joint. It is the primary stabilizer against tibial caudal subluxation (drawer movement) and combines with the cranial ligament to limit internal tibial rotation and hyperextension.[62]

Little is known about the handling of ruptures of this ligament because it is a relatively uncommon injury. Most cases are due to severe trauma and are accompanied by rupture of the medial collateral and cranial cruciate ligaments. Medial meniscal injury is also common in this situation. Isolated caudal cruciate ruptures do occur, however. It has been suggested that the caudal cruciate is not functionally significant because the normal standing angle of the dog's stifle tends to work against caudal drawer motion,[73] and experimental severing of the ligament by Harari and co-workers did not create any functional or pathological changes in seven dogs observed postoperatively for six months.[74] In the absence of any clinical series reports it is difficult for the clinician to decide on the best method of handling a case. Our approach is to try to surgically stabilize an isolated injury only in working and sporting dogs or when the injury occurs in conjunction with other ligament injuries of the stifle.

CLINICAL SIGNS

Demonstration of caudal drawer motion is fundamental to diagnosing this injury. This can be complicated by the concomitant injuries mentioned.

Testing for caudal drawer motion can produce confusing results because the tibia seems always to be subluxated caudally at rest from the pull of the hamstring muscles. Therefore, what may appear to be cranial drawer motion is actually the reduction of tibial subluxation. From this reduced position, we can then demonstrate caudal motion. Therefore, unlike testing for cranial motion, it is more important to note the relative position of the thumbs as they grasp the femur and tibia *before* motion is applied to the tibia (see Chapter 15).

With cranial drawer motion, the sequence is as follows:

1. Tibial reduced position.
2. Cranial drawer position.
3. Reduced position.

With the caudal drawer motion, the sequence is:

1. Tibial caudal drawer position.
2. Reduced position.
3. Caudal drawer position.

Caudal drawer motion is always more prominent in flexion than extension because the collateral ligaments limit motion in extension.

DIAGNOSIS

Radiographs are important in caudal cruciate injuries because of these injuries' frequent association with other traumatic injuries and because of a higher percentage of avulsion injuries than with the cranial cruciate. This is probably due to the fact that the caudal ligament is larger and stronger than the cranial and therefore resists rupture but predisposes to avulsion.

SURGICAL TREATMENT

Little has been documented concerning clinical management of caudal cruciate injuries. No really satisfactory technique exists for large, active dogs. The technique shown here (Fig. 20–30) is satisfactory for small breeds and cats but is not always as useful in large breeds. Avulsion injuries are well stabilized by wire or screw fixation (Fig. 20–31). Repair of collateral and meniscal injuries is described next.

Technique for a Ruptured Ligament

A medial or lateral arthrotomy is combined with approaches to the medial and lateral caudal compartments of the stifle joint.[5] Fragments of ligament are excised and meniscectomy is performed when indicated. The joint capsule is then sutured and collateral ligament repairs are made if needed. Stabilization is commenced on the medial side with placement of mattress sutures (size 2–0 to 0 nonabsorbable material), to imbricate the caudomedial joint capsule (Fig. 20–30A). A large imbricating suture of size 0 to 3 braided polyester material or heavy monofilament nylon (see three-in-one technique above) is then placed from the medial half of the proximal patellar ligament to a hole drilled through the caudomedial corner of the tibia (Fig. 20–30B). This suture is tied tightly, with drawer motion reduced and the stifle positioned at the standing angle.

Similar sutures are placed on the lateral aspect of the joint (Fig. 20–30C), but the large suture is anchored around the fibular head. The fibular nerve should be protected during suture placement. A fascia lata transfer is also used on the lateral side. The strip is based on the lateral side of the patella and is long enough to be pulled around the head of the fibula and sutured to itself.

The fascia strip and large imbricating sutures are similar to those used in the technique of DeAngelis and Betts.[75] However, they are positioned more distally at the patellar end to more closely approximate the angle of caudal ligament. Imbrication of the caudomedial and lateral joint capsule is based on the technique of Hohn and Newton for cranial cruciate rupture.[73]

AFTERCARE ■ No splint is used unless the medial collateral ligament was repaired. Exercise is severely restricted for four weeks, then gradually increased through the eighth week.

Technique for Avulsion

Most avulsions occur at the *femoral origin* of the ligament and are easily accessible for lag screw or wire fixation (Fig. 20–31A). If the fragment is large enough, fixation with a lag screw is preferred (Fig. 20–31B). Wire fixation can also be used if the bone fragment is small. The wire should pass through the ligament close to the fragment and then pass through bone tunnels to the medial condylar cortex, where it is twisted tightly (Fig. 20–31C). Another fixation method involves placing two or three Kirschner wires through the fragment at diverging angles. These pins should penetrate the opposite condylar cortex.

Avulsion of the *tibial insertion* is treated similarly, although the fragment is much more difficult to expose. Best exposure is probably afforded by the approach to the caudomedial compartment of the joint.[5] The medial head of the gastrocnemius muscle and popliteal vessels must be strongly retracted.

AFTERCARE ■ A Thomas splint (see Fig. 1–11) or long lateral splint (see Fig. 19–12) is maintained for four weeks, and exercise is severely restricted. After splint removal, activity is slowly increased through the eighth week.

Meniscal Injuries

Unlike the situation in humans, damage to the meniscal cartilages of the dog and cat rarely occurs as a primary injury; in almost all cases, one or more stifle ligaments are torn or stretched. Most commonly, the caudal horn of the medial meniscus is damaged as a result of the cranial tibial drawer motion that results from rupture of the cranial cruciate ligaments. Because the medial meniscus is firmly attached to the tibia by the caudal tibial ligament and to the medial collateral ligament, it moves with the tibia. Cranial drawer motion displaces the caudal horn cranial to the femoral condyle and subjects the caudal horn to injury as a result of crushing and shear forces. Cranial drawer

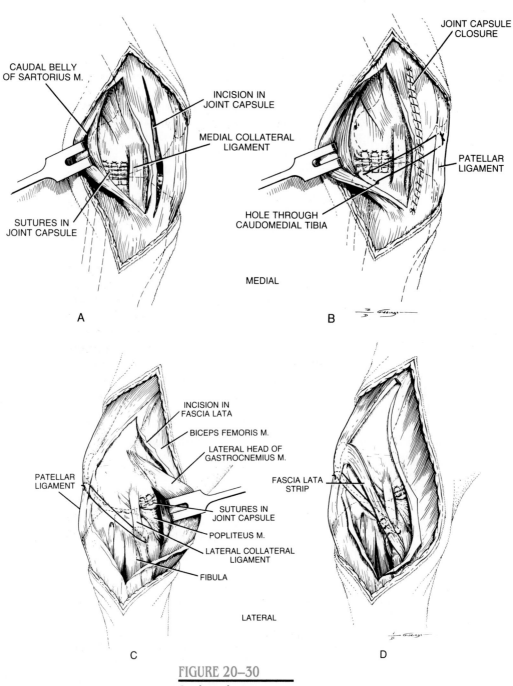

CAUDAL BELLY
OF SARTORIUS M.

INCISION IN
JOINT CAPSULE

MEDIAL COLLATERAL
LIGAMENT

SUTURES IN
JOINT CAPSULE

A

JOINT CAPSULE
CLOSURE

HOLE THROUGH
CAUDOMEDIAL TIBIA

PATELLAR
LIGAMENT

MEDIAL

B

INCISION IN
FASCIA LATA

BICEPS FEMORIS M.

LATERAL HEAD OF
GASTROCNEMIUS M.

PATELLAR
LIGAMENT

SUTURES IN
JOINT CAPSULE

POPLITEUS M.

LATERAL COLLATERAL
LIGAMENT

FIBULA

LATERAL

C

FASCIA LATA
STRIP

D

FIGURE 20–30

See legend on opposite page

motion in extension is much more injurious to the meniscus and joint capsule than is drawer motion in flexion.[76] Isolated tears of the lateral meniscus have been seen by us, but rarely.

Various types of lesions develop in damaged menisci[77] (Fig. 20–32). Caudal longitudinal tears and detachment as well as folding with variable degrees of shredding of the caudal medial horn are the most commonly seen abnormalities. The incidence of meniscal injuries following rupture of the cranial cruciate ligament can run as high as 53 percent.[78] This incidence reflects a predominance of chronic cases as seen in a referral practice. Early surgical repair of the cruciate injury results in a much lower incidence of meniscal injury.

CLINICAL SIGNS AND DIAGNOSIS

A clicking or snapping sound during weight-bearing or palpation is the classic clinical sign associated with meniscal lesions. It is diagnostic when present, but its absence does not rule out the diagnosis. Palpation is more likely to produce a click in an unsedated animal. Minimal drawer motion in an acutely swollen stifle may indicate that the displaced meniscus is acting as a wedge to prevent drawer motion.[78] The chronic lameness due to cranial cruciate ligament rupture that suddenly worsens is usually the result of secondary meniscal tearing. Similarly, meniscal injury should be suspected in the relatively acute cruciate rupture with significant degenerative joint disease.

Radiography has not been a reliable method of diagnosis in this condition. Arthroscopy will undoubtedly become important at some point, but at present, it is not useful for routine examination of the canine stifle joint. Surgical exploration remains the most common and useful method of definitive diagnosis.

TREATMENT

Meniscectomy

INDICATIONS

Considerable controversy surrounds the question of meniscectomy in humans and in animals. A more conservative approach is becoming evident as growing

---

FIGURE 20–30

Rupture of the caudal cruciate ligament. (A) The left stifle has been exposed by a medial approach to the stifle joint combined with an approach to the medial collateral ligament and caudomedial compartment of the joint.[5] The caudomedial joint capsule has been imbricated with mattress sutures of nonabsorbable material (size 3/0–0) placed vertically to the joint caudal to the medial collateral ligament. (B) Following closure of the joint capsule, a heavy gauge (size 0–4) braided polyester suture is placed between the proximal patellar ligament and a drill hole in the caudomedial corner of the proximal tibia. This suture is tightened with the stifle at a normal standing angle and with drawer motion reduced. (C) The skin is retracted laterally to allow incision of the fascia lata and retraction of the biceps femoris. This reveals the lateral collateral ligament and caudolateral joint capsule.[5] The joint capsule is imbricated caudal to the lateral collateral ligament and a heavy-gauge braided polyester suture is placed around the head of the fibula to the proximal patellar ligament. This suture is tied tightly with the stifle in a normal standing angle. (D) For further augmentation, a strip of fascia lata may be dissected free proximally and left attached to the lateral border of the patella distally. This strip is passed around the fibular head, pulled taut, and then sutured to itself and to the surrounding fascia.

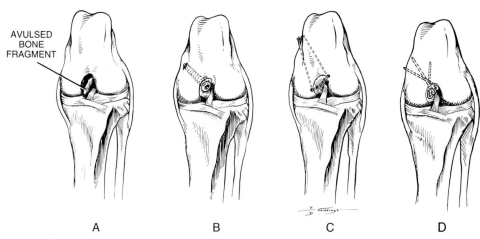

AVULSED
BONE
FRAGMENT

A   B   C   D

FIGURE 20–31

Avulsion of the femoral origin of the caudal cruciate ligament. (A) A fragment of bone with the attached ligament has been avulsed from the medial femoral condyle. (B) A lag screw has been used to fix the fragment. A lateral approach to the stifle gives best exposure.[5] (C) Stainless steel wire (20 to 22 gauge) is threaded through the ligament close to the bone fragment. Two parallel holes are drilled at opposite points on the edge of the femoral defect; the wire is passed through these holes, then twisted on the medial surface of the condyle. (D) Three Kirschner wires can be inserted at diverging angles to stabilize the fragment.

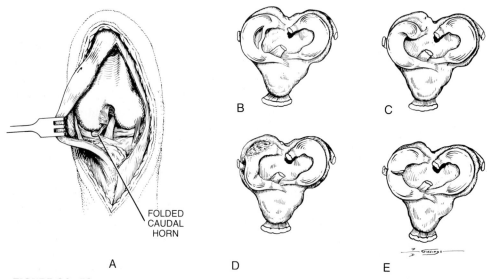

B   C

FOLDED
CAUDAL
HORN

A   D   E

FIGURE 20–32

Lesions of the medial meniscus. (A) Folded caudal horn. (B) Longitudinal (bucket-handle) tear. (C) Medial peripheral detachment. (D) Caudomedial peripheral detachment with shredding of the cartilage. (E) Transverse tear.

numbers of arthroscopic examinations in humans indicate the human knee to be quite capable of normal function in the presence of minor meniscal injuries.[79] Stone and associates[76] have pointed out that abnormal position of the medial meniscus (owing to drawer motion) does not necessarily indicate meniscal damage. Because damaged meniscal cartilage does not heal, removal of the tissue may often be the best treatment, but it seems reasonable to remove only menisci that exhibit severe derangement such as:

1. Folding that cannot be reduced.
2. Crushing and erosion with longitudinal parenchymal tears.
3. Torn tibial ligaments.
4. Extensive peripheral detachment.

Partial meniscectomy to remove damaged tissue is indicated to remove very small areas of semidetached cartilage. This must be done carefully to avoid injury to articular cartilage.

The rationale behind removal of the damaged meniscus is that a fibrocartilaginous meniscus will regenerate to replace the removed meniscus. Such regeneration originates in vascular fibrous connective tissue of the joint capsule and is complete within seven months. All meniscus cartilage has to be removed for this fibroplasia to develop. Controversy surrounds the quality of the cartilage that develops. In one report, the cartilage was histologically similar to that of the normal meniscus.[80] Minimal signs of degenerative joint disease were seen in these experimental dogs following meniscectomy. Other experimental work has demonstrated a structure that was only one-third the size of the normal meniscus and was morphologically and biochemically inferior to meniscus cartilage.[24]

TECHNIQUE

A medial arthrotomy[5] is preferred for medial meniscectomy because it provides better exposure and allows a transverse joint incision if exposure from the medial parapatellar incision proves inadequate. Visualization of the caudal meniscal horns is aided by joint instability. If the cranial cruciate is torn, cranial drawer motion is produced by placing a curved hemostat or small Hohman retractor in the intercondylar space and hooking it over the caudal edge of the tibial plateau. This allows the tibia to be levered into the drawer position. Flexion of the joint is also useful for increasing visualization of the caudal meniscal horns.

Total medial meniscectomy begins by cutting of the intermeniscal and cranial tibial ligaments (Fig. 20–33A,B).[78] All cutting is done with great care to avoid injury to articular cartilage of the tibia and femur. Number 11 and 15 blades or No. 64 Beaver miniblades (R. Beaver, Inc., Belmont, MA) are the most useful sizes for the procedure. A Kocher forceps or meniscus clamp (Ascott Enterprises, Missassauga, Ontario) is attached to the freed cranial horn. It is pulled laterally (axially) while the medial joint capsule is retracted medially (abaxially). The meniscus is dissected away from the joint capsule with the blade in a vertical position to avoid cutting the medial collateral ligament (Fig. 20–33C). Dissection continues caudal to the medial collateral as strong traction is applied to the clamped meniscus in a craniolateral direction. Cutting the caudal synovial attachment is the most difficult part of

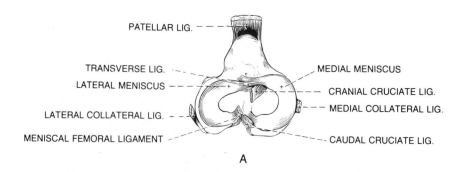

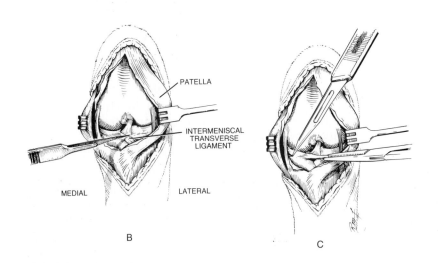

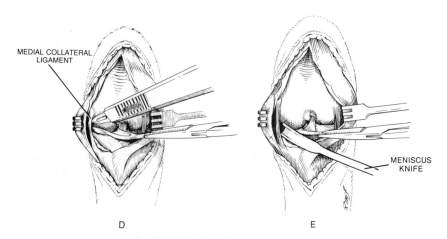

FIGURE 20–33

See legend on opposite page

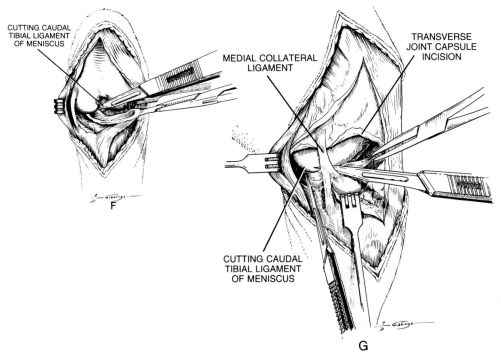

FIGURE 20-33

Medial meniscectomy.[78] (A) Menisci and meniscal ligaments of the left stifle joint, dorsal aspect. (From Evans HE, Christensen GC: Miller's Anatomy of the Dog. 2nd ed. Philadelphia, W. B. Saunders Company, 1979, p. 262. By permission). (B) The left stifle has been exposed by a medial parapatellar approach.[5] The cranial tibial and intermeniscal ligaments are severed. (C) Strong craniolateral traction is applied to the meniscus, and the medial joint capsule is retracted to allow dissection of the cranial horn free from the joint capsule. The scalpel blade is oriented vertically to avoid cutting the medial collateral ligament. (D) Continued traction allows the caudal joint capsule attachments to be cut. (E) A small curved meniscus knife (Veterinary Instrumentation, Sheffield, England; Jorgensen Laboratories Inc, Loveland, Colorado) simplifies freeing the meniscus caudal to the collateral ligament. (F) The caudal tibial ligament of the meniscus is cut with the blade held parallel to the tibia. (G) For additional exposure of the caudal peripheral attachments, a medial transverse joint incision is made from the parapatellar incision, extending caudally deep to the medial collateral ligament. Caudal capsular attachments can be easily cut, but care must be taken to avoid the popliteal vessels. The meniscus is dissected free of the deep portion of the medial collateral ligament. The caudal tibial meniscal ligament is cut, as in F. The capsule is closed with mattress sutures.

the procedure and may require additional exposure, as discussed below. A small curved meniscus knife (Veterinary Instrumentation, Sheffield, England; Jorgensen Laboratories, Loveland, CO) greatly simplifies this part of the surgery. The knife is worked around the periphery of the meniscus, freeing it from the synovial membrane and collateral ligament. If these attachments can be freed at this point (Fig. 20–33D), the entire meniscus can be pulled cranially and the caudal tibial ligament can be cut (Fig. 20–33F) to free the meniscus.

If additional exposure is required, a medial transverse joint incision is made from the medial collateral ligament cranially to join the parapatellar incision (Fig. 20–33F). The medial collateral ligament is elevated to allow the incision to be extended caudally deep to it. The meniscus is dissected away from the caudal joint capsule and medial collateral ligament. Care is taken to avoid the popliteal vessels immediately caudal to the capsule. After the caudal capsular attachments are freed, the caudal tibial ligament is cut as described above to free the meniscus.

AFTERCARE ■ No specific aftercare is required for meniscectomy. The care is usually dictated by repair of associated ligament damage. Heavy exercise should be withheld for six months, if possible, to allow for regeneration of the meniscus before extreme stress is placed on the joint. Hannan and associates[24] have demonstrated a chondroprotective effect by polysulfated glycosaminoglycan (Arteparon, Luitpold Werk, Munich, FRG; Adequan, Luitpold Pharmaceutical Inc., Shirley, NY) following experimental meniscectomy. Dosage of 2 mg/kg body weight subcutaneously three times per week for three weeks, then twice weekly until the dogs were killed at 23 weeks, significantly improved the biochemical and morphological parameters studied in articular cartilage.

Collateral Ligament Injuries

Ligament injuries that overstress the structure and damage ligament fibers are known as sprains (see Chapter 19). Such injuries may be minor (first degree) or more severe, with stretching and rupture of ligament fibers (second degree); or they may result in tearing or avulsion of the ligament (third degree).[81] Only third-degree and some second-degree injuries require surgical therapy.

Damage to collateral ligaments of the canine stifle occurs relatively infrequently. Severe injury is usually associated with traumatic incidents, such as being hit by an automobile or direct blows. Meniscal and cruciate damage should always be suspected with any collateral ligament injury severe enough to produce instability of the joint.

An understanding of the functional anatomy of these ligaments is necessary to diagnose the resulting instability.[82] Both ligaments are taut in extension and function with the cruciate ligaments to prevent internal tibial rotation. In extension, the collateral ligaments are the primary stabilizers of lateral (valgus) and medial (varus) angulation of the tibia. In flexion, the lateral ligament relaxes and allows internal tibial rotation to be limited only by the cruciates while the medial ligament remains taut and limits external tibial rotation. Since the cruciates do not limit external tibial rotation, the medial collateral is the primary stabilizer of this motion.

CLINICAL SIGNS

Injury to the medial ligament is more common than injury to the lateral side. Tearing of the cranial cruciate and medial meniscus commonly accompanies the collateral damage. Joint effusion and tenderness with no weight-bearing are the obvious signs. Tibial angulation is checked with the joint in extension, and any drawer motion is reduced. Varus instability is present with lateral laxity, and valgus instability is present with medial laxity. When the medial collateral is completely torn, marked external tibial rotation is possible with the stifle flexed.

Physical examination will usually provide the diagnosis, but radiographs with the joint stressed to accentuate the instability are often useful.

Injuries that produce observable instability in large, active dogs should be surgically repaired as early as possible. Even if the ligament is grossly intact and even if it heals by fibroplasia, it will always remain loose and will allow joint laxity.

Stretched ligaments (second-degree injury) are tightened by suture imbrication, torn ligaments are sutured, and avulsed ligaments are reattached or synthetically replaced (Fig. 20–34; see also Figs. 19–6 and 19–7). Exposure of either ligament is readily done, either primarily or during an approach to the stifle joint.[5] Collateral ligaments of the stifle, especially the lateral ligament, must always be sutured or reattached with the stifle in extension to prevent shortening of the ligament, which either limits extension or overstresses the repair when the animal extends the joint.

AFTERCARE ■ All injuries are immobilized in a Thomas splint (see Fig. 1–11) or long lateral splint (see Fig. 19–12) for four weeks, followed by two more weeks of leash-only exercise. Activity can be slowly increased after seven or eight weeks.

Luxation of the Stifle Joint

Total derangement of the knee, with rupture of all four major ligaments, is a disastrous injury seen on occasion. Cats appear to suffer a higher incidence than do dogs. Vascular integrity of the limb distal to the stifle must be carefully evaluated as the popliteal vessels may become entrapped by the tibial luxation.

More commonly seen is injury of the cranial and caudal cruciate and medial collateral ligaments. Also damaged to varying degrees are the secondary restraints of the joint such as joint capsule, menisci, and patellar ligament. Additionally, most have a variety of other traumatic injuries such as fractures or ruptured viscera. Despite the magnitude of this injury, good function can be obtained if a meticulous repair is made of each injury.[83] Paramount to attempting such repairs is a thorough preoperative assessment of the stifle joint. Such an examination can be done adequately and humanely only under general anesthesia in this circumstance. Owing to the multiple derangements of the joint, palpation can be confusing, and the diagnoses reached must always be regarded as presumptive.

Surgery should start with a thorough exploration of the joint, and this requires adequate surgical exposure. Meniscal injuries in this instance do not often require meniscectomy; most damage is usually done to meniscofemoral or meniscotibial ligaments or the joint capsule attachments. These can usually be sutured and should be done first, while the exposure is greatest. The collateral ligament injury should be stabilized next, as this will restore basic

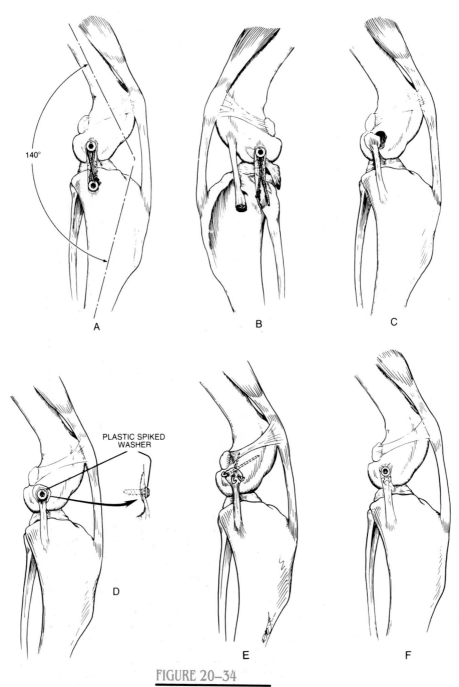

PLASTIC SPIKED
WASHER

FIGURE 20–34

See legend on opposite page

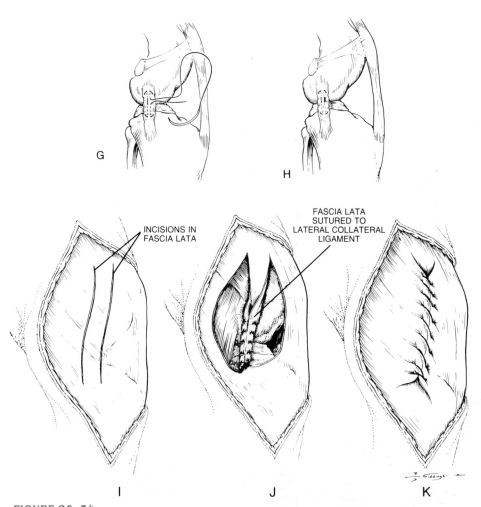

INCISIONS IN
FASCIA LATA

FASCIA LATA
SUTURED TO
LATERAL COLLATERAL
LIGAMENT

FIGURE 20–34

Surgical repair of collateral ligament injuries. (A) A midportion medial collateral tear has been sutured, using a locking loop pattern (see Fig. 19–1). The ligament repair is protected by heavy-gauge (0–3) braided polyester suture placed between two bone screws placed in the origin and insertion areas. This suture is tied with the joint extended or at a standing angle. (B) A midportion lateral collateral tear has been sutured as in A. Only one bone screw is needed, since a bone tunnel drilled in the fibula functions well for the distal insertion of the protective suture. (C) Avulsion of the origin of the medial collateral ligament. (D) The avulsion has been secured using a plastic spiked washer on a 3.5-mm screw. (E) Reattachment is also possible with three diverging Kirschner wires placed through the fragment. (F) This tear close to the origin of the medial collateral ligament was sutured with a locking loop pattern, and the suture was then secured around a bone screw. When possible, a bone tunnel can be used rather than a screw, as in B. (G) A stretched ligament is being imbricated by means of a modified locking loop suture pattern. (H) Tying the suture results in shortening of the ligament between the suture loops. (I) Fascia lata reinforcement of a lateral collateral ligament injury[51] commences by elevating a strip of fascia that is left attached at each end. (J) The fascia is sutured to the repaired ligament. (K) The fascial defect is sutured.

alignment to the joint and simplify the remaining surgery. Stabilization of the cruciate instability follows. The authors have usually used extra-articular methods, but Hulse and Shires attribute much of their success in these problems to intra-articular stabilization.[83] Extra-articular repair of the cruciate ligament injuries and postoperative support with transarticular external skeletal fixators was successful in 13 cases reported by Aron.[84] The final step is careful imbrication of all available joint capsule and periarticular tissue to further stabilize the joint.

Aftercare consists of exercise limitation as described above for each of the individual procedures. Surprisingly good function has been seen in these patients, both by us and others.[83, 84] A consistent finding is reduction of 30 to 40 degrees in range of motion in the stifle joint. Arthrodesis is a possible option for a chronically unstable and painful joint, but amputation results in better overall function of the animal.

Osteochondritis Dissecans of the Femoral Condyle

The pathophysiology of osteochondrosis and osteochondritis dissecans (OCD) is discussed in Chapter 18.

The shoulder joint is most commonly involved, but the stifle is occasionally involved and is often overlooked. OCD is seen in all large breeds of dogs, especially the retrievers. Signs are usually first noted at 5 to 7 months of age. Early surgical treatment is indicated to remove loose cartilage and minimize osteoarthrosis. The prognosis is more guarded than for lesions of the shoulder, but about 75 percent will be normally functional if surgical treatment is done at an early age. Some degree of osteoarthrosis is to be expected.

CLINICAL SIGNS

Lameness varies from minimal to severe. Measurement of the diameter of the thigh muscles may demonstrate evidence of mild disuse atrophy. Palpation of the joint is not often rewarding, although very slight drawer motion movement may be noted if muscle atrophy is present. Joint effusion can often be noted. If a joint mouse has formed from detachment of the cartilage flap, popping or crepitus can be present.

DIAGNOSIS

Radiographs are always necessary for diagnosis, and technically high-quality films are necessary to detect a small lesion. Mediolateral and caudocranial views are needed, the latter in two different degrees of flexion-extension. Lesions are most commonly found on the medial aspect of the lateral femoral condyle (Fig. 20–35), although the medial condyle can be affected. Slight flattening of the articular surface and subchondral sclerosis are the most common findings.

SURGICAL TREATMENT

Either a lateral or medial parapatellar approach provides adequate exposure (Fig. 20–36A).[5] The cartilage flap is excised, and the edges of the defect are

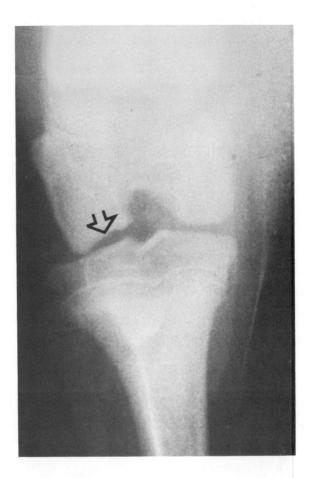

FIGURE 20–35

Osteochondritis dissecans lesion (*arrow*) of the lateral femoral condyle; caudocranial view.

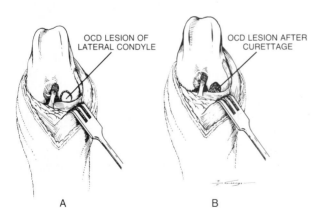

A   B

FIGURE 20–36

Osteochondritis dissecans of the femoral condyles. (*A*) A lesion of the lateral femoral condyle has been exposed by a medial parapatellar approach.[5] (*B*) The cartilage flap has been excised, and the edges of the lesion are debrided by curettage.

trimmed to make a clean vertical border (Fig. 20–36B). The edges of the lesion are trimmed to make certain that the cartilage left is firmly adhered to the subchondral bone. Multiple drilling of the defect with a Kirschner wire may aid in early revascularization of a sclerotic lesion. Occasionally, the cartilage defect will damage the underlying meniscus and necessitate meniscectomy.

AFTERCARE ■ Close confinement for four weeks followed by gradual resumption of normal activity is advised.

Avulsion of the Proximal Tendon of the Long Digital Extensor Muscle

Although it occurs infrequently, avulsion of the origin of the long digital extensor (LDE) muscle is a disabling injury resulting in severe degenerative joint disease.[85] Avulsion is a disease of skeletally immature, long-legged breeds such as sighthounds and Great Danes in the age range of 5 to 8 months, but rupture of the tendon can occur in mature animals, especially those with lateral patellar luxation.

The LDE muscle originates in the extensor fossa of the lateral femoral condyle. The tendon crosses the joint and passes deep to the cranial tibial muscle through a sulcus in the proximolateral tibia. It is apparently not important to stability of the stifle joint. The detached bony fragment rapidly

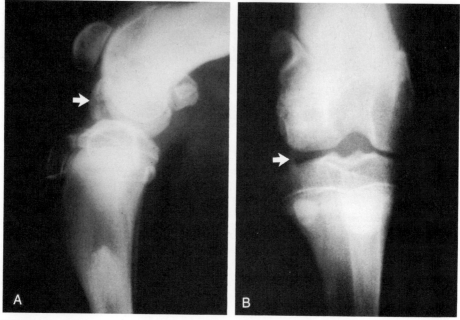

FIGURE 20–37

Avulsion of the long digital extensor (LDE) tendon of origin from the lateral femoral condyle. *(A)* The avulsed osteochondral fragment that was the origin of the tendon can be seen opposite the arrow in the cranial compartment of the stifle joint; mediolateral view. *(B)* The fragment can also be seen in the lateral aspect of the joint in the craniocaudal view, but it is less obvious.

hypertrophies to several times its original size. The injury rarely is associated with known significant trauma. Surgical treatment produces gratifying results if performed before degenerative joint disease becomes evident.

CLINICAL SIGNS

Pain and joint effusion are seen immediately after the injury. Pain is most pronounced in the craniolateral aspect of the joint. Lameness is variable and subsides quickly. Loss of toe function does not seem to be a common problem. Firm thickening of the lateral joint area is evident within two to three weeks, and pressure applied over this area may produce pain and crepitus.

DIAGNOSIS

Radiographs of the stifle in flexed lateral and caudocranial views reveal an opaque density within the joint (Fig. 20–37). On the lateral view, the opacity is seen cranial to the femoral condyle and distal to the extensor fossa. The caudocranial view reveals the calcified mass to be just lateral to the femoral condyle. The radiographic size of the mass is much less than actual size since a portion of it is cartilaginous and secondarily fibrotic.

SURGICAL TREATMENT

Reattachment of the avulsed fragment is the treatment of choice in recent injuries. If the fragment is so hypertrophic that the outline of the original fragment is no longer discernible, it is better to detach the bone fragment and reattach the tendon to adjacent soft tissue.

Exposure of the lesion is by way of a lateral approach to the stifle joint.[5] The avulsion is immediately visible when the joint capsule is incised (Fig. 20–38A). If the injury is recent and the avulsed fragment is not hypertrophied or covered with granulation tissue, it is reattached with a 3.5- or 4.0-mm lag screw and plastic spiked washer (Fig. 20–38B) (Synthes [USA], Paoli, PA). Three diverging Kirschner wires can also serve as fixation.

Because the tendon is not important in stabilizing the joint, it is better to excise hypertrophic bone than to try reattachment and chance a delayed or fibrous union. This removes the mechanical irritation of the hypertrophic fragment. The bone can be cut free and the tendon can be attached to the joint capsule or fascia of the cranial tibial muscle (Fig. 20–38C).

AFTERCARE ■ Special precautions are not needed. Two weeks of house confinement and leash exercise are needed for soft-tissue healing.

Luxation of the Proximal Tendon of the Long Digital Extensor Muscle

This unusual problem, wherein the tendon displaces caudally out of the tibial sulcus, causes variable clinical signs. The dog may show marked lameness, with the leg occasionally not bearing weight,[86] or there may be no lameness

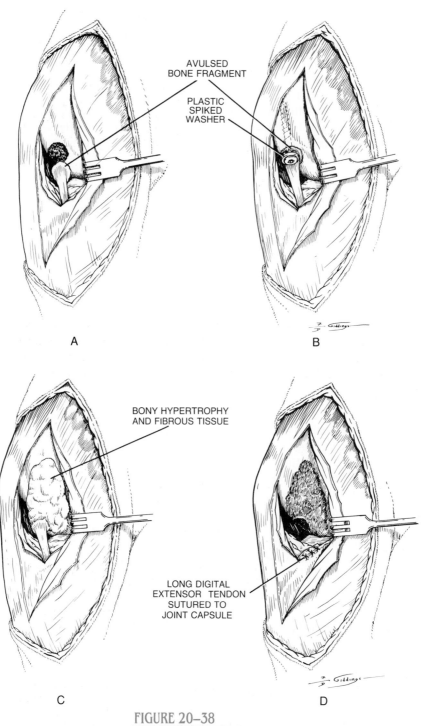

AVULSED
BONE FRAGMENT

PLASTIC
SPIKED
WASHER

A

B

BONY HYPERTROPHY
AND FIBROUS TISSUE

LONG DIGITAL
EXTENSOR TENDON
SUTURED TO
JOINT CAPSULE

C

D

FIGURE 20–38

See legend on opposite page

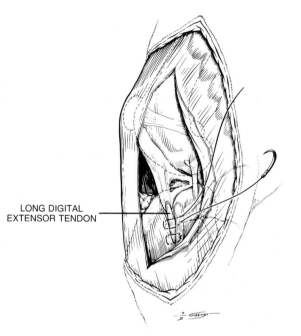

FIGURE 20–39

Luxation of the proximal tendon of the long digital extensor muscle. Two mattress sutures are placed across the tibial sulcus to prevent luxation of the tendon.

LONG DIGITAL
EXTENSOR TENDON

at all but a clicking sound accompanying each step. This sound mimics a meniscal click and often can be produced on palpation by flexing the stifle while pushing proximally on the foot to simulate weight-bearing and can be felt by placing a hand on the limb while the animal is walking. Surgical repair carries a good prognosis.

SURGICAL TREATMENT

Although an acute injury may respond to external immobilization for two to three weeks, most cases are chronic when seen and require surgery.

A vertical skin incision is made between the tibial tubercle and the fibula. Dissection will easily reveal the tendon and the tibial sulcus. Nonabsorbable sutures are used to create a "roof" over the sulcus to trap the tendon (Fig. 20–39). If possible, the suture is placed through a bone tunnel along the edge of the sulcus. Where there are no suitable points for bony anchorage, the suture is placed through periosteum and fascia. In some instances, it may be necessary to deepen the sulcus to obtain adequate reduction of the tendon.

AFTERCARE ■ External immobilization is not required; exercise should be restricted for two to three weeks.

FIGURE 20–38

Avulsion of the tendinous origin of the long digital extensor muscle. (A) A fresh avulsion fracture has been exposed by a lateral approach to the femur. The bone fragment and attached tendon have pulled away from the femur. (B) A 4.0-mm lag screw and plastic spiked washer (Synthes [USA], Paoli, PA) has been used to attach the avulsed fragment. (C) An example of a case of several weeks' duration, with bony hypertrophy and fibrous tissue covering the avulsed fragment. The bone fragment is not reattached in this situation. (D) The hypertrophic avulsed fragment has been resected and the tendon sutured to the joint capsule. The fascia of the cranial tibial muscle can also be used for attaching the tendon.

Arthrodesis of the Stifle Joint

A general discussion of indications for and principles of arthrodesis is found in Chapter 19. Strict attention to detail to establish proper joint angle and rigid internal fixation is necessary for success.

Arthrodesis of the stifle is an alternative to amputation for severely comminuted intra-articular fractures, acute total luxation, chronic luxation or subluxation from a variety of causes, severe osteoarthritis, and severe patellar luxations that have not responded to conventional repair.

Function of the limb is markedly affected; however, when the fusion is at the proper angle (135 to 140 degrees in the dog and 120 to 125 degrees in the cat), function is satisfactory for pet animals. With fusion, the limb is sometimes circumducted, especially at faster gaits when the limb becomes relatively too long compared with the opposite limb. Knuckling of the toes may also occur at these times. Overall function of the fused limb is not as good in most dogs as with amputation. Bone plate fixation is the most suitable fixation for large breeds and is useful in all sizes of animals (see Fig. 20–40). Lag screws and tension band wire are suitable for small- to medium-sized animals (see Fig. 20–41A). Pins with tension band wire are satisfactory in cats and small breeds (see Fig. 20–41B).

SURGICAL TECHNIQUE
Bone Plate[33]

Because of the large size of the contact surfaces at the fusion site, it is difficult to change the angle of the joint after the initial cut to remove articular cartilage and subchondral bone without sacrificing large amounts of bone and thus shortening the limb. It is therefore worth the effort to do very precise planning of the initial ostectomy cuts.

A bilateral approach is made to the stifle, and the tibial tuberosity is osteotomized to allow proximal retraction of the entire quadriceps group.[5] The meniscal cartilages are completely excised. Although the collateral ligaments can be sacrificed at this time, maintaining them simplifies intraoperative manipulation of the limb. Kirschner wires are driven into the distal femur and proximal tibia, perpendicular to the long axis of each bone (wires 1 and 2, Fig. 20–40A). Both of these pins should lie in the sagittal midline plane of the limb. The selected joint angle is subtracted from 180 degrees to obtain the complementary angle. In the illustrated case, the chosen angle is 140 degrees and the complementary angle is 40 degrees. Since bone can easily be removed from both the femur and tibia, a 20-degree wedge of bone is removed from each. The plane of these ostectomies is parallel to Kirschner wires placed at angles of 20 degrees to the original wires (wires 3 and 4, Fig. 20–40A).

The initial ostectomies are performed with an osteotome (Fig. 20–40B) or an oscillating saw held parallel to pins 3 and 4. The popliteal vessels must not be severed. Rongeurs or a rasp is used to smooth the contact surfaces. Once the proper angle has been established, the bones are temporarily stabilized with two Kirschner wires placed in an "X" fashion (Fig. 20–40C). Pins 1, 2, 3, and 4 should be maintained in the sagittal midline plane during placement of the "X" pins to ensure that the lower limb is not rotated; the pins are then removed.

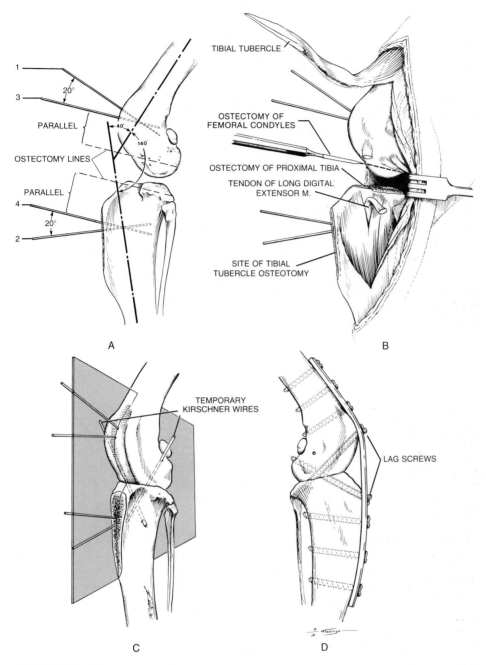

TIBIAL TUBERCLE

OSTECTOMY OF
FEMORAL CONDYLES

OSTECTOMY OF PROXIMAL TIBIA

TENDON OF LONG DIGITAL
EXTENSOR M.

SITE OF TIBIAL
TUBERCLE OSTEOTOMY

PARALLEL

OSTECTOMY LINES

PARALLEL

TEMPORARY
KIRSCHNER WIRES

LAG SCREWS

A

B

C

D

FIGURE 20–40

Arthrodesis of the stifle by bone plate fixation. (A) Planning of the ostectomies. Kirschner wires 1 and 2 are placed perpendicular to the femoral and tibial shafts. The joint angle chosen—140 degrees—has a complementary angle of 40 degrees. Dividing this by two gives a result of 20 degrees, so that pins 3 and 4, placed at an angle of 20 degrees to pins 1 and 2, are parallel to the ostectomy lines desired. (B) The tibial ostectomy is complete. The femoral cut is made with an osteotome held parallel to pin 3. An oscillating saw can also be used. (C) The joint is temporarily fixed by crossed pins. Kirschner wires 1 through 4 are kept in alignment with the sagittal plane to prevent rotation of the lower limb. The wires are removed after the crossed pins are placed. (D) A bone plate is contoured after removing sufficient tibial crest to allow good contact. Screws 3 and 6 are placed first in a dynamic compression plate (Synthes [USA], Paoli, PA) to supply compression, or a separate compression device can be used in the tibia. At least one lag screw should cross the joint, and two are preferable, as shown here.

A bone plate that will allow at least four screws in each fragment is contoured to the cranial bone surfaces. Some of the tibial tuberosity and crest is removed to allow better contact of the plate (Fig. 20–40D). At least one screw should be lagged across the contact surfaces after compression is obtained with the plate screws inserted in a dynamic compression plate (Synthes [USA], Paoli, PA) or with a separate compression device. The tibial tuberosity is pinned to one side of the plate in such a position that the patella does not contact the plate. Alternatively, the patella may be excised. The X-pins can be removed or left in place. Bone graft is not needed because of the large contact surfaces of the femur and tibia.

AFTERCARE ■ Most dogs and cats do not require external support of the limb. Because the plate is functioning as a tension band, it provides very rigid fixation. However, because the plate is angled and because there is a natural fulcrum at the stifle joint, the plate or screws may break if activity is excessive. External support of the limb should be used if there is any question about the owner's ability to restrict the animal's activity. About eight weeks is required for radiographic signs of fusion, and activity should be restricted during this period. Fracture of the tibia at the distal end of the plate sometimes occurs and is probably a good reason to remove the plate six to nine months postsurgically. Pins, wires, and screws are not removed unless they loosen.

Screw and Pin Fixation

These procedures begin as just described above. After the contact surfaces are prepared, lag screws or pins are placed in an X fashion across the joint (Fig. 20–41A,B). The pins or screws must penetrate the tibial cortices for best holding power. Pins 1, 2, 3, and 4 are removed. A pin is then driven from the proximal trochlear sulcus into the proximal tibia emerging on the cranial cortex distal to the tibial crest. A hole is drilled transversely through the

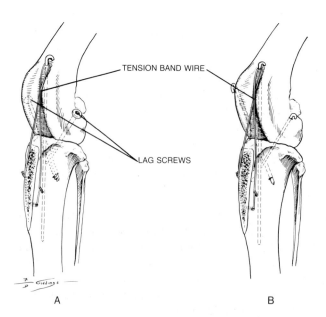

TENSION BAND WIRE

LAG SCREWS

A   B

FIGURE 20–41

Arthrodesis of the stifle by lag screw or pin fixation. *(A)* After the contact surfaces are prepared, crossed lag screws are placed from the femoral condyles to the proximal tibia. A small pin is driven from the proximal trochlear sulcus into the proximal tibia, and a tension band wire is placed from the head of the pin to the tibial crest. *(B)* Pins can be substituted for lag screws in small dogs and cats.

proximal tibial crest and a tension band wire (size 18 to 22 gauge, 1.0 to 0.6 mm) is placed between the pin and the tibial crest.

AFTERCARE ■ External support using a Thomas splint (see Fig. 1–11) or a long lateral splint (see Fig. 19–12) is advisable for four weeks postoperatively. Exercise is severely restricted until radiographs show advanced fusion, usually about 8 to 10 weeks postoperatively.

THE TARSUS AND METATARSUS

Ligamentous injuries of the tarsus resulting in varying degrees of instability are relatively common in athletic breeds because of the propulsive force supplied by the hind legs. Unlike those of the carpus, tarsal injuries are more apt to be caused by spontaneous overstress rather than by outside traumatic forces.

Conservative treatment of second- and third-degree ligamentous injuries by cast immobilization is not recommended because permanent instability is the usual result.[81] Aggressive surgical treatment is much more rewarding, but it does require a good working knowledge of the anatomy of the region. Unfortunately, the official terminology of the tarsus differs markedly from that in current popular use.

Anatomy of the Tarsus

The bones of the tarsus are arranged in several levels, with a complex arrangement of ligaments (see Figs. 8–1 and 20–42). The joint between the tibia and fibula and the talus and calcaneus is the *tarsocrural* joint, often called the tibiotarsal, talocrural, or hock joint. *Intertarsal* joints include all articulations between tarsal bones, with four of them named specifically:

1. *Talocalcaneal joint.* The joint between the talus and calcaneus.
2. *Talocalcaneocentral joint.* This joint is primarily an articulation between the talus and central tarsal bone, but the joint capsule is continuous with the calcaneus.
3. *Calcaneoquartal joint.* The joint between the calcaneus and the fourth tarsal. This joint and the talocalcaneocentral joint collectively are popularly known as the *proximal intertarsal joint.* This name is useful to the surgeon because of the awkwardness of the official names.
4. *Centrodistal joint.* The joint between the central tarsal bone and the distal numbered tarsal bone. The popular name is the distal intertarsal joint.
5. *Tarsometatarsal joints.* The joints between the distal tarsal and metatarsal bones.

The most common injuries involve the collateral ligaments of the tarsocrural joint (Fig. 20–42A–D) and the plantar ligaments and tarsal fibrocartilage (Fig. 20–42D). Both collateral ligaments have long and short parts. The long parts serve to limit extension, and the short parts prevent hyperflexion. The plantar ligaments and tarsal fibrocartilage are tension bands that limit extension of the intertarsal and tarsometatarsal joints. The remaining ligaments are much smaller and shorter, connecting individual bones.

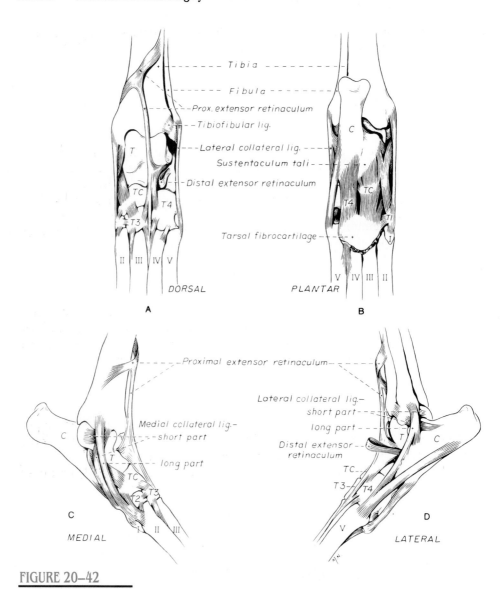

FIGURE 20–42

Ligaments of the left tarsus. *(A)* Dorsal aspect. *(B)* Plantar aspect. *(C)* Medial aspect. *(D)* Lateral aspect. C = calcaneus; T1, T3, T4 = first, third, fourth tarsals; T = talus; I through V = metatarsals; TC = central tarsal. (All from Evans HE, Christensen GC: Miller's Anatomy of the Dog, 2nd ed. Philadelphia, W. B. Saunders Company, 1979, pp. 265, 267. By permission).

As in the carpus, directional terms used in the proximal portions of the limb are not used in the tarsus. Distal to the tarsocrural joint, *cranial* becomes *dorsal* and *caudal* becomes *plantar.*

Surgical Approaches

Several approaches to various areas of the tarsus have been described.[5] Because there are no muscles covering these bones except on the plantar side, approaches are generally made directly over the area of interest. Deep structures such as tendons, vessels, and nerves are isolated and retracted as needed.

Injuries of the Tarsus and Metatarsus

CLINICAL SIGNS

Many tarsal injuries are a result of overstress of ligamentous structures and occur without a history of known trauma. Sudden exertion, such as jumping, can be sufficient to damage plantar ligaments and cause a hyperextension injury. Affected animals are usually nonweight-bearing, have variable swelling in the tarsal region, and show gross instability of the tarsus. The limb is commonly carried in flexion. Palpation will usually be sufficient to localize the area of probable injury.

DIAGNOSIS

Radiographs are necessary to verify the diagnosis and to localize the damage. Stress radiographs will show the area of instability. Standard dorsoplantar and lateral or medial views, plus obliques, will also identify avulsions and other fractures. Nonscreen film or fine-detail screens are essential.

TARSOCRURAL LUXATION AND SUBLUXATION

Many complete luxations of this joint are accompanied by fracture of one or both malleoli, and internal fixation of the fractures results in stability of the joint. Treatment of such injuries is described in Chapter 8.

Rupture or avulsion of the collateral ligaments (Fig. 20–43A,B) produces

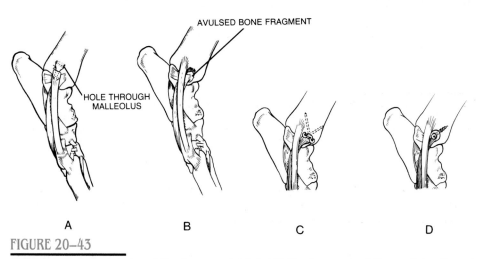

AVULSED BONE FRAGMENT

HOLE THROUGH MALLEOLUS

A   B   C   D

FIGURE 20–43

Collateral ligament injuries of the tarsocrural joint. (A) The long part of the medial collateral ligament is torn near its origin on the malleolus. A hole is drilled through the malleolus, and a locking loop suture is passed through this hole to pull the ligament against the bone. (B) An avulsion of the origin of the short part of the medial collateral ligament. (C) Diverging Kirschner wires used to stabilize the avulsed fragment. (D) Lag screw fixation is ideal if the fragment is large enough to allow screw placement.

subluxation. Medial injuries allow valgus (lateral) deviation of the foot, and lateral injuries allow varus (medial) angulation. These deviations are easily palpated and confirmed radiographically. Rupture of just the long or short part of the ligament produces only moderate instability and may be difficult to diagnose preoperatively.

Surgical Technique

Principles of treatment are similar to those described in Chapter 19, such as imbricating, suturing, reattaching, or replacing ligaments as indicated. It is important to repair both the long and short part of the ligament in order to achieve good function. Reattachment of the long part of the ligament is illustrated in Figure 20–43A. A bone tunnel is used in the malleolus to anchor the suture. An avulsion of the short part is depicted in Figure 20–43B,C, fixed with a small lag screw. Another method of fixation is the placement of three diverging Kirschner wires passed through the fragment into the tibia. Capturing a small fragment and holding it with stainless steel wire is illustrated in Figure 20–29.

If good repair or reattachment of the ligament is not possible, the repair can be augmented by synthetic ligaments (Fig. 20–44B,C).

AFTERCARE ■ Ligamentous repairs are protected with a short lateral splint for four to six weeks followed by an elastic bandage for an additional two weeks (see Chapter 19). Exercise is restricted to leash walking until eight weeks, then gradually increased to normal at 10 to 12 weeks.

SHEARING INJURY OF THE TARSUS

This abrasion injury occurs when the dog's lower limb is run over by the tire of an automobile with its brakes locked attempting to avoid the animal. Soft tissues in contact with the pavement are simply ground away, often eroding skin, muscle, ligaments, and even bone. The medial tarsal and metatarsal region is most commonly affected, with the medial malleolus and collateral ligaments often completely destroyed (Fig. 20–44A,B). One or more tarsal or metatarsal joints may be open and various amounts of debris are ground into all the tissues. The lateral side is less commonly involved and represents a less serious injury than a comparable injury on the medial side. Owing to the fact that the dog normally stands with a few degrees of valgus (lateral) deviation of the hindpaw, ligamentous stability of the medial side of the tarsus and metatarsus is much more critical than on the lateral aspect.

Best results are obtained by treating these wounds in an open manner, with early stabilization of the joints and any accompanying fractures. Skin grafting is delayed and indicated only where granulation tissue does not adequately close the skin, which is a rare occurrence. Early or delayed arthrodesis is indicated in those cases for which it is not possible to restore reasonable joint function. Variables to be considered in choosing a plan of action are:

1. Assuming that the joint(s) can be stabilized, is there enough articular surface to allow good function? Loss of bone in the tarsocrural articulation is critical. If the answer is no, arthrodesis is indicated.

2. What will the owner accept as reasonable function? A large, active breed presents different problems from a small and sedentary animal. In the former, aggressive ligamentous repair, augmentation, or replacement is necessary, while in the latter case it may be possible to obtain good results by very conservative methods. Stabilization of joints by scar tissue may well provide adequate support in the smaller and less active animals, but it rarely will support the tension loads of the medial side in large, athletic individuals.

3. How will support for the joints or fractured bones be provided? Regardless which approach is taken to the ligamentous instability, the involved joints must be stabilized during the healing period. Because of the necessity for daily bandage changes for 2 to 3 weeks when treating these large open wounds, the use of conventional casts or splints is difficult. External skeletal fixation devices have greatly aided in solving this problem.

Treatment

Initial debridement must be meticulous but not too aggressive, with emphasis on removal of obviously dead tissue and foreign matter from both soft tissue and joint spaces. Copious irrigation with Ringer's or saline solution is very important at this time. Addition of 10 percent povidone iodine or 0.2 percent chlorhexidine is favored by some. After adequate debridement, it may be possible to partially close the wound by suturing skin. This can be helpful, but care must be taken to:

1. Leave adequate open area for unimpeded wound drainage. Placement

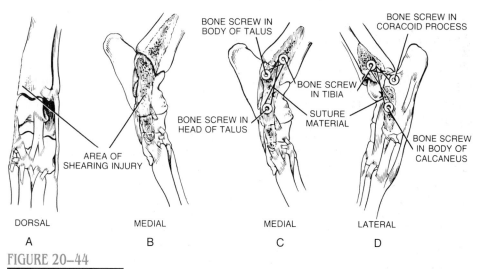

FIGURE 20–44

Shearing injury of the tarsus. (*A* and *B*) The medial malleolus and medial aspects of the proximal tarsal bones have been ground away, resulting in instability and valgus deformity. (*C*) Placement of medial synthetic ligaments.[87] The proximal screw is placed as distally as possible while the tibial cochlea is avoided. One screw is placed in the body of the talus to simulate the short part of the ligament, and another screw is placed in the head of the talus to simulate the long ligament. Two strands of size 0–2 braided polyester suture are placed between each of the screws and tied with the short portion taut in flexion and the long portion taut in extension. (*D*) Placement of lateral synthetic ligaments.[87] Placement is similar to that of the medial side, with the screws placed in the coracoid process and base of the calcaneus.

of Penrose or tube drains under the sutured skin is usually advisable for 2 to 5 days.

2. Avoid closing skin under tension. Serious circulatory stasis develops owing to the tourniquet-like effect of excessive skin tension in the lower limbs.

Several debridements over a number of days may be necessary to adequately remove all devitalized tissue owing to the difficulty in determining viability of badly traumatized tissue.

If there are portions of ligaments, joint capsule, or other tissues that can be sutured to support the joint and to close the synovial membrane, this should be done. Monofilament or synthetic absorbable suture is most trouble free. Re-establishment of the tibiotarsal collateral ligament complex is usually hampered by loss of bone, and small bone screws may have to be used to anchor the synthetic ligament. There is a tendency is to use monofilament wire in this contaminated area, but heavy braided suture is a much more functional ligament and has resulted in very few problems related to suture sinus drainage tracts. Three bone screws are positioned to mimic the normal ligaments as closely as possible (Fig. 20–44C,D). Precise placement of these bone screws for attachment of heavy braided polyester suture and adequate soft-tissue debridement are necessary for successful treatment.[87] The proximal screw is placed as distally in the tibia as possible, bearing in mind that the tibial cochleae is recessed a considerable distance into the distal tibia and can be seen by stressing the tarsus to open the joint. The screw must not enter the joint. The distal screws are placed to simulate the insertion points of the long and short parts of the collateral ligaments.

Medially (Fig. 20–44C), both screws are placed in the talus, the proximal one in the body. This screw should be angled slightly distad to avoid the trochlear sulcus of the talus. The distal screw is placed in the head of the talus, approximately halfway between the base of the medial trochlear ridge and the distal articular surface. Laterally (Fig. 20–44D) the screws are similarly placed in the calcaneus. The proximal screw goes into the base of the coracoid process, and the distal screw is placed halfway between the distal base of the coracoid process and the distal articular surface. Double strands of heavy braided polyester suture (size 0–2) are placed between the screws. The short ligament should be moderately taut in flexion and the long portion taut in extension. The sutures are tied tightly enough to stabilize the joint, but motion without binding should still be possible. The long ligament is tied with the joint in extension, and the short with the joint flexed. Washers can be used on the screws to prevent the suture from slipping over the head of the screw.

Treatment of the open wound is simplified by use of transarticular external skeletal fixation (Kirschner-Ehmer splint) to stabilize the joint (Fig. 20–45A, B). Fixation is maintained until granulation tissue has covered the defect, usually three to four weeks. Sterile laparotomy sponges soaked in povidone iodine or chlorhexidine solution are loosely bandaged to the limb for several days, and debridement is repeated daily or every other day until all dead tissue is removed. The wound must be kept moist and provision made for adequate drainage of exudate.[88] Moist gauze with copious absorbent padding and dressing changes are used daily until healthy granulation covers the wound. At this point, nonadherent dressings, either dry or with antibacterial ointments, and minimal absorbent padding are used in place of the moist dressings. Intervals between dressing changes can gradually be spread out as discharge lessens. The wound must be kept protected until it is well epithelialized, which may take up to 10 to 12 weeks.

Aftercare

When granulation tissue completely covers the wound, but not before three weeks postoperatively, the external fixator is removed. An elastic support bandage should be maintained for another three weeks with very restricted activity. Normal exercise is not allowed until the 8th to 12th week, depending on the stability achieved. Loosening of the bone screws and skin irritation from the screw head are both indications for removing the screws. This should not be done before three to four months postoperatively if possible. Failure to stabilize the joint adequately will result in degenerative joint disease and poor function. In such a situation arthrodesis offers the best chance of restoring function.

OSTEOCHONDRITIS DISSECANS OF THE TALUS

OCD occurs in the same canine population as do the other manifestations of osteochondrosis, although the Rottweiler is overrepresented (see Chapter 18). The disease may be bilateral and may affect either the medial (most common)

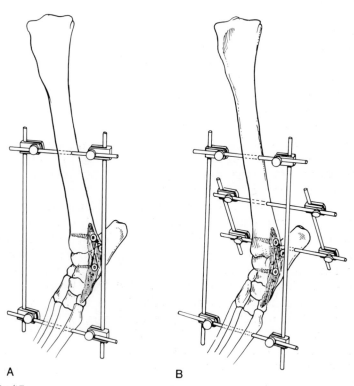

A　　　　　　　　　　B

FIGURE 20–45

(A) A simple external skeletal fixation splint used to support and protect a medial tarsocrural ligament repair in small breeds. (B) A stiffer external fixator frame for support of ligamentous repair in large breeds.

or lateral ridge of the talus. Early surgical removal of the semidetached cartilage flap is essential for good results. Degenerative joint disease may ensue after surgery because of instability or incongruity of the joint following removal of a large flap. If the flap is large enough to be stabilized, every effort should be made to do so in order to minimize postoperative instability.

Clinical Signs

Hindlimb lameness is characterized by a shortened stride. Often there is hyperextension at the tarsocrural joint. Medial joint effusion and thickening of the tarsus on the medial aspect of the joint develop as degenerative changes progress within the joint. Less effusion and soft-tissue changes are appreciated when the lateral ridge of the talus is involved. Pain may be manifested on flexion and extension of the joint, which may also show a decreased range of motion in flexion. Crepitus is occasionally present.

Diagnosis

Radiographs in the extended dorsoplantar and flexed lateral position will reveal a defect in the medial ridge of the trochlea (Figs. 20–46A,B and 20–47). Free ossicles may also be seen occasionally. Lateral lesions are much more difficult to demonstrate owing to the superimposition of the calcaneus in conventional craniocaudal views. Caudocranial-mediolateral oblique views are usually helpful (Fig. 20–46C). Lateral lesions are seen predominantly in Rottweilers.

Surgical Technique

A medial approach to the joint with osteotomy of the malleolus is necessary in some large lesions for adequate exposure. There may be problems in

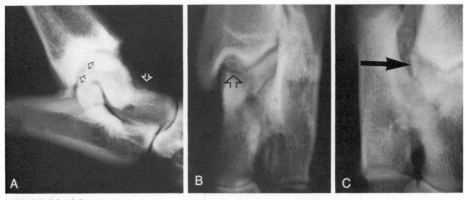

FIGURE 20–46

Osteochondritis dissecans of the talus. (A) In this chronic case many signs of degenerative joint disease are present, such as osteophytes and subchondral sclerosis. Note the flattening of the ridge of the talus (black arrows) and the free osteochondral fragment within the joint (white arrow); lateromedial view. (B) A large fragment can be seen on the medial ridge of the talus in this craniocaudal-lateromedial oblique view. (C) A displaced fragment of the lateral ridge of the talus is visualized in this caudocranial-mediolateral oblique view.

FIGURE 20–47

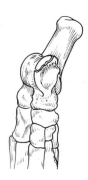

Osteochondritis dissecans lesion on the medial ridge of the talus. The lesion can be located anywhere on the ridge but is most likely to be centrally placed, as here, or more proximally.

achieving proper osteotomy, reduction, and stabilization of the malleolus owing to the inflammatory proliferation of soft tissues present in chronic cases. Therefore we find it helpful to explore the joint with arthrotomies cranial and caudal to the collateral ligament.[5] If exposure is inadequate owing to lesion size or position, the malleolus must then be osteotomized. When screw fixation of the osteotomy is anticipated, predrilling the screw hole in the malleolus prior to osteotomy ensures accurate reduction and fixation of the malleolus. Lag screw fixation of a lateral ridge fragment is facilitated by a medial malleolar osteotomy approach, as is visualization of a proximal ridge lesion.[89] If the lesion cannot be fixed in place, the loose cartilage fragment is removed and minimal curettage is performed, in order to minimize the amount of instability produced.

AFTERCARE ■ A snug, padded bandage is maintained for two weeks, and normal exercise is not allowed until four to six weeks postoperatively.

PROGNOSIS ■ Surgical treatment of osteochondritis dissecans of the talus resulted in a worse score for function and radiographic changes than did nonsurgical treatment in one small series of cases (11 dogs, 17 joints: 11 surgical, 6 nonsurgical).[90] All dogs had significant degenerative joint disease clinically and radiographically. Although numbers are few in this series, the message is clear: Surgical treatment must be done early, and the lesion must be small for surgical treatment to be worthwhile. In any case the prognosis is not encouraging, and the owner should be forewarned regarding long-term function of the dog.

LUXATION OF THE TENDON OF THE SUPERFICIAL DIGITAL FLEXOR MUSCLE

Spontaneous rupture of the medial or lateral retinaculum of this tendon as it crosses the tuber calcanei allows the tendon to luxate medially or laterally.[86] The Sheltie and Collie breeds seem overrepresented in our cases.

Surgical repair that is made before extensive fibrosis develops is very successful. Chronic tendinitis can cause marked changes in the tendon and decrease chances for success.

Clinical Signs

Lameness is not dramatic and may be intermittent. Moderate swelling on either side of the calcaneus can be noted, and a distinct popping sensation

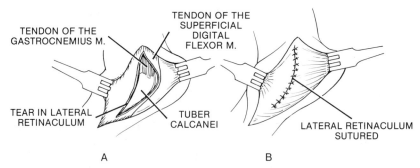

TENDON OF THE
GASTROCNEMIUS M.

TENDON OF THE
SUPERFICIAL
DIGITAL
FLEXOR M.

TEAR IN LATERAL
RETINACULUM

TUBER
CALCANEI

LATERAL RETINACULUM
SUTURED

A   B

FIGURE 20–48

(A) Medial luxation of the tendon of the superficial digital flexor muscle follows tearing of the lateral retinaculum at the calcaneus. (B) Surgical repair consists of suturing the retinaculum with nonabsorbable suture material.

will be felt as the hock is flexed and extended. The tendon can sometimes be palpated in the luxated position and then reduced as the hock is extended. Flexion then results in reluxation.

Surgical Repair

An incision is made along the calcaneus on the side opposite the direction of the luxation, curving from the distal calcanean tendon toward the calcaneus (Fig. 20–48). The tendon is reduced, and interrupted nonabsorbable sutures are placed from the edge of the tendon to adjoining retinacular tissue to maintain the tendon in the reduced position.

AFTERCARE ■ A short lateral splint is applied for three weeks (see Chapter 19). Normal exercise can be resumed four weeks postoperatively.

PROGNOSIS ■ Good function can be expected. We have seen Shelties break down in the opposite limb within a few weeks of the first injury.

AVULSION OF THE GASTROCNEMIUS TENDON

The common calcanean tendon, or Achilles' mechanism, consists of three tendons that insert on the tuber calcanei of the talus: the gastrocnemius; the common tendon of the biceps femoris, semitendinosus, and gracilis muscles; and the tendon of the superficial digital flexor muscle.

The gastrocnemius tendon is the largest of this group and the most powerful extensor of the tarsocrural joint. It can be avulsed from the tuber by normal activity, without outside trauma. Most injuries develop during running and presumably occur as the animal pushes off the limb with the foot firmly planted. Affected dogs are primarily from the large sporting and working breeds and are usually 5 years of age and up.

These facts suggest that degenerative changes in the tendon may play a part in the pathogenesis of this injury, but this is only speculative at this time. Very few reports exist on this condition.[91] Owing to contracture of the muscle, any attempt at nonsurgical treatment will invariably result in permanent deformity. It is necessary to surgically reattach the tendon to the bone to restore function.

Clinical Signs

The lameness seen with this injury is severe and nonweight-bearing for several days, but within one to two weeks the animal starts using the leg again. During weight-bearing at this time the stifle will be seen to be slightly extended, the tarsocrural (hock) joint moderately flexed, and the digits are flexed.

The position of the digits result in a crab-like stance. Because the superficial digital flexor tendon is intact, it is forced to take a longer course to reach the digits when the hock joint is flexed beyond the normal standing angle. The result is as if the digital flexor muscle was contracted, and so the digits stay flexed during weight-bearing. They can easily be manually extended if the tarsocrural joint is extended with the stifle flexed.

Shortly after the injury regional edema and pain predominate the physical findings. Later the region becomes engulfed in fibroplasia and the gastrocnemius muscle contracts. Often, careful palpation will reveal the end of the tendon 2 to 3 cm proximal to the tuber and deep to the superficial digital flexor tendon. The distal end of the tendon mushrooms and becomes very firm on palpation owing to the fibroplasia. Eventually the gap between the tuber and the tendon becomes filled with fibrous tissue and gives the impression during palpation that the tendon is intact. Radiographs are useful at this time in establishing the diagnosis.

Radiographic Signs

During the acute phase, edema of the soft tissues will be appreciated, and it may be possible to visualize the retracted tendon if soft-tissue radiographic technique is used. Small avulsed bone fragments near the tuber calcanei are diagnostic (Fig. 20–49A). More chronic cases have visible roughening of the tuber and increased soft-tissue density in the region between the tuber and the retracted tendon (Fig. 20–49B).

Surgical Technique

A lateral paramedian approach is made over the distal tendon and tuber calcanei.[5] The lateral retinaculum of the superficial digital flexor tendon is incised to allow medial retraction of the tendon. In acute injuries the avulsed end of the gastrocnemius tendon will be immediately evident. The tendon is debrided to create a smooth end for suturing. In chronic cases considerable debridement is necessary to free the tendon and tuber from the fibroplasia. The tuber should be cleared of all tissue prior to suturing and the tendinous end should be resected proximally until normal tendinous tissue is identified. With moderate tension it should be just possible to bring the cut end into apposition with the tuber when the stifle and hock joints are at normal standing angles.

Medial and lateral bone tunnels are drilled from the center of the tuber toward the medial and lateral cortices (Fig. 20–50B,C). These holes should emerge in an area where they will not interfere with gliding of the superficial

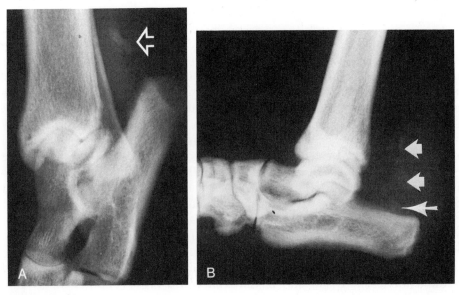

FIGURE 20-49

Avulsion of the tendon of the gastrocnemius muscle at the tuber calcanei. *(A)* A large bone fragment is visible here. The position of the fragment is an indication of how far the tendon has retracted. *(B)* Two avulsed bone fragments are seen with the retracted tendon *(broad arrows)*. A roughened area on the tuber calcanei *(narrow arrow)* indicates the area of avulsion. Marked soft tissue density in the area suggests a chronic course.

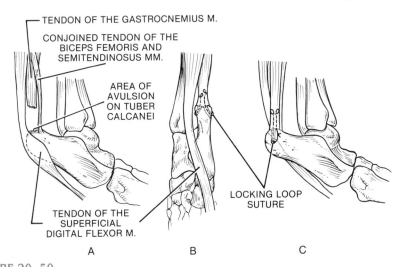

FIGURE 20-50

(A) Avulsion of the tendon of the gastrocnemius muscle from the tuber calcanei. Note that the tendon of the superficial digital flexor muscle and the conjoined tendons of the biceps femoris and semitendinosus muscles are intact and partially support the tarsocrural joint. *(B and C)* The tendon of the gastrocnemius muscle is reattached to the tuber calcanei with locking-loop sutures (see Fig. 19–1) of size 0–2 nonabsorbable suture secured through bone tunnels in the calcaneus.

digital flexor tendon. Locking-loop sutures (see Fig. 19–6) are placed medially and laterally in the tendon. Suture material should be large, size 0 to 2, and preferably monofilament nylon or polypropylene for ease of handling in the tendon. Braided polyester is also acceptable, but monofilament stainless steel wire should be avoided as it will quickly fracture owing to movement in this area. One end of each suture is then passed through a bone tunnel, the hock is extended and the stifle flexed to relax the gastrocnemius, and each suture is tied over the bone to its opposite end. The retinaculum of the superficial digital flexor tendon is sutured as in Figure 20–48B, and the remaining tissues are closed in layers.

AFTERCARE ■ A short leg lateral splint (see Fig. 19–13) is applied for four weeks. It is not necessary to immobilize the stifle joint. The splint is followed by a Robert Jones bandage (see Fig. 19–17) for 7 to 10 days. Exercise is severely restricted until eight weeks postoperatively, then slowly increased to normal at 12 weeks.

PROGNOSIS ■ Very good function has been obtained in our cases. Considerable periosteal bony proliferation has been seen in some, but this abates and remodels with time and does not cause permanent changes.

TARSOCRURAL ARTHRODESIS

Indications for arthrodesis of the hock joint are not uncommon in small animal practice under these circumstances:

1. Severe shearing injury.
2. Degenerative joint disease (most commonly due to osteochondritis dissecans).
3. Chronic instability or hyperextension.
4. Comminuted intra-articular fractures.
5. Irreparable injury of the calcanean tendon apparatus.
6. Sciatic nerve palsy when combined with transposition of the long digital extensor tendon.[92]

Assuming there are no disease conditions of the hip or stifle, function of the fused limb is satisfactory. These joints must flex more than normal to compensate for fusion at the hock level. If they do not function normally, the leg will be circumducted markedly during the forward swing phase of gait. As with all arthrodeses, additional strain is placed on adjacent joints and may lead to degenerative joint disease, particularly in the more distal tarsal joints.

Surgical fusion of this joint is a severe challenge to the surgeon because of the magnitude and orientation of the forces of weight-bearing. Additionally, the small size of the bones of the tarsus impose limitations on the size and shape of implants used in internal fixation. Failure rates, as high as 50 percent in our hands,[93] have led us to be much more aggressive in using more and larger implants and in supporting them with external casts and splints until fusion is certain. It also seems useful to promote fusion of the talocalcaneal joint by curettage and crossing of the joint by one of the screws or pins. Lag screw, bone plate, and external skeletal fixation techniques are all applicable when properly executed.

Surgical Technique

SCREW FIXATION

Single lag screw fixation is suitable only for cats and dogs under 8 to 10 kg body weight. All others should receive two screws. The joint is approached medially by malleolar osteotomy.[5] The malleolus and medial collateral ligaments are detached, and the bone is cut into very small chips with a rongeur and used as bone graft to supplement autogenous cancellous bone from the proximal tibia.

The functional angle for dogs is typically between 135 and 145 degrees; in cats it is 115 to 125 degrees. This angle should be carefully checked in the opposite limb preoperatively. In Figure 20–51A, the angle chosen is 135 degrees; the complementary angle is 45 degrees. Since it is most convenient to cut the distal tibia at 90 degrees to its long axis, the talus is cut at a 45-degree angle to the axis of the tarsus-foot. Considerable bone must be removed from the tibia because of the depth of the cochlea. The cartilage can also be removed with power burs, curettes, or rongeurs by following the bony contours (Fig. 20–51B).

In some cases the fibula will prevent apposition of the tibia and talus after bone and cartilage removal. It is then necessary to resect the lateral malleolus or perform a supramalleolar section of the fibula through a separate short lateral incision.

Initial fixation is obtained by two Kirschner wires driven across the contact surfaces in a plantarolateral direction (Fig. 20–51C). Drilling for the lag screw can then proceed without motion of the contact surfaces. Screws of 4.5 mm are appropriate for animals of 15 to 18 kg or larger, and 3.5-mm screws are ideal for smaller animals. Full-threaded screws are preferred because of their ease of removal.

The glide hole is drilled in the tibia first (Fig. 20–51C,D). The tap hole is then drilled through the talus and calcaneus. Placement of 4.5-mm screws is illustrated in Figure 20–51. The glide hole is started at a point on the tibia 2 to 2.5 cm from the end of the bone and at an angle of 15 to 20 degrees from the tibial sagittal plane. The hole is measured with the depth gauge and is tapped, and a screw of appropriate length is inserted and tightened (Fig. 20–5E,F). An alternate technique consists of drilling the 3.2-mm tap hole first, then enlarging the tibial hole with the 4.5-mm glide drill. A second hole is drilled from the cranial aspect of the distal tibia into the tuber calcanei with a tap drill sized for the screw diameter selected. Soft tissue in the space between the distal tibia and calcaneus must be protected. *Both* bones are tapped and the screw is inserted. This positional screw protects the lag screw from bending loads. In dogs over 10 kg body weight it is preferable to insert two screws across the joint (Fig. 20–51G). In this situation a single Kirschner wire is placed between the two screws. Autogenous cancellous bone graft (Chapter 3) is packed into and around the contact surfaces. The Kirschner wires are left in place.

AFTERCARE ■ External support is *imperative* to prevent bending loads on the screws. A short lateral splint or cylinder cast (see Figs. 19–10, 19–13) is maintained for six to eight weeks, or until radiographic signs of fusion are evident. Exercise is severely restricted until radiographic fusion, then slowly

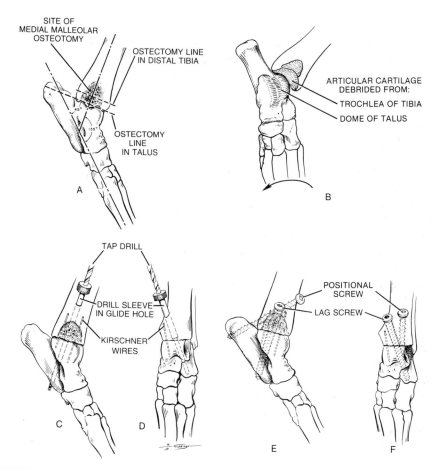

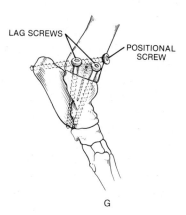

FIGURE 20–51

Arthrodesis of the tarsocrural joint by screw fixation. (A) The angle chosen here for the fusion is 135 degrees. The complementary angle of 45 degrees also describes the angle to be cut through the talus, since the tibia is best cut 90 degrees to its axis. The joint is exposed medially by a malleolar osteotomy.[5] (B) An alternative method of removing articular cartilage involves debridement with a power bur or curettes, following the normal contour of the articular surface. (C and D) Temporary fixation is obtained by two Kirschner wires placed across the joint at an angle. A 4.5-mm (or 3.5-mm) glide hole has been drilled, and the 3.2-mm (or 2.0-mm) tap drill is inserted through a drill sleeve. The drill penetrates the plantarolateral cortex of the calcaneus near its base. (E and F) The hole is tapped and a screw of appropriate length and diameter is inserted. A second hole is drilled from the cranial aspect of the distal tibia into the tuber calcanei with a tap drill sized for the screw diameter selected. Soft tissue in the space between the distal tibia and calcaneus must be protected. Both bones are tapped and the screw inserted. (G) In dogs over 10 kg body weight it is preferable to insert two screws across the joint. In this situation a single Kirschner wire is placed between the two screws.

increased to return to normal six weeks later. Implants should be removed routinely about six months postoperatively. Because of bending loads exerted on the fusion site, micromotion eventually results in screw breakage, which causes irritation and pain. Fully threaded screws are more easily removed than are partially threaded cancellous screws.

BONE PLATE FIXATION

Tarsocrural arthrodesis with a *cranially* placed bone plate is possible if one screw is placed through the plate and into the calcaneus to act as a positional screw (Fig. 20–52). All four cortices are tapped, as the purpose of this screw is to prevent bending loads on the plate. Care must be taken to avoid extending the plate beyond the proximal intertarsal joint. Autogenous cancellous bone graft (Chapter 3) is packed around the arthrodesis site before closing the soft tissues. Aftercare is identical to that described above for screw fixation.

Tarsocrural arthrodesis with a *laterally* placed plate (Fig. 20–53) is possible only with a plate that allows a large number of screws/unit of length, such as the AO/ASIF Veterinary Cuttable Plate (Synthes [USA], Paoli, PA). Because the plate is loaded on edge, it is very resistant to the bending loads of this joint. Despite this mechanical advantage, such techniques have not been satisfactory in the past owing to inability to place a sufficient number of screws distal to the arthrodesis site.[93] The Veterinary Cuttable Plate (VCP) solves this difficulty by the number of screw holes available. Additionally the plates are available in both 1 and 1.5 mm thickness and can be stacked to increase their thickness and stiffness.

In Figure 20–53 a 1.5-mm thick plate and 2.7-mm screws are used, following the method of Sumner-Smith and Kuzma.[94] The distal one-third of the fibula is resected, and the joint surfaces are prepared as in Figure 20–51. A lag screw (3.5- to 6.5-mm diameter) is placed across the joint to provide compression at the arthrodesis site, from the calcaneus distally, through the talus, and into the tibia proximally (Fig. 20–53A). Drilling the glide hole from the talus to the calcaneus before reduction ensures accurate placement of this

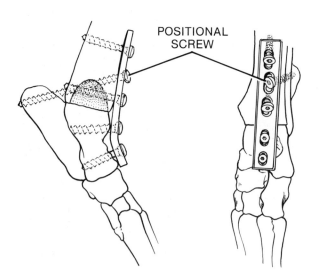

POSITIONAL SCREW

FIGURE 20–52

Tarsocrural arthrodesis with a cranially placed bone plate is possible if one screw is placed through the plate and into the calcaneus to act as a positional screw. All four cortices are tapped. Care must be taken to avoid extending the plate beyond the proximal intertarsal joint.

hole. In small breeds, the lag screw may be passed from the distal plate hole. The plate is molded to the tibia and around the calcaneus distally, where a sharp bend and slight twist are necessary to fit the bone closely.

Screw placement starts distally with two screws in the calcaneus. The next screw is placed in the distal tibia and is positioned eccentrically in the plate hole to provide compression. Two more screws are similarly placed in the tibia, taking care to avoid the lag screw. The rest of the screws are placed in the center of the plate holes, and the lag screw is retightened. Autogenous cancellous bone graft (Chapter 3) is packed around the arthrodesis site before closing the tissues.

Aftercare is exactly as described above for screw fixation.

EXTERNAL SKELETAL FIXATION

Fixation by means of the Kirschner-Ehmer apparatus (Fig. 20–54) is particularly applicable to open or shearing injuries of the hock. Open luxation with comminuted fractures of the tibial trochlea or condyles of the talus is also a relatively common injury best treated by arthrodesis. Minimal metal at the area of contamination lessens infection problems, and all the metal can easily be removed.

The contact surfaces are prepared as already described after adequate soft-tissue debridement (see Fig. 20–51A). A Steinmann pin is driven through the calcaneus and talus into the distal tibia with the joint at the desired angle (Fig. 20–54A). If the pin follows the medullary canal, it is driven into the proximal metaphyseal region. If the pin penetrates the tibial cortex, it is driven completely through the cortex and is cut about 1 cm from the calcaneus.

An alternative method consists of driving the pin from the proximal tibia as described for fracture repair in Chapter 7. After penetrating the calcaneus, the pin is pulled from the distal end until the proximal end is below the proximal articular surface of the tibia. Transfixation pins are driven through

FIGURE 20–53

Tarsocrural arthrodesis with a laterally placed plate is possible only with a plate that allows a large number of screws/unit of length, such as the AO/ASIF Veterinary Cuttable Plate (Synthes [USA], Paoli, PA). Here, a 1.5-mm thick plate and 2.7-mm screws are used, following the method of Sumner-Smith and Kuzma.[94] At least one screw must cross the joint as a lag screw, to provide compression at the arthrodesis site. The distal one-third of the fibula is resected to allow lateral placement of the plate, which is molded around the calcaneus distally.

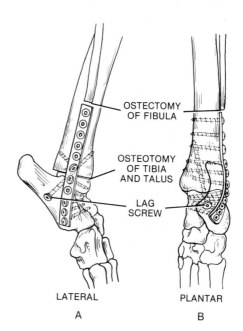

OSTECTOMY OF FIBULA

OSTEOTOMY OF TIBIA AND TALUS

LAG SCREW

LATERAL

A

PLANTAR

B

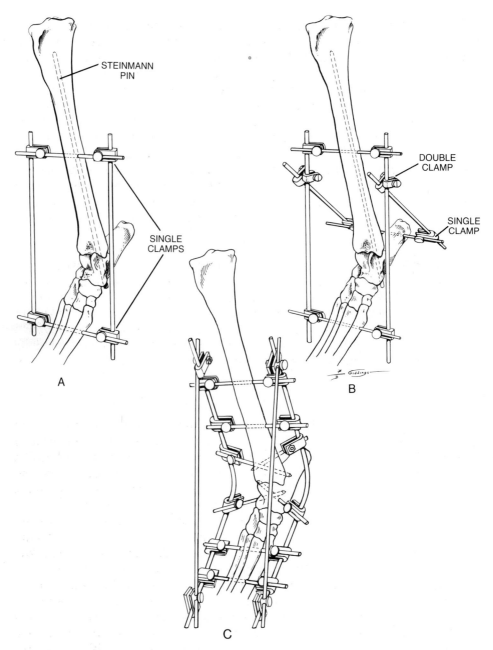

FIGURE 20–54

Arthrodesis of the tarsocrural joint by external skeletal fixation. (A) The joint surfaces are prepared as in Figure 20–51A or B. A Steinmann pin is driven from the calcaneus into the proximal tibia with the joint at the selected angle. Transfixation pins are driven through the tibia and metatarsal bones. These pins are connected with bilateral rods secured by single clamps. (B) Additional stability in large dogs is provided by a second transfixation pin in the calcaneus. This pin is connected to the first set of connecting rods with single clamps distally and double clamps proximally. (C) When no intramedullary pin is used, a more rigid frame is used to prevent bending loads at the arthrodesis site. One of the easier methods is shown here, using a curved connecting rod to eliminate the need for double clamps. Using half pins for the middle sets of fixation pins simplifies the problem of fitting the pins to the connecting rods on both sides when drill guides are not available. At least one of the fixation pins should cross the tarsocrural joint to neutralize shear forces.

the tibia and through the bases of the metatarsals. These pins are connected by single clamps and connecting rods. A large autogenous cancellous bone graft taken from the proximal tibia will significantly speed healing and can be used in a contaminated site. Fixation can be made even more rigid in large breeds by placing a transfixation pin through the calcaneus, and connecting it with double clamps to the proximal ends of the other connecting rods (Fig. 20–54B). When no intramedullary pin is used, and in larger breeds, a more rigid frame is used to prevent bending loads at the arthrodesis site. One of the easier methods is shown in Figure 20–54C, using a curved connecting rod to eliminate the need for double clamps. Using half pins for the middle sets of fixation pins simplifies the problem of fitting the pins to the connecting rods on both sides when drill guides are not available. At least one of the fixation pins should cross the tarsocrural joint to control shearing motion at the arthrodesis site.

AFTERCARE ■ This apparatus allows open treatment of soft-tissue injuries, as for shearing injuries. Healing of the arthrodesis will be slow and fixation may need to be maintained for 10 to 12 weeks or until radiographic signs of fusion are present. Exercise should be restricted to the house, a small pen, or a leash until the apparatus is removed. The transfixation pins are removed when good fusion is present, but the Steinmann pin should be left in place for four to six months to absorb some of the bending stress on the arthrodesis.

HYPEREXTENSION WITH SUBLUXATION OF THE PROXIMAL INTERTARSAL JOINT

This is a common injury of the tarsus in small animals. The majority of affected animals have no history of known trauma. Although hyperextension (dorsiflexion) is seen in all breeds of dogs, the Shetland sheepdog[94A] and Collie seem to be predisposed, while the injury is apparently unrecorded in the cat. Affected animals fall into two groups: highly athletic animals such as racing greyhounds or coursing dogs, and obese, poorly conditioned dogs.

Although the entire proximal intertarsal joint is affected, the primary instability is at the calcaneoquartal joint. Stability of the talocentral joint distinguishes this injury from complete luxation, described below (Fig. 20–56). Tearing or avulsion of the plantar ligament between the fourth tarsal and calcaneus (Fig. 20–55A,B) is the primary injury. Loss of this tension band structure results in a characteristic hyperextension and variable degrees of plantigrade stance. Primary repair of the soft-tissue injury or cast fixation is rarely successful and arthrodesis of the calcaneoquartal joint is recommended. Arthrodesis of this joint causes little functional disability, although racing animals rarely return to the track. The tension band wire fixation described here is applicable to any size animal and is relatively simple to perform.

Clinical Signs

The degree of plantigrade stance varies, the worst cases appearing to be standing on the calcaneus bone, while many have only 30 to 40 degrees of angulation. Pain and soft-tissue swelling are not severe, and most animals tolerate palpation with little show of resentment. The joint is unstable only on the plantar aspect. Complete luxation with more general instability can occur and is discussed later in the chapter.

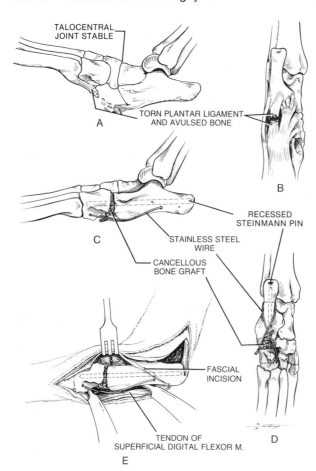

TALOCENTRAL
JOINT STABLE

TORN PLANTAR LIGAMENT
AND AVULSED BONE

A

B

C

RECESSED
STEINMANN PIN

STAINLESS STEEL
WIRE

CANCELLOUS
BONE GRAFT

FASCIAL
INCISION

D

TENDON OF
SUPERFICIAL DIGITAL FLEXOR M.

E

FIGURE 20–55

Arthrodesis of the calcaneoquartal joint for hyperextension with subluxation of the proximal intertarsal joint. *(A and B)* Tearing or avulsion of the plantar ligament of the calcaneoquartal joint allows hyperextension (dorsiflexion) at the proximal intertarsal joint. *(C and D)* The joint is exposed by a plantarolateral approach with medial retraction of the superficial digital flexor tendon.[5] The calcaneoquartal joint cartilage is debrided, and an autogenous cancellous bone graft is inserted. A tension band wire (18–20 gauge) is placed between the calcaneus and plantar tubercle of the fourth tarsal but not tightened. A small Steinmann pin (⁵⁄₆₄ to ⅛ inch in diameter) is driven through the calcaneus into the fourth tarsal and then countersunk beneath the cartilage of the tuber calcanei. The tension band wire is now tightened. *(E)* Plantarolateral view of the completed fixation. The superficial digital extensor tendon is retracted medially.

Diagnosis

A mediolateral radiograph, with the joint stressed in extension, will confirm the site of instability and may demonstrate avulsed fragments of bone from either the fourth tarsal bone or the base of the calcaneus (Fig. 20–55A). Note that the talocentral joint remains unaffected by the instability of the calcaneoquartal joint.

Surgical Technique

The joint is exposed by a plantarolateral approach, with medial retraction of the tendon of the superficial digital flexor.[5] Fragments of the torn or avulsed ligament are excised to allow access to the joint. Articular cartilage is debrided on the joint surfaces with a pneumatic surgical bur or by curettage. A hole is drilled transversely through the midportion of the calcaneus and the plantar tubercle of the fourth tarsal bone (Fig. 20–55C,D). An 18 to 20 gauge (1.0 to 0.8 mm) stainless steel wire is threaded through both holes in a figure-8 manner. A pilot hole for the intramedullary pin is drilled through the shaft of the calcaneus, favoring the dorsal aspect of the medullary canal. This hole is best made with a bone drill rather than a pin because of the extreme hardness of this bone. Autogenous cancellous bone graft from the proximal tibia is placed into the joint space with the joint extended to open it. A single pin (from ⁵⁄₆₄ to ⅛ inch [1.9 to 3.2 mm] in diameter) is started at the proximal calcaneus and driven to the distal end of the fourth tarsal bone. The pin is retracted 1 cm, cut, and countersunk beneath the surface of the tuber calcanei to protect the superficial digital flexor tendon.

The tension band wire is now tightened by twisting in both halves of the figure 8 (Fig. 20–55D,E). The twists are cut and bent flat against the bone. The lateral retinaculum of the superficial digital flexor tendon is sutured as in Figure 20–48B to prevent its luxation and the skin is closed routinely.

AFTERCARE ■ Although external casts or splints are not required, a padded bandage is useful during the first postoperative week. Exercise is restricted to the house, a small pen, or a leash until radiographic signs of fusion are noted, usually six to eight weeks postoperatively. At this time, activity can be slowly increased to normal at 12 weeks.

HYPEREXTENSION WITH LUXATION OF THE PROXIMAL INTERTARSAL JOINT

A much less common injury than subluxation, this luxation (Fig. 20–56A) is usually a result of severe trauma and may be complicated by fractures of the tarsal bones. Arthrodesis of the joint is the preferred method of fixation, since primary repair of the ligaments is fruitless. Function is excellent with this fusion. Because the entire proximal intertarsal joint is involved, bone plate fixation results in more stable fixation of the talocalcaneal portion of the joint than does tension band wire fixation as shown in Figure 20–55. This method can be modified to provide additional stability of the talocalcaneal joint by adding the medial screw and wire fixation shown in Figure 20–57D and E. External skeletal fixators are also adaptable to this procedure.

Clinical Signs and Diagnosis

This condition is differentiated from subluxation by instability of the joint in all planes and is confirmed radiographically by marked dorsal displacement of the distal segment rather than hinging at the dorsal aspect of the proximal intertarsal joint.

Surgical Technique: Bone Plate Fixation

The joint is exposed by a lateral incision from the tuber calcanei to the base of the metatarsals. Articular cartilage is removed from the entire joint. The lateral side of the base of the calcaneus must be flattened to allow firm seating of the bone plate. This may involve sacrifice of a portion of the insertion of the long part of the lateral collateral ligament, which can be reattached by a suture running beneath the plate.

A 7-hole plate of a 3.5- or 2.7-mm screw size is typically used (see Fig. 20–56B,C). Three screws are placed proximally, one penetrating the calcaneus and talus and the rest attached only to the calcaneus. One screw spans the tarsus distal to the proximal intertarsal joint, and three screws are placed in metatarsals 4 and 5. Autogenous cancellous bone graft (Chapter 3) is used in the joint space.

AFTERCARE ■ External support is advisable because the plate is not in the tension band position. A short lateral splint or cylinder cast (see Figs. 19–10 and 19–

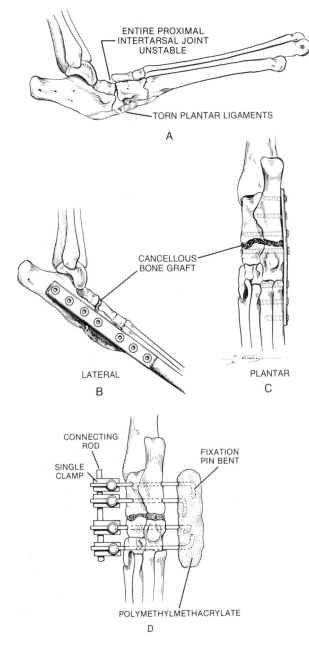

ENTIRE PROXIMAL
INTERTARSAL JOINT
UNSTABLE

TORN PLANTAR LIGAMENTS

A

CANCELLOUS
BONE GRAFT

LATERAL

B

PLANTAR

C

CONNECTING
ROD

SINGLE
CLAMP

FIXATION
PIN BENT

POLYMETHYLMETHACRYLATE

D

FIGURE 20–56

Arthrodesis for hyperextension with luxation of the proximal intertarsal joint. *(A)* Complete luxation is differentiated from subluxation by marked dorsal displacement of the distal tarsus at the proximal intertarsal joint. *(B* and *C)* Following curettage of the proximal intertarsal joint. Bone plate fixation requires smoothing of the lateral surface of the calcaneus and base of the fifth metatarsal. Plates are usually of the 3.5- or 2.7-mm screw size. At least three screws are placed in the calcaneus. The No. 3 screw is angled to engage the head of the talus, and number 4 screw spans the tarsus. The distal screws are placed in metatarsals 4 and 5. *(D)* External skeletal fixation is applicable to this surgery. Illustrated are both the use of conventional clamp fixation *(left)*, and the use of polymethylmethacrylate dental tray cement as a connecting rod *(right)*. Fixation pins are bent for more stability in the cement. See text for details.

13) is maintained until radiographic signs are present, usually six to eight weeks.

Because the plate crosses the tarsometatarsal joint, it will always loosen as a result of joint motion, which causes the metatarsal screws to migrate. The plate should be left in place at least four months, preferably six months. If the distal metatarsal screws loosen before this, it is advisable to remove them, but the tarsal screws should be left in until four to six months have passed.

Loss of blood supply to the skin as a result of the original or surgical trauma may lead to skin necrosis over the plate. This should be treated as an open granulating wound, with the plate left in place. The plate is removed about four months postoperatively if fusion is good, and the skin defect is grafted or allowed to granulate.

Surgical Technique: External Skeletal Fixator

Stabilization of this arthrodesis is also possible by means of an external skeletal fixator (Kirschner-Ehmer splint, Kirschner Medical Inc., Timonium, MD). This method is advantageous when there are open wounds associated with the injury and when bone plate fixation is not available. The fixation pins can be connected conventionally with clamps, as on the left side of Figure 20–56D, or by means of polymethylmethacrylate cement (dental tray cement or hoof repair acrylic), as on the right side of Figure 20–56D.

The joint is approached from a dorsal incision centered over the joint, and articular cartilage is removed by power bur or curettage. Autogenous cancellous bone from the proximal tibia is placed in the joint space (see Chapter 3). Two fixation pins are placed transversely in the calcaneus and talus. If the fixation will use connecting clamps, care must be taken to ensure that the pins are spaced widely enough to allow placement of the clamps.

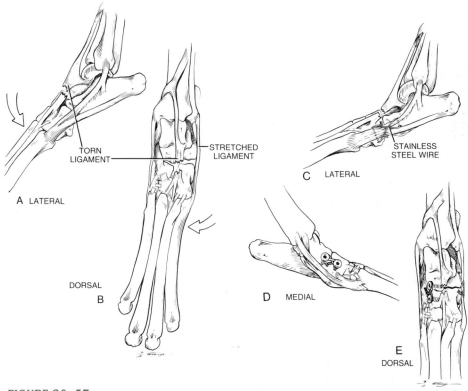

FIGURE 20–57

Surgical repair of proximal intertarsal subluxation with dorsal instability. (A and B) Excessive flexion and often varus deformity occur when the dorsal ligaments are ruptured. (C) Lateral instability is stabilized with stainless steel wire (20 to 22 gauge) placed through drill holes in the bony prominences of the distolateral calcaneus and proximolateral fourth tarsal bones. (D and E) Dorsomedial instability is stabilized by placing stainless steel wire (20 to 22 gauge) between screws placed in the base of the talus and central tarsal bones.

Two more pins are placed distally in the tarsal bones. If there is not sufficient room to place both pins in the tarsus, the distal pin is driven through the bases of the metatarsal bones. The pins are then connected by clamps or cement. If cement is to be used, the fixation pins are bent at a right angle at the protruding end in order to give more surface contact for the cement. The latter is mixed until reaching a dough-like consistency, then molded into a rod approximately ¾-inch (2 cm) diameter and hand packed onto the fixation pins. The arthrodesis site must be stabilized until the cement has hardened, typically 8 to 10 minutes from the start of mixing.

AFTERCARE ■ The animal is closely confined and the fixator maintained until radiographic signs of bony fusion are well defined. This will typically take 8 to 10 weeks. Exercise is slowly returned to normal four weeks after fixator removal.

PROXIMAL INTERTARSAL SUBLUXATION WITH DORSAL INSTABILITY

This injury is much less common than hyperextension at the proximal intertarsal joint. Although the primary damage is to the dorsal ligaments (Fig. 20–57A,B), there is often a medial or lateral instability, with varus deformity resulting from lateral instability being very common.

The condition is evidently caused by overstress (that is, self-induced), because outside trauma is rarely reported by the owner, although some animals have sustained this injury while climbing woven wire fences. Diagnosis of the condition can be difficult because the subluxation can be demonstrated only by palpation. The dog stands normally because the plantar ligaments are intact, but instability creates inflammation and pain in the joint and causes a mild lameness, which is worse if there is medial or lateral instability superimposed.

Because the dorsal ligaments do not function as tension bands, conservative treatment by casting for three to four weeks is often effective if there is no medial or lateral laxity. The smaller the patient, the more likely is conservative treatment to succeed. In larger breeds and in athletic animals, surgical treatment is more commonly indicated.

Clinical Signs and Diagnosis

There are few clinical signs with this condition other than a mild hindlimb lameness. A physical examination will reveal abnormal flexion at the proximal intertarsal joints. Medial and lateral stability should be tested, and stress-position radiographs should be made to confirm the physical findings. Figure 20–57A,B illustrates dorsolateral instability.

Surgical Technique

Primary surgical repair is indicated when dorsal ligamentous instability is complicated by medial or lateral instability. Surgery becomes even more important in a large athletic dog.

Stabilization from both the medial and lateral sides is usually indicated. The areas are approached by incisions directly over the areas. Medial and dorsal instability can be eliminated by placing stainless steel wire of 20 to 22 gauge (0.8 to 0.6 mm) between screws placed in the talus and central tarsal bones (Fig. 20–57D,E). Articular cartilage of the proximal intertarsal joint is debrided before screw placement, and suturing of any available ligament fragments is useful. Bone grafting is not routinely needed. If there is significant lateral instability, a tension band wire can be added laterally (Fig. 20–57C). Bony projections are available on both the distal calcaneus and proximal fourth tarsal to allow bone tunnels to be drilled for wire placement. Stainless steel wire of 20 to 22 gauge (0.8 to 0.6 mm) is used for the tension band.

AFTERCARE ■ A short lateral splint (see Fig. 19–13) is applied for four weeks, with activity restricted through eight weeks postoperatively. If the joint does not completely fuse, the screw may loosen and back out, thus requiring removal.

LUXATION OF THE HEAD OF THE TALUS

This is an infrequent but very disabling injury (Fig. 20–58A) that is difficult to repair if it is not diagnosed early. Surgical stabilization is quite successful and is indicated in most animals, but closed reduction and casting have been satisfactory in cats and small dogs.

Clinical Signs and Diagnosis

Considerable swelling and deformity of the proximodorsal tarsus is evident, with lameness typified by the animal's carrying the leg. Because of possible concurrent damage of the insertion of the medial collateral ligament, the tarsus should be evaluated for medial instability. Radiographs are necessary to confirm the diagnosis.

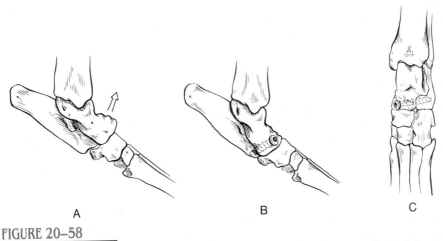

A   B   C

FIGURE 20–58

Luxation of the talus. (A) The head of the talus luxates dorsally. There may also be injury to the insertion of the medial collateral ligament. (B and C) A positional screw is placed distally in the talus to avoid the tarsal sinus. The screw is driven into the calcaneus.

Surgical Technique

The bone is exposed by a proximal extension of the approach to the central tarsal bone.[5] The head of the talus can be reduced after the proximal intertarsal joint is opened by flexion and lateral (varus) stress on the metatarsus. A positional screw is placed between the talus and calcaneus and is placed as distally as possible in the talus to avoid crossing the tarsal sinus (Fig. 20–58B,C). If medial instability remains at the talocentral joint, joint cartilage of the calcaneocentral joint is debrided, and a second bone screw is placed in the medial side of the central tarsal bone. Stainless steel wire is placed around the head of both screws and tightened, similar to the procedure illustrated for distal intertarsal instability in Figure 20–57D,E.

AFTERCARE ■ A short lateral splint (see Fig. 19–13) is applied and maintained for four weeks. Exercise is limited through the eighth postoperative week.

FRACTURE-LUXATION OF THE CENTRAL TARSAL BONE

Unlike most fractures of the central tarsal bone, which are almost exclusively a fracture of the racing greyhound (see Chapter 8), fracture-luxation of this bone (Fig. 20–59) is seen sporadically in all breeds. Fracture of the bone occurs at the plantar tubercle, which remains attached to the plantar ligaments, while the rest of the bone displaces dorsomedially. Closed reduction and cast fixation are rarely successful, and surgical stabilization is always advisable. Good function can be anticipated.

Clinical Signs and Diagnosis

Protrusion of the bone is readily palpable because there is minimal soft-tissue swelling. If the bone is luxated completely out of contact with the talus and distal tarsal bones, mild varus deformity and hyperextension may be noted. Radiographs confirm this diagnosis.

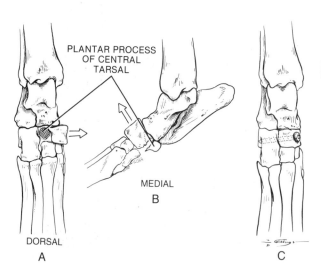

PLANTAR PROCESS OF CENTRAL TARSAL

MEDIAL

B

DORSAL

A

C

FIGURE 20–59

Fracture-luxation of the central tarsal bone. (A) The central tarsal luxates dorsomedially. (B and C) Fixation is by means of a positional screw through the central tarsal into the fourth tarsal bone. A threaded Kirschner wire or small pin may be substituted in small dogs.

Surgical Technique

The bone is approached by an incision directly dorsal to it.[5] The bone is reduced by flexing and lateral bending at the joint. A positional screw is directed laterally into the fourth tarsal bone. A further illustration of placement of this screw is found in Figure 8–11. Threaded Kirschner wire has been successfully substituted for the bone screw in toy breeds.

AFTERCARE ■ A short lateral splint (see Fig. 19–13) is applied and maintained for four weeks. Exercise is limited through the eighth postoperative week.

DISTAL INTERTARSAL SUBLUXATION WITH DORSOMEDIAL INSTABILITY

This injury (Fig. 20–60A) can be seen in isolation or combined with hyperextension at the proximal intertarsal joint or tarsometatarsal luxation with dorsal instability. Cast fixation has been disappointing in our experience, and we advise surgical stabilization. The technique shown here is combined with proximal intertarsal arthrodesis when this condition is concurrent with hyperextension.

Clinical Signs and Diagnosis

Valgus deformity resulting from dorsomedial ligamentous instability can be appreciated on palpation. Soft-tissue swelling is minimal. Radiographs in the stressed position confirm the site of instability and should be studied carefully for fractures of the fourth tarsal bone, a frequent complication.

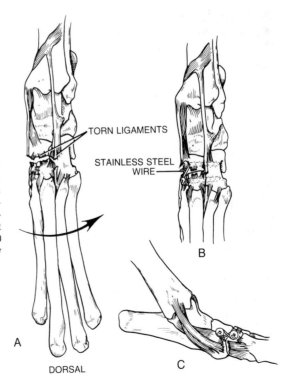

FIGURE 20–60

Distal intertarsal subluxation with dorsomedial instability. *(A)* Valgus deformity is evident following rupture of the medial and dorsal ligaments of the centrodistal joint. *(B and C)* Bone screws are placed through the central and distal tarsals into the fourth tarsal. Articular cartilage of the centrodistal joint is debrided, and stainless steel wire (20 to 22 gauge) is looped around the screw heads and tightened.

TORN LIGAMENTS

STAINLESS STEEL WIRE

A

DORSAL

B

C

Surgical Technique

The area is exposed by a distomedial extension of the approach to the central tarsal bone.[5] Articular cartilage is removed from the centrodistal joint. Bone screws are placed from the central and second tarsal bones laterally into the fourth tarsal bone. Stainless steel wire, 20 to 22 gauge (0.8 to 0.6 mm) is looped around the screw heads and twisted tightly (Fig. 20–60B,C).

AFTERCARE ■ A short, lateral splint (see Fig. 19–13) is applied and maintained for four weeks. Exercise is limited through the eighth postoperative week.

HYPEREXTENSION WITH SUBLUXATION OF THE TARSOMETATARSAL JOINTS

This injury (Fig. 20–61A) is not as common as proximal intertarsal hyperextension. The plantar tarsal fibrocartilage is torn in this situation. As with other hyperextension injuries, conservative treatment by cast fixation is virtually never successful. Arthrodesis of the tarsometatarsal joints is the best treatment and yields good results and virtually normal function is anticipated.

Clinical Signs and Diagnosis

This condition seems to be more often related to known trauma than does proximal intertarsal hyperextension; thus, more soft-tissue swelling is seen. The injury often happens when an animal becomes tangled in a wire mesh fence while attempting to climb it. Pain is not marked, and most animals will attempt weight-bearing within a few days, with a typically plantigrade stance.

Radiographs taken with hyperextension stress readily confirm the injury (Fig. 20–61A). In some cases, more complete luxation with plantar displacement of the bases of one or more metatarsal bones will be seen. Rarely are all four metatarsals completely luxated.

Surgical Technique

The joints are exposed by means of a plantar approach.[5] The superficial and deep digital flexor tendons are alternately retracted medially and laterally to allow debridement of articular cartilage of the joints. These joints do not form a straight line across the tarsus; therefore, each one must be curetted independently.

FIGURE 20–61

Hyperextension of the tarsometatarsal joints. *(A and B)* Rupture of plantar tarsal fibrocartilage removes the tension band support for the joint and allows hyperextension to develop. *(C and D)* Arthrodesis by pin and tension band wire. A plantar approach is used to expose the joint for cartilage debridement.[5] Stainless steel wire (18 to 20 gauge) is placed through bone tunnels in the distal calcaneus and proximal metatarsals. The Steinmann pin ($5/64$ to $1/8$ inch in diameter) is driven into the fourth metatarsal and recessed into the calcaneus to prevent damage to the superficial digital flexor tendon. *(E and F)* Lateral bone plate fixation for arthrodesis. Two screws in the fourth tarsal bone and three screws in the metatarsals are minimum for this situation. In large breeds, bending loads on the medial side are neutralized with screw and wire fixation. External support in a cast or splint is necessary. *(G)* External skeletal fixation is applicable to this surgery. Illustrated are both the use of conventional clamp fixation *(left)*, and the use of polymethylmethacrylate dental tray cement as a connecting rod *(right)*. Fixation pins are bent for more stability in the cement. See text for details.

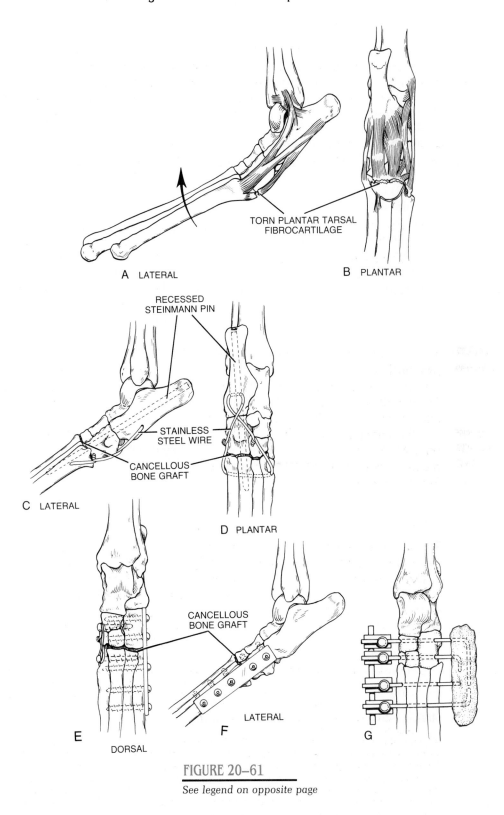

A LATERAL

B PLANTAR

TORN PLANTAR TARSAL
FIBROCARTILAGE

RECESSED
STEINMANN PIN

STAINLESS
STEEL WIRE

CANCELLOUS
BONE GRAFT

C LATERAL

D PLANTAR

CANCELLOUS
BONE GRAFT

E

DORSAL

F

LATERAL

G

FIGURE 20–61

See legend on opposite page

Several fixation techniques are adaptable to this condition. A *pin and tension band wire method* works well and requires minimal equipment (Fig. 20–61C,D). Transverse holes for the wire (18 to 20 gauge) are drilled in the bases of the calcaneus and the metatarsal bones. The wire must be placed deep to the superficial digital flexor tendon. Because of the collective "quarter-moon" cross-sectional shape of the proximal metatarsal bones, it is unlikely that the drill will go through more than three of the four bones. A small bases of the calcaneus and the metatarsal bones. The wire must be placed the calcaneus, across the fourth tarsal bone, and into the base of metatarsal IV. It is then retracted 1 cm, cut short, and countersunk beneath the cartilage of the tuber calcanei. It is worthwhile to predrill a hole in the calcaneus for the pin with a bone drill. Autogenous cancellous bone graft (Chapter 3) is packed into the joint space before the wire is tightened. Because the pin crosses the calcaneoquartal joint, spontaneous fusion of the joint often follows.

Lateral plate fixation (Fig. 20–61E,F) also provides excellent stabilization. A five-hole plate of appropriate size is attached to the fourth, central, and distal tarsal bones proximally and to the metatarsals distally. Again, rarely will more than three of the metatarsals be engaged by any drill hole. A lateral bony projection of the base of metatarsal V will have to be removed to allow seating of the plate. Addition of wire and screw fixation medially is indicated in large breeds. Autogenous cancellous bone grafting (Chapter 3) of the joint spaces is advisable.

Stabilization of this arthrodesis is also possible by means of an *external skeletal fixator* (Kirschner-Ehmer splint, Kirschner Medical Inc., Timonium, MD). This method is advantageous when there are open wounds associated with the injury and when bone plate fixation is not available. The fixation pins can be connected conventionally with clamps as on the left side of Figure 20–61G or by means of polymethylmethacrylate cement (dental tray cement or hoof repair acrylic), as on the right side of Figure 20–61G.

The joint is approached and articular cartilage is removed by power bur or curettage as described above. Autogenous cancellous bone from the proximal tibia is placed in the joint space (see Chapter 3). Two fixation pins are placed transversely in the distal tarsal bones. If the fixation will use connecting clamps, care must be taken to ensure that the pins are spaced widely enough to allow placement of the clamps. Three more pins are placed distally in the metatarsal bones. The pins are then connected by clamps or cement. If cement is to be used, the fixation pins are bent at a right angle at the protruding end in order to give more surface contact for the cement. The latter is mixed until reaching a dough-like consistency, then molded into a rod approximately ¾ inch (2 cm) in diameter and hand packed onto the fixation pins. The arthrodesis site must be stabilized until the cement has hardened, typically 8 to 10 minutes from the start of mixing.

AFTERCARE ▪ External casting is not needed with the tension band wire or external fixator technique, but it is advised with bone plating because the plate is not in a tension band position. A short lateral splint (see Fig. 19–13) or the external fixator is maintained until radiographic signs of fusion are noted, usually 8 to 10 weeks postoperatively. Exercise should be severely limited through this period and is slowly returned to normal four weeks after splint or fixator removal.

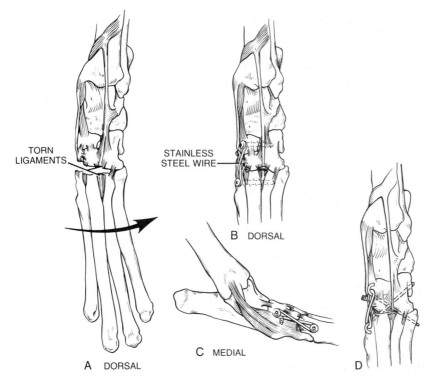

TORN
LIGAMENTS

STAINLESS
STEEL WIRE

B DORSAL

C MEDIAL

A DORSAL

D

FIGURE 20–62

Tarsometatarsal subluxation with dorsomedial instability. *(A)* Valgus deformity develops as a result of disruption of the dorsomedial tarsometatarsal ligaments. *(B* and *C)* A direct medial approach exposes the affected joints, and articular cartilage is removed. Bone screws are placed in the central and fourth tarsal and metatarsals 2, 3, and 4. Stainless steel wire (20 to 22 gauge) is placed around the screw heads and tightened. *(D)* Support can also be provided with Kirschner wires and a tension band wire placed between the pins.

TARSOMETATARSAL SUBLUXATION WITH DORSOMEDIAL INSTABILITY

Although angular displacement may not appear severe with this injury (Fig. 20–62A), it is nonetheless a disabling problem. This is because the medial tarsus is the tension side, and attempted weight-bearing further aggravates valgus deviation. Cast fixation generally yields poor results, but simple surgical repair carries a good prognosis.

Clinical Signs and Diagnosis

This injury is rarely spontaneous, most of the time being directly attributable to trauma; thus, it may be associated with other local or remote injuries. The instability can be appreciated on palpation but probably cannot be differentiated from distal intertarsal subluxation. Radiographs of the animal in the stressed position are necessary to confirm the diagnosis.

Surgical Technique

A medial incision is made directly over the affected joints. Articular cartilage is debrided in the second and third tarsometatarsal joints. Bone screws are placed in the central-fourth tarsal and in the bases of metatarsals II and IV. Stainless steel wire (20 to 22 gauge, 0.8 to 0.6 mm) is looped around the screw heads and tightened. A second technique applicable here is cross pinning of the tarsometatarsal joint with Kirschner wires (Fig. 20–62D). A tension band wire placed between the pins provides good stability.

AFTERCARE ■ A short lateral splint (see Fig. 19–13) is applied and maintained for three weeks. Exercise is limited throughout the eighth postoperative week. The pins may migrate after active weight-bearing starts and should be removed in this circumstance.

TARSOMETATARSAL SUBLUXATION WITH DORSAL INSTABILITY

As with dorsal instability at the proximal intertarsal level, this injury (Fig. 20–63) is apparently self-induced in most cases; it is rarely associated with known trauma. It is perhaps one of the lesser tarsal injuries, often responding to cast fixation for three to four weeks. The larger the dog and the more instability present, the greater is the need for surgical treatment. All chronic cases should undergo operation.

Clinical Signs and Diagnosis

History and clinical signs are similar to those of proximal intertarsal dorsal instability, that is, a rather vague and intermittent lameness. Because the deformity is not seen when the dog is standing, palpation to exert flexion stress is important in diagnosis. Radiographs showing the stress position will confirm the site of instability.

Surgical Technique

Paired medial and lateral incisions expose the joints. Small pins or Kirschner wires are driven from the proximal metatarsals into the tarsal bones in an "X" fashion (Fig. 20–63B,C). It is best not to cross the proximal intertarsal joint with the pins. Each pin is driven to the desired depth, retracted 1 cm, and cut 1 cm from the bone. A hook is bent in the pin and is then tapped back against the bone. Pins can also be driven in the opposite direction, from the tarsus into the metatarsals. Alternatively, combined medial and lateral screw and wire fixation as in Figure 20–62D can be used.

AFTERCARE ■ A short-leg lateral splint (see Fig. 19–13) is maintained for four weeks. Exercise is restricted through eight weeks postoperatively. The pins will almost certainly migrate when active weight-bearing starts; they should then be removed.

LUXATION AND SUBLUXATION OF THE METATARSOPHALANGEAL AND INTERPHALANGEAL JOINTS

These injuries are identical to those of the forefoot (see Chapter 21, Figs. 21–40 and 21–44). Amputation of the toes and arthrodesis at the proximal interphalangeal joint are illustrated in Figures 21–42 and 21–44.

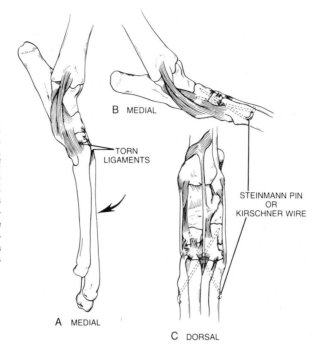

FIGURE 20-63

Tarsometatarsal subluxation with dorsal instability. (A) Flexion deformity can be induced from tearing of the dorsal ligaments of the tarsometatarsal joints. (B and C) Cross pinning through paired medial and lateral incisions is sufficient to stabilize this condition. The pins should be seated close to the bones to prevent skin irritation. These pins can also be driven from the tarsus in the opposite direction.

REFERENCES

1. Basher AWP, Walter MC, Newton CD: Coxofemoral luxation in the dog and cat. Vet Surg 15:356, 1986.
2. Bone DL, Walker M, Cantwell HD: Traumatic coxofemoral luxation in dogs: Results of repair. Vet Surg 13:263, 1984.
3. Harari J, Smith CW, Rauch LS: Caudoventral hip luxation in two dogs. J Am Vet Med Assoc 185:312, 1984.
4. Thacher C, Schrader SC: Caudal ventral hip luxation in the dog: A review of 14 cases. J Am Anim Hosp Assoc 21:167, 1985.
5. Piermattei DL, Greeley RG: An Atlas of Surgical Approaches to the Bones of the Dog and Cat, 2nd ed. Philadelphia, W. B. Saunders Company, 1979.
6. DeAngelis M, Prata R: Surgical repair of coxofemoral luxation in the dog. J Am Anim Hosp Assoc 9:175, 1973.
7. Allen SW, Chambers JN: Extracapsular suture stabilization of canine coxofemoral luxation. Cont Ed 8:457, 1986.
8. Braden TD, Johnson ME: Technique and indications of a prosthetic capsule for repair of recurrent and chronic coxofemoral luxations. Vet Comp Orthop Traum 1:26, 1988.
9. Piermattei DL: A technique for surgical management of coxofemoral luxations. Small Anim Clin 3:373, 1963.
10. Piermattei DL: Fabrication of an improved toggle pin. Vet Med/Sm Anim Clin 60:384, 1964.
11. Gendreau CL, Rouse GP: Surgical manage-

ment of the hip. Proc Am Anim Hosp Assoc 42:393, 1975.
12. Hunt CA, Henry WB: Transarticular pinning for repair of hip dislocation in the dog: A retrospective study of 40 cases. J Am Vet Med Assoc 187:828, 1985.
13. Herron MR: Atraumatic ventral coxofemoral luxation in dogs (Abstr). Vet Surg 15:123, 1986.
14. Wadsworth PL, Lesser AS: Use of muscle transfer to prevent reluxation of the hip: Two case reports. Proc Vet Orthop Soc 14th Annual Meeting, 1986.
15. Corley EA: Hip dysplasia: A report from the Orthopedic Foundation for Animals. Sem Vet Med Surg 2:141, 1987.
16. Riser WH, Newton CD: Canine hip dysplasia as a disease. In Bojrab MJ (ed): Pathophysiology in Small Animal Surgery. Philadelphia, Lea & Febiger, 1981, pp. 618–623.
17. Lust G, Rendano VT, Summers BA: Canine hip dysplasia: Concepts and diagnosis. J Am Vet Med Assoc 187:638, 1985.
18. Lanting FL: Canine Hip Dysplasia and Other Orthopedic Diseases. Loveland, Colorado, Alpine Publications, Inc., 1981.
19. Olewski JM, Lust G, Rendano VT, et al: Degenerative joint disease: Multiple joint involvement in young and mature dogs. Am J Vet Res 44:1300, 1983.
20. Rendano VT, Ryan G: Canine hip dysplasia evaluation. J Vet Radiol 26:170, 1985.
21. Bardens JW: Palpation for the detection of

joint laxity. Proc Canine Hip Dysplasia Symposium and Workshop, Orthopedic Foundation for Animals, St Louis, 1972:105–109.

22. Wright PJ, Mason TA: The usefulness of palpation of joint laxity in puppies as a predictor of hip dysplasia in a guide dog breeding programme. J Small Anim Pract 18:513, 1977.

23. Barr ARS, Denny HR, Gibbs C: Clinical hip dysplasia in growing dogs: The long-term results of conservative management. J Small Anim Pract 28:243, 1987.

24. Hannan N, Ghosh P, Bellenger C, Taylor T: Systemic administration of glycosaminoglycan polysulfate (Arteparon) provides partial protection of articular cartilage from damage produced by meniscectomy in the canine. J Orthop Res 5:47, 1987.

25. Bardens JW, Hardwick H: New observations in the diagnosis and cause of hip dysplasia. Vet Med/Small Anim Clin 63:238, 1968.

26. Slocum B, Devine T: Pelvic osteotomy technique for axial rotation of the acetabular segment in dogs. J Am Anim Hosp Assoc 22:331–338, 1986.

27. Slocum B, Devine T: Pelvic osteotomy in the dog as treatment for hip dysplasia. Sem Vet Med Surg 2:107–116, 1987.

28. Schrader SC: Triple osteotomy of the pelvis and trochanteric osteotomy as a treatment for hip dysplasia in the immature dog: The surgical technique and results of 77 consecutive operations. J Am Vet Med Assoc 189:659–665, 1986.

29. Hauptman J, Prieur WD, Butler HC, Guffy MM: The angle of inclination of the canine femoral head and neck. Vet Surg 8:74, 1979.

30. Walker TL, Prieur, WD: Intertrochanteric femoral osteotomy. Sem Vet Med Surg 2:117–130, 1987.

31. Montavon PM, Hohn RB, Olmstead ML, et al: Inclination and anteversion angles of the femoral head and neck in the dog. Vet Surg 14:277, 1985.

32. Prieur WD: Double hook plate for intertrochanteric osteotomy in the dog. Synthes Veterinary Bulletin 1:1–4, 1984.

33. Brinker WO, Hohn RB, Prieur WD: Manual of Internal Fixation in Small Animals. Berlin, New York, Springer-Verlag, 1984.

34. Leger L, Sumner-Smith G, Gofton N, et al: A.O. hook plate fixation for metaphyseal fractures and corrective wedge osteotomies. J Small Anim Pract 23:209–216, 1982.

35. Olmstead ML, Hohn RB, Turner TT: Technique for total hip replacement. Vet Surg 10:44, 1981.

36. Olmstead M: Total hip replacement. Vet Clin N Am 17:943, 1987.

37. Berzon JL, Howard PE, Covell SJ, et al: A retrospective study of the efficacy of femoral head and neck excisions in 94 dogs and cats. Vet Surg 9:88, 1980.

38. Lippincott CL: Excision arthroplasty of the femoral head and neck utilizing a biceps femoris muscle sling. Part two: The caudal pass. J Am Anim Hosp Assoc 20:377, 1984.

39. Mann FA, Tanger CH, Wagner-Mann C, et al: A comparison of standard femoral head and neck excision and femoral head and neck excision using a biceps femoris muscle flap in the dog. Vet Surg 16:223, 1987.

40. Gendreau C, Cawley AJ: Excision of the femoral head and neck: the long term results of 35 operations. J Am Anim Hosp Assoc 13:605, 1977.

41. Gambardella PC: Legg-Calvé-Perthes disease in dogs. In Bojrab MJ (ed): Pathophysiology in Surgery. Philadelphia, Lea & Febiger, 1981, pp. 625–630.

42. Ljunggren GL: Legg-Perthes disease in the dog. Acta Orthop Scand (suppl)95:7, 1967.

43. Pidduck H, Webbon PM: The genetic control of Perthes disease in toy poodles—A working hypothesis. J Small Anim Pract 19:729, 1978.

44. Lee R, Fry PD: Some observations of the occurrence of Legg-Calvé-Perthes disease (coxaplana) in the dog, and an evaluation of excision arthroplasty as a method of treatment. J Small Anim Pract 10:309, 1969.

45. Ljunggren GL: Conservative vs surgical treatment of Legg-Perthes disease. Anim Hosp 2:6, 1966.

46. Putnam RW: Patellar luxation in the dog. M.Sc. Thesis. Presented to the faculty of graduate studies, University of Guelph, Ontario, Canada, January 1968.

47. Priester WA: Sex, size, and breed as risk factors in canine patellar dislocation. J Am Vet Med Assoc 160:740, 1972.

48. Johnson ME: Feline patellar luxation: A retrospective case study. J Am Anim Hosp Assoc 22:835, 1986.

49. Singleton WB: The surgical correction of stifle deformities in the dog. J Small Anim Pract 10:59, 1969.

50. Flo GF, Brinker WO: Fascia overlap procedure for surgical correction of recurrent medial luxation of the patella in the dog. J Am Vet Med Assoc 156:595, 1970.

51. Rudy RW: Stifle joint. In Archibald J (ed): Canine Surgery, 2nd ed., Santa Barbara, American Veterinary Publications, 1974, pp. 1104–1159.

52. Vierheller RC: Surgical correction of patellar ectopia in the dog. J Am Vet Med Assoc 134:429, 1959.

53. Slocum B, Slocum DB, Devine T, et al: Wedge recession for treatment of recurrent luxation of the patella. Clin Orthop Rel Res 164:48, 1982.

54. Boone EG, Hohn RB, Weisbrode SR: Trochlear recession wedge technique for patellar luxation: An experimental study. J Am Anim Hosp Assoc 19:735, 1983.

55. Flo GL: Surgical correction of a deficient trochlear groove in dogs with severe congenital patellar luxations utilizing a carti-

lage flap and subchondral grooving. M.S. Thesis, Michigan State University, East Lansing, Mich., 1969.

56. Whittick WG: Canine Orthopedics. Philadelphia, Lea & Febiger, 1974, pp. 319–321.

57. Brinker WO, Keller WE: Rotation of the tibial tubercle for correction of luxation of the patella. MSU Vet 22:92, 1962.

58. Singleton WB: The diagnosis and treatment of some abnormal stifle conditions in the dog. Vet Rec 69:1387, 1957.

59. Willauer CC, Vasseur PB: Clinical results of surgical correction of medial luxation of the patella in dogs. Vet Surg 16:31, 1987.

60. Vasseur PB, Pool RR, Arnoczky SP, et al: Correlative biomechanical and histologic study of the cranial cruciate ligament in dogs. Am J Vet Res 46:1842, 1985.

61. Paatsama S: Ligament injuries in the canine stifle joint. A clinical and experimental study. Thesis. Royal Veterinary College, Stockholm, 1952.

62. Arnoczky SP, Marshall JL: The cruciate ligaments of the canine stifle: An anatomical and functional analysis. Am J Vet Res 38:1807, 1977.

63. Arnoczky SP: The cruciate ligaments: The enigma of the canine stifle. J Small Anim Pract 29:71, 1988.

64. Arnoczky SP, Torzilli PA, Marshall JL: Biomechanical evaluation of anterior cruciate ligament repair in the dog. An analysis of the instant center of motion. J Am Anim Hosp Assoc 13:553, 1977.

64A. Pond MJ, Campbell JR: The canine stifle joint. I. Rupture of the anterior cruciate ligament. An assessment of conservative and surgical management. J Small Anim Pract 13:1, 1972.

65. Vasseur PB: Clinical results following conservative management for rupture of the cranial cruciate ligament in dogs. Vet Surg 13:243, 1984.

66. Flo G: Modification of the lateral retinacular imbrication technique for stabilizing cruciate ligament injuries. J Am Anim Hosp Assoc 11:570, 1975.

67. Dulisch M: Suture reaction following extra-articular stifle stabilization in the dog—Part I: A retrospective study of 161 stifles. J Am Anim Hosp Assoc 17:569, 1981.

68. Smith GK, Torg JS: Fibular head transposition for repair of cruciate-deficient stifle in the dog. J Am Vet Med Assoc 187:375, 1985.

69. Piermattei DL, Moore RW: A preliminary evaluation of a modified over-the-top procedure for ruptured cranial cruciate ligament in the dog. 8th Annual Conference, Veterinary Orthopedic Society, Snowbird, Utah, 1981.

70. Arnoczky SP, Tarvin GB, Marshall JL, Saltzman B: The over-the-top procedure, a technique for anterior cruciate ligament substitution in the dog. J Am Anim Hosp Assoc 15:283, 1979.

71. Tarvin GB, Arnoczky SP: Incomplete rupture of the cranial cruciate ligament in a dog. Vet Surg 10:94, 1981.

72. Scavelli TD, Schrader SC, Matthiesen DT: Incomplete rupture of the cranial cruciate ligament of the stifle joint in 25 dogs (abstract). Vet Surg 18:80, 1989.

73. Hohn RB, Newton CD: Surgical repair of ligamentous structures of the stifle joint. In Bojrab MJ (ed): Current Techniques in Small Animal Surgery, Philadelphia, Lea & Febiger, 1975, pp. 470–479.

74. Harari J, Johnson AL, Stein LF, et al: Evaluation of experimental transection and partial excision of the caudal cruciate ligament in dogs. Vet Surg 16:151, 1987.

75. DeAngelis MP, Betts CW: Posterior cruciate ligament rupture. J Am Anim Hosp Assoc 9:447, 1973.

76. Stone EA, Betts CW, Rudy RL: Folding of the caudal horn of the medial meniscus secondary to severance of the cranial cruciate ligament. Vet Surg 9:121, 1980.

77. Flo G, DeYoung D, Tvedten H, et al: Classification of meniscal injuries in the canine stifle based upon gross pathological appearance. J Am Anim Hosp Assoc 19:325, 1983.

78. Flo GL, DeYoung D: Meniscal injuries and medial meniscectomy in the canine stifle. J Am Anim Hosp Assoc 14:683, 1978.

79. Goodfellow J: He who hesitates is saved (editorial). J Bone Joint Surg 62–B:4, 1980.

80. DeYoung D, Flo GL, Tvedten H: Experimental medial meniscectomy in dogs undergoing cranial cruciate ligament repair. J Am Anim Hosp Assoc 16:639, 1980.

81. Farrow CS: Sprain, strain, and contusion. Vet Clin N Am 8:169, 1978.

82. Vasseur PB, Arnoczky SP: Collateral ligaments of the canine stifle joint: Anatomic and functional analysis. Am J Vet Res 42:1133, 1981.

83. Hulse DA, Shires P: Multiple ligament injury of the stifle joint in the dog. J Am Anim Hosp Assoc 22:105, 1986.

84. Aron D: Traumatic dislocation of the stifle join: Treatment of 12 dogs and one cat. J Am Anim Hosp Assoc 24:333, 1988.

85. Pond MJ: Avulsion of the extensor digitorum longus muscle in the dog: A report of four cases. J Small Anim Pract 14:785, 1973.

86. Bennett D, Campbell JR: Unusual soft tissue orthopaedic problems in the dog. J Small Anim Pract 20:27, 1979.

87. Aron DN: Prosthetic ligament replacement for severe tarsocrural joint instability. J Am Anim Hosp Assoc 23:41, 1987.

88. Swaim SF: Management and bandaging of soft tissue injuries of dog and cat feet. J Am Anim Hosp Assoc 21:329, 1985.

89. Van Ee RT, Gibson K, Roberts ED: Osteochondritis dissecans of the lateral ridge of the talus in a dog. Am Vet Med Assoc 193:1284, 1988.

90. Smith MM, Vasseur PB, Morgan JP: Clinical evaluation of dogs after surgical and non-

surgical management of osteochondritis dissecans of the talus. J Am Vet Med Assoc 187:31, 1985.

91. Bonneau NH, Olivieri M, Breton L: Avulsion of the gastrocnemius tendon in the dog causing flexion of the hock and digits. J Am Anim Hosp Assoc 19:717, 1983.

92. Lesser A, Solimen SS: Experimental evaluation of tendon transfer for the treatment of sciatic nerve paralysis in the dog. Vet Surg 9:72, 1980.

93. Klause SE, Piermattei DL, Schwarz PD: Tarsocrural arthrodesis: Complications and recommendations. Vet Comp Ortho & Traum 12:119, 1989.

94. Sumner-Smith G, Kuzma A: A technique for arthrodesis of the canine tarsocrural joint. J Small Anim Pract 30:65, 1989.

94A. Campbell JR, Bennett D, Lee R: Intertarsal and tarso-metatarsal subluxation in the dog. J Small Anim Pract 17:427, 1976.

95. Cardinet GH, Guffy MM, Wallace LJ: Canine hip dysplasia: Effects of pectineal tenotomy on the coxofemoral joints of German shepherd dogs. J Am Vet Med Assoc 164:591, 1974.

96. Bowen JM, Lewis RE, Kneller SK, et al: Progression of hip dysplasia in German shepherd dogs after unilateral pectineal myotomy. J Am Vet Med Assoc 161:899, 1972.

97. Olmstead MR: Lateral luxation of the patella. In Bojrab MJ (ed): Pathophysiology in Surgery. Philadelphia, Lea & Febiger, 1981, pp. 638–640.

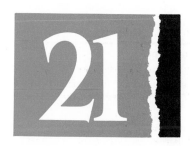

Diagnosis and Treatment of Orthopedic Conditions of the Forelimb

Forelimb Lameness

Following a history and lameness examination as described in Chapter 15, it is usually possible to localize the cause of lameness with some degree of accuracy. Following this comes the exercise of constructing a list of possible diagnoses and working through them until the correct one is found. The following listing is not exhaustive, but it includes the problems that are seen regularly.

FORELIMB LAMENESS IN LARGE BREED, SKELETALLY IMMATURE DOGS

General/Multiple
- Trauma—fracture, luxation
- Panosteitis
- Hypertrophic osteodystrophy
- Cervical cord lesion—vertebral instability

Shoulder Region
- Osteochondritis dissecans of humeral head

Elbow Region
- Osteochondritis dissecans of medial trochlear ridge
- Ununited anconeal process
- Fragmentation of medial coronoid process
- Avulsion and calcification of the flexor tendons of the medial epicondyle
- Subluxation due to premature physeal closure

Carpal Region
- Subluxation/valgus or varus deformity due to premature physeal closure
- Valgus deformity due to retained cartilage cores in the ulna

FORELIMB LAMENESS IN LARGE BREED, SKELETALLY MATURE DOGS

General/Multiple
- Trauma—fracture, luxation, muscle and nerve injuries
- Panosteitis
- Cervical cord lesion—disk, tumor, vertebral instability
- Brachial plexus tumor
- Bone or cartilage tumor
- Hypertrophic osteoarthropathy

Shoulder Region
- Osteochondritis dissecans of humeral head
- Degenerative joint disease, primary or secondary
- Contracture of infraspinatus muscle
- Tenosynovitis of biceps brachii tendon
- Luxation

Elbow Region
- Degenerative joint disease, primary or secondary
- Fragmentation of medial coronoid process
- Avulsion injury of medial epicondyle
- Subluxation due to premature physeal closure
- Luxation

Carpal Region
- Ligamentous instability/hyperextension
- Subluxation due to premature physeal closure
- Degenerative joint disease, primary or secondary
- Inflammatory joint disease

FORELIMB LAMENESS IN SMALL BREED, SKELETALLY IMMATURE DOGS

General/Multiple
- Trauma—fracture, luxation
- Atlantoaxial luxation

Shoulder Region
- Congenital luxation

Elbow Region
- Congenital luxation
- Subluxation due to premature physeal closure

Carpal Region
- Subluxation due to premature physeal closure

Forelimb Lameness

FORELIMB LAMENESS IN SMALL BREED, SKELETALLY MATURE DOGS

General/Multiple
- Trauma—fracture, luxation, muscle and nerve injuries
- Cervical cord lesion—disk, tumor
- Brachial plexus tumor
- Hypertrophic osteoarthropathy

Shoulder Region
- Degenerative joint disease, primary or secondary
- Medial luxation, nontraumatic

Elbow Region
- Degenerative joint disease, primary or secondary
- Subluxation due to premature physeal closure

Carpal Region
- Degenerative joint disease, primary or secondary
- Inflammatory joint disease
- Subluxation due to premature physeal closure

THE SHOULDER

Luxations of the Shoulder

Luxations of the shoulder are relatively uncommon in the dog. Obviously traumatic luxations are seen in all breeds, but the toy poodle and sheltie show a particular propensity to develop medial luxations (Fig. 21–1) without any history of obvious trauma. At the time of presentation, many of these animals have a history of lameness of several months' duration. This suggests some genetic predisposition. Most luxations—perhaps 75 percent—are medial, and a large proportion of the remainder are lateral (see Fig. 21–3). Cranial and caudal luxations are seen only occasionally (see Figs. 21–5 and 21–7). Although the tendons of the parascapular muscles have long been thought of as the primary stabilizers of the shoulder joint, it was found experimentally that cutting the tendons that cross the shoulder joint resulted in minimal changes in joint motion, whereas cutting the joint capsule and glenohumeral ligaments caused marked alteration of joint motion.[1] This suggests that careful

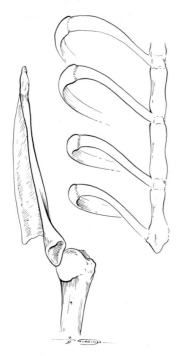

FIGURE 21–1

Medial luxation of the left shoulder (ventrodorsal view).

imbrication suturing of the capsule and associated ligaments should be an important part of any surgical repair.

The leg is usually carried with the elbow flexed and adducted and the lower limb abducted and supinated in the case of the medial luxation. In a lateral luxation the position is similar except that the lower limb is adducted. On palpation, the relative positions of the acromial process and the greater tubercle are the keys to determining the position of the humeral head relative to the glenoid. These points can be palpated on the normal limb and then compared with the affected limb. Clinical signs and physical examination are usually diagnostic; but as with any skeletal injury, diagnosis should always be confirmed radiographically in order to eliminate the possibility of bone injuries such as fractures. Stress radiography has been suggested as an objective method of measuring instability in this joint.[51] The presence of a severely eroded glenoid resulting from chronic luxation or the presence of a dysplastic glenoid or humeral head greatly reduces the probability of a successful reduction. Congenital luxations are usually irreducible because of severe malformations of both the glenoid and humeral head.

If the injury is seen within a few days following the dislocation, and particularly if there is a known history of trauma, it is probably always worthwhile to attempt closed reduction and immobilization of the limb for approximately two weeks. If the joint is relatively stable following reduction, there is a good chance that this type of treatment will be successful. If the joint remains unstable following reduction or if the luxation recurs while the leg is in the sling, surgical treatment is always indicated.

MEDIAL LUXATION

Prosthetic ligaments and imbrication techniques have not been as successful as methods for transposing the biceps tendon. Medial transposition and tenodesis[2] of the biceps tendon create a stabilizing lateral force on the humeral head. If the glenoid is not of normal size and shape, surgical stabilization will usually fail. Treatment in this situation is excision arthroplasty (see Fig. 21–10) or arthrodesis (see Fig. 21–11).

Surgical Technique

The shoulder joint is exposed by the approach to the craniomedial region of the shoulder joint.[3] Typically, the tendon of insertion of the subscapularis muscle will be found torn at its insertion on the lesser tubercle. If this has happened, the tendon may have retracted a considerable distance and can be difficult to identify. The tendon should be tagged with a suture when it is identified to assist in later suturing. If the joint capsule is not torn, open it carefully to inspect the joint, for it is important to save as much as possible for suturing. Careful assessment of the medial labrum of the glenoid and the lateral side of the humeral head is necessary. If the labrum is worn, the probability of successful stabilization is markedly reduced. If there is sufficient chondromalacia of the humeral head articular cartilage owing to rubbing on the medial labrum, degenerative joint disease changes could limit long-term success even if the joint is stabilized. Arthrodesis or excision arthroplasty (see below) is probably indicated in these circumstances.

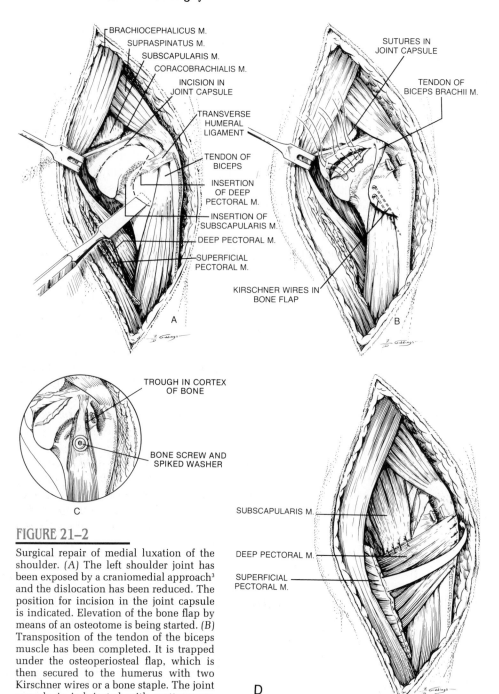

BRACHIOCEPHALICUS M.
SUPRASPINATUS M.
SUBSCAPULARIS M.
CORACOBRACHIALIS M.
INCISION IN
JOINT CAPSULE
TRANSVERSE
HUMERAL
LIGAMENT
TENDON OF
BICEPS
INSERTION
OF DEEP
PECTORAL M.
INSERTION OF
SUBSCAPULARIS M.
DEEP PECTORAL M.
SUPERFICIAL
PECTORAL M.

A

SUTURES IN
JOINT CAPSULE
TENDON OF
BICEPS BRACHII M.
KIRSCHNER WIRES IN
BONE FLAP

B

TROUGH IN CORTEX
OF BONE
BONE SCREW AND
SPIKED WASHER

C

SUBSCAPULARIS M.
DEEP PECTORAL M.
SUPERFICIAL
PECTORAL M.

D

FIGURE 21-2

Surgical repair of medial luxation of the shoulder. *(A)* The left shoulder joint has been exposed by a craniomedial approach[3] and the dislocation has been reduced. The position for incision in the joint capsule is indicated. Elevation of the bone flap by means of an osteotome is being started. *(B)* Transposition of the tendon of the biceps muscle has been completed. It is trapped under the osteoperiosteal flap, which is then secured to the humerus with two Kirschner wires or a bone staple. The joint capsule is imbricated with mattress sutures of heavy absorbable material. *(C)* Another method of attachment is the use of a plastic spiked washer and bone screw (Synthes [USA], Paoli, PA). The bone beneath the tendon is cut to form a shallow trough to encourage early attachment of the tendon. *(D)* The deep pectoral muscle has been advanced and sutured to the origin of the superficial pectoral muscle. The superficial pectoral muscle is advanced craniolaterad until it can be sutured to the fascia of the acromial head of the deltoideus muscle. The subscapularis muscle is attached to the proximal border of the deep pectoral muscle and to any humeral periosteum or fascia available.

If the articular surfaces are in good condition and the luxation is recent, it may be possible to stabilize the joint by suture of the joint capsule and the subscapularis tendon (Fig. 21–2B, D). If this does not appear to be a viable option, tenodesis of the biceps tendon is carried out.

The transverse humeral ligament is transected over the biceps tendon (Fig. 21–2A) and the tendon is mobilized from the bicipital groove after incising the joint capsule as needed. A crescent-shaped flap of bone is elevated from the lesser tubercle with an osteotome. The bone flap should hinge on the periosteum along its cranial edge. Bone, and sometimes articular cartilage, is curetted from underneath the flap to accommodate the tendon. The tendon is transposed to lie under the flap and is held in place by Kirschner wires driven through the flap into the humerus (Fig. 21–2B). An alternative method of tenodesis is illustrated in Figure 21–2C. The tendon is bluntly split and a bone screw and spiked washer (Synthes [USA], Paoli, PA) are used to fix the tendon to the bone in a shallow trough in the cortex. Removal of some cortical bone allows the tendon to heal to the bone more readily than if it were simply attached to the periosteal surface.

Joint capsule and medial glenohumeral ligament imbrication is accomplished by mattress or cruciate sutures of synthetic absorbable material. If the joint seems unstable when the humerus is externally rotated (thus turning the humeral head medially), a derotational suture to temporarily tether the humerus is helpful. Large-gauge nonabsorbable monofilament or braided polyester is anchored to the medial labrum of the glenoid by a bone tunnel or bone screw. A bone tunnel is then drilled through the greater tubercle in the region of the transverse humeral ligament. After passing the suture through the tunnel, it is tied moderately taut with the humerus *internally* rotated. Joint capsule and medial glenohumeral ligament imbrication is accomplished by mattress or Lembert sutures of absorbable material.

The deep pectoral muscle is sutured to the superficial pectoral muscle, and the subscapularis muscle is advanced as far cranially as possible and sutured to the deep pectoral muscle (Fig. 21–2D). The superficial pectoral muscle is pulled across the cranial border of the humerus and sutured to the acromial head of the deltoideus muscle. The effect of these transpositions is to tighten the muscles and to reinforce medial support of the joint. The remaining tissues are closed in layers.

AFTERCARE ■ The limb is supported in a foreleg (Velpeau) sling for 14 days (see Fig. 19–16). Exercise is restricted for four weeks. Passive flexion-extension exercise may be needed following removal of the sling, supplemented with swimming when possible.

PROGNOSIS ■ Hohn and colleagues[2] reported an overall 93 percent success rate (15 cases) for the tenodesis procedure applied to both medial and lateral luxations. Vasseur's group reported 40 percent (two cases) of their medial luxation cases had normal gaits, 20 percent (one case) had occasional limping, and 40 percent (two cases) had persistent limping following the tenodesis procedure.[4] If cases are carefully selected, and those with wearing of the glenoid or humeral head are eliminated, it is likely that these figures could be improved.

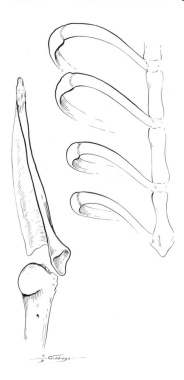

FIGURE 21–3

Lateral luxation of the left shoulder (ventrodorsal view).

LATERAL LUXATION

Lateral luxations (Fig. 21–3) are more often seen in larger breeds of dogs and are usually traumatic in origin. As such, they are more amenable to closed reduction when seen within a few days of the injury. Fixation after a closed reduction is by means of a spica splint (see Fig. 19–11) rather than a Velpeau sling, which tends to turn the humeral head laterally. For surgical treatment of irreducible or chronic luxations, biceps tenodesis can again be used to stabilize the joint.[2] If the tendon is moved laterally, it creates a medial force on the humeral head.

Surgical Technique

The shoulder joint is exposed by the approach to the cranial region of the shoulder joint.[3] If the joint capsule is not torn, open it carefully to inspect the joint, for it is important to save as much as possible for suturing. Careful assessment of the lateral labrum of the glenoid and the medial side of the humeral head is necessary. If the labrum is worn, the probability of successful stabilization is markedly reduced. These changes are less likely seen here than in medial luxations because of the more acute nature of most lateral luxations. If there is sufficient chondromalacia of the articular cartilage of the humeral head owing to rubbing on the lateral labrum, degenerative joint disease changes could limit long-term success even if the joint is stabilized. Arthrodesis or excision arthroplasty (see below) is probably indicated in these circumstances.

If the articular surfaces are in good condition and the luxation is recent, it may be possible to stabilize the joint by suture of the lateral joint capsule (see Fig. 21–8). If this does not appear to be a viable option, tenodesis of the biceps tendon is carried out.

The transverse humeral ligament is transected over the biceps tendon, and the joint capsule is incised as needed to allow lateral transposition of the tendon (Fig. 21–4A). In order to transpose the tendon lateral to the crest of the greater tubercle, it may be necessary to rongeur or curette a trough at the proximal end of the tubercular osteotomy site (Fig. 21–4B). The tendon is then held lateral to the tubercle, which is then reattached to the humerus with Kirschner wires; in large breeds, pins and a tension band wire, or bone screws are used (Fig. 21–4C). Several sutures are placed between the biceps tendon and the deltoideus fascia. The joint capsule is imbricated with mattress or Lembert sutures. The superficial pectoral muscle is moved craniolaterally to allow attachment to the fascia of the deltoideus and biceps muscles.

AFTERCARE ■ A foreleg spica splint (see Fig. 19–11) is maintained for 14 days. Exercise is restricted for four weeks. Passive flexion-extension exercise may be needed following removal of the splint, supplemented with swimming when possible.

PROGNOSIS ■ In one series of six cases treated by lateral transposition of the biceps, five dogs had normal function and one limped occasionally at follow-up.[4]

CRANIAL LUXATION

In our experience, cranial luxation, a relatively rare injury, is always the result of trauma. The biceps tendon can again be used for the stabilization of this infrequent luxation (Fig. 21–5). It is transposed cranially and thus is under increased tension and tends to hold the humeral head more tightly within the glenoid.[5]

Surgical Technique

The shoulder is exposed by the cranial approach to the shoulder joint.[3] An incision is made in the transverse humeral ligament over the biceps tendon, and a trough is cut on the osteotomy surface on the crest and in the tubercle to accommodate the biceps tendon. If, as a result of tension, the tendon cannot be positioned within the osteotomy site on the humerus, sufficient bone is removed from the proximal osteotomy site to form a slight trough there (Fig. 21–6A). The tubercle is replaced and attached with Kirschner wires; in large breeds, pins and a tension band wire are used (Fig. 21–6B). Screw fixation should probably be avoided to prevent injury to the tendon. The joint capsule is imbricated with mattress or Lembert sutures.

AFTERCARE ■ The limb is supported in either a foreleg spica splint or Velpeau sling for 10 to 14 days (see Fig. 19–11). Exercise is restricted for 4 weeks. Passive flexion-extension exercise may be necessary after removal of the external fixation, and swimming is encouraged.

CAUDAL LUXATION AND SUBLUXATION

Like cranial luxation, this injury occurs infrequently and may be either a self-induced or traumatic injury. Hyperextension of the joint is the probable cause.

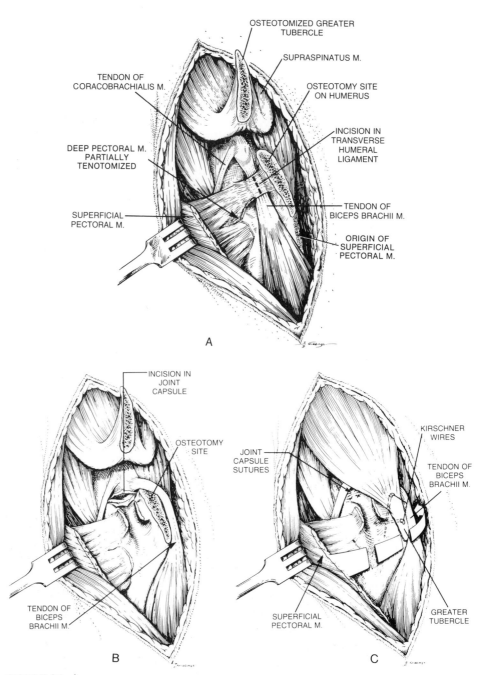

FIGURE 21–4

Surgical repair of lateral luxation of the shoulder. *(A)* The left shoulder has been exposed by a cranial approach.[3] The greater tubercle of the humerus has been osteotomized, and the incision is marked in the transverse humeral ligament. *(B)* The joint capsule has been incised to aid in moving the biceps tendon lateral to the greater tubercle osteotomy site. A small area of the proximal osteotomy site has been removed to ease positioning of the biceps tendon. *(C)* The greater tubercle is pinned back to its original site by two Kirschner wires or bone screws, thus trapping the biceps tendon laterally. The joint capsule is imbricated with mattress sutures, and the superficial pectoral muscle is attached to the fascia of the acromial head of the deltoideus and the biceps muscles.

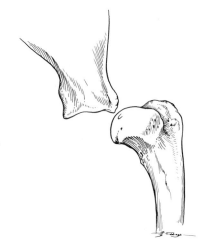

FIGURE 21–5

Cranial luxation of the left shoulder (mediolateral view).

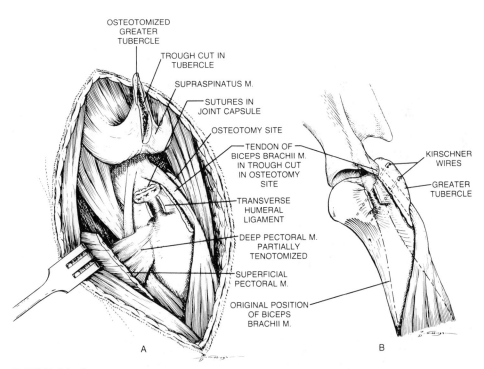

OSTEOTOMIZED
GREATER
TUBERCLE

TROUGH CUT IN
TUBERCLE

SUPRASPINATUS M.

SUTURES IN
JOINT CAPSULE

OSTEOTOMY SITE

TENDON OF
BICEPS BRACHII M.
IN TROUGH CUT
IN OSTEOTOMY
SITE

TRANSVERSE
HUMERAL
LIGAMENT

DEEP PECTORAL M.
PARTIALLY
TENOTOMIZED

SUPERFICIAL
PECTORAL M.

ORIGINAL POSITION
OF BICEPS
BRACHII M.

KIRSCHNER
WIRES

GREATER
TUBERCLE

A

B

FIGURE 21–6

Surgical repair of cranial luxation of the shoulder. (A) The left shoulder has been exposed by a cranial approach.[3] The transverse humeral ligament has been cut, and the biceps tendon has been transposed cranially to lie in a trough created in the tubercular osteotomy site and in the tubercle itself. The joint capsule is imbricated with mattress sutures. (B) The tubercle is reattached to the osteotomy site with two Kirschner wires holding the biceps tendon in a position that creates impaction of the humeral head in the glenoid.

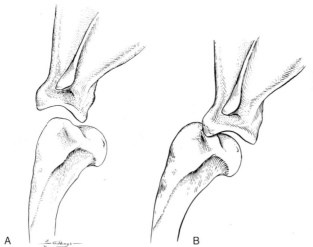

FIGURE 21–7

Caudal luxation and subluxation of the shoulder. *(A)* Caudal luxation of the left shoulder (lateromedial view). *(B)* Caudal subluxation of the left shoulder (lateromedial view). The joint space is increased caudally as extension stress is applied to the joint.

The luxation may be total, as shown in Figure 21–7*A*, or subluxated. In the latter case, the joint space between the humeral head and the caudoventral rim of the glenoid is increased on extension-stress radiographs (Fig. 21–7*B*). Imbrication of the lateral and caudolateral joint capsule has worked well in these cases.

Surgical Technique

CAUDAL LUXATION ■ The shoulder joint is exposed by a craniolateral approach with osteotomy of the acromial process.[3] The joint capsule will be at least partially torn but may need to be opened farther to allow access to the joint. After inspection for intra-articular damage, the humeral head is reduced and the craniolateral and caudolateral joint capsule is imbricated with mattress or Lembert sutures of synthetic absorbable material (Fig. 21–8).

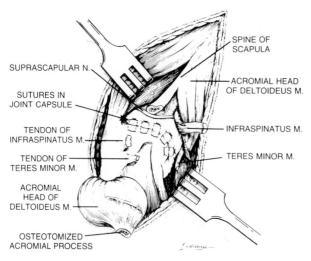

SPINE OF SCAPULA

SUPRASCAPULAR N.

SUTURES IN JOINT CAPSULE

TENDON OF INFRASPINATUS M.

TENDON OF TERES MINOR M.

ACROMIAL HEAD OF DELTOIDEUS M.

OSTEOTOMIZED ACROMIAL PROCESS

ACROMIAL HEAD OF DELTOIDEUS M.

INFRASPINATUS M.

TERES MINOR M.

·FIGURE 21–8

Caudal luxation of the shoulder. The left shoulder has been exposed by a craniolateral approach with an osteotomy of the acromial process.[3] The infraspinatus and teres muscles have been freed by tenotomy. Mattress sutures of heavy-gauge absorbable suture have been used to imbricate the joint capsule as far cranially and caudally as possible, following the line of the rim of the glenoid.

FIGURE 21–9

Caudal subluxation of the shoulder. The left shoulder has been exposed by a caudolateral approach.[3] The caudolateral joint capsule has been imbricated with mattress sutures of heavy-gauge absorbable suture. The suture line follows the rim of the glenoid as far caudad as possible, taking care to avoid the caudal circumflex humeral artery.

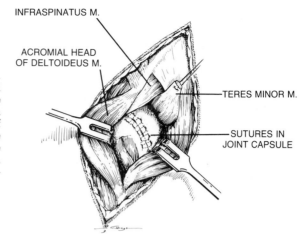

INFRASPINATUS M.

ACROMIAL HEAD
OF DELTOIDEUS M.

TERES MINOR M.

SUTURES IN
JOINT CAPSULE

CAUDAL SUBLUXATION ■ The shoulder is exposed by a caudolateral approach.[3] The caudolateral joint capsule is imbricated with mattress or Lembert sutures of synthetic absorbable material (Fig. 21–9).

AFTERCARE ■ The limb is supported in a foreleg (Velpeau) sling for 14 days (see Fig. 19–16). Exercise is restricted for four weeks. Passive flexion-extension exercise may be needed following removal of the sling.

Excision Arthroplasty

In some cases, the glenohumeral joint cannot be reconstructed adequately. This is due most commonly to excessive wear of the medial labrum of the glenoid as a result of chronic medial luxation. Gunshot wounds on occasion damage the articular surfaces in such a way that nothing resembling normal joint function can result. The traditional method of treatment in these situations has been arthrodesis, which is technically demanding and requires bone-plating equipment in most cases.

An alternative salvage procedure is resection of the glenoid and a portion of the humeral head based on the method of Parkes.[6] This procedure has been modified by us to include partial excision of the humeral head in an attempt to provide a larger vascular surface. We postulate that this will result in a more rapid and proliferative fibroplasia and hence earlier stability of the pseudoarthrosis.

SURGICAL TECHNIQUE

The joint is exposed by the approach to the craniolateral region of the shoulder by osteotomy of the acromial process.[3] The joint capsule is opened widely and the tendon of the biceps muscle is detached from the supraglenoid tubercle (Fig. 21–10A). With care taken to protect the suprascapular nerve, ostectomies are made in the glenoid and humeral head (Fig. 21–10B) with an osteotome or high-speed pneumatic surgical bur. The glenoid ostectomy is made obliquely to bevel the edge. The deep (medial) edge is longer than the

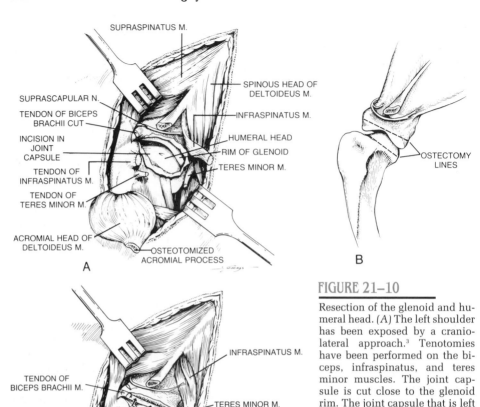

SUPRASPINATUS M.

SPINOUS HEAD OF DELTOIDEUS M.

SUPRASCAPULAR N.

TENDON OF BICEPS BRACHII CUT

INCISION IN JOINT CAPSULE

TENDON OF INFRASPINATUS M.

TENDON OF TERES MINOR M.

ACROMIAL HEAD OF DELTOIDEUS M.

INFRASPINATUS M.

HUMERAL HEAD

RIM OF GLENOID

TERES MINOR M.

OSTEOTOMIZED ACROMIAL PROCESS

A

OSTECTOMY LINES

B

TENDON OF BICEPS BRACHII M.

INFRASPINATUS M.

TERES MINOR M.

JOINT CAPSULE

C

FIGURE 21–10

Resection of the glenoid and humeral head. (A) The left shoulder has been exposed by a craniolateral approach.[3] Tenotomies have been performed on the biceps, infraspinatus, and teres minor muscles. The joint capsule is cut close to the glenoid rim. The joint capsule that is left attached to the humeral head is preserved. (B) Positions of both ostectomy lines. (C) Both ostectomies have been completed. The teres minor muscle has been pulled medially where it has been sutured to the biceps tendon, which has previously been sutured to the fascia of the supraspinatus muscle. Accessible joint capsule from the humeral head is sutured to the teres minor. A small notch may be cut in the base of the spine of the scapula to allow the suprascapular nerve to be positioned more proximally if it is too near the ostectomy. The infraspinatus is reattached to its insertion, and the acromial process is wired to the spine more proximally than normal.

superficial edge. The caudal circumflex humeral artery must also be protected during the ostectomy process.

A notch is cut in the base of the spine of the scapula to allow the suprascapular nerve to be displaced proximally. The infraspinatus is reattached, but the teres minor muscle is pulled medially between the two ostectomy surfaces and sutured to the biceps tendon and medial joint capsule (Fig. 21–10C). Whatever joint capsule is available is then pulled into the "joint space" and sutured to the teres minor muscle and biceps tendon. The purpose of these maneuvers is to interpose soft tissue between the ostectomies and hasten formation of a fibrous false joint. It may be necessary to wire the acromial process to the scapular spine more proximally than normal in order to remove laxity in the deltoideus muscle created by the ostectomies, which shorten the distance between the acromial osteotomy site and the insertion of the muscle.

AFTERCARE ■ The limb is not immobilized postoperatively. Early, gentle use of the limb is encouraged by leash walking. More vigorous activity is forced starting 10 days postoperatively, and swimming is encouraged. Early activity stimulates the fibrosis necessary to create a false joint without any bony contact.

PROGNOSIS ■ It must be appreciated that this is a salvage procedure and that normal function of the limb is not to be expected. Moderate, pain-free exercise capability is the objective, and it usually is achieved. A slight limp and some atrophy of the shoulder girdle muscles are expected.

Thirteen cases have been reported in two series.[7, 8] Good to excellent pain-free function was noted in each case. One case had bilateral surgery for chronic medial luxations of the shoulders, and, at six months postoperatively, the animal was using both limbs at all times and bore about 80 percent of normal weight on the limbs.

Arthrodesis of the Shoulder Joint

Surgical fusion of the shoulder joint results in remarkably little functional disability because of the extreme mobility of the scapula. This scapular motion compensates for loss of motion in the shoulder joint. This is not to indicate that use of the limb is normal but that enough function remains for active use of the limb. In one study, the only gait abnormalities noted were limited circumduction and inability to advance the limb quickly when running.[50]

Indications for arthrodesis of the shoulder are most commonly comminuted fractures of the glenoid, neck of the scapula, or head of the humerus. Additionally, chronic medial luxation of the shoulder joint often results in severe erosion of the glenoid and humeral head, making surgical repair impossible. Severe degenerative joint disease is a legitimate but uncommon indication. As with all arthrodeses, this is a mutilating operation and should be considered only as a last-resort salvage procedure. It is important that other joints of the limb be normal if this procedure is done.

SURGICAL TECHNIQUE

A combined craniolateral and cranial approach to the shoulder joint is performed with osteotomy of both the acromial process and the greater tubercle (Fig. 21–11A).[3] This widely exposes the joint and allows the joint capsule to be opened for debridement of cartilage on both articular surfaces.

The biceps tendon is detached at the supraglenoid tubercle, and the suprascapular nerve is protected during cartilage removal along the lines shown in Figure 21–11B. Creating flat surfaces eliminates shear stress at the bone surfaces, especially when compression is exerted. The greater tubercle region of the humerus is contoured with rongeurs or saw to provide a gentle curve on a line from the spine of the scapula to the cranial aspect of the humerus. A small intramedullary pin or Kirschner wire is driven from the cranial humeral cortex into the glenoid with the shoulder at a functional angle of about 105 degrees (Fig. 21–11C). An 8- to 10-hole plate is contoured to fit the cranial surface of the humerus and the dorsocranial junction of the spine

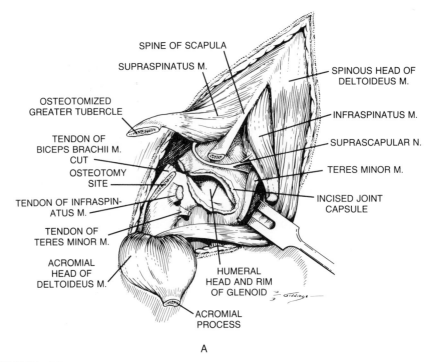

SPINE OF SCAPULA

SUPRASPINATUS M.

SPINOUS HEAD OF
DELTOIDEUS M.

OSTEOTOMIZED
GREATER TUBERCLE

INFRASPINATUS M.

TENDON OF
BICEPS BRACHII M.
CUT
OSTEOTOMY
SITE

SUPRASCAPULAR N.

TENDON OF INFRASPIN-
ATUS M.

TERES MINOR M.

INCISED JOINT
CAPSULE

TENDON OF
TERES MINOR M.

ACROMIAL
HEAD OF
DELTOIDEUS M.

HUMERAL
HEAD AND RIM
OF GLENOID

ACROMIAL
PROCESS

A

FIGURE 21–11

Arthrodesis of the shoulder joint. (A) The left shoulder has been exposed by a combined cranial and craniolateral approach.[3] The biceps tendon has been detached from the supraglenoid tubercle, and the joint capsule is opened.

with the body of the scapula. Some torsion of the plate will be necessary in order to make it fit the junction of the spine and the body of the scapula. The reconstruction plate (Synthes [USA], Paoli, PA) is especially suitable for this procedure because it is more easily contoured than conventional plates. The plate must either pass over the suprascapular nerve with sufficient room for the nerve or be placed underneath the nerve. In attaching the plate, thought must be given to placing at least one screw in lag fashion across the debrided bone surfaces to create compression. As shown in Figure 21–11C, the third screw hole was chosen.

One or two cancellous screws can be used to advantage in the humeral head. (Some types of plates do not accept cancellous screws except at the end holes.) The pin can be removed after the plate is attached. The bone removed from the greater tubercle during the contouring process is used as a bone graft in and around the joint (Fig. 21–11D). The biceps tendon is reattached to the fascia of the supraspinatus muscle or to the cortex of the humerus medial to the plate using a bone screw and spiked washer (see Fig. 21–14B, C). The osteotomized greater tubercle is attached to the humerus lateral to the plate with a screw or pins. The soft tissues are closed routinely in layers.

Aftercare

The shoulder is immobilized in a spica splint for four weeks (see Fig. 19–11). Radiographic signs of fusion should be noted between 6 and 12 weeks

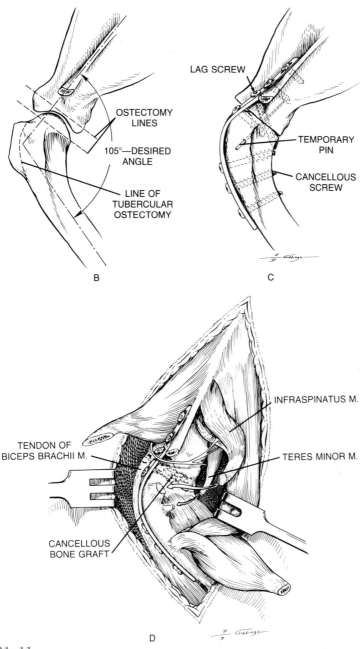

FIGURE 21–11

Continued (B) With the joint positioned at a functional angle of 105 to 110 degrees, ostectomies of the glenoid and humeral head are performed to remove articular cartilage and produce flat opposing surfaces. The greater tubercle is further ostectomized to provide a gentle curve from the humeral neck to the cranial cortex. (C) A small pin is driven across the joint to hold the bones at the correct angle while the plate is contoured and attached, after which the pin is removed. At least one screw must be a lag screw between the scapula and the humerus. (D) Bone graft obtained from the greater tubercle is placed around the opposed bones. The biceps tendon is sutured to the supraspinatus muscle fascia. The osteotomized portion of the tubercle attached to the supraspinatus muscle is pinned or screwed lateral to the plate, and the rest of the tissues are closed routinely.

postoperatively, at which time the splint is removed and the dog allowed to return to normal activity over a four-week period.

Osteochondritis Dissecans of the Humeral Head

A general discussion of osteochondrosis is found in Chapter 18. In the shoulder joint, the disease is manifested as a fragment of cartilage that becomes partially or fully detached from the caudocentral aspect of the humeral head, usually opposite the caudoventral rim of the glenoid. The cartilage flap usually remains attached to normal cartilage along the cranial edge of the flap; however, it may become free within the joint, in which case it usually becomes lodged in the caudoventral pouch of the joint capsule.

Free cartilage fragments within the joint usually are resorbed, but some may remain viable and even grow in size, since they are nourished by synovial fluid. Others become attached to synovial membrane, where they can become vascularized and undergo partial ossification; they are then called *ossicles*. Those cartilage fragments that lodge in the caudal joint usually do not create clinical signs unless they grow in size sufficient to irritate the synovial membrane (see Fig. 18–2). However, any fragments that migrate to the bicipital tendon sheath often produce clinical lameness.[9]

CLINICAL SIGNS AND HISTORY

Dogs of the large breeds are most commonly affected in a 2:1 to 3:1 male:female ratio. Various studies have reported bilateral involvement between 27 and 68 percent.[10–13] Many dogs showing bilateral radiographic signs will be clinically lame in only one limb. It is worth noting that when an animal is markedly lame in one leg, it is difficult to assess lameness in the contralateral leg. It is likely that those animals diagnosed radiographically as bilateral in reality are showing only the signs of osteochondrosis in one shoulder and never develop a loose cartilage flap. This supposition is supported by a clinical series in which only 20 percent of the bilaterally affected animals needed surgical treatment.[12]

Although most animals first show clinical signs between 4 and 8 months of age, some will present much later, at 2 to 3 years of age. In these cases, the owners have simply ignored, or did not notice, the early lameness. Lameness is often first noted after severe exercise, but it may be insidious in onset. A shortening of the swing phase of gait leads to atrophy of the spinatus and deltoid muscles. This is a constant finding if lameness has been present more than 2 to 3 weeks. The change of gait is most noticeable at a walk. Pain on palpation is variable and is more often noted on severe extension than flexion or rotation. Crepitus is also variable. Clinical signs are most notable after rest that has been preceded by heavy exercise.

DIAGNOSIS

Diagnosis is based on radiographic confirmation of a typical defect in the humeral head (see Fig. 18–2). Arthrography is a valuable tool in confirming the presence of a cartilage flap or joint mouse and is particularly valuable in

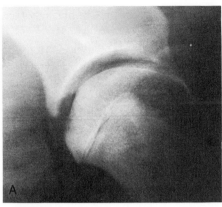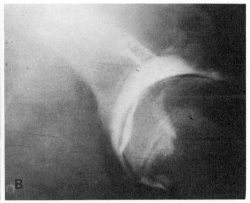

FIGURE 21–12

Osteochondritis dissecans of the humeral head. *(A)* A flattening of the subchondral bone of the caudal aspect of the humeral head can be appreciated here, but there is no visible indication of the presence or absence of a cartilage flap. This could simply be the manifestation of osteochondrosis. *(B)* This contrast arthrogram shows dye filling of the joint space and a filling defect that represents the cartilage flap.

those cases that appear to have bilateral lesions as judged by plain films. This technique is underused in diagnosing and evaluating dogs for surgical treatment.[14] Virtually any intravenous or myelographic contrast agent can be used if it is diluted to less than 100 mg iodine/ml diluent; an 8.4 percent concentration of technical grade metrizamide (33 mg iodine/ml) was found to be very satisfactory by Muhumuza.[15] Suter and Carb recommended a 30 to 40 percent solution of contrast media.[16] Depending on body size, 2 to 4 ml is injected into the shoulder joint with aseptic precautions. Two milliliters of diatrizoate meglumine (Renografin-76, Squibb Diagnostics, New Brunswick, NJ) injected intra-articularly into large joints without dilution has worked well (RH Wrigley, personal communication, 1989). As can be seen in Figure 21–12, the dye outlines cartilage flaps if they are present.

TREATMENT

Varying opinions have been expressed regarding surgical versus nonsurgical treatment of this condition. As experience has been gained, a more aggressive surgical approach has become evident. Although some animals do recover spontaneously, this can happen only if the flap breaks loose and is absorbed in the joint cavity. Furthermore, this process may take 9 to 12 months, and bilaterally affected animals are unlikely to recover to the point of clinical soundness.[10] An additional little-appreciated danger is that the loose cartilage flap may survive within the joint, as described above. Large ossicles cause severe inflammatory changes and degenerative joint disease. We have retrieved such ossicles from 3- and 4-year-old dogs. If the flap never breaks free, a similar deterioration of the joint occurs. We have removed partially attached flaps in 3-year-old dogs.

Surgical treatment has yielded much more uniformly good results in our experience as well as in the studies of others.[13, 17] Not only is the final outcome more predictable but soundness is achieved within one to two months, and late degenerative changes are less probable. As stated in Chapter 18, we recommend surgery if:

1. Lameness has persisted more than six weeks.
2. The animal is over 7 to 8 months of age.
3. The cartilage flap or joint mouse is confirmed radiographically, regardless of the animal's size.

Osteochondroplasty of the Humeral Head

The aim of surgery is to remove cartilage flaps still attached and to remove all fragments of free cartilage from within the joint. Removal of the cartilage allows a fibrocartilage scar to fill the defect and seal the edges of the articular cartilage bordering the defect.

The choice of surgical approach is variable. The caudolateral approach[3] or variations of it have generally worked well for us if an assistant is present. A humeral head retractor (Scanlan Surgical Instruments, Inc., Englewood, CO) is useful for exposure of the lesion. If we work alone, the more generous exposure of the craniolateral approach with osteotomy of the acromial process[3] is preferable, lessening the need for retraction. However, this is a longer procedure and is associated with more postoperative morbidity.

The caudolateral approach provides adequate visualization of the lesion if the joint capsule is adequately retracted and if the leg is severely internally rotated (Fig. 21–13A). A scalpel blade or small curved osteotome is used to cut the cartilage flap free (Fig. 21–13B, C). Irregular and undermined loosened areas of cartilage at the periphery of the lesion should be trimmed and smoothed to create vertical walls with a curette. Curettage of the floor of the lesion should be very cautiously done to minimize removal of subchondral bone. There is often a film of unorganized material covering the lesion. This can be gently scraped to expose the bone. There may be merit in *forage*, the technique of drilling multiple holes in the bed of the lesion with a Kirschner wire. This creates vascular channels to the subchondral bone and hastens ingrowth of fibrous tissue in the defect. The caudal cul-de-sac of the joint cavity must always be explored for free fragments of cartilage. Exposure of this area is enhanced by a small Hohmann retractor and by flexing the shoulder and elbow (Fig. 21–13D). The final step is forceful lavage of the joint to flush out small cartilage fragments. If cartilage fragments have been identified in the bicipital tendon sheath, they will have to be removed by a cranial approach, as they cannot be exposed from a caudolateral approach.[3]

AFTERCARE ■ Seroma formation is more common with shoulder surgery than with virtually any other canine surgery. This is perhaps due to the extreme amount of sliding motion of the skin and subcutis in this region over the muscle fascia. The only prevention is enforced rest for the first 10 to 14 postoperative days. A Velpeau sling (see Fig. 19–16) may be indicated for some hyperactive animals. Small seromas clear spontaneously in two to five weeks; large ones are treated with hot packs. They can be safely aseptically aspirated by two weeks postoperatively. If not resolving by three weeks, they are drained with Penrose drains for one week.

From three through six weeks postoperatively, very minimal activity

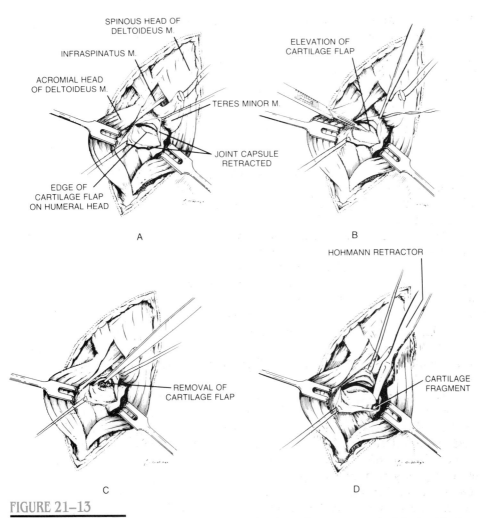

FIGURE 21–13

Osteochondroplasty of the humeral head for osteochondritis dissecans. *(A)* The left shoulder has been exposed by a caudolateral approach.[3] The lateral edge of the cartilage flap is visible after retraction of the joint capsule by stay sutures. *(B)* The cartilage flap is elevated from the humeral head by sharp dissection. *(C)* When the flap has been sufficiently elevated, it can be cut free along its cranial border. *(D)* The caudal cul-de-sac of the joint capsule is retracted with a small Hohmann retractor to allow removal of any free cartilage fragments.

(house confinement or leash) is suggested, following which exercise is gradually increased to normal at two to three months postoperatively.

Arthroscopy

Successful treatment of osteochondritis dissecans in 23 shoulder joints in 21 dogs has been reported by Person.[18] Force plate evaluation showed objective signs of improvement in gait in nine of 10 dogs seen postoperatively for follow-up. This method of treatment may well see much more application in the future but, at the present time, is not widely used.

Tenosynovitis of Biceps Tendon

This disease process is a common cause of forelimb lameness in medium to large breed dogs that are usually middle aged or older. There is some predilection for animals that are not physically well conditioned.

ANATOMY AND PATHOPHYSIOLOGY

After originating on the supraglenoid tubercle the tendon of the biceps brachii muscle passes distally through the intertubercular groove of the humerus, where it is stabilized by the transverse humeral ligament. The muscle inserts distally on the radius and ulna, and its main function is flexion of the elbow. It has little involvement in stabilizing the normal shoulder joint.[1] The tendon is surrounded by a synovial sheath that is an extension of the glenohumeral joint capsule. This sheath extends distally just beyond the transverse humeral ligament. There is no bursa associated with this tendon.

This injury is a *strain* injury to the tendon of the biceps brachii. These injuries are discussed in Chapter 19 in more detail. The mechanism of injury to the biceps tendon can either be direct or indirect trauma or simple overuse. Thus the pathological changes range from partial disruption of the tendon (grade 3 strain) to chronic inflammatory changes, including dystrophic calcification. Pathological changes also can be secondary to other diseases such as osteochondritis dissecans, where joint mice migrate to the synovial sheath and create an acute synovitis.[9] Thus it can be seen that the initial irritating source usually initially affects either the tendon or the synovial membrane individually, but soon the inflammatory process involves the opposite member. Proliferation of fibrous connective tissue and adhesions between the tendon and sheath limits motion and causes pain.[19]

HISTORY AND CLINICAL SIGNS

An inciting traumatic incident may be recalled by the owner, but usually the onset of the disease is insidious, and many cases will be of several months' duration when presented. The lameness is subtle and intermittent and worsens with exercise. Since the pain is present only during gliding motion of the tendon, there is no hesitation to bear weight on the limb; therefore there is little change in the stance phase of gait.[19] The swing phase of locomotion is limited because the shoulder joint is guarded by limiting the amount of extension and flexion.

Atrophy of the spinati muscle group is soon evident, but more distal muscles appear normal in size. Shoulder pain on manipulation is not a constant finding, especially in chronic cases. Pain is elicited by applying deep digital pressure over the tendon in the intertubercular groove region while simultaneously flexing the shoulder and extending the elbow.

DIAGNOSIS

Although the history and clinical signs are suggestive, further diagnostic tests are necessary for confirmation of the diagnosis. Diseases that have initially been confused with tenosynovitis in our experience include osteosarcoma, chondrosarcoma, and neurofibromas that involve the brachial plexus. Plain radiographs are useful to survey the joint for avulsion fractures in the region of the supraglenoid tubercle, calcification in the biceps tendon, and osteophytes in the intertubercular groove. Contrast arthrography is useful in some cases, although in the majority of cases it will not be essential to the diagnosis. Nevertheless, arthrograms (see discussion in Osteochondritis Dissecans section above) will outline the tendon and disclose synovial hyperplasia, tendon rupture, and joint mice. This procedure is therefore often useful in deciding which cases need surgical, rather than medical, treatment.

Synovial fluid analysis should be routinely performed but often fails to disclose much information. The fluid is typically normal or shows signs of mild inflammatory disease (viscous fluid, clear to hazy, with less than 5000 white blood cells/μl). (See also Table 17–2.) Any signs of sepsis, such as turbid fluid, would be a contraindication to arthrography or intra-articular corticosteroid therapy, which is discussed below.

Definitive diagnosis of bicipital tenosynovitis is often not possible, and the diagnosis is backed into by eliminating other causes of lameness. Proof of the diagnosis often depends on response to treatment.

TREATMENT

In acute cases the treatment is aimed at reducing inflammation in the affected structures before the pathological changes become irreversible. Rest and anti-inflammatory nonsteroidal drug therapy (see Chapter 17) are often sufficient. Strict confinement for four to six weeks is needed for resolution, and premature return to activity will almost ensure a chronic disease state. Systemic treatment with either nonsteroidal or corticosteroidal drugs has been unsuccessful in chronic cases in our hands. Intra-articular corticosteroid treatment can be successful in this disease if there are no mechanical causes, such as joint mice, and when the pathological changes are not too well established. There is no way of knowing if this is the case initially, so treatment is always given on a trial basis unless the injury is relatively acute and uncomplicated.

Arthrocentesis must be done with aseptic technique, and we prefer 1.5-inch, 22-gauge spinal needles. Less accidental trauma is done to the articular cartilage with these short-bevel needles with stylets. The joint is entered from the acromial process, with the needle directed toward the glenoid and angled slightly cranially. Synovial fluid is aspirated and immediately observed for turbidity. If the fluid is off color or the viscosity markedly changed, a complete examination of the fluid is completed before injecting the joint to protect against corticosteroid injection into a septic joint. If there are no contraindications, 20 to 40 mg of prednisolone acetate (Depo-Medrol, Upjohn Co., Kalamazoo, MI) is injected. This is followed by strict confinement for two weeks and light activity the third week. If the lameness has been markedly improved but not eliminated, a second injection is given at three weeks. If this is not curative, the dog should have surgical treatment. Return of the lameness several months or years later is not uncommon, and many will respond again to injection.

Surgical treatment is recommended for dogs that do not respond to medical treatment or those in which a mechanical problem is found initially. The goal of surgical treatment is elimination of movement of the biceps tendon in the inflamed tendon sheath, and this is accomplished by tenodesis of the bicipital tendon.

Surgical Technique

The tendon is exposed by a cranial approach to the shoulder joint.[3] The transverse humeral ligament and joint capsule are opened to expose the tendon and the intertubercular groove, which often has osteophytes along each edge (Fig. 21–14A). Partial rupture of the tendon near its origin is not uncommon. Joint mice are searched for and removed, and the tendon is transected near the supraglenoid tubercle. The tendon is reattached to the humerus distal to the groove by a bone screw and spiked washer (Synthes [USA], Paoli, PA), as shown in Figure 21–14B, or the tendon can be pulled through a bone tunnel in the greater tubercle and then sutured to the supraspinatus muscle (Fig. 21–14C). There is no loss of stability to the shoulder joint apparent from this procedure.[1] A section of the tendon should be saved for histopathological examination.

AFTERCARE ■ The limb is supported in a Velpeau sling and the animal closely confined for three weeks. Exercise is allowed to slowly increase to normal at six weeks postoperatively.

PROGNOSIS ■ About two thirds of the cases we have seen are treated medically, and approximately two thirds of these are cured by the treatment. The remainder of this group is divided between those that are treated again medically and those that do not respond and require surgical treatment. Those treated surgically early respond better than those that are operated on late. Normal gait and use of the leg return in 50 to 60 percent of the dogs, and the remainder stay variably lame, undoubtedly owing to chronic degenerative joint disease. Medical management of this problem is discussed in Chapter 17. Surgical treatment of this problem in man is variably reported to be 50 to 94 percent successful.[20, 21]

Rupture of the Tendon of the Biceps Brachii Muscle

The same forces that would cause an avulsion of the supraglenoid tubercle in the young dog (see Fig. 9–3) cause rupture of the tendon of the biceps near its origin on the tubercle in the mature dog. Initially, there is pain and effusion in the cranial shoulder joint region. Although the animal will exhibit an obvious lameness on the affected limb, flexion of the elbow joint is not obviously impaired. It is not usually possible to palpate the area of rupture in the tendon digitally because of swelling of tissues. Partial rupture is not uncommonly a cause of biciptal tenosynovitis.

Arthrography is essential in diagnosis.[15, 18] The contrast media may not allow actual visualization of the ruptured tendon, but a filling defect tends to support the clinical diagnosis. Plain films may demonstrate a slight laxity in the joint, but this is not consistent.

Because repair of the tendon is difficult, and because there are no adverse effects from detaching the biceps tendon,[1] the treatment of choice is tenodesis.

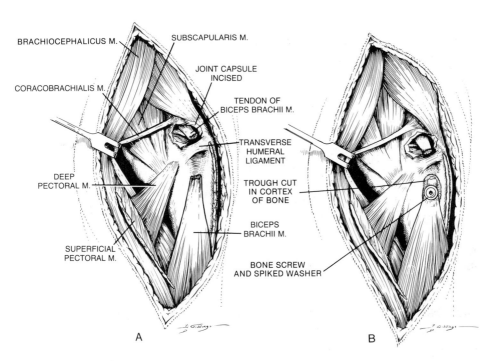

BRACHIOCEPHALICUS M.

SUBSCAPULARIS M.

JOINT CAPSULE INCISED

CORACOBRACHIALIS M.

TENDON OF BICEPS BRACHII M.

TRANSVERSE HUMERAL LIGAMENT

DEEP PECTORAL M.

TROUGH CUT IN CORTEX OF BONE

BICEPS BRACHII M.

SUPERFICIAL PECTORAL M.

BONE SCREW AND SPIKED WASHER

A

B

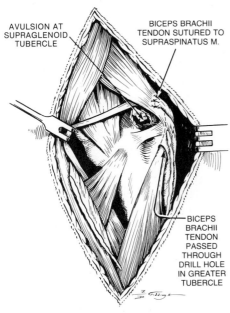

AVULSION AT SUPRAGLENOID TUBERCLE

BICEPS BRACHII TENDON SUTURED TO SUPRASPINATUS M.

BICEPS BRACHII TENDON PASSED THROUGH DRILL HOLE IN GREATER TUBERCLE

C

FIGURE 21–14

Tenodesis of the biceps brachii tendon. (A) The tendon is exposed by a craniolateral approach to the shoulder.[3] The tendon is cut near the supraglenoid tubercle and again distal to the intertubercular groove. (B) With the elbow flexed, the tendon is fixed to the humerus in a position that creates some tension on the muscle. After curettage of the periosteum, the tendon is bluntly split and attached to the humerus with a bone screw and an AO/ASIF plastic spiked washer (Synthes [USA], Paoli, PA). (C) A second method of attaching the tendon is illustrated. The tendon is cut free from the tubercle but is not cut again distally as above. A hole is drilled laterally through the greater tubercle, and the tendon is brought through the bone tunnel and sutured to the insertion of the supraspinatus muscle.

This method is described in the section, Tenosynovitis of Biceps Tendon (above).

Fibrotic Contracture of the Infraspinatus Muscle

This condition is a cause of shoulder lameness in hunting or working dogs. Electrophysiological and histological studies have indicated infraspinatus contracture to be a primary muscle disorder rather than a neuropathy. Affected muscle shows degeneration and atrophy with fibrous tissue replacement. The cause of this syndrome is hypothesized as an acute traumatic event that results in incomplete rupture of the infraspinatus muscle, leading to fibrotic contracture.[22] Although the trauma is usually self-induced, outside sources may also be the cause of injury.

Usually, there is a history of a sudden onset of lameness during a period of heavy activity such as hunting. Lameness and tenderness in the shoulder region gradually disappear in a 10- to 14-day period, to be replaced by a chronic lameness developing three to four weeks later. At this time, the animal elicits no pain but is completely unable to rotate (pronate) the shoulder joint internally. This results in a stance with the elbow adducted and the foot abducted (Fig. 21–15A). The lower limb swings in a lateral arc as the foot is advanced during the stride. There is atrophy of the infraspinatus muscle on palpation; when the limb is forcibly pronated, the proximal border of the scapula becomes more prominent as it abducts from the thorax. Radiographs are usually normal. Although rare, the condition can be bilateral.

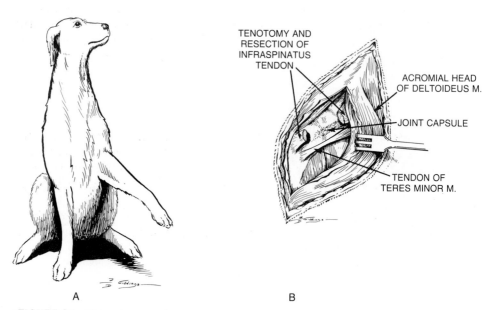

A   B

FIGURE 21–15

Fibrotic contracture of the infraspinatus muscle. (A) Typical sitting posture of a dog with infraspinatus contracture. The lower limb is permanently externally rotated and therefore shortened. (B) The left shoulder has been exposed by the craniolateral approach by tenotomy of the infraspinatus muscle.[3] The tendon is dissected free of the joint capsule until the shoulder moves freely; then about 1 cm of the tendon is excised.

Treatment consists of tenotomy and excision of part of the tendon of insertion of the infraspinatus muscle on the greater tubercle of the humerus. The tendon is exposed by the approach to the craniolateral region of the shoulder joint by tenotomy of the infraspinatus muscle.[3] The approach is modified only in that the joint capsule is not opened. The belly of the infraspinatus is inspected to confirm its fibrosis and contracture, following which the tendon is severed. If necessary, the tendon may be dissected from the joint capsule following tenotomy in order to allow a complete range of motion (Fig. 21–15B). About 1 to 1.5 cm of tendon is excised. It is occasionally necessary to incise the fibrotic joint capsule, which is then left open. A distinct "pop" is often felt when the last of the adhesions is broken down. Full range of motion is immediately restored.

Aftercare/Prognosis

Dogs routinely walk immediately with no constraint of the limb. Leash exercise can be resumed immediately and normal activity in 10 to 14 days. These animals uniformly return to normal stability and use of the limb.[23]

Fibrotic Contracture of the Supraspinatus Muscle

Although only a single case of this condition appears to have been reported,[24] the clinical signs were identical to those described for infraspinatus contracture. The dog responded well to sectioning of the tendon of insertion of the supraspinatus muscle. It would thus seem important to inspect both spinatus muscles for evidence of fibrosis and contracture before either tendon is sectioned.

Dorsal Luxation of the Scapula

Multiple ruptures and tearing of the insertions of the serratus ventralis, trapezius, and rhomboideus muscles on the cranial angle and dorsal border of the scapula allow the scapula to move dorsally on weight-bearing. Onset of clinical lameness is usually acute and is often directly associated with jumps and falls.

Considerable soft-tissue swelling is evident for several days after injury. Mobility of the scapula is easily demonstrated and is diagnostic. This uncommon problem is seen in both dogs and cats.

SURGICAL TECHNIQUE

The objective of surgical repair is to attach the scapula to a suitable rib with heavy stainless steel wire and to reattach as many muscles as possible.[25] An inverted L-shaped incision is made along the cranial and dorsal borders of the scapula. If any portions of the trapezius, serratus, or rhomboideus muscle insertions are intact, they are cut sufficiently to allow lateral retraction of the

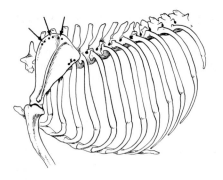

FIGURE 21–16

Dorsal luxation of the scapula. Heavy stainless steel wire is used to secure the caudal border of the scapula to an adjacent rib. Alternatively, holes are drilled through the cranial angle and vertebral border (*arrows*) to allow suturing to the serratus ventralis muscle.

scapula so that its caudal angle and caudal borders can be visualized. Two holes are drilled from a medial to lateral direction through the caudal border of the scapula, close to the caudal angle (Fig. 21–16). Stainless steel wire of 20 to 22 gauge is carefully placed around an adjacent rib with the ends placed through the scapular holes, then pushed laterally through the muscles. The wire is twisted until dorsal movement of the scapula is minimized, but still possible. All muscular insertions are sutured to the extent possible, and all tissues are closed in layers.

It is sometimes possible to eliminate the wire suture and simply attach muscle to the scapula through holes drilled near the cranial angle.

AFTERCARE ■ The scapula is immobilized in either a Velpeau sling (see Fig. 19–16) or a spica splint (see Fig. 19–11) for two weeks. Exercise is gradually increased to normal in the two weeks after sling or splint removal.

THE ELBOW

Traumatic Luxation of the Elbow

Because of the bony anatomy of the region, virtually all elbow luxations are lateral (Fig. 21–17A,B). The large square caudodistal corner of the medial

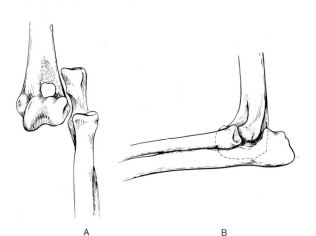

FIGURE 21–17

Lateral luxation of the elbow. (A) Craniocaudal view. (B) Latero-medial view. Note that in this case the anconeus is completely luxated.

A   B

epicondyle of the humerus prevents the ulna from moving medially, whereas the rounded shape of the lateral epicondyle permits the anconeal process to clear the lateral epicondylar crest when the elbow is flexed more than 90 degrees. When medial luxations are seen, they are usually accompanied by severe ligamentous damage.

CLINICAL SIGNS

The general appearance of an animal with a lateral luxation is distinct, although it is similar to that distinguishing the infraspinatus contracture shown in Figure 21–15A. Palpation easily differentiates the condition, with the laterally displaced radius and ulna being quite prominent. The antebrachium and foot are abducted, and the elbow is flexed. There is usually marked pain and resistance to flexion and extension. Because of elbow flexion, the foot does not touch the ground when the animal is either standing or sitting.

DIAGNOSIS

Although the basic diagnosis can be made by physical examination, radiographs in two planes are necessary to look for associated fractures and avulsion of ligaments.

TREATMENT

Closed Reduction

Virtually all lateral luxations can be reduced closed during the first few days after injury. Muscle contracture makes later reduction more difficult.

With the animal under general anesthesia, firm palpation is used to establish the position of the humeral condyles relative to the radius and ulna. In some cases, the anconeal process will still be inside (medial to) the lateral epicondylar crest. In such a situation, medial pressure is maintained on the olecranon while the elbow is flexed to 100 to 110 degrees. Medial pressure is then placed on the radial head to force it over the humeral capitulum to the reduced position. If medial pressure on the radial head does not bring about reduction, additional pressure can be exerted by slightly extending the joint to lock the anconeal process inside the lateral epicondylar crest. The antebrachium should then be twisted inward (pronated) and adducted, causing the radial head to slip medially relative to the fixed fulcrum of the anconeus.[26]

If the anconeus lies lateral to the lateral epicondyle, an additional step is required. With the elbow flexed to 100 to 110 degrees, the antebrachium is twisted inward (pronated) to force the anconeus inside the lateral condyle (Fig. 21–18A). The joint is extended slightly, then flexed while medial pressure on the radial head is continued. With pronation, the radial head can be forced over the capitulum (Fig. 21–18B).

Following reduction, evaluation of ligamentous damage is necessary. Although most luxations can be reduced closed, a few will require open reduction.

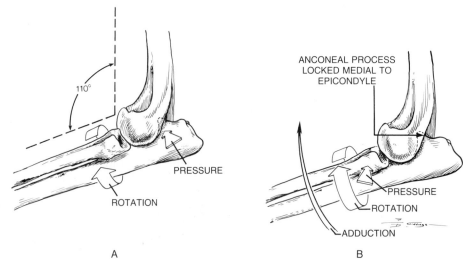

FIGURE 21-18

Closed reduction of lateral luxation of the elbow. *(A)* With the elbow flexed to 100 to 110 degrees, the antebrachium is twisted internally and the joint is slightly extended to lock the anconeal process inside the lateral epicondyle. *(B)* Continuous medial pressure is maintained on the radial head while the antebrachium is internally twisted. Gradual flexion and adduction of the antebrachium forces the radial head medially, using the anconeal process as a fulcrum.

Examination of Collateral Ligaments

The collateral ligaments of the elbow are illustrated in Figure 21–19*A* and *B*. These ligaments are intimately associated with the tendons of origin of the extensor (lateral) and flexor (medial) muscles and may be difficult to differentiate from these tendons at surgery.

The ligaments are evaluated by the method of Campbell.[26] After reduction, the elbow and carpus are both flexed to 90 degrees. Rotation of the paw laterally and medially causes similar rotation of the radius and ulna, which are constrained at the elbow by the collateral ligaments. If these ligaments are intact, lateral rotation of the paw is possible to about 45 degrees and medial rotation to about 70 degrees. If the lateral collateral is severed or avulsed, the paw can be rotated *medially* to about 140 degrees. If the medial ligament is damaged, the paw can be rotated *laterally* to about 90 degrees. In both cases, the paw rotation is about double the normal and can be compared with the opposite limb.

Excessive movement indicates damage to the collateral ligaments, and a decision must be made as to whether surgical treatment is indicated. If the joint is easily reluxated, the decision for surgical repair is simple to make. If the joint is reasonably stable despite the signs of ligament damage mentioned, the decision is more difficult. Immobilization will allow healing by fibrosis of periarticular soft tissues and may provide sufficient stability for smaller breeds, especially if they are not athletic or working animals. Conversely, surgical treatment is more often indicated in larger and more active animals.

Open Reduction

The elbow is exposed by the approach to the head of the radius and lateral compartments of the elbow joint.[3] Organized hematoma and shreds of ligament

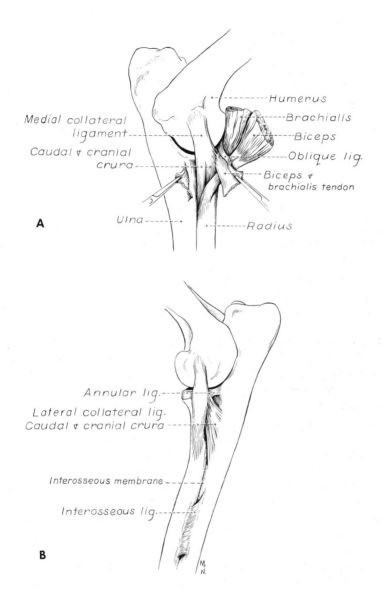

FIGURE 21–19

Collateral ligaments of the elbow. (A) Medial ligaments of the left elbow. (B) Lateral ligaments of the left elbow. (A and B from Evans HE, Christensen GC: Miller's Anatomy of the Dog, 2nd ed. Philadelphia, W. B. Saunders Company, 1979. By permission.)

muscle and joint capsule are cleaned from the joint. The procedure then continues as for a closed reduction. It may be necessary to use a smooth-surfaced instrument such as closed scissor blades or a bone lever to pry the radial head into the reduced position. Because of the inevitable damage to articular cartilage, this maneuver should be avoided if possible.

If reduction is still not possible, it may be necessary to extend the exposure by performing the caudal approach with osteotomy of the olecranon process.[3] It also allows debridement of granulation and scar tissue in chronic cases. This relieves the tension exerted by the triceps muscle and simplifies reduction. Following reduction, necessary repairs are performed as explained in the following discussion.

Repair of Ligaments

The surgical principles governing repair of ligamentous injuries are discussed in Chapter 19. Stretched ligaments are plicated (shortened), torn ligaments are sutured, and avulsed ligaments are reattached. Occasionally, ligaments are totally replaced or supplemented with various synthetic materials, although this is rarely necessary in the elbow.

Figure 21–20 illustrates repair of the lateral collateral ligaments. The elbow is approached laterally, with transection of the tendinous origin of the ulnaris lateralis[3] (Fig. 21–20A). The ligament is sutured or reattached to the bone (Fig. 21–20B). The adjacent extensor muscles are plicated with mattress sutures in the tendinous areas (Fig. 21–20C). Similar repairs are done medially if both ligaments are damaged. If the ligaments are torn near their distal insertions, they can be attached by suturing to the annular ligament. Damage in the midportion of the ligament is handled by suturing, using the locking loop suture described in Chapter 19.

Aftercare

CLOSED OR OPEN REDUCTION WITH NO LIGAMENT DAMAGE ■ The elbow is most stable when moderately extended to about the normal standing angle of 140 degrees. Because the elbow joint is very prone to lose range of motion as a result of periarticular fibrosis when completely immobilized, a soft splint (such as the modified Robert Jones dressing, see Fig. 19–17) is useful. Five to seven days is usually sufficient immobilization if exercise is restricted to the house or leash for two more weeks. Passive flexion-extension exercises are started immediately after removal of the dressing.

CLOSED REDUCTION WITH LIGAMENT DAMAGE ■ More rigid postoperative immobilization is needed in this situation despite the risk of joint stiffness. A spica splint (see Fig. 19–11) or Thomas splint (see Fig. 1–11) is maintained for two weeks. Passive flexion-extension exercise is important following splint removal. Exercise is restricted to the house or leash for three to four more weeks.

LIGAMENT DAMAGE SURGICALLY REPAIRED ■ Aftercare is similar to that above for ligament damage, except that the splint is maintained for three weeks.

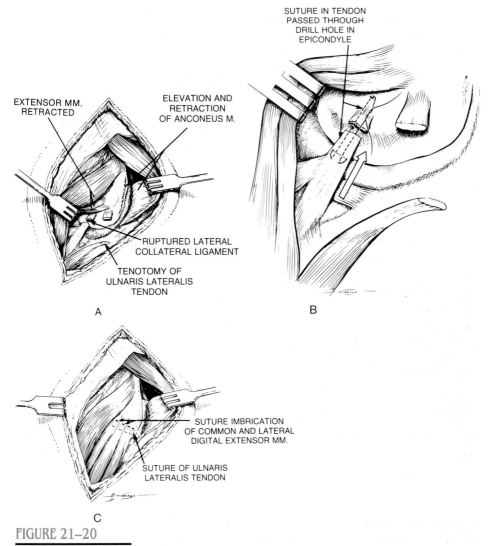

EXTENSOR MM.
RETRACTED

ELEVATION AND
RETRACTION
OF ANCONEUS M.

RUPTURED LATERAL
COLLATERAL LIGAMENT

TENOTOMY OF
ULNARIS LATERALIS
TENDON

A

SUTURE IN TENDON
PASSED THROUGH
DRILL HOLE IN
EPICONDYLE

B

SUTURE IMBRICATION
OF COMMON AND LATERAL
DIGITAL EXTENSOR MM.

SUTURE OF ULNARIS
LATERALIS TENDON

C

FIGURE 21–20

Surgical repair of lateral collateral ligaments of the elbow. (A) The left elbow has been exposed by a lateral approach with tenotomy of the ulnaris lateralis. Retraction of the other extensor muscles exposes the torn ligament. (B) The ligament has been torn close to the humerus. A locking loop suture has been placed in the tendon. One end of the suture is passed through a bone tunnel in the epicondyle to allow the ligament to be pulled to the bone. (C) The common and lateral digital extensors are imbricated with mattress sutures, and the ulnaris lateralis is sutured.

Developmental Abnormalities Affecting the Elbow Joint

Disturbed growth resulting from premature physeal closure of either the radius or ulna can produce subluxation of the elbow. Treatment of these problems is covered in Chapter 14.

Congenital luxation of the elbow is seen on occasion. Hypoplasia or aplasia of the medial collateral ligament is the primary deformity. This leads to osseous changes consisting of hypoplasia of the coronoid and anconeal processes and a shallow trochlear notch. The proximal ulna is typically deviated laterally and dorsocranially as it rotates 45 to 90 degrees.[27]

Extensive arthroplastic procedures have produced functional joints in one series of six cases.[28] In neonates, closed reduction and stabilization for seven to ten days by means of a pin driven from the olecranon into the distal humerus has also been successful in our hands. In older pups (12 to 16 weeks old), open approach is necessary for reduction. The ulna is osteotomized distal to the trochlear notch and then the humeroulnar joint is reduced. Small pins or Kirschner wires are used to cross-pin the ulna to the humeral condyles. The limb is supported in a splint until the pins are removed in two to three weeks. Failure to achieve functional repair will require amputation or arthrodesis.

Ununited Anconeal Process

This condition is found primarily in large breed dogs, especially German shepherds, Basset Hounds, and the St. Bernard. It is characterized by failure of the ossification center of the anconeus to fuse with the olecranon by 5 months of age. Instability or detachment of the process leads to inflammatory changes and eventual osteoarthrosis of the elbow joint. The condition can be bilateral.

Hayes and associates[29] observed a positive association between risk and adult body weight; they suggested that in addition to familial genetics and hormonal factors, growth plate trauma associated with rapid or long periods of growth might be involved in the etiology. Olsson[30] has suggested that this condition is a manifestation of osteochondrosis, that is, a failure of endochondral ossification. This theory is further discussed in Chapter 18.

In an intensive study, Wind found a developmental incongruity of the trochlear notch of the ulna that was associated with the development of ununited anconeal process (UAP), fragmented coronoid process (FCP), and osteochondritis dissecans of the medial humeral condyle (OCD).[31] In affected breeds a slightly elliptical trochlear notch with a decreased arc of curvature develops that is too small for the humeral trochlea. This results in major points of contact in areas of the anconeal process and medial coronoid process and little or no contact in other areas of the trochlea (see Fig. 21–21B). The overall incidence of isolated UAP in Wind's study of 825 dogs was 0.2 percent, and UAP combined with FCP and OCD was 3 percent.[32] Although the German shepherd is noted for the occurrence of UAP, Wind found the incidence of isolated UAP to be only 1 percent, but 17 percent in combination with FCP and OCD.

CLINICAL SIGNS

Clinical signs are usually not apparent before 7 to 8 months of age. The signs consist initially of only a slight limp, with the lower limb and elbow slightly abducted. The swing phase of gait is limited by reduced motion at the elbow joint, which is virtually locked. The elbow circumducts laterally during the swing phase of gait. The dog stands and sits with the paw externally rotated, and the toes often seem widespread. Crepitus on flexion-extension is more likely in older animals; joint effusion is also noticeable. Effusion causes puffiness in the area between the lateral epicondyle and the ulna.

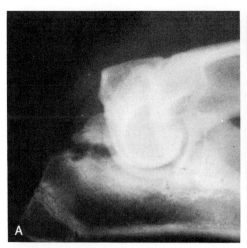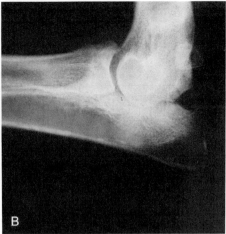

FIGURE 21–21

(A) Extreme flexion of the elbow permits good visualization of this ununited anconeal process in a 6-month-old dog. Note the wide lucent zone dividing the olecranon from the anconeal process (mediolateral view). (B) In this 24-month-old dog the anconeal process has become completely detached and is seen at the proximal extent of the caudal joint capsule. Signs of joint incongruency and secondary degenerative joint disease are evident (mediolateral view).

DIAGNOSIS

Clinical signs, age, and breed form the basis for a provisional diagnosis; however, this must be radiographically confirmed. Both elbows should be examined. Acute flexion of the elbow moves the anconeus distal to the medial epicondyle and facilitates visualization (Figs. 21–21 and 21–22). Considerable arthritic changes in the form of osteophytes may be visible throughout the joint and are best visualized from the craniocaudal view.

TREATMENT

Surgical Excision

Removal of the process is the most widely practiced method of treatment. Although it is unquestionably true that the joint is mildly unstable with the anconeous removed, it is much better to remove the source of inflammation and degenerative changes. In a series of 19 operations on 16 dogs, with an average follow-up of 19.5 months, good function was noted in most cases despite some loss of range of motion, crepitus, and arthritic changes.[33] Early removal—before marked arthrosis—produces the best results.

FIGURE 21–22

Ununited anconeal process (lateromedial view).

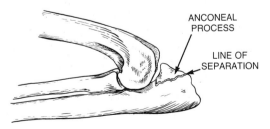

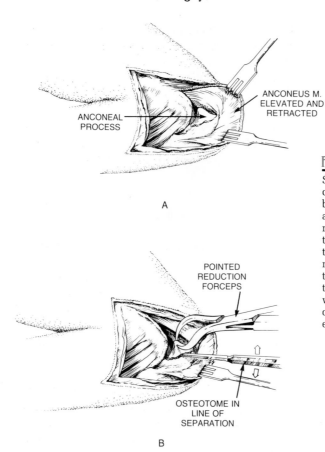

ANCONEUS M.
ELEVATED AND
RETRACTED

ANCONEAL
PROCESS

A

POINTED
REDUCTION
FORCEPS

OSTEOTOME IN
LINE OF
SEPARATION

B

FIGURE 21–23

Surgical removal of ununited anconeal process. *(A)* The left elbow has been exposed by an approach to the caudal compartment of the elbow joint.[3] With the anconeus muscle retracted, the anconeus is visualized. *(B)* A narrow osteotome is being used to free the anconeal process from the ulna. Grasping the process with a small pointed bone forceps aids in removing the process.

The elbow is exposed by a lateral approach to the caudal compartment of the elbow[3] (Fig. 21–23A). Considerable synovial hyperplasia may need to be resected in order to visualize the anconeus adequately. Usually, the process is still attached to the ulna by a fibrous union and must be sharply dissected to free it. This is usually done with a narrow osteotome or periosteal elevator (Fig. 21–23B). Grasping the process with a small pointed bone clamp or towel forceps aids in removing it from the joint. The anconeal process may be completely free within the joint, particularly in older dogs. In such cases, it may migrate to the proximal portion of the joint. It usually is not well attached and can be removed quite easily.

Screw Fixation

Repair of the ununited anconeal process by screw fixation has been advocated.[34] It is true that when a lag screw is properly placed, the process will heal. The difficulty in this approach lies in properly placing the screw. The primary consideration is that the process must be perfectly positioned or it will interfere with one of the humeral condyles on extension of the elbow. The wobble induced by such interference results in fatigue fracture of the screw. Screw fixation has the best chance of success in the animal that is presented early, between 5½ and 6 months of age. In this circumstance the process is still firmly attached to the ulna and has not moved. This will ensure that fixation of the process will be in an anatomically perfect position. The screw is placed from the caudal side of the ulna by first drilling a tap hole from the process caudally through the ulna, and then drilling a glide hole from the caudal ulnar side. This eliminates having the screw head in the joint as the original technique described.[34]

AFTERCARE ■ Those animals with significant joint effusion tend to have slow soft-tissue healing. Immobilizing the joint in a modified Robert Jones dressing (see Fig. 19–17) for seven to ten days aids significantly in preventing seromas and dehiscence.

Osteochondritis Dissecans of the Medial Humeral Trochlear Ridge

Osteochondritis dissecans (OCD) affects the medial trochlear ridge of the humerus, sometimes bilaterally, in the same dog populations that are affected by OCD of the shoulder. Although retrievers, Bernese mountain dogs, and rottweilers between the ages of 5 to 8 months are the most commonly affected, many other large breeds are affected as well. (A general discussion of osteo-chondrosis is found in Chapter 18.)

Wind found a developmental incongruity of the trochlear notch of the ulna that was associated with the development of ununited anconeal process (UAP), fragmented coronoid process (FCP), and osteochondritis dissecans of the medial humeral condule (OCD).[31] In affected breeds a slightly elliptical trochlear notch with a decreased arc of curvature develops that is too small for the humeral trochlea. This results in major points of contact in areas of the anconeal process and medial coronoid process and little or no contact in other areas of the trochlea. The incidence of FCP and OCD (which were not separated in this study) was 16 percent.[32]

CLINICAL SIGNS

Affected dogs show a foreleg lameness or stiffness and stilted gait starting between the ages of 5 to 8 months. Lameness is intensified by exercise and is often most prominent immediately after resting. Pain may be elicited by deep palpation over the medial collateral ligament or by stressing the ligament by flexing the carpus 90 degrees and rotating the foot laterally. Pain may also be evident on hyperflexion or extension of the joint. Crepitus is occasionally elicited in dogs over one year of age, when osteoarthrosis will be sufficiently advanced to produce palpable thickening of the joint on the medial aspect.

DIAGNOSIS

The radiographic diagnosis of OCD of the elbow joint has been well described by Olsson.[35] A subchondral defect can be seen on the cranial articular surface of the medial aspect of the humeral trochlea in the craniocaudal projection (Fig. 21–24A,B). Sclerosis of the medial condyle is often present near the lesion. Roughening of the medial epicondylar surface is an early sign. The lesion is radiographically visible by the age of 5 to 6 months.[35] Later in the

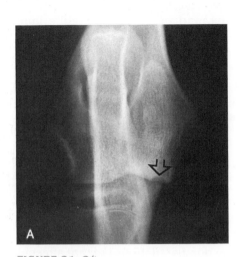

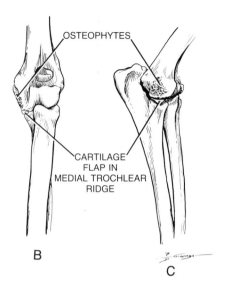

OSTEOPHYTES

CARTILAGE
FLAP IN
MEDIAL TROCHLEAR
RIDGE

B

C

FIGURE 21–24

Osteochondritis dissecans of the medial humeral trochlear ridge. *(A)* A subchondral defect *(arrow)* is seen on this craniocaudal view of the right limb. *(B)* Similar changes are seen here in the trochlear ridge of the left limb, and, in addition, osteophytes are present on the medial epicondyle. *(C)* Although the cartilage flap is seen in this drawing, it is rarely seen radiographically owing to superimposition of the condyles.

disease, osteophyte production is apparent in many areas of the joint. The lateral view also allows visualization of discontinuity of the medial trochlea (Fig. 21–24C). In dogs older than 9 to 10 months, osteophytes will be seen on the anconeus and radial head. Both elbows should be examined. Fragmented coronoid process (see below) is not uncommonly seen concurrently with osteochondritis.

TREATMENT

Treatment consists of surgical excision of cartilage flaps and removal of loose cartilage from the joint. Good results are obtained only if surgery is done before degenerative joint disease is well established. This means roughly that animals operated on after 9 months of age have a progressively poorer prognosis.

Surgical Technique

The elbow is approached from the medial aspect.[36] This simple muscle-separating approach gives adequate exposure. Some prefer an osteotomy of the medial epicondyle.[3] The epicondyle is fixed with a lag screw. Drilling for placement of the lag screw before osteotomy of the epicondyle ensures accurate replacement of the epicondyle and simplifies the drilling process.

Removal of the cartilage flap is easily accomplished with either approach because the usual location of the lesion is in the center of the surgical field (Fig. 21–25). Sharp excision frees partially attached flaps. Curettage should be just sufficient to clean the edges of the lesion. The joint should be thoroughly searched for free fragments of cartilage before the closure.

FIGURE 21-25

Surgical treatment of osteochondritis dissecans of the medial humeral condyle. The left elbow has been exposed by a medial approach with osteotomy of the epicondyle.[3] The pronator teres and flexor carpi radialis muscles and the medial collateral ligament are attached to the osteotomized bone. The cartilage flap is being elevated with a scalpel.

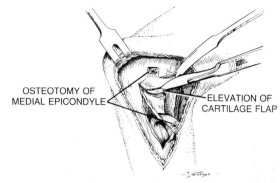

OSTEOTOMY OF MEDIAL EPICONDYLE

ELEVATION OF CARTILAGE FLAP

AFTERCARE ■ Close confinement for four weeks allows fibroplasia to fill the cartilage defect.

Fragmented Medial Coronoid Process

The breeds of animals affected, clinical manifestations, and etiopathology of the fragmented coronoid process (FCP) are similar to those found for OCD of the humeral trochlea. Indeed, these conditions coexist in 37 percent of cases.[37] Like OCD, this lesion is often considered to be part of the osteochondrosis complex,[37] but trauma[38] or growth discrepancies between the radius and ulna have been proposed as causes.

Wind found a developmental incongruity of the trochlear notch of the ulna that was associated with the development of ununited anconeal process (UAP), fragmented coronoid process (FCP), and osteochondritis dissecans of the medial humeral condyle (OCD).[31] In affected breeds a slightly elliptical trochlear notch with a decreased arc of curvature develops, which is too small for the humeral trochlea. This results in major points of contact in areas of the anconeal process and medial coronoid process and little or no contact in other areas of the trochlea. The incidence of FCP and OCD (which were not separated in this study) was 16 percent, and the incidence of FCP with UAP was 3 percent.[32]

Surgical excision of loose cartilage or bony fragments before significant arthrosis develops affords a good prognosis, but later surgery in the presence of marked arthrosis is not as successful.[38] This is verified by our own experience. The fragmented coronoid process frequently causes a "kissing" lesion on the medial aspect of the humeral condyle. This lesion is a cartilage abrasion and is difficult to distinguish from an old OCD lesion, especially in older dogs.

CLINICAL SIGNS

There is little to clinically differentiate FCP from OCD of the elbow. Pain on flexion-extension of the elbow and lateral rotation of the paw is a little more consistent in FCP. In dogs older than 10 to 11 months, joint effusion and general thickening resulting from osteophyte production are also more evident.

DIAGNOSIS

Radiographic examination of the elbow is important despite the fact that radiographic signs of the FCP are often nonspecific. Excessive osteoarthrosis and superimposition of the radial head and coronoid process make identification of the FCP difficult. Craniocaudal, flexed mediolateral, and 25-degree craniocaudal-lateromedial views with the elbow flexed 30 degrees and the lower leg slightly internally rotated are necessary for diagnosis.[35,38] Osteophyte production is more dramatic with FCP than with OCD. This is seen first on the anconeal process in the flexed mediolateral view, as are osteophytes on the cranial radial head and humeral condyles (Figs. 21–26A and 21–27B). The medial epicondyle shows marked roughening, as sometimes does the medial

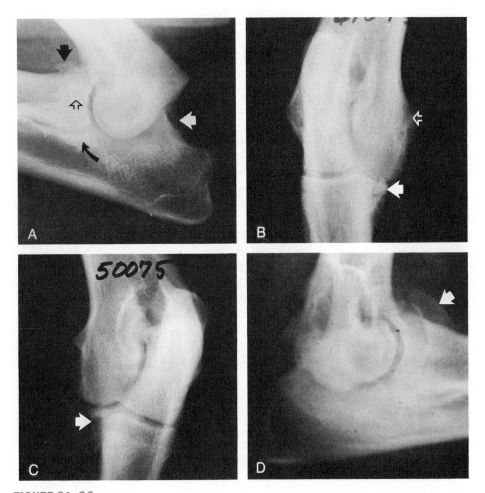

FIGURE 21–26

Fragmentation of the medial coronoid process of the ulna. (A) Mediolateral view. Osteophytes are noted on the anconeal process (white arrow) and the radial head (large black arrow). Sclerosis of the ulna (curved black arrow) is evident, and the coronoid process (open black arrow) cannot be visualized superimposed on the radial head. (B) Craniocaudal-lateromedial oblique view. Osteophytes are also seen on the medial epicondyle (open white arrow), and the nondisplaced coronoid fragment is uncharacteristically well visualized (solid arrow). (C) Craniocaudal-lateromedial oblique view. This coronoid is large and obviously displaced. (D) A large intra-articular ossicle (arrow) and multiple severe degenerative changes are noted in this 8-year-old dog. The underlying pathology was fragmentation of the coronoid process (mediolateral view).

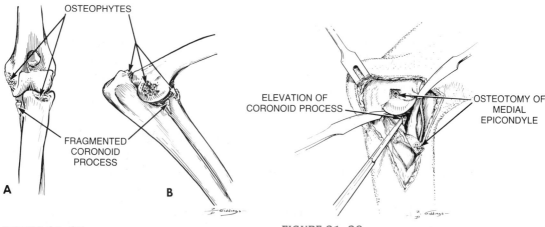

FIGURE 21-27

Fragmented coronoid process. (A) Osteophyte production is evident on the medial epicondyle and a displaced fragmented process is noted on this craniocaudal view. There is typically a faint erosion of the articular cartilage of the humeral condyle opposite the site of the fragmented process. The process may not be displaced in all cases. (B) In this mediolateral view, osteophytes are present on the anconeus and cranial radial head. The fragmented process can be seen here, but radiographically it is superimposed on the radial head.

FIGURE 21-28

Surgical treatment of fragmented medial coronoid process. The left elbow has been exposed by a medial approach with osteotomy of the epicondyle.[3] The coronoid process is being elevated with a small osteotome.

surface of the ulna near the coronoid. Both of these areas are best visualized in the craniocaudal views (Fig. 21–26B,C). Although the detached process may be seen on any view, the oblique projection offers the least obstructed view. Older dogs may have bizarre degenerative changes (Fig. 21–26D). This disease often is not radiographically diagnosable until about 7 months of age because it is often an inferred diagnosis based on the secondary osteophytes.

Although radiographic signs may be suggestive, definitive diagnosis often depends on arthrotomy. This should be undertaken immediately on any young large breed animal that shows persistent lameness and radiographic signs of osteoarthritis or joint effusion.

SURGICAL TECHNIQUE

Exposure of the joint is identical to that for OCD, discussed above (Fig. 21–28). Sharp adduction and internal rotation of the antebrachium are helpful in increasing exposure of the process. In most cases the process is loose enough to be readily apparent, but in some it is necessary to exert force on the process in order to find the cleavage plane. Older dogs with secondary osteophytes present different problems. In these the medial aspect of the process may be overgrown with osteophytes sufficiently to cover the cleavage plane and may give the process sufficient stability so that it is not easily moved. It is necessary to remove the osteophytes by rongeurs before the FCP can be appreciated.

Because of the possibility of slight malarticulation owing to discrepancies between the ulna and humeral condyle,[31,32] Olsson advised removal of the base of the medial coronoid so there is no possibility of contact with the condyle (SE Olsson, personal communication, 1988). The joint is carefully inspected for OCD lesions and then irrigated to remove cartilage fragments before closure.

AFTERCARE/PROGNOSIS ■ Confinement is advisable for four weeks before returning the dog to normal activity. The outlook for function is good if the FCP is removed before secondary degenerative joint disease (DJD) is well established. These animals will have recognizable signs of DJD later in life but usually function well, as the changes are not as severe as in untreated cases (see Fig. 21–26D). This means that those animals operated on at 7 to 9 months have the best outlook; the prognosis declines rapidly when surgery is delayed past 12 months.

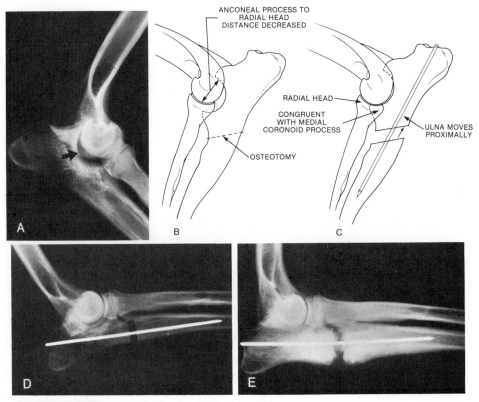

FIGURE 21–29

Incongruity of the elbow in the growing dog; the ulna is too short relative to the radius. (A) This mediolateral radiograph of elbow region illustrates that the trochlear notch (arrow) is not congruent with the radial head, resulting in subluxation of the humeroulnar joint. (B) Drawing illustrates the changes seen radiographically in A. Note the position and angle of the osteotomy. (C) Following osteotomy of the ulna the proximal ulna is free to move proximally due to muscular forces. (D) Postoperative radiograph of the case shown in A. Note the congruity of the trochlear notch of the ulna and the humeral condyles. A transverse osteotomy was performed here. (E) Three weeks postoperatively the ulnar gap is being bridged by callus, and the humeroulnar joint is congruent. Normal exercise can be resumed. (B and C, from Gilson SD, Piermattei DL, Schwarz PD: Treatment of humeroulnar subluxation with a dynamic proximal ulnar osteotomy. A review of 13 cases. Vet Surg 18:114, 1989. By permission.)

Elbow Incongruity in the Growing Dog

Intermittent forelimb lameness of moderate intensity may be seen occasionally in the immature Basset Hound, Welsh Corgi, and other chondrodystrophied breeds. If physical examination and lameness evaluation suggest the elbow joint as the source of lameness, the joint should be evaluated for asynchronous growth of the radius and ulna. This results in the ulna being either too short relative to the radius (Fig. 21–29A,B) or the radius being too short relative to the ulna (Fig. 21–30A,B), and thus differs from the trochlear notch incongruity described by Wind,[31,32] although the effects can be similar when the ulna is too short. This situation is by far the more common problem, and very similar changes are seen in the elbows of animals suffering from premature closure of the distal ulnar growth plate due to injury. These problems are discussed in Chapter 14. In the cases under consideration here, there is usually no evidence of injury to the growth plates that can be identified, and the cause of the asynchronous growth is not known.

RADIOGRAPHIC FINDINGS

Mediolateral projections with the joint in approximately 90 degrees of flexion are most useful (Figs. 21–29A and 21–30A), although the craniocaudal view should also be examined. Varying degrees of degenerative changes will be seen, depending on the age of the animal. Ununited anconeal process may be seen concurrently in breeds such as the Basset Hound that are prone to this problem.

SURGICAL TECHNIQUE

The objective of surgical treatment when the ulna is too short is to re-establish normal articulation of the humeroulnar joint. This can be done by a lengthening osteotomy of the ulna with rigid internal fixation. The difficulty with this is knowing when the ulna is in perfect alignment with the humeral condyles. A very small malalignment could lead to cartilage abrasion and late degenerative joint disease. By allowing the muscular forces to affect the proximal ulna, a dynamic reduction is achieved, which has a much better chance of being truly anatomical (Fig. 21–29B,C). The length of the limb is unaffected by this procedure. The surgery is very simple and has produced good results.[40]

When the radius is too short a dynamic reduction can be achieved by shortening the ulna. If enough ulna is removed to allow the radial head to contact the lateral humeral condyle, muscular forces will seat the head anatomically, and the humeroradial joint is re-established (Fig. 21–30B,C). The potential drawback in this procedure is that the limb is shortened, and if there is pre-existing shortening owing to severe physeal arrest, the end result could affect limb function. In this situation, lengthening with internal fixation as discussed in Chapter 14 would be indicated.

In either procedure discussed below it is important that the intramedullary pin used be *nonthreaded*, since it is critical that bone be able to slide on the pin to achieve dynamic reduction.

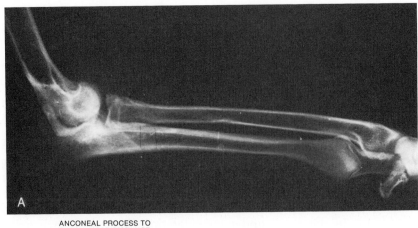

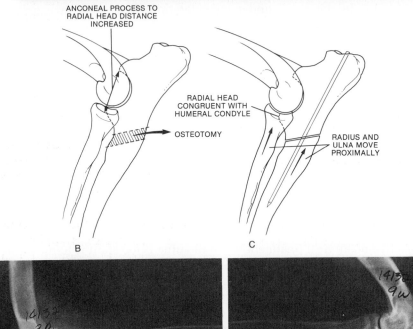

FIGURE 21–30

Incongruity of the elbow in the growing dog; the radius is too short relative to the ulna. (A) This mediolateral radiograph of elbow region illustrates a gap between the humeral condyle and the radial head, resulting in subluxation of the humeroradial joint. (B) Illustrated here are the changes seen in A and the site for the ulnar ostectomy. (C) Following ostectomy, the radius and distal ulna are pulled into reduction by muscular forces. (D) In the postoperative radiograph the gap between the humeral condyle and the radial head has been partially reduced. An overly generous section was removed from the ulna. (E) At nine weeks postoperatively the ulna has healed and the humeroradial joint is congruent. (B and C, from Gilson SD, Piermattei DL, Schwarz PD: Treatment of humeroulnar subluxation with a dynamic proximal ulnar osteotomy. A review of 13 cases. Vet Surg 18:114, 1989. By permission.)

The ulna is exposed by a caudal approach to the proximal shaft of the ulna.[3] The joint capsule is incised on both sides of the ulna in the distal trochlear notch area. An oblique osteotomy of the ulna is performed distal to the trochlear notch (see Fig. 21–29B). This cut should be made with a Gigli wire saw or power saw as an osteotome may split this hard bone. Typically the osteotomy will spontaneously gap open as the cut in the bone is completed, illustrating the dynamic muscular forces working on the proximal ulna. If such is not the case, a periosteal elevator is used to break down the interosseous membrane until the proximal ulna can be moved by forcing the osteotomy gap open. A small nonthreaded intramedullary pin or Kirschner wire, .062 to 3/32 inch diameter (1.6 to 2.4 mm), is driven from the tuber olecrani across the osteotomy and seated into the midshaft region of the bone (Fig. 21–29C,D). The oblique osteotomy and the pin protect against angular displacement of the tuber from triceps muscle forces.

If the radius is too short in relation to the ulna, a similar approach is made to the proximal ulna. An ostectomy of the ulna distal to the trochlear notch is performed instead of a simple osteotomy (Fig. 21–30B,C). The width of the removed bone must be sufficient to allow the radius and distal ulna to move proximally until the radial head articulates normally with the lateral aspect of the humeral condyle. Some narrowing of the gap will be seen postoperatively (Fig. 21–30D). A pin is driven as in the previous case.

AFTERCARE/PROGNOSIS ■ With either type surgery it is important that early active weight-bearing of the limb be achieved. A padded bandage is applied and nonsteroidal anti-inflammatory drugs (see discussion in Chapter 17) are administered to help achieve this by reducing pain and inflammation. Leash walking and limited free exercise are encouraged. Radiographic evaluation of healing should be pursued and the dog not returned to full activity until clinical union of the ulna is achieved (Figs. 21–29E and 21–30E).

If surgery is done before degenerative joint disease is established, good results can be expected.[40]

Avulsion and Calcification of the Flexor Tendons of the Medial Epicondyle

Fragments of bone embedded in the flexor muscles of the medial epicondyle and associated with forelimb lameness have been reported using a variety of descriptive terms. Ljunggren and associates reported an island of bone off the distal end of the medial epicondyle in an 8-month-old German shepherd dog and described this as *ununited medial epicondyle*.[41] The term *dystrophic calcification* was used by Henry to describe calcification within the joint capsule distal to the medial epicondyle.[42] Recently Zontine and associates proposed a new hypothesis to explain these clinical observations.[43] They did not observe any cases that met all the criteria for an ununited epicondyle, but rather found that cases in young dogs were avulsions of the tendinous origin of the humeral head of the flexor carpi ulnaris or the superficial digital flexor muscles. The avulsed fragment is viable bone, with periosteal blood supply from the muscles, and therefore these fragments may grow in size with time and become much larger than the original defect in the epicondyle (Fig. 21–31A,B). In dogs with joint incongruity or other intra-articular pathology, dystrophic calcification of these tendons develops in response to the chronic inflammation (Fig. 21–31C,D). The calcified areas do not grow as large as in

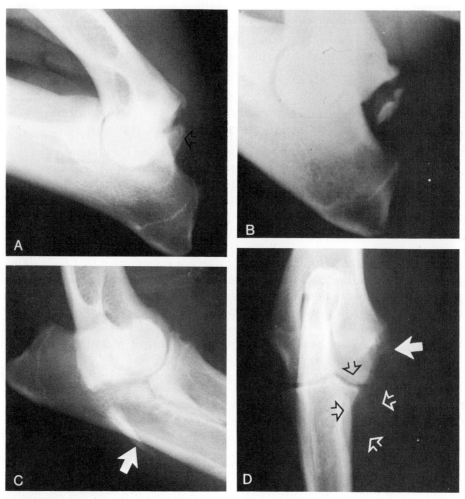

FIGURE 21–31

Avulsion and calcification of the flexor tendons of the medial epicondyle as defined by Zontine and associates.[43] (A and B) Traumatic avulsion of the medial epicondyle in two young dogs. The detached fragments are much larger than can be accounted for by defects in the epicondyle and represent avulsed bone fragments that have undergone further growth and calcification (mediolateral views). (C) Dystrophic calcification within flexor tendon (arrow) in the presence of joint incongruity. Note sclerosis of the trochlear notch area of the ulna and osteophytes on the radial head (mediolateral view). (D) Same dog as in C, craniocaudal view. The calcified area, outlined by the open arrows, is poorly visualized in this view. Osteophytosis of the epicondyle is present (solid arrow).

the previous situation. Both of these problems are found primarily in the same large breeds as are subject to the various manifestations of osteochondrosis.

HISTORY, CLINICAL SIGNS, AND DIAGNOSIS

Young dogs with traumatic avulsions develop signs of acute forelimb lameness between 5 and 8 months of age. Tenderness on palpation and joint effusion are prominent early but rapidly diminish. Older dogs with dystrophic calcification have a much more slowly developing and intermittent lameness with few local signs. Despite their size the bony masses are difficult to palpate.

Radiographic examination is essential for diagnosis. Examples of both problems are shown in Figure 21–31.

SURGICAL TECHNIQUE

Surgical excision of the bone fragments is necessary for relief of clinical signs. The fragments are not readily visible during exploration and have to be located with a sharp probe. The muscle is bluntly separated to expose the bone, which is then sharply dissected from the muscle. It is very easy to miss one of the smaller fragments, and if it is an avulsed fragment, the bone mass can continue to grow since it has a periosteal blood supply.

Aftercare/Prognosis

A padded bandage is used postoperatively to prevent hematoma and edema. Complete rest for three weeks is needed for healing of the musculotendinous tissues. Relief from lameness is complete if all the fragments are removed. Return of lameness in the future could indicate continued growth of a small fragment missed during the surgery.[43] If dystrophic calcification is secondary to joint instability or fragmented coronoid, the long-term prognosis will probably be determined by the primary problem.

Arthrodesis of the Elbow

Arthrodesis is an alternative to amputation for severely comminuted intra-articular fractures, chronic luxation or subluxation from a variety of causes, and severe osteoarthritis. High radial nerve palsy has also been suggested as an indication.[39] Elbow arthrodesis is a very disabling fusion and should be considered only when the owner refuses amputation. Amputation will provide better overall function than arthrodesis.

Strict attention to detail to establish proper joint angles and rigid internal fixation are necessary for success. Although a variety of fixation methods have been described, multiple-screw or bone plate fixation has yielded the best results in our experience. (See Chapter 19 for discussion of indications for and principles of arthrodesis.)

SURGICAL TECHNIQUE

Bone Plate Fixation

The joint is exposed by a combined caudal approach with osteotomy of the olecranon process and the lateral approach to the elbow (Fig. 21–32A). An

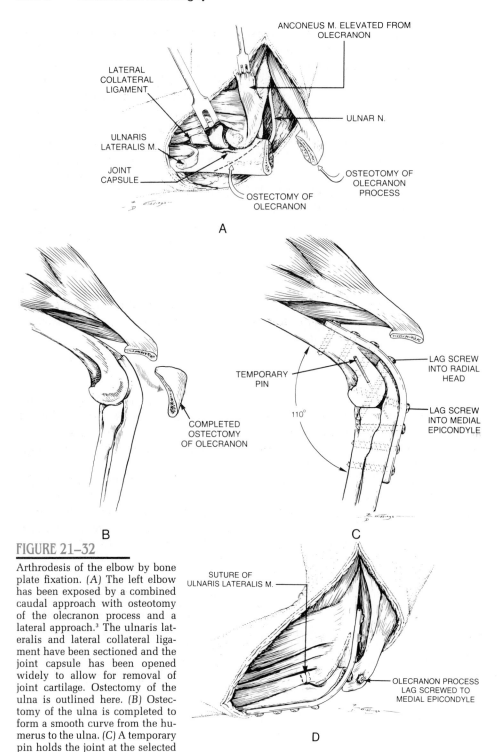

ANCONEUS M. ELEVATED FROM OLECRANON

LATERAL COLLATERAL LIGAMENT

ULNAR N.

ULNARIS LATERALIS M.

JOINT CAPSULE

OSTEOTOMY OF OLECRANON PROCESS

OSTECTOMY OF OLECRANON

A

COMPLETED OSTECTOMY OF OLECRANON

B

TEMPORARY PIN

LAG SCREW INTO RADIAL HEAD

LAG SCREW INTO MEDIAL EPICONDYLE

110°

C

SUTURE OF ULNARIS LATERALIS M.

OLECRANON PROCESS LAG SCREWED TO MEDIAL EPICONDYLE

D

FIGURE 21–32

Arthrodesis of the elbow by bone plate fixation. (A) The left elbow has been exposed by a combined caudal approach with osteotomy of the olecranon process and a lateral approach.[3] The ulnaris lateralis and lateral collateral ligament have been sectioned and the joint capsule has been opened widely to allow for removal of joint cartilage. Ostectomy of the ulna is outlined here. (B) Ostectomy of the ulna is completed to form a smooth curve from the humerus to the ulna. (C) A temporary pin holds the joint at the selected angle, and the plate is contoured. A minimum of four plate holes for each bone is required. One screw is lagged through the plate and lateral epicondyle into the radial head and a second through the plate and ulna into the medial epicondyle. (D) The olecranon process is lag-screwed to the humerus medial to the plate, and the ulnaris lateralis tendon sutured. The anconeus muscle has been excised.

ostectomy of the ulna is done to provide a smooth curve from the caudal humeral shaft to the caudal ulnar shaft with the joint at the functioning angle, usually 110 degrees (Fig. 21–32B). The lateral joint capsule is opened widely to allow the radius and ulna to be rotated medially and thus expose the interior of the joint. Articular cartilage is removed from all congruent surfaces of the radial head, humeral condyles, and trochlear notch of the ulna. The humeral capitulum is flattened to fit against the radial head.

A temporary pin is driven across the joint to hold it at the selected angle, and an 8- to 10-hole bone plate is contoured to the caudal surfaces of the ulna and humerus (Fig. 21–32C). The proximal ulna may have to be flattened slightly to allow good seating of the plate. One screw can be placed as a lag screw through the plate and lateral epicondyle into the radial head. Ideally, a second lag screw is lagged through the plate and ulna into the medial epicondyle. The rest of the screws are tapped in both cortices, and the pin is removed.

Autogenous cancellous bone graft from the proximal humerus and the ulnar ostectomy is packed into and around the joint. The olecranon process is attached medial to the plate by a lag screw (Fig. 21–32D). The anconeus muscle is detached from the humerus and the ulnaris lateralis tendon sutured. The remaining tissues are closed in layers.

Lag Screw Fixation

This technique requires less surgical exposure and less operating time and eliminates the cost of a large bone plate.[44] The joint is exposed by the lateral approach to the elbow.[3] Additional extensor muscles and the lateral collateral ligament are cut to widely expose the joint (Fig. 21–33A). Articular cartilage is debrided as detailed previously.

A temporary pin is placed across the joint to maintain the desired angle. Screw No. 1 is placed as a lag screw from the lateral condyle to the radial head (Fig. 21–33B,C). The second screw is lagged from the olecranon process into the humerus just proximal to the supratrochlear foramen. The third screw is a lag screw from the ulna into the medial condyle. Screw No. 4 is a positional screw, threaded into the ulna and the center of the condyles. The pin is removed. Autogenous cancellous bone graft from the proximal humerus is packed into and around the joint, the extensor and anconeus muscles are sutured, and the remaining tissues are closed in layers.

Aftercare ■ A spica splint is applied and maintained for four weeks (see Fig. 19–11). Exercise is restricted for four more weeks, at which time radiographic signs of fusion should be noted and exercise can gradually be returned to normal.

THE CARPUS

The carpus and foot constitute a complex and highly critical structure. The larger and more athletic the animal, the more devastating are injuries in this area. The horseman's cliché of "no feet, no horse" can also be applied to the dog. There is a tendency to treat ligamentous injuries of the carpus very

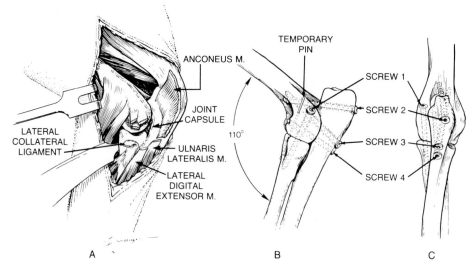

FIGURE 21–33

Elbow arthrodesis with lag screw fixation. *(A)* The left elbow has been exposed by a lateral approach. The ulnaris lateralis, lateral digital extensor, and lateral collateral ligament have been sectioned, allowing the joint capsule to be opened widely. Removal of articular cartilage follows. *(B)* A temporary pin fixes the joint at the desired angle, and the screws are placed in order. Screws Nos. 1, 2, and 3 are lag screws, and screw No. 4 is a positional screw, threaded in both bones. *(C)* Caudal view of the screw placement.

conservatively, with cast immobilization, and to hope for sufficient fibroplasia to stabilize the joint. Although this may be moderately successful in small and inactive breeds, it rarely restores full function in large breeds. Randomly oriented collagen in scar tissue cannot withstand tensile stress and soon breaks down, leaving the joint permanently unstable. Such instability soon leads to degenerative joint disease, as described in Chapter 17.

Anatomy of the Carpus

The bones of the carpus are arranged in a proximal and distal row (Fig. 21–34A,C), with three joint levels: the antebrachiocarpal, the middle carpal, and the carpometacarpal. The middle carpal is often referred to as the *intercarpal joint*, but this term properly describes the joints between carpal bones of a given level.

Ligaments of the carpus are generally short, none spanning all three joints, and most crossing only one joint level, connecting individual carpal bones (Fig. 21–34A–D). On the palmar side of the carpus, the joint capsule is well developed and blends with the palmar carpal fibrocartilage and ligaments.

Surgical Approaches

The carpal joints are opened on the dorsal aspect of the midline, elevating and retracting the carpal extensor tendons medially and the digital extensor

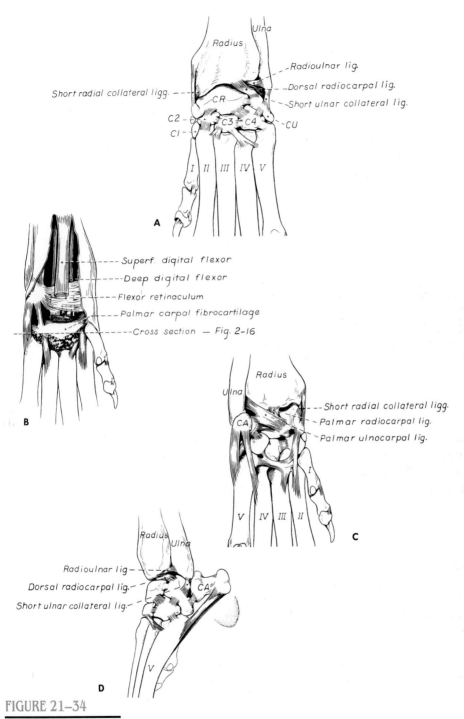

FIGURE 21–34

Ligaments of the carpus. (A) Ligaments of the left carpus, dorsal aspect. CR = radial carpal; CU = Ulnar carpal; C-1 to C-4 = First, second, third, fourth carpals; I to V = Metacarpals. (B) Superficial ligaments of the left carpus, palmar aspect. (C) Deep ligaments of the left carpus, palmar aspect. CA = Accessory carpals; I to V = Metacarpals. (D) Ligaments of the left carpus, lateral aspect. CA = Accessory carpal; V = Metacarpal V. (A–D from Evans HE, Christensen GC: Miller's Anatomy of the Dog, 2nd ed. Philadelphia, WB Saunders Company, 1979. By permission).

tendons laterally.[3] The synovial capsule must be incised at each individual joint space because the synovium is adherent to each carpal bone. The palmar ligaments and carpal fibrocartilage can be exposed by an incision slightly medial to the midline. The flexor retinaculum is incised medial to the deep digital flexor tendon, which is then retracted laterally.

Surgery of the lower limbs can be done with a tourniquet, as explained in Chapter 8. Lack of oozing hemorrhage greatly simplifies and speeds surgery. The penalty is increased postoperative swelling.

Clinical Signs of Injury

Most carpal luxations occur as a result of a fall or jump, but automobile trauma is also common. Affected limbs are non–weight-bearing, have variable swelling and joint effusion in the carpal region, and show gross instability of the carpus. The limb is commonly carried in abduction and flexed at the elbow and carpus. Palpation will usually be sufficient to localize the area of probable injury.

Diagnosis of Injury

Radiographs are necessary to verify the diagnosis and to localize the damage. Stress radiographs will show the area of instability. Standard cranial and lateral or medial views, plus obliques, will also identify avulsions and other fractures. Nonscreen film or fine-detail screens are essential.

Luxation of the Antebrachiocarpal Joint

Total luxation of the antebrachiocarpal joint is, fortunately, a rare injury (Fig. 21–35). Such total disruption of the ligamentous structure is disastrous. Panarthrodesis (see Figs. 21–44 and 21–45) is usually the only means of restoring function. Fusion of the antebrachiocarpal joint only has not been successful in our hands.

Subluxation of the Antebrachiocarpal Joint

The most commonly injured ligaments at this joint level are the radial collaterals, resulting in medial instability and valgus (lateral) deformity of the foot (Fig. 21–36). Because the dog normally stands with the foot in valgus by a few degrees, the medial ligaments are always under tension. Injuries to the lateral ligaments are both less common and less serious because they are not subject to as much tension stress.

SURGICAL TECHNIQUE

The long radial collateral ligament is important primarily when the joint is in extension. The short ligament limits and stabilizes mainly in flexion. Because the carpus slides in a dorsopalmar direction during flexion and extension, the

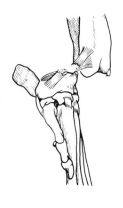
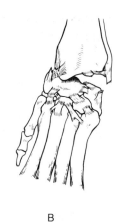

A   B

FIGURE 21–35

Luxation of the antebrachiocarpal joint. All the ligaments of the carpus are disrupted.

function of these ligaments is complex. An attempt is always made to suture the ligaments, but this is particularly difficult in the short ligament.

The area is exposed by a medial incision directly over the area. The ligaments are found immediately deep to the antebrachial fascia. Bolstering a suture repair of the ligaments with synthetic material is usually advisable. Bone tunnels are drilled in the medial prominence of the radial carpal bone and in the radius (Fig. 21–36B,C). Braided polyester suture, size 0 to 2, is passed through these holes in a manner that simulates both the long and short ligaments. Although stainless steel wire is commonly advised for such application, its use is not recommended for situations in which it is subject to alternate stretching and relaxation. Wire will quickly fatigue and break under such conditions and should only be used when it is under a continuous tension stress. The suture is tightened until the joint is stable but still mobile, then tied. The knot can be oversewn with fine wire or lightly seared with

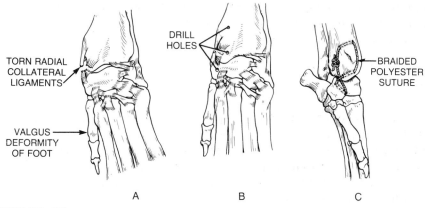

A   B   C

FIGURE 21–36

Subluxation of the antebrachiocarpal joint resulting from tearing of the radial collateral ligaments. (A) Valgus deformity of the foot develops from medial instability. (B and C) Synthetic braided suture is threaded through bone tunnels placed in the radial carpal bone and radius to simulate both the long and short ligaments. An attempt is made to suture the ligaments, which have been omitted in these views for greater clarity.

electrocoagulation to prevent untying. Earley has reported success in the use of autogenous tissue, such as the abductor pollicis longus or flexor carpi radialis tendons, in replacing the radial collateral ligaments.[45] The tendons are placed through bone tunnels in a fashion similar to that used for the synthetic material.

AFTERCARE ■ The carpus is immobilized in 10 to 15 degrees of flexion in a caudal splint (see Fig. 19–14) for four to six weeks. Strict confinement is continued through the eighth week, with a firm padded bandage in place after splint removal. A slowly progressive increase in exercise is then allowed, starting with leash walking, then short periods of free exercise.

This program is slowly increased in intensity for another four to six weeks, at which point most patients are able to return to near normal activity.

Luxation of the Radial Carpal Bone

A relatively rare condition, luxation of the major bone of the carpus is possible following a jump or fall. The radial carpal bone pivots 90 degrees medially and dorsopalmar, coming to rest against the distopalmar rim of the radius (Fig. 21–37A,B).

CLINICAL SIGNS

Severe lameness is always present with abduction of the limb and elbow flexion. Swelling is not remarkable, and the joint is not easily movable. Pain and crepitus are usually elicited by palpation, which easily reveals the displaced bone and a depression in its normal area.

TREATMENT

Surprisingly, the bone can often be reduced closed if seen soon after injury. Functional stability is unlikely to result, however, because of damage to the radial collateral ligaments. Although splint fixation for a few weeks may well be justified in a toy or small breed, many patients will require surgical stabilization.

Surgical Technique

The joint is exposed by a dorsal midline approach.[3] The following is a modification of the repair described by Punzet.[46] The lateromedial rotation is corrected first, and the bone is rotated in a palmodorsal direction to reduce it. A small pin is placed from the medial nonarticulating surface of the bone into the ulnar carpal bone. The pin is cut short and countersunk into the articular cartilage. A synthetic radial collateral ligament is constructed as detailed previously (see Fig. 21–36B,C). The remaining ligament is sutured if possible.

AFTERCARE ■ The carpus is immobilized in 10 to 15 degrees of flexion in a caudal splint (see Fig. 19–14) for four to six weeks. Strict confinement is continued through the eighth week, with a firm padded bandage in place after

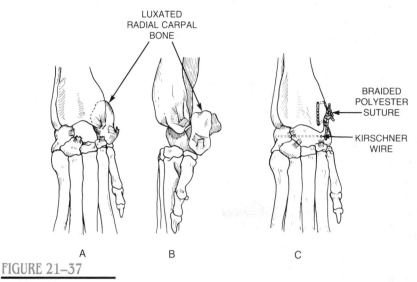

FIGURE 21–37

Luxation of the radial carpal bone. (*A* and *B*) Dorsal and medial views illustrating the palmaro-medial luxation of the radial carpal bone. The bone is rotated 90 degrees medially and dorsopalmar. (*C*) The bone is reduced, and a Kirschner wire is driven through the bone into the ulnar carpal. Synthetic radial collateral ligaments stabilize the medial side of the joint.

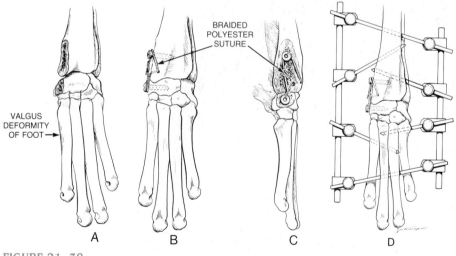

FIGURE 21–38

Shearing injury of the medial carpus. (*A*) The radial styloid process and medial aspect of the radial carpal bone and the associated collateral ligaments have been ground away. (*B* and *C*) Bone screws provide anchor points for the synthetic ligament of braided polyester suture. Placement of the screws and bone tunnel closely mimic the normal ligament. (*D*) In order to simplify open treatment of soft tissues, the joint is stabilized in 10 degrees of flexion with external skeletal fixation (Kirschner-Ehmer splint). The connecting rods are bent to allow the desired amount of extension.

splint removal. A slowly progressive increase in exercise is then allowed, starting with leash walking, then short periods of free exercise.

This program is slowly increased in intensity for another four to six weeks, at which point most patients are able to return to near normal activity.

Shearing Injury of the Carpus

This abrasion injury occurs when the dog's lower limb is run over by the tire of an automobile with its brakes locked attempting to avoid the animal. Soft tissues in contact with the pavement are simply ground away, often eroding skin, muscle, ligaments, and even bone. The medial carpal and metacarpal regions are most commonly affected, with the radial styloid process and radial collateral ligaments often completely destroyed (Fig. 21–38A). One or more carpal or metacarpal joints may be open, and various amounts of debris are ground into all the tissues. The lateral side is less commonly involved and represents a less serious injury than a comparable injury on the medial side. Owing to the fact that the dog normally stands with a few degrees of valgus (lateral) deviation of the forepaw, ligamentous stability of the medial side of the carpus and metacarpus is much more critical than on the lateral aspect.

Best results are obtained by treating these wounds in an open manner, with early stabilization of the joints and any accompanying fractures. Skin grafting is delayed and indicated only where granulation tissue does not adequately close the skin, a rare occurrence. Early or delayed arthrodesis is indicated in those cases where it is not possible to restore reasonable joint function. Variables to be considered in choosing a plan of action are:

1. Assuming that the joint(s) can be stabilized, is there enough articular surface to allow good function? Loss of bone in the tarsocrural articulation is critical. If the answer is no, arthrodesis is indicated.
2. What will the owner accept as reasonable function? A large active breed presents problems different from those of a small and sedentary animal. In the former, aggressive ligamentous repair, augmentation, or replacement is necessary, while in the latter case it may be possible to obtain good results by very conservative methods. Stabilization of joints by scar tissue may well provide adequate support in the smaller and less active animals, but it rarely will support the tension loads of the medial side in large athletic individuals.
3. How will support for the joints or fractured bones be provided? Regardless of which approach is taken to the ligamentous instability, the involved joints must be stabilized during the healing period. Because of the necessity for daily bandage changes for two to three weeks when treating these large open wounds, the use of conventional casts or splints is difficult. External skeletal fixation devices have greatly aided in solving this problem.

TREATMENT

Initial debridement must be meticulous but not too aggressive, with emphasis on removal of obviously dead tissue and foreign matter from both soft tissue and joint spaces. Copious irrigation with saline or Ringer's solution is very important at this time. Addition of 10 percent povidone iodine or 0.2 percent chlorhexidine is favored by some. After adequate debridement, it may be possible to partially close the wound by suturing skin. This can be helpful, but care must be taken to:

1. Leave adequate open area for unimpeded wound drainage. Placement of Penrose or tube drains under the sutured skin is usually advisable for two to five days.
2. Avoid closing skin under tension. Serious circulatory stasis develops owing to the tourniquet-like effect of excessive skin tension in the lower limbs.

Several debridements over a number of days may be necessary to adequately remove all devitalized tissue because of the difficulty in determining viability of badly traumatized tissue.

If there are portions of ligaments, joint capsule, or other tissues that can be sutured to support the joint and to close the synovial membrane, this should be done. Monofilament or synthetic absorbable suture is most trouble free. Re-establishment of the radial collateral ligament complex is usually hampered by loss of bone, and small bone screws may have to be used to anchor the synthetic ligament. There is a tendency to use monofilament wire in this contaminated area, but heavy braided suture is a much more functional ligament and has resulted in very few problems related to suture sinus drainage tracts. Two bone screws are positioned to mimic the normal ligaments as closely as possible (Fig. 21–38B,C). Precise placement of these bone screws for attachment of heavy braided polyester suture and adequate soft-tissue debridement are necessary for successful treatment. The sutures are tied tightly enough to stabilize the joint, but motion without binding should still be possible. Washers can be used on the screws to prevent the suture from slipping over the head of the screw.

Treatment of the open wound is simplified by use of transarticular external skeletal fixation (Kirschner-Ehmer splint) to stabilize the joint (Fig. 21–38D). Fixation is maintained until granulation tissue has covered the defect, usually three to four weeks. Sterile laparotomy sponges soaked in povidone iodine or chlorhexidine solution are loosely bandaged to the limb for several days, and debridement is repeated daily or every other day until all dead tissue is removed. The wound must be kept moist and provision made for adequate drainage of exudate.[47] Moist gauze with copious absorbent padding and dressing changes are used daily until healthy granulation covers the wound. At this point, nonadherent dressings, either dry or with antibacterial ointments, and minimal absorbent padding are used in place of the moist dressings. Intervals between dressing changes can gradually be spread out as discharge lessens. The wound must be kept protected until it is well epithelialized, which may take up to 10 to 12 weeks.

Aftercare

When granulation tissue completely covers the wound, but not before three weeks postoperatively, the external fixator is removed. A firm elastic support bandage should be maintained for another three weeks with very restricted activity. Normal exercise is not allowed until the eighth to 12th week, depending on the stability achieved. Loosening of the bone screws and skin irritation from the screw head are both indications for removing the screws. The screw in the radial carpal bone is particularly prone to loosening because of its motion. This should not be done before three to four months postoperatively if possible.

Failure to adequately stabilize the joint will result in degenerative joint disease and poor function. In such a situation arthrodesis offers the best chance of restoring function. See the discussion below regarding arthrodesis.

Middle Carpal Luxation and Subluxation

LUXATION

Complete disruption of the middle carpal joint is unusual but does occur, as illustrated in Figure 21–39. This is a combined antebrachiocarpal and middle carpal luxation because the ulnar carpal remains attached to the distal carpal bones in this 10-pound mixed terrier. In this case, the foot has twisted laterally (supination) about 60 degrees. A closed reduction was performed, and the lower limb was splinted for six weeks. Spontaneous ankylosis of the middle carpal joint adequately stabilized the carpus in this small animal.

It is highly unlikely that adequate stability would occur in a larger animal that was treated conservatively. Hyperextension of the middle carpal joint would almost always develop, necessitating partial arthrodesis of the carpus (see Figs. 21–42 and 21–43). Because of the complexity of the injury, primary repair and stabilization of a complete luxation—although technically possible—are not very feasible.

SUBLUXATION

Subluxation of the middle carpal joint, with medial instability, is a much more common problem. Ligamentous disruption between the radial carpal

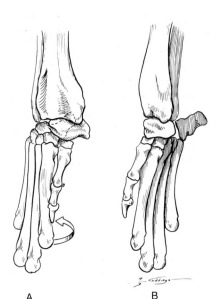

FIGURE 21–39

Middle carpal joint luxation, right limb. (A) This is actually a combined middle and antebrachiocarpal luxation because the ulnar carpal bone has remained with the distal carpals. The foot has supinated 60 degrees. Dorsal view. (B) Medial view showing supination of the foot.

A   B

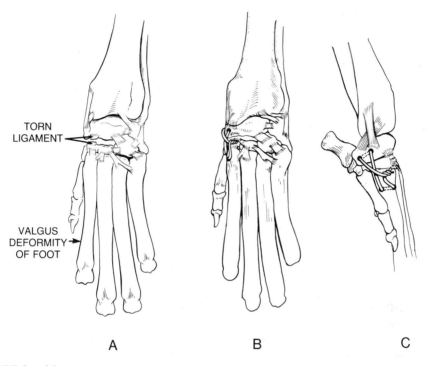

TORN
LIGAMENT

VALGUS
DEFORMITY
OF FOOT

A   B   C

FIGURE 21–40

Middle carpal joint subluxation with medial instability. Left limb, dorsal view. (*A*) Ligaments are torn between the radial carpal and carpal 2. (*B* and *C*) Bone tunnels are drilled in the palmaromedial process of the radial carpal bone and in the base of metacarpal II. Stainless steel wire of 20 to 22 gauge (0.8 to 0.6 mm) is threaded through the holes in figure-eight fashion and the wire tightened enough to eliminate the valgus instability.

and carpal 2 and occasionally between carpal 2 and metacarpal II results in valgus deformity of the foot (Fig. 21–40A).

Less easily appreciated is the fact that the palmaromedial ligaments or carpal fibrocartilage is often damaged, with resultant hyperextension (see discussion below). This hyperextension affects only the medial half of the carpus and therefore is not as dramatic as the examples shown below. The mediolateral projection stress radiographs mentioned below (Fig. 21–41) will need to be taken with slight internal rotation (pronation) of the paw to demonstrate hyperextension in this situation. If hyperextension is *not* present, the repair can proceed as described here. If hyperextension *is* present, the medial wire augmentation repair described here is performed, plus a partial arthrodesis of the medial half of the middle carpal and carpometacarpal joints (Fig. 21–42) is preferred. The Kirschner wires seen in Figure 21–42 are placed in metacarpals II and III in this case.

Surgical Technique

The incision for the dorsal approach to the carpus is positioned dorsomedially on the carpus.[3] If a partial arthrodesis is to be performed concurrently, it is done first. See the discussion below for details.

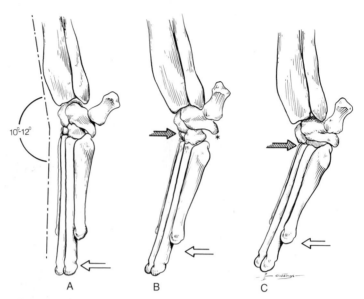

FIGURE 21–41

Stress radiographs for diagnosis of carpal hyperextension. Left limb, lateral views. *(A)* Lateral view of a normal carpus with the foot stressed *(open arrow)* to maximal extension of 10 to 12 degrees. *(B)* Lateral view of hyperextension at the middle carpal joint *(closed arrow)*. Note the gap between the palmar process of the ulnar carpal bone *(star)* and the base of metacarpal V. *(C)* Lateral view of hyperextension at the carpometacarpal level *(closed arrow)*.

The wire placement proceeds by exposure of the medial aspect of the joint. A bone tunnel is drilled through the palmaromedial process of the radiocarpal bone and through the base of metacarpal II (Fig. 21–40B,C). Stainless steel wire, 18 to 22 gauge (1 to 0.6 mm), is threaded through the holes in figure-8 fashion. The valgus deformity is reduced and the wire tightened until the instability is abolished. Care must be taken to turn the twisted end of the wire closely against the bone to minimize skin irritation. Closure of the skin completes the procedure.

FIGURE 21–42

Partial arthrodesis of the carpus with pin fixation. *(A)* The carpus is exposed by a dorsal midline incision.[3] The middle carpal, carpometacarpal, and intercarpal joints are debrided of articular cartilage. *(B)* Slots are burred in the dorsal cortex of metacarpals III and IV in the distal third of the bones. Kirschner wire (0.045 or 0.062 inch) is introduced into the medullary canal in the manner of a Rush pin. *(C)* An alternative method of placing the Kirschner wires is to drive them from the metacarpophalangeal joints proximally. Two pins are placed and driven to the base of metacarpals III and IV. *(D)* Autogenous cancellous bone graft is placed in all the prepared joint spaces. The carpus is flexed 90 degrees, and palmar and proximal pressure on the metacarpal bones is applied to correctly position the carpal bones relative to the metacarpals. The Kirschner wires are now driven into the proximal row of carpal bones as deeply as possible without penetrating the articular surface. *(E)* Both pins are seated, and the protruding end is bent into a hook shape and cut off. *(F)* Pins placed at the metacarpophalangeal joint are also bent to a hook shape and cut off.

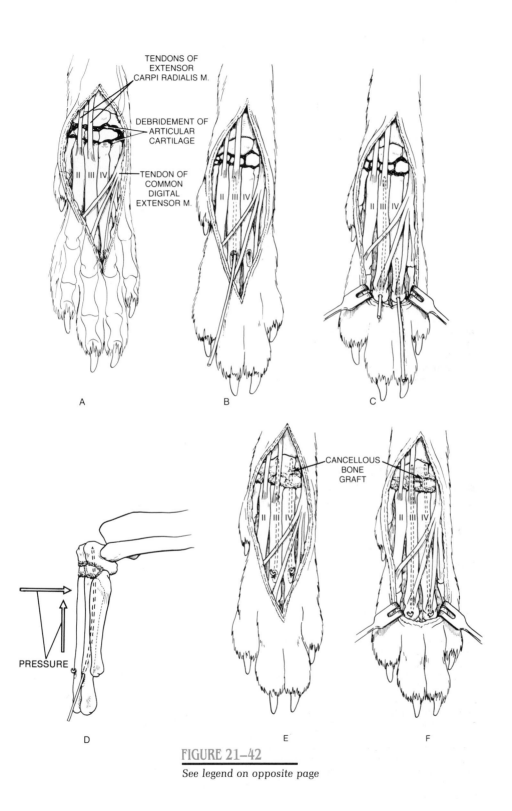

TENDONS OF
EXTENSOR
CARPI RADIALIS M.

DEBRIDEMENT OF
ARTICULAR
CARTILAGE

II III IV

TENDON OF
COMMON
DIGITAL
EXTENSOR M.

II III IV

II III IV

A   B   C

PRESSURE

CANCELLOUS
BONE
GRAFT

II III IV

II III IV

D   E   F

FIGURE 21–42

See legend on opposite page

AFTERCARE ■ The carpus is immobilized in 10 to 15 degrees of flexion in a caudal splint (see Fig. 19–14) for four to six weeks. Strict confinement is continued through the eighth week, with a firm padded bandage in place after splint removal. A slowly progressive increase in exercise is then allowed, starting with leash walking, then short periods of free exercise. This program is slowly increased in intensity for another four to six weeks, at which point most patients are able to return to near normal activity. If a partial arthrodesis was done, use the aftercare routine for that procedure.

Hyperextension of the Carpus

Among the most serious injuries to the canine carpus, hyperextension is also one of the more common, occurring in midsize and large breeds of dogs after falls and jumps. The structures responsible for maintaining the normal 10 to 12 degrees of carpal extension are the palmar ligaments and palmar carpal fibrocartilage (see Fig. 21–34B–D). It is commonly held that hyperextension of the carpus is a result of tendon injury, but in fact the only tendon that bears on carpal stability in extension is the flexor carpi ulnaris, which inserts on the accessory carpal bone. Sectioning of this tendon results in very slight hyperextension at the antebrachiocarpal joint. Diagnosis of this problem is relatively easy because there will be either a laceration of the skin or, in the case of spontaneous rupture or avulsion (rare), palpable evidence of soft-tissue inflammation.

HISTORY AND CLINICAL SIGNS

Invariably there is a history of injury caused by a fall or jump. If there is no history of injury and hyperextension has developed slowly, immune-mediated joint disease may be the cause (see Chapter 17).

Surprisingly, minimal signs of pain and inflammation are associated with hyperextension injuries. Animals commonly will attempt weight-bearing within a few days. A seal-like or plantigrade stance is characteristic but variable in appearance. Some animals may be walking on their carpal pads, but others may show only 20 to 30 degrees of extension.

DIAGNOSIS

In order to select the proper treatment, it is important to know at which joint level the injury has occurred. In our experience, the distribution of injuries has been as follows:

1. Antebrachiocarpal, 10 percent.
2. Middle carpal, 28 percent.
3. Carpometacarpal, 46 percent.
4. Combined middle and carpometacarpal, 16 percent.

Definition of the joint level is possible only by radiographic examination. A medial or lateral exposure is made with the limb stressed to maximal carpal extension (see Fig. 21–41). In chronic injuries, varying degrees of bony proliferation will be present where the more proximal bones override the distal bones. In *chronic* middle carpal instability, the radial and ulnar carpal bones pivot in a palmar direction, their dorsodistal edges coming to rest on the base of the metacarpals, creating a wide gap between the craniodorsal surface of the radius and the radial carpal bone.

Panarthrodesis (fusion of all three joint levels) has been the most widely practiced method of treating carpal hyperextension, regardless of the joint level involved.[48] This has been a satisfactory method of treatment, with 97 percent of owners reporting improvement in gait and 74 percent reporting normal use of the limb[48]; nevertheless, it destroys a normal joint (antebrachiocarpal) and requires the use of bone-plating equipment (see Figs. 21–44 and 21–45) or external skeletal fixators (see Fig. 21–38D).

It is our belief that partial arthrodesis (fusion of the middle carpal and carpometacarpal joints only) is a better approach for those injuries that involve only the middle and distal joints (Figs. 21–42 and 21–43). With this technique, flexion of the major joint of the carpus—the antebrachiocarpal joint—is maintained, and gait is affected little. Conversely, in chronic cases with marked degenerative joint disease, panarthrodesis will yield better results.

Progress has been reported by Earley in primary repair of these injuries, using heavy stainless steel wire to reconstruct damaged ligaments and palmar carpal fibrocartilage.[45] Fibrocartilage is torn in the carpometacarpal injury. Perhaps this method will eventually replace arthrodesis as a treatment for hyperextension, but it has not been useful in our hands.

Conservative treatment by splinting in flexion or hyperextension seems

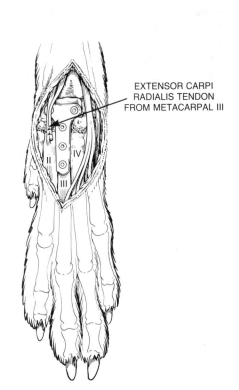

EXTENSOR CARPI
RADIALIS TENDON
FROM METACARPAL III

FIGURE 21–43

Partial arthrodesis of the carpus using T-plate fixation. The plate is attached to the distal end of the radial carpal bone, the screws angling proximally. The first screw in the long end of the plate is placed in carpal 3, and the other two screws in the third metacarpal. The tendon of the extensor carpi radialis inserting on metacarpal III has been transposed to metacarpal II and is sutured there. Left limb, dorsal view.

to have little application, since virtually all animals will break down again following return to weight-bearing. Patients with mild hyperextension at the antebrachiocarpal level and smaller animals are the best candidates for treatment by splintage. Arthrodesis can be performed later if necessary.

Two basic types of arthrodesis are performed in the carpal region. Panarthrodesis involves surgical fusion of all three joint levels, the antebrachiocarpal, the middle carpal, and the carpometacarpal. Partial arthrodesis involves fusion of only the middle and distal joints.

Partial Arthrodesis

Partial, or subtotal, arthrodesis involves surgical fusion of only the middle level and carpometacarpal joints. The function of the carpus remains essentially normal in this technique because there is little motion normally present in these joint levels. The antebrachiocarpal joint, which is responsible for virtually all flexion of the carpus, remains functional.

The major indication for partial arthrodesis is hyperextension of the middle carpal and carpometacarpal joint levels, these cases comprising 90 percent of all hyperextension injuries of the carpus. Both joints are fused when either is injured because of the technical difficulty of fusing either individually. On occasion, instability will develop medially at either of these joints and will not respond to treatment (see Fig. 21–40); these cases could also be considered for partial arthrodesis.

PIN FIXATION

A dorsal midline approach to the carpus is made with the incision extending distally to the level of the metacarpophalangeal joints (see Fig. 21–42A).[3] A tourniquet can be used. Preparations are made to collect a cancellous bone graft from the proximal humerus of the same limb (see Chapter 3). Articular cartilage of the middle carpal, intercarpal, and carpometacarpal joints is debrided with a curette or air turbine drill. Care is taken to preserve the insertions of the extensor carpi radialis tendon on the proximal ends of metacarpals II and III. If the air turbine drill is available, slots are burred through the distal cortex of metacarpals III and IV at the level of the distal third of the shaft (see Fig. 21–42B).

Kirschner wires (0.045 or 0.062 inch, 1.2 or 1.6 mm) are introduced through the slots into the medullary canal in the manner of a Rush pin and driven proximally into the base of the metacarpal bone (see Fig. 21–42C). Autogenous cancellous graft is collected from the proximal humerus and packed into the debrided joint spaces.

With the carpus held in extreme flexion to reduce the subluxation of the middle carpal or carpometacarpal level, pins are driven proximally into the radial carpal bone (see Fig. 21–42D). The pins must not penetrate the proximal articular cartilage of the radial carpal bone. The pins are then bent to form a hook at the distal end and cut off, after which the hook is rotated flat against the bone (see Fig. 21–42E).

If no air drill is available, it is difficult to cut slots in the metacarpal bones; the pins are thus driven from the metacarpophalangeal joint proximally into the shaft of the bone similarly to pinning a metacarpal fracture (see Fig.

12–16). The pins should enter the bone slightly dorsal to the articular cartilage of the distal end of the metacarpal bone. After the pins are seated in the radial carpal bone, the distal ends are bent to form a hook, cut off, and rotated flat against the bone (see Figs. 21–42C,F).

T-PLATE FIXATION

A small T plate (Synthes Ltd. [USA], Paoli, PA) can also be used for partial arthrodesis. The joint is exposed, prepared, and bone grafted as detailed previously for pin fixation. The plate is attached to the distodorsal surface of the radial carpal bone (see Fig. 21–43) and is placed as far distally on the radial carpal bone as possible in order to avoid interference with the cranial rim of the radius. The two screws in the radial carpal bone are angled proximally to allow the plate to be properly positioned.

The distal portion of the plate must lie over the third metacarpal bone. This necessitates cutting the tendon of insertion of the extensor carpi radialis. It is sutured to the insertion of its paired tendon on metacarpal II. The two distal screws in the plate are placed in metacarpal III. The most proximal screw is either placed in carpal 3, as shown in Figure 21–43, or in the base of metacarpal III.

AFTERCARE ■ A padded support bandage is applied for several days, and after swelling has subsided, a molded splint or short leg cylinder cast (see Figs. 19–10 and 19–14) is applied to the caudal surface of the limb. This support is maintained until radiographic signs of fusion are noted, typically six to eight weeks later. If the pins were driven from the metacarpophalangeal joint, they should be removed before allowing exercise. A gradual return to normal exercise is allowed over the next four weeks.

Panarthrodesis

Indications for panarthrodesis are primarily those that involve the antebrachiocarpal joint: polytrauma, such as fractures or multiple ligamentous injuries, degenerative joint disease, and hyperextension injuries at this level. Arthrodesis for brachial plexus paralysis is not recommended because of the poor elbow function and self-mutilation of the foot that usually occur. It does not appear to be practical to fuse only the antebrachiocarpal level; therefore, when this level must be fused, the other two levels are also fused. Fusion of only the antebrachiocarpal joint is technically possible, but the stress placed on the metacarpal and carpometacarpal joints disposes them to increased laxity and degenerative changes. It should be remembered that because there is very little motion in the middle and distal joints of the carpus, fusion of the antebrachiocarpal level effectively destroys all motion in the carpus.

Either bone plate or external skeletal fixation can be applied for stabilization of this fusion. Plate fixation was originally applied dorsally,[48] but this position is mechanically unsound since the plate is not on the tension side of the carpus and is therefore subject to bending forces. The plate will loosen or break unless the carpus is supported in a cast or splint until fusion is radiographically verified. A palmar position for the plate is obviously mechanically superior and has been found to be useful by Chambers and

Bjorling.[49] External skeletal fixators can be applied in a variety of configurations and are especially valuable in the presence of open injuries.

DORSAL BONE PLATE FIXATION

A dorsal midline approach from the level of the distal radius to the midmetacarpal level[3] is used after a tourniquet has been placed. Preparations are made to collect a cancellous bone graft from the same limb (see Chapter 3). Articular cartilage of the antebrachiocarpal, the middle carpal, the carpometacarpal, and the intercarpal joints is debrided with a curette or air turbine drill. The tendons of the extensor carpi radialis on metacarpals II and III can be sacrificed. After debridement of articular cartilage of all three joint levels (Fig. 21–44A), a seven-hole compression plate, usually for 3.5-mm screws, is applied to the dorsal surface of the distal radius, bridging the carpus, and attaching distally to the third metacarpal (Fig. 21–44B). Three screws are placed in the distal radius, one in the radial carpal bone, and three in the third metacarpal bone. The distal screw must be placed first in order to center the plate over metacarpal III and so ensure that the screws will be centered in this rather narrow bone. The self-compressing load position is used for the first two screws in the radius and metacarpal III in order to compress all the joint levels. The plate is contoured to produce about 10 degrees of extension in the carpus (Fig. 21–44C,D). Autogenous cancellous bone from the proximal humerus is used to pack all the joint spaces and space beneath the plate. The extensor carpi radialis tendons are sutured to joint capsule in the area.

AFTERCARE ■ A short, molded palmar splint (see Fig. 19–14) is maintained until radiographic signs of fusion are noted, usually six to eight weeks. Exercise is gradually returned to normal over the following four weeks.

If function of the limb is good, most plates will need to be removed in six to 12 months because of loosening or irritation. The metacarpal bones are supple enough to bend slightly during weight-bearing, and this may cause loosening of the distal screws. Fatigue fractures of metacarpal III occur at the end of the plate on occasion. The plate should be removed and the foot splinted until bone healing is well advanced, usually about four weeks.

PALMAR BONE PLATE FIXATION[49]

A palmaromedial approach to the distal radius and carpus is used to expose the area.[3] Preparations are also made to collect a cancellous bone graft from the proximal humerus of the same limb (see Chapter 3). Ligaments, palmar carpal fibrocartilage, and joint capsule are sharply dissected from the distal radius and carpal bones. Articular cartilage of all joint levels is removed by powered burs or curettes. Any bony prominences that prevent close contact of the plate and bone are removed in preparation for attaching an appropriate-size plate. This is usually a 3.5-mm screw and self-compressing plate in large breed dogs, and it should be long enough to place three screws in the radius and in metacarpal III.

The carpus is positioned in normal extension (10 to 12 degrees), and a Kirschner wire is drilled from the distal radius into the carpus to temporarily maintain the desired angle while the plate is contoured to fit the palmar

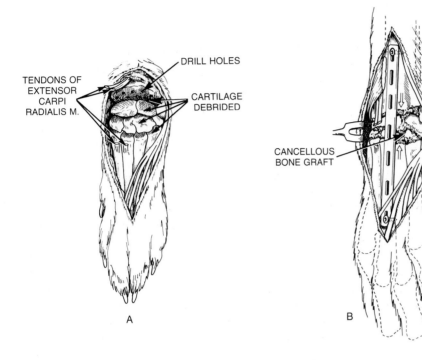

FIGURE 21–44

Panarthrodesis of the carpus with a dorsal plate. *(A)* The left carpus has been exposed by a dorsal midline incision,[3] and the tendons of the extensor carpi radialis severed at metacarpals II and III. Removal of articular cartilage is eased by maximum flexion of the joint. Multiple drill holes penetrate the distal radius to aid in vascularization. *(B)* A seven- or eight-hole bone plate is contoured to provide 10 to 12 degrees of carpal extension (see *D*) and is attached distally to the third metacarpal and proximally to the radius. The abductor pollicis longus muscle must be cut to seat the plate on the radius proximally. The screws in this dynamic compression plate (Synthes Ltd. [USA], Paoli, PA) are placed in the load position to produce compression. It is important that the distal screw be placed first, in order to center the plate on metacarpal III. Autogenous cancellous bone graft is packed into the joint spaces. *(C and D)* The bone plate is completely attached, with three screws in the radius, three in the third metacarpal, and one in the radial carpal bone. Autogenous cancellous bone graft is used to pack the joint spaces and under the plate. Note that about 10 degrees of carpal extension have been maintained.

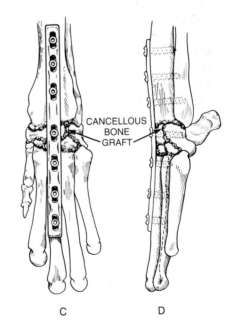

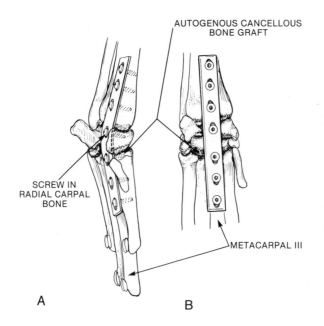

AUTOGENOUS CANCELLOUS
BONE GRAFT

SCREW IN
RADIAL CARPAL
BONE

METACARPAL III

A

B

FIGURE 21–45

Carpal panarthrodesis with a palmar plate.[49] A palmaromedial approach to the distal radius and carpus[3] is made to allow plate placement on the distal radius and metacarpal bone III. Autogenous cancellous bone graft is used in the prepared articular surfaces. Plate size for large breed dogs is typically 2.7 to 3.5 mm.

surface of the distal radius and metacarpal III (Fig. 21–45). The plate is attached first at the distal hole to ensure that the screw holes in metacarpal III will be centered in this narrow bone. The plate is then attached using the self-compressing load position for the first two screws in the radius and metacarpal III in order to compress all the joint levels. Cancellous bone graft is added to the joint surface areas and the Kirschner wire removed before closing the tissues in layers.

AFTERCARE ■ A padded support bandage is applied for several days, and after swelling has subsided, a molded splint (see Fig. 19–14) is applied to the caudal surface of the limb. This splint is maintained until radiographic signs of fusion are noted, typically six to eight weeks later. A gradual return to normal exercise is allowed over the next four weeks. If the animal can be closely confined, and if the use of a splint presents difficulties in treatment of soft-tissue wounds, it is possible to dispense with use of the splint.

External Skeletal Fixation

There are occasions when it is desirable to perform panarthrodesis of the carpus in the face of actual or potential infection. Open comminuted fractures and severe shearing injuries are the most common indications. Early arthrodesis will help in management of the soft-tissue injury by providing stabilization of the area, thus improving blood supply and optimizing the local defense reaction. Considerable time and expense are also saved. In this situation, the Kirschner-Ehmer splint configuration shown in Figure 21–38D, and variations, can be used to advantage to stabilize the joint after preparation of the joint surfaces, as described previously. Autogenous cancellous bone graft (see Chapter 3) can be safely used in the presence of infection but should be withheld if there is frank suppuration. In this circumstance the graft will be washed out of the site by the exudate and therefore wasted. It is more useful to wait until healthy granulation has covered the area and then elevate the granulation tissue and insert the graft.

AFTERCARE ■ Bone healing in open injuries will probably be delayed, and the splint will have to be maintained for 10 to 12 weeks. Radiographic fusion in closed injuries will usually be attained by eight weeks. If bone pins loosen before fusion is radiographically visible, the pins can be either replaced or removed and followed with a few more weeks of immobilization in a short leg cast (see Fig. 19–10).

Luxation of the Metacarpophalangeal and Interphalangeal Joints

Luxation or subluxation of the phalanges can occur at any joint level (Fig. 21–46), but the distal interphalangeal joint is the most commonly involved. These injuries are confined almost exclusively to racing greyhounds and working dogs. In greyhounds, the toe is usually luxated to the left side, that is, the inside of the track. In other breeds, the distribution is more random.

These are serious injuries for a running or working dog and should not be dismissed lightly. Aggressive surgical repair has yielded much better results than more conservative approaches, such as closed reduction and splintage. Many of these animals end up with instability of the joint and chronic degenerative changes in the joints that slow them markedly or leave them reluctant to traverse hard ground.

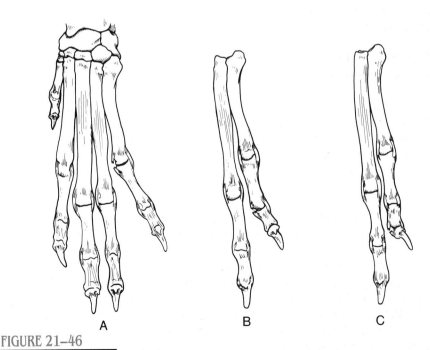

A   B   C

FIGURE 21–46

Luxation and subluxation of the phalanges. (A) Lateral subluxation of the metacarpophalangeal joint with rupture of the medial collateral ligaments. (B) Lateral subluxation of the proximal interphalangeal joint with rupture of the medial collateral ligaments. (C) Lateral subluxation of the distal interphalangeal joint with rupture of the medial collateral ligaments.

Surgical treatment by suture repair of collateral ligaments and joint capsule (Fig. 21–47) works best when performed within the first 10 days after injury. Fibroplasia of these structures makes accurate suturing more difficult after 10 days. Failure to stabilize the joint leaves only the alternatives of amputation (Figs. 21–48 and 21–49) or arthrodesis (Fig. 21–50). Amputation of the second or fifth toe at any joint level is not too serious in most dogs, but in the middle toes the results are not as good because they are the main weight-bearing digits. The more distal the amputation is, the better the prognosis. Although amputations usually give good results in working animals, the outcome in racing animals is more difficult to predict; some animals will run well and some will not.

Arthrodesis is a rational approach to metacarpophalangeal and proximal interphalangeal chronic instability in the racing animal. The most precise and predictable method of arthrodesis involves the use of "mini-plates" and 2.0-

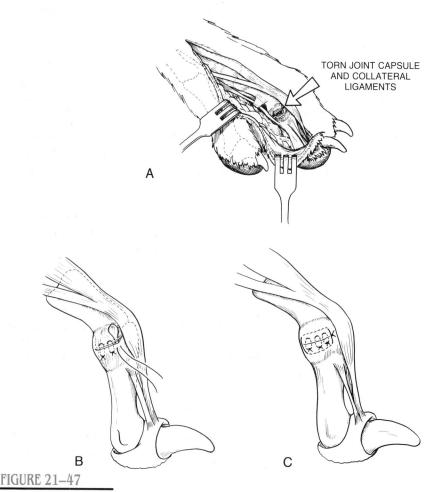

FIGURE 21–47

Suture repair of proximal interphalangeal subluxation. (A) The affected joint is exposed by a dorsal incision, with reflection of tissues on the side of the instability.[3] Tearing of joint capsule and collateral ligaments can be seen below the arrow. (B) Three mattress sutures of 4–0 monofilament or synthetic absorbable material are placed across the torn capsule and collateral ligaments. (C) A purse-string–like suture encompasses the other sutures.

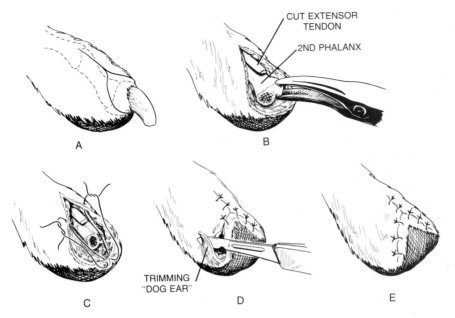

FIGURE 21–48

Amputation at the middle or distal interphalangeal joint. The procedure is drawn for the distal interphalangeal joint but does not differ in principle from a middle joint amputation. (A) The skin incision encircles the nail, sparing the digital pad, and continues proximally over the bones for a short distance. The incision shown would have to be extended proximally a short distance to expose the middle joint. (B) Soft tissue is sharply dissected away from the bone to be removed, and disarticulation is performed at the desired level. Rongeurs are used to remove the condylar portion of the remaining phalanx. (C) Skin sutures are placed to create a Y-shaped incision and to pull the pad over the cut end of the bone. (D) Excess skin is trimmed to allow smooth skin closure. (E) Skin suturing has been completed.

or 1.5-mm bone screws (Fig. 21–50A). Kirschner wires and a tension band wire are also applicable (Fig. 21–50B). Very little functional disability results from such a fusion, and joint pain is obviously banished.

CLINICAL SIGNS

Lameness is usually absent to minimal at a walk when the animal is presented. Only when the dog is worked at faster gaits does it become evident that the dog is favoring a foot. Swelling, pain, and crepitus are not prominent, but the instability can be appreciated by careful palpation. The interphalangeal joints must be extended when palpating for stability.

DIAGNOSIS

Confirmation of the clinical diagnosis by radiographs is essential to rule out fractures and to allow identification of avulsions, which are treated as shown in Figure 12–19. Both total luxations and subluxations are seen.

TREATMENT

Suture Repair of Interphalangeal Luxation

The interphalangeal joint is exposed through a dorsal incision[3] (Fig. 21–47A). The torn joint capsule and collateral ligaments are visible beneath the skin.

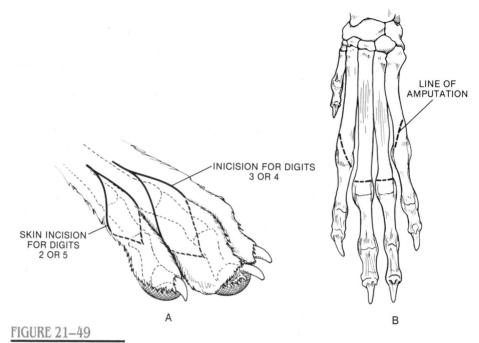

INICISION FOR DIGITS
3 OR 4

SKIN INCISION
FOR DIGITS
2 OR 5

LINE OF
AMPUTATION

A   B

FIGURE 21–49

Amputation at the metacarpophalangeal (or metatarsophalangeal) joint. *(A)* Skin incisions are designed to remove the digital pad, and when sutured, they both create a straight line. *(B)* After disarticulating to remove the phalanges, the metacarpal bone is amputated at the indicated level. Beveling the medial and lateral bones improves the cosmetic appearance, especially on the lateral side.

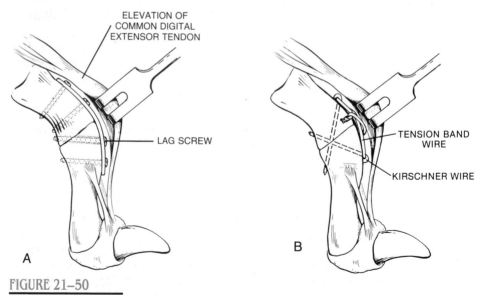

ELEVATION OF
COMMON DIGITAL
EXTENSOR TENDON

LAG SCREW

TENSION BAND
WIRE

KIRSCHNER WIRE

A   B

FIGURE 21–50

Arthrodesis of the proximal interphalangeal joint. Similar technique can be employed at the metacarpophalangeal (or metatarsophalangeal) joint. *(A)* An AO/ASIF straight Mini-Plate (Synthes [USA], Paoli, PA) has been contoured over the dorsal surface of the proximal and middle phalangeal bones after removing articular cartilage at the joint. Mini L-Plates (AO/ASIF) can also be applied medially or laterally. Screws of 1.5 to 2.0 mm diameter are used to attach the plate. One screw has been lagged across the joint through the plate. *(B)* Kirschner wires and a tension band wire can also be used to stabilize this arthrodesis.

Three mattress sutures of 4-0 monofilament or synthetic absorbable suture material are placed vertically to the tear in the capsule and collateral ligaments (Fig. 21–47B). These sutures are then encompassed within a single large "purse-string" suture, as shown in Fig. 21–47C. Occasionally, the extensor tendon apparatus will be slightly luxated as a result of tearing of its retinaculum. A few sutures are placed in the edge of the tendon and joint capsule to stabilize it.

After reduction of total luxations, usually only one side of the joint is unstable and that side is sutured. If both sides of the joint are loose after reduction, suture repair is performed bilaterally.

AFTERCARE ■ A molded plastic bivalve splint (see Fig. 19–15) is applied to the foot for three weeks. Following splint removal, exercise is severely limited for one week, after which activity is slowly resumed to normal six weeks postoperatively.

Amputation of a Toe

The surgical principles of toe amputation vary little with the joint level involved. The skin incision is made to preserve the pad when amputation is at the interphalangeal level (Fig. 21–48A), but the toe pad is removed for a metacarpophalangeal amputation (Fig. 21–49A).

The joint is disarticulated by sharp dissection, which also involves section of both the flexor and extensor tendons. It is desirable to remove the palmar sesamoids when amputation occurs at the metacarpophalangeal joint. The distal end of the proximal remaining bone is always removed. In the case of a distal interphalangeal amputation, the distal third of the middle phalanx is removed to provide more soft tissue between the skin and bone end (Fig. 21–48B). When amputating at the metacarpophalangeal level, the condyle is removed when metacarpal III or IV is involved, but bones II and V are beveled for a more cosmetic closure (Fig. 21–49B). Skin suturing may involve removal of skin "dog ears" to result in smooth skin closure (Fig. 21–48D,E).

AFTERCARE ■ A snug padded bandage is maintained for 10 days, and normal activity is not resumed until three weeks postoperatively.

Arthrodesis of Metacarpophalangeal or Proximal Interphalangeal Joints

The joint is exposed by a mid-dorsal approach.[3] The extensor tendon is reflected to one side by incising its retinaculum at the joint capsule. The joint is opened and articular cartilage removed by rongeurs, conforming the surfaces to get good contact at the functional angle, which is judged by an adjacent toe. A four- or five-hole, straight "mini-plate" (Synthes Ltd. [USA], Paoli, PA) is contoured to the dorsal surface of the bone and attached with 2.0- or 1.5-mm screws (Fig. 21–50A). An attempt is made to lag-screw across the joint with at least one screw. Bone grafting is not necessary. Alternatively, Kirschner wires can be driven across the joint and the joint compressed with a tension band wire (Fig. 21–50B).

AFTERCARE ■ A molded bivalve splint (see Fig. 19–15) is maintained for six weeks, at which time radiographic signs of healing should be seen. Exercise is slowly increased for two to three weeks before full activity is allowed.

REFERENCES

1. Vasseur PB, Pool RR, Klein BS: Effects of tendon transfer on the canine scapulohumeral joint. Am J Vet Res 44:811, 1983.
2. Hohn RB, Rosen H, Bohning RH, Brown SG: Surgical stabilization of recurrent shoulder luxation. Vet Clin North Am 1:537, 1971.
3. Piermattei DL: An Atlas of Approaches to the Bones of the Dog and Cat, 3rd ed. Philadelphia, W. B. Saunders Company, in preparation.
4. Vasseur PB: Clinical results of surgical correction of shoulder luxation in dogs. J Am Vet Med Assoc 182:503, 1983.
5. DeAngelis M, Schwartz A: Surgical correction of cranial dislocation of the scapulohumeral joint in a dog. J Am Vet Med Assoc 156:435, 1970.
6. Parkes L: Excision of the glenoid. Presented at 3rd Annual Meeting of Veterinary Orthopedic Society, Aspen, Colorado, 1976.
7. Breucker KA, Piermattei DL: Excision arthroplasty of the canine scapulohumeral joint: Report of three cases. Vet Comp Orthop Traum 3:134, 1988.
8. Franczuski D, Parkes LJ: Glenoid excision as a treatment in chronic shoulder disabilities: Surgical technique and clinical results. J Am Anim Hosp Assoc 14:637, 1988.
9. LaHue TR, Brown SG, Roush JC, et al: Entrapment of joint mice in the bicipital tendon sheath as a sequela to osteochondritis dissecans of the proximal humerus in dogs: A report of six cases. J Am Anim Hosp Assoc 24:99, 1988.
10. Vaughan LC, Jones DGC: Osteochondritis dissecans of the head of the humerus in dogs. J Small Anim Pract 9:283, 1968.
11. Griffiths RC: Osteochondritis dissecans of the canine shoulder. J Am Vet Med Assoc 12:1733, 1968.
12. Smith CW, Stowater JL: Osteochondritis dissecans of the canine shoulder joint: A review of 35 cases. J Am Anim Hosp Assoc 11:658, 1975.
13. Harrison JW, Hohn RB: Osteochondritis dissecans. In Bojrab MJ (ed): Current Techniques in Small Animal Surgery. Philadelphia, Lea & Febiger, 1975, pp 504–509.
14. Storey EC: Prognostic value of arthrography in canine osteochondrosis (osteochondritis) dissecans. Vet Clin North Am 8:301, 1978.
15. Muhumuza L, et al: Positive contrast arthrography—a study of the humeral joints in normal beagle dogs. Vet Radiol 29:157, 1988.
16. Suter PF, Carb AV: Shoulder arthrography in dogs—radiographic anatomy and clinical application. J Small Anim Pract 10:407, 1969.
17. Birkeland R: Osteochondritis dissecans in the humeral head of the dog. Nord Vet Med 19:294, 1967.
18. Person M: Arthroscopic treatment of osteochondritis dissecans in the canine shoulder. Vet Surg 18:175, 1989.
19. Lincoln JD, Potter K: Tenosynovitis of the biceps brachii tendon in dogs. J Am Anim Hosp Assoc 20:385, 1984.
20. Becker DA, Cofield RH: Tenodesis of the long head of the biceps brachii for chronic bicipital tendinitis. J Bone Joint Surg 71-A:376, 1989.
21. Post M, Benca P: Primary tendinitis of the long head of the biceps. Clin Orthop Rel Res 246:117, 1989.
22. Pettit GD, Chatburn CC, Hegreberg GA, Meyers KM: Studies on the pathophysiology of infraspinatus muscle contracture in the dog. Vet Surg 7:8, 1978.
23. Bennett RA: Contracture of the infraspinatus muscle in dogs: A review of 12 cases. J Am Anim Hosp Assoc 22:481, 1986.
24. Bennett D, Campbell JR: Unusual soft tissue orthopaedic problems in the dog. J. Small Anim Pract 20:27, 1979.
25. Hoerlein BF, Evans LE, Davis JM: Upward luxation of the canine scapula—A case report. J Am Vet Med Assoc 136:258, 1960.
26. Campbell JR: Luxation and ligamentous injuries of the elbow of the dog. Vet Clin North Am 1:429, 1971.
27. Bingel SA, Riser WH: Congenital elbow luxation in the dog. J Small Anim Pract 18:445, 1977.
28. Milton JL, Horne RD, Bartels JE, Henderson RA: Congenital elbow luxation in the dog. J Am Vet Med Assoc 175:572, 1979.
29. Hayes HM, Selby LA, Wilson GP, Hohn RB: Epidemiologic observations of canine elbow disease (Emphasis on dysplasia). J Am Anim Hosp Assoc 15:449, 1979.
30. Olsson SE: Osteochondrosis in the dog. In Kirk RW (ed): Current Veterinary Therapy VI. Philadelphia, W. B. Saunders Company, 1977, pp 880–886.
31. Wind AP: Elbow incongruity and developmental elbow diseases in the dog: Part I. J Am Anim Hosp Assoc 22:711, 1986.
32. Wind AP, Packard ME: Elbow incongruity and developmental elbow diseases in the dog: Part II. J Am Anim Hosp Assoc 22:725, 1986.
33. Sinibaldi KR, Arnoczky SP: Surgical removal of the ununited anconeal process in

the dog. J Am Anim Hosp Assoc 11:192, 1975.

34. Herron MR: Ununited anconeal process—A new approach to surgical repair. Mod Vet Pract 51:30, June 1970.

35. Olsson SE: The early diagnosis of fragmented coronoid process and osteochondritis dissecans of the canine elbow joint. J Am Anim Hosp Assoc 19:616, 1983.

36. Probst CW, Flo GL, McLoughlin MA, et al: A simple medial approach to the canine elbow for treatment of fragmented coronoid process and osteochondritis dissecans. J Am Anim Hosp Assoc 25:331, 1989.

37. Olsson SE: Osteochondrosis of the elbow joint in the dog: Its manifestations, indications for surgery, and surgical approach. Arch Am Coll Vet Surg 6:46, 1977.

38. Berzon JL, Quick CB: Fragmented coronoid process: Anatomical, clinical, and radiographic considerations with case analyses. J Am Anim Hosp Assoc 16:241, 1980.

39. Moore RW, Withrow SJ: Arthrodeses. Compend Cont Ed 3:319, 1981.

40. Gilson SD, Piermattei DL, Schwarz PD: Treatment of humeroulnar subluxation with a dynamic proximal ulnar osteotomy. A review of 13 cases. Vet Surg 18:114, 1989.

41. Ljunggren G, Cawley AJ, Archibald J: The elbow dysplasias in the dog. J Am Vet Med Assoc 148:887, 1966.

42. Henry WB: Radiologic diagnosis and surgical management of fragmented medial coronoid process in dogs. J Am Vet Med Assoc 184:799, 1984.

43. Zontine WJ, Weitkamp RA, Lippincott CL: Redefined type of elbow dysplasia involving calcified flexor tendons attached to the medial humeral epicondyle in three dogs. J Am Vet Med Assoc 194:1082, 1989.

44. Brown SG: Elbow arthrodesis. Presented at the 5th Annual Surgical Forum, Am Coll Vet Surgeons, Chicago, 1976.

45. Earley T: Canine carpal ligament injuries. Vet Clin North Am 8:183, 1978.

46. Punzet G: Luxation of the os carpi radiale in the dog–pathogenesis, symptoms and treatment. J Small Anim Pract 15:751, 1974.

47. Swaim SF: Management and bandaging of soft tissue injuries of dog and cat feet. J Am Anim Hosp Assoc 21:329, 1985.

48. Parker RB, Brown SG, Wind AP: Pancarpal arthrodesis in the dog: A review of forty-five cases. Vet Surg 10:35, 1981.

49. Chambers JN, Bjorling DE: Palmar surface plating for arthrodesis of the canine carpus. J Am Anim Hosp Assoc 18:875, 1982.

50. Fowler DJ, Presnell KR, Holmberg DL: Scapulohumeral arthrodesis: Results in seven dogs. J Am Anim Hosp Assoc 24:667, 1987.

51. Puglisi TA, Tanger CH, Green RW, et al: Stress radiography of the canine humeral joint. J Am Anim Hosp Assoc 24:235, 1988.

PART III

Miscellaneous Diseases of the Musculoskeletal System

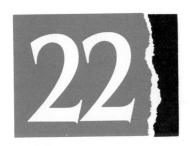

Disease Conditions in Small Animals

Eosinophilic panosteitis is a rather common disease of long bones in large breeds of young dogs, especially the German shepherd. The disease also has been called osteomyelitis, enostosis, fibrous osteodystrophy, juvenile osteomyelitis,[1] and "Eo Pan" by breeders.

Although this disease causes severe lameness, it is self-limiting, and there is no permanent aftermath. Therefore, because the condition gets better "by itself," intensive investigations of the various stages of this disease have been lacking. Many contradictions exist as to its clinical features.

The etiology of eosinophilic panosteitis is unknown, although infection, metabolic disease, endocrine dysfunction, allergy, autoimmune mechanisms, parasitism, and hereditary factors have been postulated.[1]

Clinical Signs

The clinical picture is that of a healthy dog with lameness of acute onset but no history of trauma. Males are affected four times more often than females.[2] The lameness may be marked, and often the dog will "carry" or favor the limb. This lameness may last a few days to several weeks.[2] In about 53 percent of cases, other limbs have become involved, thereby characterizing the condition as causing a "shifting leg lameness."[3] These recurring bouts usually subside by the time the animal reaches 2 years of age.[1, 4] However, dogs up to 5 years of age have incurred "Eo Pan."[3, 4]

Examination

Gentle palpation along the distal, middle, and proximal areas of long bones may elicit exquisite pain when the involved area is reached, even in stoic animals. This reaction may consist of crying out, wincing, pulling the leg away, or, occasionally, snapping at the examiner. When palpating, the clinician's fingers should push aside muscle bundles (especially of the humerus and femur) so that bone is reached prior to squeezing. This avoids misinterpretation arising from hurting normal muscle tissue trapped in the palpation.

Depending on when thorough veterinary attention is sought and how elaborate the workup completed, other factors may be present, such as fever,[1, 2] muscle atrophy,[2] eosinophilia,[1, 2] decreased activity, and inappetence. Others have disclaimed the occurrence of fever,[3] muscle atrophy,[1, 3] and eosinophilia.[3] Eosinophilia has been reported to be seen only in the first two days of clinical signs.[1]

Radiographic Signs

Radiograpically, the disease may be separated into three stages.[3] Often, the clinician sees the case in the middle phase and the other stages only during extensive studies of this condition.

EARLY PHASE ■ Although the limb may be asymptomatic, radiographic changes may be detected during a survey of all the long bones. These consist of blurring and accentuation of trabecular patterns, best seen at the proximal and distal ends of the diaphysis (Fig. 22–1). The contrast between the cortex and medullary canals is diminished. In some cases, a few granular densities are seen.

MIDDLE PHASE ■ Patchy, mottled, sclerotic-looking densities appear, especially around the nutrient foramen in the early stages (Fig. 22–2). In some cases, the entire diaphysis is involved; in others, there may be only pea-sized lesions (Fig. 22–3). In a third of Eo Pan cases, the periosteum becomes involved. Initially, a subtle roughening appears that becomes more dense within one or two weeks and eventually becomes as dense as the cortex (Figs. 22–2 and 22–3).

LATE PHASE ■ In the process of recovery, the medullary canal attains normal density while the coarse trabecular pattern remains. In about a third of the cases, the cortex remains thicker than normal. A few granular densities may be present. It may require several months for these changes to disappear completely. In general, the lesions affect the central part of the radius, the proximal third of the ulna, the distal and central parts of the humerus, the proximal third of the tibia, and the central and proximal parts of the femur.

Histopathology

Histopathologic findings[3] of the lesions consist of accentuation of osteoblastic and fibroblastic activity in the periosteum, endosteum, and marrow. Fibrosis occurs in the marrow. There is evidence of neither acute or chronic inflammation nor malignancy. In highly mature lesions, the cortical thickening consists of thickened lamellar bone with haversian systems, whereas in

FIGURE 22–1

FIGURE 22–2

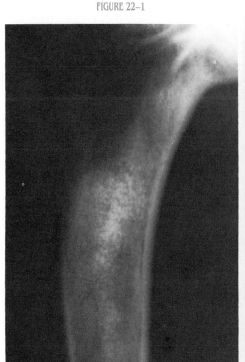

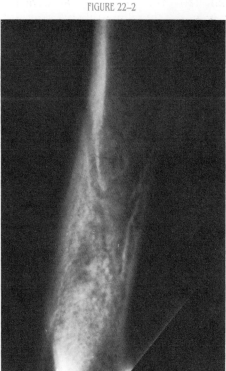

FIGURE 22–1

Early stage of eosinophilic panosteitis in the humerus of a 9-month-old male German shepherd. Granular densities are seen.

FIGURE 22–2

Middle stage of eosinophilic panosteitis with increased densities around the nutrient foramen in a 6-month-old male Great Pyrenees. Note the periosteal thickening caudal to the foramen.

immature lesions, cellular fiber bone is present with many osteoblasts and osteoclasts.

Differential Diagnosis

Differential diagnosis includes osteochondritis dissecans, fragmented coronoid process, un-united anconeal process, hip dysplasia, cruciate disease, coxofemoral luxation, and fractures. When there is a shifting leg lameness, other conditions such as rheumatoid arthritis, systemic lupus erythematosus (SLE), or bacterial endocarditis must be considered. The diagnosis of Eo Pan is determined by palpation and radiography.

Treatment

Treatment is symptomatic to relieve pain by using aspirin, corticosteroids, and other agents. None of these has been documented to hasten the resolution of the condition.[1]

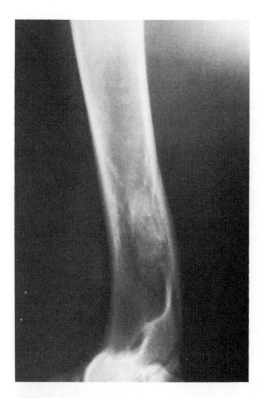

FIGURE 22-3

Middle stage of eosinophilic panosteitis showing a small sclerotic area in the distal humerus of a 6-month-old German shepherd. Note the thickened caudal cortex adjacent to the sclerotic patch.

NUTRITIONAL DISORDERS

Although nutritional problems affecting bone and muscle are beyond the scope of this text,[1, 5–10] some clinical situations that may confront the orthopedist are considered.

Clinical Problems

There are three common problems we see: obesity, consequences of the all-meat diet, and oversupplementation in large and giant breeds of dogs.

OBESITY

Although obesity has not been proved to cause osteoarthritis, at least in mice,[11] common sense tells us that excessive weight on injured or congenitally deformed joints or spinal conditions can affect musculoskeletal performance. Prevention of obesity is obviously accomplished more readily than treatment. If the veterinary clinician observes patients gaining weight, or if an animal has a potential for arthritis or back problems or becomes neutered, the client should be warned to watch the animal's weight carefully and to cut back food intake before weight gain becomes unmanageable.

If an animal is obese, the endocrine system, especially the thyroid, should be examined. For a "diet," we usually recommend cutting the total daily caloric intake by one third to one half in order to reduce the animal's weight.

Canine vitamin supplementation may be administered to alleviate the owner's apprehension concerning dietary restriction. Often, if the owner is sincere and conscientious, decreasing the amount of presently fed food by one third to one half is all that is necessry. Owners (even those who are themselves overweight) seem to understand and accept "the more weight your pet carries, the more it abuses its bad joint, which could potentially hasten joint destruction, necessitating surgery or leading to a painful life." When this does not seem to be effective, prescribed reducing diets may be tried. Our usual goal is to achieve a conformation in which there is an observable indentation along the flank region and ribs, which should be individually palpable. Some clients may need to be told, "Your dog needs to lose four pounds," instead of these guidelines. For a lighter-weight breed, the owner may monitor progress using a bathroom scale at home.

THE ALL-MEAT DIET

Publicity concerning all-meat diets has been widespread enough that the syndrome is rarely seen today. Low in calcium and high in phosphorus, this diet has the tendency to cause secondary nutritional hyperparathyroidism (SNH), a condition in which the parathyroids are stimulated to secrete parathormone. This hormone increases the resorption of calcium from bone in order to maintain proper serum levels. In the young animal, the result may be loss of skeletal density and thinning of the bone cortex. Lameness or pathological fracture may result (Fig. 22–4). In an adult animal that is fed an all-meat diet, the process is slow and can result in osteopenia. Treatment

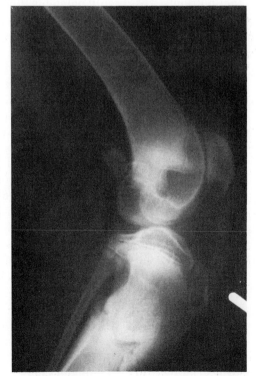

FIGURE 22–4

Five-month-old male Gordon setter with pathological fracture of the tibia from secondary nutritional hyperparathyroidism. Note the thin cortices of the femur. This dog was fed a balanced home diet by a breeder using egg shells (which are not absorbed in the canine intestine) for the calcium source.

involves feeding the animal a balanced commercial diet as well as supplementation with calcium.

HYPERNUTRITION AND OVERSUPPLEMENTATION

The most perplexing nutritional problem facing the orthopedist is presented when a breeder asks the veterinary clinician to test serum calcium and phosphorus levels in a young dog of large or giant breed that has poor bony conformation. Although it may appear that improper nutrition is to blame, this may or may not be the answer. A few points are worth emphasizing in this regard. In giant breeds, the phosphorus may be twice as high in the dog 3 to 6 months old as in the adult (8.7 mg/100 ml versus 4.2 mg/100 ml). The calcium may be slightly higher in a younger animal (11.1 mg/100 ml versus 9.9 mg/100 ml for an adult).[5] In those dogs with known dietary excesses or imbalances of calcium and phosphorus, the serum calcium and phosphorus levels usually are in the normal range as a result of the dog's homeostatic mechanisms, if the parathyroid gland is working properly. More sensitive indicators of dietary imbalance are the quantities of calcium and phosphorus excreted in the urine over 24 hours and the creatinine clearance ratios.

Most commercial dry dog foods contain the proper quantities of and balance between calcium and phosphorus. People owning large breeds feel that this commercial diet may be good for the normal "run-of-the-mill" dog, but not for their dog, which is going to be large. Often the owner feeds a mixture of foods suggested by the breeder, for whom the diet produced champions. These mixtures include vitamins, dicalcium phosphate, bone meal, high-protein cereals, meat, milk, cottage cheese, eggs, wheat germ, and other nutrients. This highly palatable diet may lead to an ingestion of excessive quantities of nutrients that can lead to a nutritional imbalance. Young Great Danes fed a balanced diet *ad libitum* had accelerated bone growth, sinking of the metacarpophalangeal joints, lateral deviation of the forepaws (valgus deformity of the carpus), cow-hocked rear limbs, enlargement of the distal radial and ulnar metaphyses, enlargements of the costochondral junctions, pain, arched backs, and inactivity. Those dogs fed two thirds of the quantity of protein and calories of the other group had slower bone growth and better conformation, and they were more active and playful.[7] It is therefore wise for the veterinarian to discuss diet with the owners of these large breeds. The importance of slow bone growth should be stressed, and the owners should be warned not to push their dogs nutritionally.

Signs of overnutrition may be mistaken for "rickets" and therefore improper acceleration of the plane of nutrition prescribed. Rickets is extremely rare and has been seen usually only under starvation or research conditions.

The valgus deformity of the carpus may correct itself when the diet is changed while the dog is still growing. Severe deformities, however, may require corrective osteotomy after skeletal maturity is complete.

Retained Cartilaginous Cores

Retained cartilaginous cores (RCC) or retained hypertrophied endochondral cartilage in the ulnar metaphysis may give an outward appearance of valgus deformity of the carpus (abduction of the foot).

These cores may extend 3 to 4 cm into the metaphysis of the ulna and on radiographs appear similar to "candlesticks" (Fig. 22–5). The cores are composed of hypertrophied hyaline cartilage cells rather than bony trabeculae.[10] This cartilage core retards the overall length of the ulna. The styloid process does not extend to the ulnar carpal bone. Therefore, lateral support of the carpus is lost and the foot abducts. Since the ulna is shortened, the normal sliding of the radius on the ulna during growth is altered and the distal radius is then bent caudally, resulting in cranial bowing of the radius (Fig. 22–6).

The cause of retained cartilaginous cores is unknown. Whether it is a form of osteochondrosis[12] or whether hypernutrition or accelerated body growth plays a role remains to be proved. When these changes are seen in a puppy, it may be advisable to decrease the plane of nutrition if it is on the high side. If the dog is mature and the deformity is severe, corrective osteotomy may be indicated.

FIGURE 22–5

FIGURE 22–6

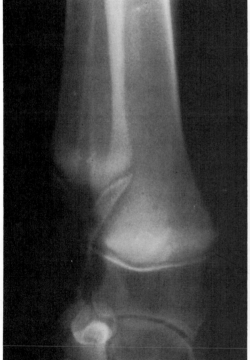
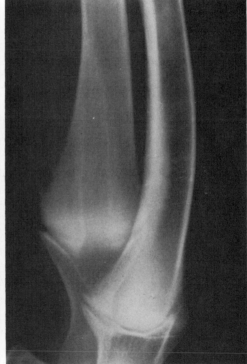

FIGURE 22–5

Four-month-old female Great Dane with painful forelegs. Note the "candlestick" core of cartilage extending from the ulnar epiphysis into the metaphysis.

FIGURE 22–6

Five-month-old male St. Bernard with increased valgus angulation of the carpus and pain elicited upon palpation of the carpus. Note the "candlestick" formation in the ulna and cranial bowing of the radius with secondary thickening of the caudal cortex (Wolff's law).

HYPERTROPHIC OSTEODYSTROPHY

Hypertrophic osteodystrophy (HO), vitamin C deficiency, or scurvy,[13] is a syndrome seen in young dogs of medium and giant breeds (Great Danes, Irish setters, boxers, Labrador retrievers). The condition is characterized by grossly observable swellings of the distal metaphyses of the radius, ulna, and tibia. This disorder has been misinterpreted by some investigators as joint swellings.

Clinical Signs

Often the dog appears to show systemic involvement with pyrexia, anorexia, pain, arched back, and reluctance to move,[1, 10] and often has a history of diarrhea the preceding week.[13] Cranial bowing of the forelegs and a valgus deformity of the carpus may occur.[4] The acute phase may last seven to 10 days[1]; however, recurrences have been seen.[13]

Radiographic Signs

Radiographically, the initial finding is a thin, radiolucent line in the metaphysis parallel to the epiphyseal plate of the radius. Secondarily, there is an extraperiosteal cuff of calcification along the metaphysis (Fig. 22–7). As the

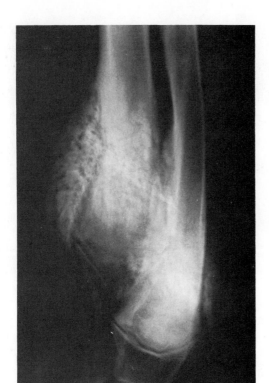

FIGURE 22–7

Six-month-old male Great Dane with extraperiosteal proliferation and calcification of the distal radius and ulna.

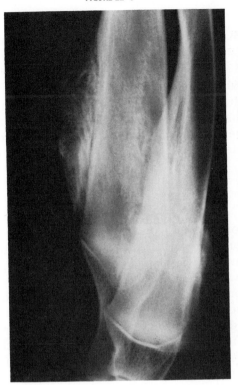
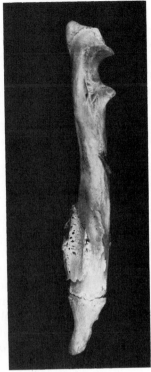

FIGURE 22–8

Same dog as shown in Figure 22–7, now 9 months old.

FIGURE 22–9

Gross specimen of the ulna shown in Figure 22–8.

dog matures, these extraperiosteal thickenings often regress (Figs. 22–8 and 22–9), but may leave a permanently thickened metaphysis.[14]

Pathogenesis

The scurvy theory arises from the radiographic similarity to scorbutic changes seen in children.[1] Whether hypertrophic osteodystrophy and scurvy are the same disease or whether vitamin C deficiency is involved at all remains to be proved.[13] The mean value of serum ascorbic acid in 18 dogs with hypertrophic osteodystrophy was only slightly below the mean of serum ascorbic acid in 28 normal young large breeds of dogs.[13] Since serum ascorbic acid levels vary with exercise, food intake, and stress, these values may be meaningless since dogs with hypertrophic osteodystrophy are under stress and anorexic.

Treatment

This disease appears to improve with whatever treatment is undertaken. In one study, 24 dogs were managed by one of these methods: no treatment, antibiotics, antibiotics and corticosteroids, or antibiotics, corticosteroids, and vitamin C. There was no statistical difference in the rates of recoveries between these treatments.[16] Most dogs recovered from systemic signs in seven to 10 days,[1, 13] whereas bony changes have required several months for resorption.[14] Death has been reported in some instances.[13] Generally, analgesics and anti-diarrheal medications are indicated.

RENAL OSTEODYSTROPHY

Although renal osteodystrophy, or "renal rickets," is infrequently seen by the orthopedist, it can occasionally produce pathological fractures or give appearance of generalized skeletal demineralization upon radiography. With renal disease, phosphorus is retained, which causes secondary hyperparathyroidism similar to that caused by nutritional imbalances or excesses of phosphorus.

When an adult dog spontaneously fractures a leg or jaw or experiences minimal trauma such as falling down two stairs, particular attention should be paid to the density of the bone on the radiograph. It is only with chronic severe kidney disease that the bone will show obvious demineralization, and usually the client would have sought veterinary attention because of the problems related to uremia.

HYPERTROPHIC PULMONARY OSTEOPATHY

Hypertrophic pulmonary osteopathy (HPO) has been known as hypertrophic pulmonary osteoarthropathy (HPOA)[15] and hypertrophic osteoarthropathy (HOA).[16] HPOA is a misnomer because the joints are not really involved, and some prefer HOA because the lung occasionally is not involved.[16]

Clinical Signs

This syndrome is characterized by lameness, reluctance to move, and firm swellings of the distal limbs. The lungs usually become involved. In a study of 60 cases, 30 percent showed thoracic disease signs prior to musculoskeletal signs.[16] Lung disease was eventually seen in 95 percent of the cases. The cause of the thoracic disease was cancer in 91 percent. *Spirocerca lupi* infestation of the esophagus and dirofilariasis can also cause HPO.

Radiographic Signs

The classic radiographic signs of HPO consist of extensive, rough periosteal formation beginning in the distal phalanges, metacarpal bones, and metatarsal bones (Fig. 22–10). Other bones may become involved (Fig. 22–11). In peracute cases with swollen limbs, the radiographs may not show the extensive periosteal changes, but such changes will be apparent within a few days.

Pathogenesis

The pathogenesis of these periosteal changes is highly speculative. Some theories include chronic anoxia, obscure toxins,[1] and autonomic neural vascular reflex mechanisms mediated by afferent branches of the vagus or intercostal nerves.[17, 18] When HPO is diagnosed, a thorough diagnostic workup, especially of the thorax, is indicated. The probability of finding a nonlethal cause is low. Lung lobectomy may allow regression of bony lesions until death occurs or until additional lung cancer intercedes.[16, 19, 20] Bony changes may take three to four months to regress after lobectomy.[20] With possible nonlethal causes (i.e., *Spirocerca lupi* infestation, dirofilariasis), the removal of the inciting cause may or may not bring about regression of HPO signs.[15, 16]

FIGURE 22–10

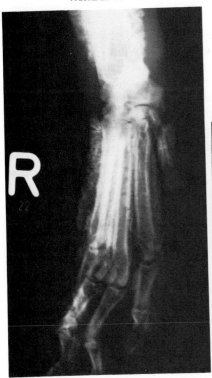

FIGURE 22–11

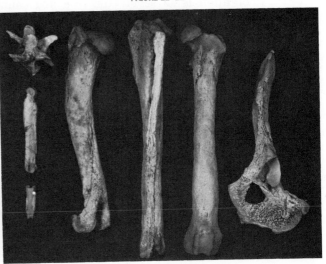

FIGURE 22–10

Phalanges, metacarpus, radius, and ulna affected with hypertrophic pulmonary osteopathy in a 5-year-old female collie mix with metastatic carcinoma to the lungs from the ovaries or uterus.

FIGURE 22–11

Gross appearance of an 8-year-old German shepherd with hypertrophic pulmonary osteopathy affecting the vertebrae, pelvis, long bones, and metacarpal and phalangeal bones.

CRANIOMANDIBULAR OSTEOPATHY

An uncommon proliferative bone disease, craniomandibular osteopathy (CMO) ("lion jaw") usually involves the mandibular rami and the tympanic bullae in Scottish, Cairn, and West Highland white terriers.[21] Other breeds that occasionally experience this condition include the Boston terrier, Labrador retriever,[22, 23] Great Dane,[24, 25] and Doberman pinscher.[26] Other bones of the head and some long bones have occasionally been involved. In some animals, only the mandibles are involved, whereas in others only the tympanic bullae seem affected.

Occurrence

The occurrence of this disease is infrequently reported in the literature. At the small animal clinic at Michigan State University only seven cases were seen in nine years (1970 to 1979), and during that time, a total of 130,000 admissions had been recorded.

Clinical Signs

The signs usually relate to pain around the mouth in growing puppies 4 to 7 months of age. Mild cases may be asymptomatic and are discovered by palpation. If the angular processes of the mandible and tympanic bullae are involved, jaw movement is diminished, even under anesthesia. Temporal and masseter muscle atrophy is apparent. Nutrition may become inadequate if the condition is so severe that the dog cannot drink liquids. The mandibular thickening may be palpable and there may be intermittent fever. However, once skeletal maturation nears (11 to 12 months of age), the pain disappears and the exostoses may even regress.

Diagnosis

Diagnosis of craniomandibular osteopathy is made on the basis of breed, signs, physical findings, and radiography.

Radiographic Signs

Radiography helps to document the condition. Changes consist of beadlike osseous proliferations of the mandible or tympanic bullae (Figs. 22–12 and 22–13). When the exostoses stop proliferating and eventually regress, the roughened borders become quite smooth. With early lesions, however, swellings may not be very radiopaque.

Histopathological Appearance

Histologically, normal lamellar bone is replaced by an enlarged coarse fiber (woven) bone. The bone marrow is replaced by a fibrous-type stroma and

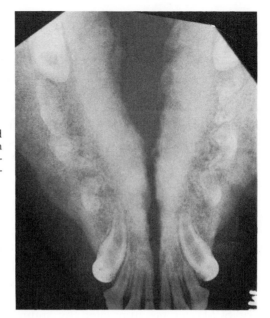

FIGURE 22–12

Open-mouth radiograph of a 6-month-old female West Highland white terrier with canine mandibular osteopathy. Note the bilateral roughened proliferations of the mandible.

some inflammation.[21] Inflammatory cells at the periphery of the invading bone have been documented and would seem to make this an inflammatory disease. However, others claim this to be a noninflammatory, nonclassifiable disease,[4, 27, 28] based upon earlier histopathological literature that may or may not have had sufficient case material to offer adequate study of the disease in various stages. Although the cause of CMO is unknown, one author has suggested possible infection (arising from the fever and histological inflammation at the periphery of the lesion), with a genetic influence, owing to its occurrence in the terrier breeds.[21]

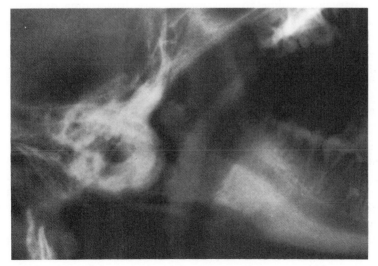

FIGURE 22–13

Proliferation of the tympanic bullae of a 7-month-old male Scottish terrier.

Treatment

Treatment is usually aimed at decreasing pain and inflammation with medication such as aspirin, cortisone, and so forth. Surgical excision of the exostoses has resulted in regrowth within three weeks in one documented case.[27] Feeding highly nutritious fluids would be important in those dogs with minimal ability to open the mouth. Euthanasia may be necessary in a very few cases.

SYNOVIAL CHONDROMETAPLASIA

Synovial chondrometaplasia (SCM) is a condition in which nodules of sclerosis, fibrocartilage, and even bone form in the synovial layer of the joint capsule, causing chronic lameness in the dog.[29] SCM has been reported in the shoulder, stifle, and hock of dogs and in the tendon sheath and bursae of horses.[29–32] SCM affects the large joints in humans.[33]

The cause of the spontaneous nodular formation is unknown, but secondary SCM can be stimulated by traumatic, degenerative, or inflammatory conditions in humans.[33]

The diagnosis is made by radiography and histological examination of the joint capsule. Multiple (10–100) joint mice seen radiographically, as well as nodular formation seen histologically, are diagnostic of the condition (Fig. 22–14). Surgical removal of loose bodies and partial synovectomy have resulted in marked improvement in most cases.[29]

SURGICAL ASPECTS OF LONG BONE NEOPLASMS

Appendicular bone tumors may be separated into three categories:

1. Primary bone tumors (osteosarcoma, chondrosarcoma, or fibrosarcoma).
2. Secondary metastatic tumors (rising most commonly from the mammary gland, lung, and prostate).[34, 35]
3. Local invasion from soft tissue tumors (such as synovial cell sarcoma).

All are malignant and carry a grave prognosis. Osteosarcoma is the most common tumor type seen in a dog's bone.

Often the presenting sign is lameness with or without systemic signs such as lethargy and anorexia. Neoplasia ought to be suspected and ruled out in the older dog with a rapidly progressive lameness (two to four weeks) as well as swelling. Palpation may reveal muscle atrophy, swelling, and increased heat and sensitivity. Neoplasia should also be suspected in dogs sustaining fractures following minimal or no trauma. Careful scrutiny of good quality radiographs is a must in such cases.

Fine detail radiography is often the best diagnostic tool to use in finding bone neoplasia, but it may be inappropriate to predict histological type based upon radiographs.[36] However, often the radiograph is very characteristic and therefore diagnostic of osteosarcoma. Biopsy in such cases is sometimes misleading owing to the lack of tumor cells in small biopsy samples. Biopsy

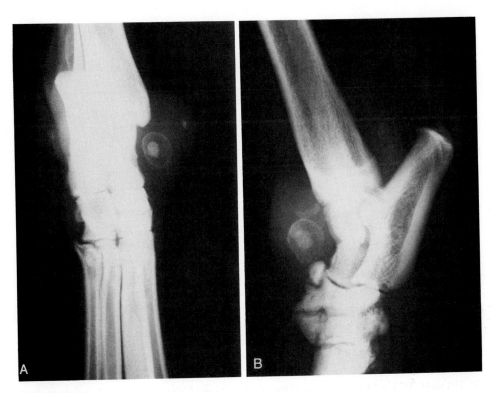

FIGURE 22-14

(A) Anteroposterior and (B) lateral radiographic views of a hock of a 1-year-old golden retriever with synovial chondrometaplasia (SCM). Note the severe soft tissue swelling and the multiple concentric loose bodies caudal to the distal tibia (in the flexor hallucis longus tendon sheath) and the talocrural joint.

should be used, however, on uncharacteristic lesions, especially if potentially curable conditions exist (e.g., infection, cysts, undifferentiated carcinoma, lymphomas, transmissible venereal tumor, and plasma cell myeloma). Biopsy is also helpful when an owner wants a more knowledgeable answer as to the probable life expectancy of his pet. Chondrosarcoma and fibrosarcoma are slow-growing, allowing slower progression until natural death.

Limb amputation is the most frequent surgical treatment in the dog and cat, with or without chemotherapy. It improves the quality of life, but 85 percent of dogs still die within eight months after amputation.[37, 38]

Recent advances in treatment of osteosarcoma in humans have increased overall survival rates to 60 to 70 percent in patients with nonmetastatic osteosarcoma.[39] However, 80 to 90 percent of humans do not have gross evidence of metastatic disease in the bone at the time of osteosarcoma diagnosis.[39] This is in contrast to our canine patients, in which 85 to 90 percent have metastatic disease when the primary tumor is removed.[38] Treatments in people include various chemotherapy regimens, pulmonary resection of metastases (often multiple surgeries), and limb salvage procedures. The goals of limb salvage procedures are to remove the tumor completely and to avoid local recurrence while reconstructing a functional extremity.[39] Endoprostheses (metal, allografts, or autoclaved autograft of resected tumor) may be inserted. However, the overall survival rates have not differed from those seen with amputation.[39]

Limb salvage in dogs has been used in selected cases and includes tumor resection and stabilization using whole cortical allografts and bone plates.[38, 40] The use of cisplatin is showing early improved survival rates with more than 50 percent of dogs living one year post treatment.[38]

REFERENCES

1. McKeown D, Archibald J: The musculo-skeletal system. In Cattcott ES (ed): Canine Medicine, 4th ed. Santa Barbara, American Veterinary Publications, Inc., 1979, pp 533–678.
2. Barrett RB, Schall WD, Lewis RE: Clinical and radiographic features of canine eosinophilic panosteitis. J Am Anim Hosp Assoc 4:94–104, 1968.
3. Bohning R Jr, Suter P, Hohn RB, Marshall J: Clinical and radiographic survey of canine panosteitis. J Am Vet Med Assoc 156:870–884, 1970.
4. Brown SG: Skeletal diseases. In Ettinger SJ (ed): Textbook of Veterinary Internal Medicine. Philadelphia, W. B. Saunders Company, 1975, pp 1715–1741.
5. Fletch SM, Smart ME: Blood chemistry of the giant breeds—bone profile. Bull Am Soc Vet Clin Pathol 2:30, 1973.
6. Morris ML: Nutrition and disease. In Cattcott EJ (ed): Canine Medicine, 4th ed. Santa Barbara, American Veterinary Publications, Inc., 1979, pp 223–252.
7. Hedhammar A, Wu FM, Krook L, et al: Oversupplementation and skeletal disease: An experimental study in growing Great Dane dogs. Cornell Vet 64(Suppl 5):32–45, 1974.
8. Krook L: Nutritional hypercalcitoninism. In Kirk RW (ed): Current Veterinary Therapy. VI. Philadelphia, W. B. Saunders Company, 1977, pp 1048–1050.
9. Krook L: Metabolic bone disease in dogs and cats. Proc Am Anim Hosp Assoc, 38th Annual Meeting, 1971, pp 350–355.
10. Riser WH, Shirer JF: Normal and abnormal growth of the distal foreleg in large and giant dogs. J Am Vet Radiol Soc VI: 50–64, 1965.
11. Moskowitz RW: Symptoms and laboratory findings in osteoarthritis. In Hollander JL (ed): Arthritis and Allied Conditions. Philadelphia, Lea and Febiger, 1972, pp 1032–1053.
12. Olsson SE: Osteochondrosis—A growing problem to dog breeders. Gaines Dog Research Progress, White Plains, NY, Gaines Dog Research Center, Summer 1976, pp 1–11.
13. Grondalen J: Metaphyseal osteodystrophy (hypertrophic osteodystrophy) in growing dogs. A clinical study. J Small Anim Pract 17:721, 1976.
14. Morgan JP: Radiology in Veterinary Orthopedics, 1st ed. Philadelphia, Lea and Febiger, 1972.
15. Thrasher JP: Hypertrophic pulmonary osteoarthropathy. J Am Vet Med Assoc 39:441–448, 1961.
16. Brodey RS: Hypertrophic osteoarthropathy in the dog: A clinicopathologic survey of 60 cases. J Am Vet Med Assoc 159:1242–1255, 1971.
17. Holling HE, et al: Hypertrophic pulmonary osteoarthropathy. J Thorac Cardiovasc Surg 46:310–321, 1963.
18. Holman CW: Osteoarthropathy in lung cancer: Disappearance after section of intercostal nerves. J Thorac Cardiovasc Surg 45:679–681, 1963.
19. Clifford DH, et al: Regression of the osseous lesions of hypertrophic pulmonary osteoarthropathy in a dog following lobectomy. J Am Anim Hosp Assoc 3:75, 1967.
20. Suter PF: Pulmonary neoplasia. In Ettinger SJ (ed): Textbook of Veterinary Internal Medicine. Philadelphia, W. B. Saunders Company, 1975, pp 754–766.
21. Riser WF, Parkes LJ, Shirer JF: Canine craniomandibular osteopathy. J Am Vet Radiol Soc 8:23–30, 1967.
22. Alexander JW, Kallfelz FA: A case of craniomandibular osteopathy in the Labrador retriever. Vet Med Small Anim Clin 70:560–563, 1975.
23. Watkins JD, Bradley R: Craniomandibular osteopathy in a Labrador puppy. Vet Rec 79:262–264, 1966.
24. Burk RL, Broadhurst JJ: Craniomandibular osteopathy in a Great Dane. J Am Vet Med Assoc 169:635–636, 1976.
25. DeVries HW, Vande Watering CC: Prednisolone in the treatment of craniomandibular osteopathy seen in a Great Dane. Neth J Vet Sci 5:123–131, 1975.
26. Watson AD, Huxtable CRR, Farrow BRH: Craniomandibular osteopathy in Doberman pinschers. J Small Anim Pract 16:11–19, 1975.
27. Pool RR, Leighton RL: Craniomandibular osteopathy in the dog. J Am Vet Med Assoc 154:657–660, 1969.
28. Jubb KVF, Kennedy PC: Bones, joints and

synovial structures. In Pathology of Domestic Animals, 2nd ed. New York, Academic Press, 1970, pp 1–100.

29. Flo GL, Stickle RL, Dunstan RW: Synovial chondrometaplasia in five dogs. J Am Vet Med Assoc 191:1417–1422, 1987.

30. Schmidt E, Schneider J: Synovial chondromatosis in the horse. Monatsschr Vet 37:509, 1982.

31. Schawalder von P: Die synoviale osteochondromatose (synoviale chondrometaplasie) biem Hund. Schweiz Arch Tierheilk 122:673–678, 1980.

32. Kirk MD: Radiographic and histologic appearance of synovial osteochondromatosis of the femorotibial bursa in a horse. A case history report. Vet Radiol 23:167–170, 1982.

33. Schajowicz F: Tumor and Tumor-like Lesions of Bones and Joints. New York, Springer-Verlag, 1981.

34. Geodegebuure SA: Secondary bone tumours in the dog. Vet Pathol 16:520–529, 1979.

35. Brodey RS, Reid CF, Sauer RM: Metastatic bone neoplasms in the dog. J Am Vet Med Assoc 148(1):29–43, 1966.

36. Probst CW, Ackerman N: Malignant neoplasia of the canine appendicular skeleton. Compendium Contin Educ 4(3):260–270, 1982.

37. Brodey RS, Abt DA: Results of surgical treatment in 65 dogs with osteosarcoma. J Am Vet Med Assoc 168:1032, 1976.

38. Withrow SJ, LaRue SM, Powers BE, et al: Osteosarcoma: New trends in treatment. In 10th Annual Kal Kan Symposium for the Treatment of Small Animal Disease, October, 1986.

39. Goorin AM, Abelson HT, Frei E: Osteosarcoma: Fifteen years later. N Engl J Med 313(26):1637–1642, 1985.

40. Vasseur PB: Limb salvage in a dog with chondrosarcoma of the tibia. J Am Vet Med Assoc 187(6):620–623, 1985.

41. O'Donoghue DH: Treatment of Injuries to Athletes. Philadelphia, W. B. Saunders Company, 1976, Chapter 4.

42. Farrow CS: Carpal sprain injury in the dog. J Am Vet Res Soc 18:38, 1977.

43. Early TD: Hyperextension injuries of the canine carpal joint. Georgia Veterinarian, 29:24, 1977.

INDEX

Note: Page numbers in *italics* refer to illustrations; page numbers followed by t refer to tables.